616.81 BKA

Textbook of Stroke Medicine

Second Edition

Textbook of Stroke Medicine

Second Edition

Edited by

Michael Brainin MD PhD
Professor and Chair, Department of Clinical Neuroscience and Preventive Medicine,
Danube University Krems, Krems, Austria

Wolf-Dieter Heiss MD PhD
Professor of Neurology, Emeritus Director, Max Planck Institute for Neurological Research and
Department of Neurology, University of Cologne, Cologne, Germany

Editorial Assistant

Susanne Tabernig MD
Vienna, Austria

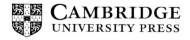
CAMBRIDGE
UNIVERSITY PRESS

CAMBRIDGE
UNIVERSITY PRESS

University Printing House, Cambridge CB2 8BS, United Kingdom

Cambridge University Press is part of the University of Cambridge.

It furthers the University's mission by disseminating knowledge in the pursuit of education, learning and research at the highest international levels of excellence.

www.cambridge.org
Information on this title: www.cambridge.org/9781107047495

Second Edition © Michael Brainin and Wolf-Dieter Heiss 2014

First Edition © Cambridge University Press 2010

Second Edition first published 2014
First Edition first published 2010

Printed in Spain by Grafos SA, Arte sobre papel

A catalog record for this publication is available from the British Library

Library of Congress Cataloging in Publication data
Textbook of stroke medicine / edited by Michael Brainin, Wolf-Dieter Heiss ; editorial assistant, Suzanne Tabernig. – Second edition.
    p. ; cm.
Includes bibliographical references and index.
ISBN 978-1-107-04749-5 (Hardback)
I. Brainin, M. (Michael), editor of compilation.   II. Heiss, W.-D. (Wolf-Dieter), 1939 December 31- editor of compilation.
III. Tabernig, Suzanne, editor of compilation.
[DNLM: 1. Stroke.   WL 355]
RC388.5
616.8′1–dc23   2013048020

ISBN 978-1-107-04749-5 Hardback

Contents

List of contributors vii
Preface ix

Section 1 – Etiology, pathophysiology, and imaging

1. **Neuropathology and pathophysiology of stroke** 1
   Konstantin-A. Hossmann and Wolf-Dieter Heiss

2. **Common causes of ischemic stroke** 33
   Bo Norrving

3. **Neuroradiology** 45
   (A) Imaging of acute ischemic and hemorrhagic stroke: CT, perfusion CT, CT angiography 45
   Patrik Michel
   (B) Imaging of acute ischemic and hemorrhagic stroke: MRI and MR angiography 49
   Jochen B. Fiebach, Patrik Michel, and Jens Fiehler
   (C) Multimodal imaging-guided acute stroke treatment based on CT and MR imaging 54
   Patrik Michel

4. **Imaging for prediction of functional outcome and for assessment of recovery** 64
   Wolf-Dieter Heiss

5. **Ultrasound in acute ischemic stroke** 82
   László Csiba

Section 2 – Clinical epidemiology and risk factors

6. **Basic epidemiology of stroke and risk assessment** 102
   Jaakko Tuomilehto

7. **Common risk factors and prevention** 119
   Michael Brainin, Yvonne Teuschl, and Karl Matz

8. **Cardiac diseases relevant to stroke** 140
   Claudia Stöllberger and Josef Finsterer

Section 3 – Diagnostics and syndromes

9. **Common stroke syndromes** 155
   Céline Odier and Patrik Michel

10. **Less common stroke syndromes** 169
    Wilfried Lang

11. **Intracerebral hemorrhage** 188
    Corina Epple, Michael Brainin, and Thorsten Steiner

12. **Subarachnoid hemorrhage** 206
    Philipp Lichti and Thorsten Steiner

13. **Cerebral venous thrombosis** 222
    Jobst Rudolf

14. **Behavioral neurology of stroke** 236
    José M. Ferro, Isabel P. Martins, and Lara Caeiro

15. **Stroke and dementia** 255
    Barbara Casolla and Didier Leys

16. **Ischemic stroke in the young and in children** 266
    Valeria Caso and Didier Leys

Section 4 – Therapeutic strategies and neurorehabilitation

17. **Stroke units and clinical assessment** 285
    Danilo Toni and Ángel Chamorro

18. **Acute therapies for stroke** 294
    Richard E. O'Brien and Kennedy R. Lees

Contents

19. **Interventional intravascular therapies for stroke** 311
Pasquale Mordasini, Jan Gralla, and Gerhard Schroth

20. **Management of acute ischemic stroke and its late complications** 326
Natan M. Bornstein and Eitan Auriel

21. **Infections in stroke** 342
Achim J. Kaasch and Harald Seifert

22. **Secondary prevention** 356
Hans-Christoph Diener, Sharan K. Mann, and Gregory W. Albers

23. **Neurorehabilitation practice for stroke patients** 371
Sylvan J. Albert and Jürg Kesselring

Index 399

Contributors

Gregory W. Albers, MD
Department of Neurology, Stanford University Medical Center, Stanford, CA, USA

Sylvan J. Albert, MD, MSc
Department of Neurology and Neurorehabilitation, Rehabilitation Centre, Valens, Switzerland

Eitan Auriel, MD
Department of Neurology, Elias Sourasky Medical Centre, Tel-Aviv, Israel

Natan M. Bornstein, MD
Department of Neurology, Elias Sourasky Medical Centre, Sackler Faculty of Medicine, Tel-Aviv University, Tel-Aviv, Israel

Michael Brainin, MD, PhD
Department of Clinical Neuroscience and Preventive Medicine, Danube University Krems, Krems, Austria

Lara Caeiro, PhD, Mcs
Department of Neurosciences, Hospital de Santa Maria and Instituto de Medicina Molecular, University of Lisboa, Portugal

Valeria Caso, MD, PhD
Department of Internal Medicine, Stroke Unit, University of Perugia, Perugia, Italy

Barbara Casolla, MD
Department of Neurology, Sapienza University, Rome, Italy

Ángel Chamorro, MD, PhD
Neurology Service, Jefe dela Unidad de Ictus Hospital Clinico, Barcelona, Spain

László Csiba, MD, PhD, DSc
Department of Neurology, University of Debrecen, Health Science Center, Debrecen, Hungary

Hans-Christoph Diener, MD, PhD
Department of Neurology, University Hospital Essen, University Duisberg Essen, Germany

Corina Epple, MD
Department of Neurology, Klinikum Frankfurt Höchst, Frankfurt, Germany

José M. Ferro, MD, PhD
Department of Neurosciences, Hospital de Santa Maria and Instituto de Medicina Molecular, University of Lisboa, Portugal

Jochen B. Fiebach, MD
Department of Neurology, Center for Stroke Research Berlin, Charité-Universitätsmedizin Berlin, Berlin, Germany

Jens Fiehler, MD
Department of Diagnostic and Interventional Neuroradiology, University Medical Center Hamburg-Eppendorf, Hamburg, Germany

Josef Finsterer, MD, PhD
Department of Internal Medicine, Krankenanstalt Rudolfstiftung, Vienna, Austria

Jan Gralla, MD, MSc
University Institute of Diagnostic and Interventional Neuroradiology, Inselspital, University of Bern, Bern, Switzerland

Wolf-Dieter Heiss, MD, PhD
Max Planck Institute for Neurological Research and Department of Neurology, University of Cologne, Cologne, Germany

Konstantin-A. Hossmann, MD, PhD
Max Planck Institute for Neurological Research, Cologne, Germany

Achim J. Kaasch, MD
Institute for Medical Microbiology, Immunology and Hygiene, Medical Center, University of Cologne, Cologne, Germany

Jürg Kesselring, MD
Department of Neurology and Neurorehabilitation, Rehabilitation Centre, Valens, Switzerland

Wilfried Lang, MD
Neurologische Abteilung, KH der Barmherzigen Brüder Wien, Vienna, Austria

Kennedy R. Lees, MD
Division of Cardiovascular and Medical Sciences, University of Glasgow and Western Infirmary, Glasgow, UK

Didier Leys, MD, PhD
Department of Neurology, Stroke Department, University of Lille, Lille, France

Philipp Lichti, MD
Department of Neurology, Klinikum Frankfurt Höchst, Frankfurt, Germany

Sharan K. Mann, MD
Department of Neurology, Stanford University Medical Center, Stanford, CA, USA

Isabel P. Martins, MD, PhD
Department of Neurosciences, Hospital de Santa Maria and Instituto de Medicina Molecular, University of Lisboa, Portugal

Karl Matz, MD
Department of Neurology, Landesklinikum Tulln, Tulln, Austria

Patrik Michel, MD
Neurology Service, Centre Hospitalier Universitaire Vaudois, University of Lausanne, Lausanne, Switzerland

Pasquale Mordasini, MD, MSc
University Institute of Diagnostic and Interventional Neuroradiology, Inselspital, University of Bern, Bern, Switzerland

Bo Norrving, MD, PhD
Department of Clinical Sciences, Division of Neurology, Lund University, Sweden

Richard E. O'Brien, MD, FRCPEdin, MBChB
City Hospitals Sunderland NHS Foundation Trust, Sunderland Royal Hospital, Sunderland, UK

Céline Odier, MD
Neurology Service, Centre Hospitalier Universitaire Vaudois, University of Lausanne, Lausanne, Switzerland

Jobst Rudolf, MD, PhD
Department of Neurology, General Hospital "Papageorgiou," Thessaloniki, Greece

Gerhard Schroth, MD
University Institute of Diagnostic and Interventional Neuroradiology, Inselspital, University of Bern, Bern, Switzerland

Harald Seifert, MD
Institute for Medical Microbiology, Immunology and Hygiene, University of Cologne, Cologne, Germany

Thorsten Steiner, MD, PhD, MME
Department of Neurology, Klinikum Frankfurt Höchst, Frankfurt, Germany and Department of Neurology, University of Heidelberg, Heidelberg, Germany

Claudia Stöllberger, MD
Department of Internal Medicine, Krankenanstalt Rudolfstiftung, Vienna, Austria

Yvonne Teuschl, PhD
Department for Clinical Neurosciences and Preventive Medicine, Danube University Krems, Krems, Austria

Danilo Toni, MD
Emergency Department Stroke Unit, Department of Neurological Sciences, University "La Sapienza," Rome, Italy

Jaakko Tuomilehto, MD, PhD
Centre for Vascular Prevention, Danube University Krems, Krems, Austria;
Diabetes Prevention Unit, National Institute for Health and Welfare, Helsinki, Finland;
King Abdulaziz University, Jeddah, Saudi Arabia; and
Instituto de Investigacion Sanitaria del Hospital Universario LaPaz (IdiPAZ), Madrid, Spain

Preface

This book is designed to improve the teaching and learning of stroke medicine in postgraduate educational programs. It is targeted at "beginning specialists," either medical students with a deeper interest or medical doctors entering the field of specialized stroke care. Therefore, the text contains what is considered essential for this readership but, in addition, goes into much greater depth, e.g. the coverage of less frequent causes of stroke, and describing the more technical facets and settings of modern stroke care.

The textbook leads the reader through the many causes of stroke, its typical manifestations, and the practical management of the stroke patient. We have tried to keep the clinical aspects to the fore, giving relative weight to those chapters that cover clinically important issues; however, the pathological, pathophysiological and anatomical background is included where necessary. The book benefits from the experience of many specialized authors, thereby providing expert coverage of the various topics by international authorities in the field. In places this leads to some differences of opinion in the approach to particular patients or conditions; as editors we have tried not to interfere with the individual character of each chapter, leaving only duplicate presentations when they were handled from different topological or didactic aspects, e.g. on genetic or rarer forms of diseases.

The development of this textbook has been triggered by the "European Master in Stroke Medicine Programme" held at Danube University in Austria. This program has been fostered by the European Stroke Organisation and has been endorsed by the World Stroke Organization. This book has been shaped by the experiences of the lecturers – most of them also leading authors for our chapters – and the feedback of our students during several runs of this course. Thus, we hope to satisfy the needs of students and young doctors from many different countries, both within and outside Europe.

Finally, we would like to thank Dr. Susanne Tabernig for her expert editorial assistance and her diligent and expert help in summarizing the chapters' contents. Thanks also to Nick Dunton and his team at Cambridge University Press for their help and patience.

Michael Brainin
Wolf-Dieter Heiss

Neuropathology and pathophysiology of stroke

Konstantin-A. Hossmann and Wolf-Dieter Heiss

The vascular origin of cerebrovascular disease

All cerebrovascular diseases (CVDs) have their origin in the vessels supplying or draining the brain. Therefore, the knowledge of pathological changes occurring in the vessels and in the blood are essential for understanding the pathophysiology of the various types of CVD and for planning of efficient therapeutic strategies. Changes in the vessel wall lead to obstruction of blood flow, by interacting with blood constituents they may cause thrombosis and blockade of blood flow in this vessel. In addition to vascular stenosis or occlusion at the site of vascular changes, disruption of blood supply and consecutive infarcts can also be produced by emboli arising from vascular lesions situated proximally to otherwise healthy branches located more distal in the arterial tree or from a source located in the heart. At the site of occlusion, opportunity exists for thrombus to develop in anterograde fashion throughout the length of the vessel, but this event seems to occur only rarely.

Changes in large arteries supplying the brain, including the aorta, are mainly caused by atherosclerosis. Middle-sized and intracerebral arteries can also be affected by acute or chronic vascular diseases of inflammatory origin due to subacute to chronic infections, e.g. tuberculosis and lues, or due to collagen disorders, e.g. giant cell arteritis, granulomatous angiitis of the central nervous system, panarteritis nodosa, and even more rarely systemic lupus erythematosus, Takayasu's arteritis, Wegener granulomatosis, rheumatoid arteritis, Sjögren's syndrome, or Sneddon and Behçet's disease. In some diseases affecting the vessels of the brain the etiology and pathogenesis are still unclear, e.g. moyamoya disease

and fibromuscular dysplasia, but these disorders are characterized by typical locations of the vascular changes. Some arteriopathies are hereditary, such as CADASIL (cerebral autosomal dominant arteriopathy with subcortical infarcts and leukoencephalopathy), in some such as cerebral amyloid angiopathy a degenerative cause has been suggested. All these vascular disorders can cause obstruction, and lead to thrombosis and embolizations. Small vessels of the brain are affected by hyalinosis and fibrosis; this "small-vessel disease" can cause lacunes and, if widespread, is the substrate for vascular cognitive impairment and vascular dementia.

Atherosclerosis is the most widespread disorder leading to death and serious morbidity including stroke [1]. The basic pathological lesion is the atheromatous plaque, and the most commonly affected sites are the aorta, the coronary arteries, the carotid artery at its bifurcation, and the basilar artery. Arteriosclerosis, a more generic term describing hardening and thickening of the arteries, includes as additional types Mönkeberg's sclerosis which is characterized by calcification in the tunica media and arteriolosclerosis with proliferative and hyaline changes affecting the arterioles. Atherosclerosis starts at young age, lesions accumulate and grow throughout life and become symptomatic and clinically evident when end organs are affected [2].

> Atherosclerosis: atheromatous plaques, most commonly in the aorta, the coronary arteries, the bifurcation of the carotid artery and the basilar artery.

The initial lesion of atherosclerosis has been attributed to "fatty streaks" and the "intimal cell mass." Those changes already occur in childhood and adolescence and do not necessarily correspond to the future sites of atherosclerotic plaques. Fatty streaks

Textbook of Stroke Medicine, Second Edition, ed. Michael Brainin and Wolf-Dieter Heiss. Published by Cambridge University Press. © Michael Brainin and Wolf-Dieter Heiss 2014.

1

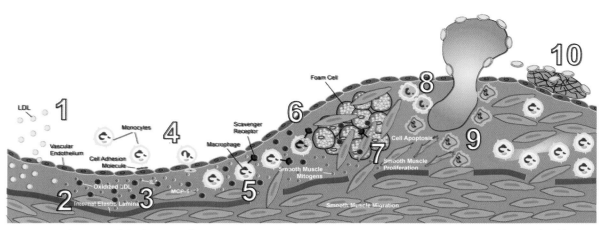

Figure 1.1. The stages of development of an atherosclerotic plaque. (1) LDL moves into the subendothelium and (2) is oxidized by macrophages and smooth muscle cells (SMC). (3) Release of growth factors and cytokines (4) attracts additional monocytes. (5) Macrophages and (6) foam cell accumulation and additional (7) SMC proliferation result in (8) growth of the plaque. (9) Fibrous cap degradation and plaque rupture (collagenases, elastases). (10) Thrombus formation. IL-1 = interlenkin-1; MCP-1 = Monocyte chemotactic protein-1. (Modified with permission from Faxon *et al.* [5].)

are focal areas of intra cellular lipid collection in both macrophages and smooth muscle cells. Various concepts have been proposed to explain the progression of such precursor lesions to definite atherosclerosis [2, 3], most remarkable of which is the response-to-injury hypothesis postulating a cellular and molecular response to various atherogenic stimuli in the form of an inflammatory repair process [4]. This inflammation develops concurrently with the accumulation of minimally oxidized low-density lipoproteins (LDLs) [5, 6], and stimulates vascular smooth muscle cells (VSMCs), endothelial cells, and macrophages [7], and as a result foam cells aggregate with an accumulation of oxidized LDL. In the further stages of artherosclerotic plaque development VSMCs migrate, proliferate, and synthesize extracellular matrix components on the luminal side of the vessel wall, forming the fibrous cap of the atherosclerotic lesion [8]. In this complex process of growth, progression, and finally rupture of an atherosclerotic plaque a large number of matrix modulators, inflammatory mediators, growth factors, and vasoactive substances are involved. The complex interactions of these many factors are discussed in the special literature [5–9].

The fibrous cap of the atherosclerotic lesion covers the deep lipid core with a massive accumulation of extracellular lipids (*atheromatous plaque*), or fibroblasts and extracellular calcifications may contribute to a *fibrocalcific lesion*. Mediators from inflammatory cells at the thinnest portion of the cap surface of a *vulnerable plaque* – which is characterized by a

larger lipid core and a thin fibrous cap – can lead to plaque disruption with formation of a thrombus or hematoma or even to total occlusion of the vessel. During the development of atherosclerosis the entire vessel can enlarge or constrict in size [10]. However, once the plaque covers >40% of the vessel wall, the artery no longer enlarges, and the lumen narrows as the plaque grows. In vulnerable plaques thrombosis forming on the disrupted lesion further narrows the vessel lumen and can lead to occlusion or be the origin of emboli. Less commonly, plaques have reduced collagen and elastin with a thin and weakened arterial wall, resulting in aneurysm formation which when ruptured may be the source of intracerebral hemorrhage (Figure 1.1).

> Injury hypothesis of progression to atherosclerosis: fatty streaks (focal areas of intra cellular lipid collection) → inflammatory repair process with stimulation of vascular smooth muscle cells → atheromatous plaque.

Thromboembolism: immediately after plaque rupture or erosion, subendothelial collagen, the lipid core, and procoagulants such as tissue factor and von Willebrand factor are exposed to circulating blood. Platelets rapidly adhere to the vessel wall through the platelet glycoproteins (GP) Ia/IIa and GP Ib/IX [11] with subsequent aggregation to this initial monolayer through linkage with fibrinogen and the exposed GP IIb/IIIa on activated platelets. As platelets are a source of nitric oxide (NO), the resulting deficiency of bioactive NO, which is an effective vasodilator, contributes to the progression of thrombosis by augmenting platelet activation, enhancing VSMC proliferation and migration, and participating in neovascularization [12]. The activated platelets also release adenosine diphosphate (ADP) and thromboxane A2 with subsequent activation of the clotting cascade. The growing thrombus obstructs or even blocks the blood flow in the vessel. Atherosclerotic thrombi are also the source for embolisms, which are the primary pathophysiological mechanism of ischemic strokes, especially from carotid artery disease or of cardiac origin.

> Rupture or erosion of atheromatous plaques → adhesion of platelets → thrombus → obstruction of blood flow and source of emboli.

Small-vessel disease usually affects the arterioles and is associated with hypertension. It is caused by subendothelial accumulation of a pathological protein, the hyaline, formed from mucopolysaccharides and matrix proteins, which leads to narrowing of the lumen or even occlusion of these small vessels. Often it is associated with fibrosis, which affects not only arterioles, but also other small vessels and capillaries and venules. Lipohyalinosis also weakens the vessel wall, predisposing for the formation of "miliary aneurysms." Small-vessel disease results in two pathological conditions: status lacunaris (lacunar state) and status cribrosus (état criblé). Status lacunaris is characterized by small irregularly shaped infarcts due to occlusion of small vessels; it is the pathological substrate of lacunar strokes and vascular cognitive impairment and dementia. In status cribrosus small round cavities develop around affected arteries due to disturbed supply of oxygen and metabolic substrate. These "criblures" together with miliary aneurysms are the sites of vessel rupture causing typical hypertonic intracerebral hemorrhages [13–16]. A second type of small-vessel disease is characterized by the progressive accumulation of congophilic, βA4 immunoreactive, amyloid protein in the walls of small- to medium-sized arteries and arterioles. Cerebral amyloid angiopathy is a pathological hallmark of Alzheimer's disease and also occurs in rare genetically transmitted diseases, e.g. CADASIL and Fabry's disease [17]. For a more detailed discussion of the etiology and pathophysiology of the various specific vascular disorders see [18–20].

> Small-vessel disease: subendothelial accumulation of hyaline in arterioles.

Types of acute cerebrovascular diseases

Numbers relating to the frequency of the different types of acute CVD are highly variable depending on the source of data. The most reliable numbers come from the in-hospital assessment of stroke in the Framingham study determining the frequency of completed stroke: 60% were caused by atherothrombotic brain infarction, 25.1% by cerebral embolism, 5.4% by subarachnoid hemorrhage, 8.3% by intracerebral hemorrhage, and 1.2% by undefined diseases. In addition, transient ischemic attacks (TIAs) accounted for 14.8% of the total cerebrovascular events [21].

Ischemic strokes result from a critical reduction of regional cerebral blood flow (rCBF) lasting beyond a critical duration, and are caused by atherothrombotic changes of the arteries supplying the brain or by emboli from sources in the heart, the aorta, or the large arteries. The pathological substrate of ischemic stroke is ischemic infarction of brain tissue, the location, extension, and shape of which depend on the size of the occluded vessel, the mechanism of arterial obstruction, and the compensatory capacity of the vascular bed. Occlusion of arteries supplying defined brain territories by atherothrombosis or embolization lead to *territorial infarcts* of variable size: they may be large – e.g. the whole territory supplied by the middle cerebral artery (MCA) – or small, if branches of large arteries are occluded or if compensatory collateral perfusion – e.g. via the circle of Willis or leptomeningeal anastomoses – is efficient in reducing the area of critically reduced flow (Figure 1.2) [14, 16]. In a smaller number of cases *infarcts* can also develop *at the borderzones* between vascular territories, when several large arteries are stenotic and the perfusion in these "last meadows" cannot be constantly maintained above the critical threshold of morphological integrity [22]. *Borderzone infarctions* are a subtype of the *low-flow* or hemodynamically induced *infarctions* which are the result of critically reduced cerebral perfusion pressure in far-downstream brain arteries. The more common low-flow infarctions affect subcortical structures within a vascular bed with preserved but marginal irrigation [23]. *Lacunar infarcts* reflect disease of the vessels penetrating the brain to supply the capsule, the basal ganglia, thalamus, and paramedian regions of the brainstem [24]. Most often they are caused by lipohyalinosis of deep arteries (small-vessel disease); less frequent causes are stenosis

3

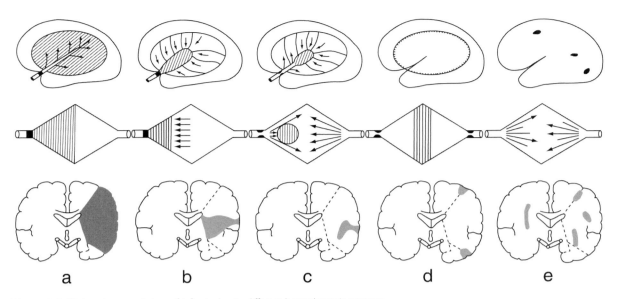

Figure 1.2. Various types and sizes of infarcts due to different hemodynamic patterns
a. Total territorial infarct due to defective collateral supply
b. Core infarct, meningeal anastomosis supply peripheral zones
c. Territorial infarct in center of supply area, due to branch occlusion
d. Borderzone infarction in watershed areas due to stenotic lesions in arteries supplying neighboring areas
e. Lacunar infarctions due to small-vessel disease. (Modified with permission from Zülch [14].)

of the MCA stem and microembolization to penetrant arterial territories. Pathologically these lacunes are defined as small cystic trabeculated scars about 5 mm in diameter, but they are more often observed on magnetic resonance images, where they are accepted as lacunes up to 1.5 cm diameter. The classic lacunar syndromes include pure motor, pure sensory, and sensorimotor syndromes, sometimes ataxic hemiparesis, clumsy hand, dysarthria, and hemichorea/hemiballism, but higher cerebral functions are not involved. A new classification of stroke subtypes is mainly oriented on the most likely cause of stroke: atherosclerosis, small-vessel disease, cardiac source, or other cause [25].

> Territorial infarcts are caused by an occlusion of arteries supplying defined brain territories by atherothrombosis or embolizations.
> Borderzone infarcts develop at the borderzone between vascular territories and are the result of a critically reduced cerebral perfusion pressure (low-flow infarctions).
> Lacunar infarcts are mainly caused by small-vessel disease.

Hemorrhagic infarctions, i.e. "red infarcts" in contrast to the usual "pale infarcts," are defined as ischemic infarcts in which varying numbers of blood cells are found within the necrotic tissue. The size can range from a few petechial bleeds in the gray matter of cortex and basal ganglia to large hemorrhages involving the cortical and deep hemispheric regions. Hemorrhagic transformation frequently appears during the second and third phase of infarct evolution, when macrophages appear and new blood vessels are formed in tissue consisting of neuronal ghosts and proliferating astrocytes. However, the only significant difference between "pale" and "red infarcts" is the intensity and extension of the hemorrhagic component, since in at least two-thirds of all infarcts petechial hemorrhages are microscopically detectable. Macroscopically, red infarcts contain multifocal bleedings which are more or less confluent and predominate in cerebral cortex and basal ganglia, which are richer in capillaries than the white matter[26]. If the hemorrhages become confluent intrainfarct hematomas might develop, and extensive edema may contribute to mass effects and lead to *malignant infarction*. The frequency of hemorrhagic infarctions in anatomical studies ranged from 18% to 42% [27], with a high incidence (up to 85% of hemorrhagic infarcts) in cardioembolic stroke [28].

Mechanisms for hemorrhagic transformation are manifold and vary with regard to the intensity of bleeding. Petechial bleeding results from diapedesis rather than vascular rupture. In severe ischemic tissue vascular permeability is increased and endothelial tight junctions are ruptured. When blood circulation is spontaneously or therapeutically restored, blood can leak out of these damaged vessels. This can also happen with fragmentation and distal migration of an embolus (usually of cardiac origin) in the damaged vascular bed, explaining delayed clinical worsening in some cases. For the hemorrhagic transformation the collateral circulation might also have an impact: in some instances reperfusion via pial networks may develop with the diminution of peri-ischemic edema at borderzones of cortical infarcts. Risk of hemorrhage is significantly increased in large infarcts, with mass effect supporting the importance of edema for tissue damage and the deleterious effect of late reperfusion when edema resolves. In some instances also the rupture of the vascular wall secondary to ischemia-induced endothelial necrosis might cause an intra-infarct hematoma. Vascular rupture can explain very early hemorrhagic infarcts and early intrainfarct hematoma (between 6 and 18 hours after stroke), whereas hemorrhagic transformation usually develops within 48 hours to 2 weeks.

> Hemorrhagic infarctions are defined as ischemic infarcts in which varying amounts of blood cells are found within the necrotic tissue. They are caused by leakage from damaged vessels, due to increased vascular permeability in ischemic tissue or vascular rupture secondary to ischemia

Intracerebral hemorrhage (ICH) occurs as a result of bleeding from an arterial source directly into the brain parenchyma and accounts for 5–15% of all strokes [29, 30]. Hypertension is the leading risk factor, but in addition advanced age, race and also cigarette smoking, alcohol consumption, and high serum cholesterol levels have been identified. In a number of instances ICH occurs in the absence of hypertension, usually in atypical locations. The causes include small vascular malformations, vasculitis, brain tumors, and sympathomimetic drugs (e.g. cocaine). ICH may also be caused by cerebral amyloid angiopathy and rarely damage is elicited by acute changes in blood pressure, e.g. due to exposure to cold. The occurrence of ICH is also influenced by the increasing use of antithrombotic and thrombolytic treatment of ischemic diseases of the brain, heart, and other organs [31, 32].

Spontaneous ICH occurs predominantly in the deep portions of the cerebral hemispheres ("typical ICH") [33]. Its most common location is the putamen (35–50% of cases). The subcortical white matter is the second most frequent location (approx. 30%). Hemorrhages in the thalamus are found in 10–15%, in the pons in 5–12%, and in the cerebellum in 7% [34]. Most ICHs originate from the rupture of small, deep arteries with diameters of 50 to 200 μm which are affected by lipohyalinosis due to chronic hypertension. These small-vessel changes lead to weakening of the vessel wall and miliary microaneurysm and consecutive small local bleedings, which might be followed by secondary ruptures of the enlarging hematoma in a cascade or avalanche fashion [35]. After active bleeding has started it can continue for a number of hours with enlargement of hematoma that is frequently associated with clinical deterioration [36].

Putaminal hemorrhages originate from a lateral branch of the striate arteries at the posterior angle, resulting in an ovoid mass pushing the insular cortex laterally and displacing or involving the internal capsule. From this initial putaminal-claustral location a large hematoma may extend to the internal capsule and lateral ventricle, into the corona radiata, and into the temporal white matter. Putaminal ICHs are considered the typical hypertensive hemorrhages.

Caudate hemorrhage, a less common form of bleeding from distal branches of lateral striate arteries, occurs in the head of the caudate nucleus. This bleeding soon connects to the ventricle and usually involves the anterior limb of the internal capsule.

Thalamic hemorrhages can involve most of this nucleus and extend into the third ventricle medially and the posterior limb of the internal capsule laterally. The hematoma may press on or even extend into the midbrain. Larger hematomas often reach the corona radiata and the parietal white matter.

Lobar (white matter) hemorrhages originate at the cortico-subcortical junction between gray and white matter and usually spread along the fiber bundles in the parietal and occipital lobes. The hematomas are close to the cortical surface and usually not in direct contact with deep hemisphere structures or the ventricular system. As atypical ICHs they are not necessarily correlated with hypertension.

5

Cerebellar hemorrhages usually originate in the area of the dentate nucleus from rupture of distal branches of the superior cerebellar artery and extend into the hemispheric white matter and into the fourth ventricle. The pontine tegmentum is often compressed. A variant, the midline hematoma, originates from the cerebellar vermis, always communicates with the fourth ventricle, and frequently extends bilaterally into the pontine tegmentum.

Pontine hemorrhages from bleeding of small paramedian basilar perforating branches cause medially placed hematomas involving the basis of the pons. A unilateral variety results from rupture of distal long circumferential branches of the basilar artery. These hematomas usually communicate with the fourth ventricle, and extend laterally and ventrally into the pons.

The frequency of recurrent ICHs in hypertensive patients is rather low (6%) [37]. Recurrence rate is higher with poor control of hypertension and also in hemorrhages due to other causes. In some instances multiple simultaneous ICHs may occur, but also in these cases the cause is other than hypertension.

In ICHs, the local accumulation of blood destroys the parenchyma, displaces nervous structures, and dissects the tissue. At the bleeding sites fibrin globes are formed around accumulated platelets. After hours or days extracellular edema develops at the periphery of the hematoma. After 4 to 10 days the red blood cells begin to lyse, granulocytes and thereafter microglial cells arrive, and foamy macrophages are formed, which ingest debris and hemosiderin. Finally, the astrocytes at the periphery of the hematoma proliferate and turn into gemistocytes with eosinophylic cytoplasma. When the hematoma is removed, the astrocytes are replaced by glial fibrils. After that period – extending to months – the residue of the hematoma is a flat cavity with a reddish lining resulting from hemosiderin-laden macrophages [34].

> Intracerebral hemorrhage (ICH) occurs as a result of bleeding from an arterial source directly into the brain parenchyma, predominantly in the deep portions of the cerebral hemispheres (typical ICH). Hypertension is the leading risk factor, and the most common location is the putamen.

Cerebral venous thrombosis (CVT) can develop from many causes and due to predisposing conditions. CVT is often multifactorial, when various risk factors and causes contribute to the development of this disorder [38]. The incidence of septic CVT has been reduced to less than 10% of cases, but septic cavernous sinus thrombosis is still a severe, however, rare problem. Aseptic CVT occurs during puerperium and less frequently during pregnancy, but may also be related to use of oral contraceptives. Among the non-infectious causes of CVT congenital thrombophilia, particularly prothrombin and factor V Leiden gene mutations, as well as antithrombin, protein C, and protein S deficiencies must be considered. Other conditions with risk for CVT are malignancies, inflammatory diseases, and systemic lupus erythematosus. However, in 20–35% of CVT the etiology remains unknown. The fresh venous thrombus is rich in red blood cells and fibrin and poor in platelets. Later on, it is replaced by fibrous tissue, occasionally with recanalization. The most common location of CVT is the superior sagittal sinus and the tributary veins.

Whereas some thromboses, particularly of the lateral sinus, may have no pathological consequences for the brain tissue, occlusion of large cerebral veins usually leads to a venous infarct. These infarcts are located in the cortex and adjacent white matter and often are hemorrhagic. Thrombosis of the superior sagittal sinus may lead only to brain edema, but usually causes bilateral hemorrhagic infarcts in both hemispheres. These venous infarcts are different from arterial infarcts: cytotoxic edema is absent or mild, vasogenic edema is prominent, and hemorrhagic transformation or bleeding is usual. Despite this hemorrhagic component heparin is the treatment of choice.

> Cerebral venous thrombosis can lead to a venous infarct. Venous infarcts are different from arterial infarcts: cytotoxic edema is absent or mild, vasogenic edema is prominent, and hemorrhagic transformation or bleeding is usual.

Cellular pathology of ischemic stroke

Acute occlusion of a major brain artery causes a stereotyped sequel of cellular alterations which evolve over a protracted period of time and which depend on the topography, severity, and duration of ischemia [39]. The most sensitive brain cells are neurons, followed – in this order – by oligodendrocytes, astrocytes, and vascular cells. The most vulnerable brain regions are hippocampal subfield CA_1, neocortical layers 3, 5, and 6, the outer segment of striate nucleus, and the Purkinje and basket cell layers of cerebellar cortex. If blood flow decreases below the threshold of energy metabolism, the primary pathology is necrosis of all cell elements, resulting in ischemic brain infarct. If ischemia is not severe enough to cause primary energy failure, or if it is of so short duration that energy metabolism recovers after reperfusion, a delayed type of cell death may evolve which exhibits the morphological characteristics of necrosis, apoptosis, or a combination of both. In the following, primary and delayed cell death will be described separately.

Primary ischemic cell death

In the core of the territory of an occluded brain artery the earliest sign of cellular injury is neuronal swelling or shrinkage, the cytoplasm exhibiting microvacuolation (MV) which ultrastructurally has been associated with mitochondrial swelling [40]. These changes are potentially reversible if blood flow is restored before mitochondrial membranes begin to rupture. One to two hours after the onset of ischemia, neurons undergo irreversible necrotic alterations (red neuron or ischemic cell change). In conventional hematoxylin-eosin-stained brain sections such neurons are characterized by intensively stained eosinophilic cytoplasma, formation of triangular nuclear pyknosis, and direct contact with swollen astrocytes (Figure 1.3). Electron-microscopically mitochondria exhibit flocculent densities which represent denaturated mitochondrial proteins. Ischemic cell change must be distinguished from artifactual dark neurons which stain with all (acid or basic) dyes and are not surrounded by swollen astrocytes [41].

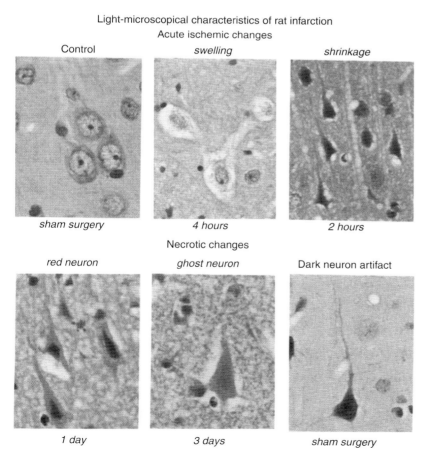

Light-microscopical characteristics of rat infarction

Acute ischemic changes

Control — sham surgery

swelling — 4 hours

shrinkage — 2 hours

Necrotic changes

red neuron — 1 day

ghost neuron — 3 days

Dark neuron artifact — sham surgery

Figure 1.3. Light-microscopical evolution of neuronal changes after experimental middle cerebral occlusion. (Modified with permission from Garcia *et al.* [126].)

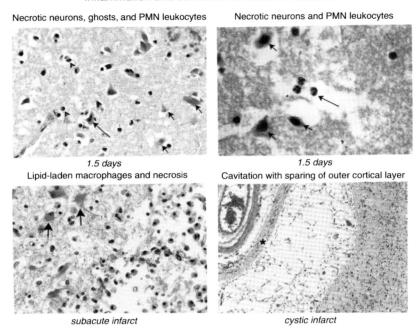

Inflammation and cavitation of ischemic infarction

Necrotic neurons, ghosts, and PMN leukocytes

Necrotic neurons and PMN leukocytes

1.5 days

Lipid-laden macrophages and necrosis

1.5 days

Cavitation with sparing of outer cortical layer

subacute infarct

cystic infarct

Figure 1.4. Transformation of acute ischemic alterations into cystic infarct. Note pronounced inflammatory reaction prior to tissue cavitation. PMN = polymorphonuclear leukocyte. (Modified with permission from Petito [39].)

With ongoing ischemia, neurons gradually loose their stainability with hematoxylin, they become mildly eosinophilic, and, after 2–4 days, transform to ghost cells with hardly detectable pale outline. Interestingly, neurons with ischemic cell change are mainly located in the periphery and ghost cells in the center of the ischemic territory, which suggests that manifestation of ischemic cell change requires some residual or restored blood flow whereas ghost cells may evolve in the absence of flow [39].

Primary ischemic cell death induced by focal ischemia is associated with reactive and secondary changes. The most prominent alteration during the initial 1–2 hours is perivascular and perineuronal astrocytic swelling, after 4–6 hours the blood–brain barrier breaks down, resulting in the formation of vasogenic edema, after 1–2 days inflammatory cells accumulate throughout the ischemic infarct, and within 1.5–3 months cystic transformation of the necrotic tissue occurs together with the development of a peri-infarct astroglial scar (Figure 1.4)

Delayed neuronal death

The prototype of delayed cell death is the slowly progressing injury of pyramidal neurons in the CA_1 sector of the hippocampus after a brief episode of global ischemia [42]. In focal ischemia delayed neuronal death may occur in the periphery of cortical infarcts or in regions which have been reperfused before ischemic energy failure becomes irreversible. Cell death is also observed in distant brain regions, notably in the substantia nigra and thalamus.

The morphological appearance of neurons during the interval between ischemia and the manifestation of delayed cell death exhibits a continuum that ranges from necrosis to apoptosis with all possible combinations of cytoplasmic and nuclear morphology that are characteristic for the two types of cell death [43]. In its pure form, necrosis combines karyorrhexis with massive swelling of endoplasmic reticulum and mitochondria, whereas in apoptosis mitochondria remain intact and nuclear fragmentation with condensation of nuclear chromatin gives way to the development of apoptotic bodies. A frequently used histochemical method for the visualization of apoptosis is terminal deoxyribonucleotidyl transferase (TdT)-mediated dUTP-biotin nick-end labeling (TUNEL assay), which detects DNA strand breaks. However, as this method may also stain necrotic neurons, a clear differentiation is not possible [44].

A consistent ultrastructural finding in neurons undergoing delayed cell death is disaggregation of ribosomes, which reflects the inhibition of protein synthesis at the initiation step of translation [45]. Light-microscopically, this change is equivalent to tigrolysis, visible in Nissl-stained material. Disturbances of protein synthesis and the associated endoplasmic reticulum (ER) stress are also responsible for cytosolic protein aggregation and the formation of stress granules [46]. In the hippocampus, stacks of accumulated ER may become visible but in other areas this is not a prominent finding.

Pathology of the neurovascular unit

The classical pathology of ischemic injury differentiates between the sensitivity of the various cell types of brain parenchyma with the neurons as the most vulnerable elements. The molecular analysis of injury evolution, however, suggests that ischemia initiates a coordinated multi-compartmental response of brain cells and vessels, also referred to as the neurovascular unit [47]. This unit includes microvessels (endothelial cells, basal lamina matrix, astrocytic endfeet, pericytes, and circulating blood elements), the cell body and main processes of astrocytes, the nearby neurons together with their axons, and supporting cells, notably microglia and oligodendrocytes. It provides the framework for the bi-directional communication between neuron and supplying microvessel. Under physiological conditions, the most prominent function is the neurovascular coupling for maintaining adequate supply of brain nutrients and clearance of waste products. Pathophysiological disturbances of microcirculation, conversely, provoke coincidental microvessel–neuron responses, possibly mediated by alterations in the matrix of the vascular and non-vascular compartments of the ischemic territory.

> Severe ischemia induces primary cell death due to necrosis of all cell elements. Not so severe or short-term ischemia induces delayed cell death with necrosis, apoptosis, or a combination of both. The neurovascular unit provides the conceptual framework for the propagation of injury from microvessels to neurons.

Animal models of stroke

According to the Framingham study, 65% of strokes that result from vascular occlusion present lesions in the territory of the MCA, 2% in the anterior and 9% in the posterior cerebral artery territories; the rest is located in brainstem, cerebellum, in watershed, or multiple regions. In experimental stroke research, this situation is reflected by the preferential use of MCA occlusion models.

Transorbital middle cerebral artery occlusion: this model was introduced in the 1970s for the production of stroke in monkeys [48] and later modified for use in cats, dogs, rabbits, and even rats. The procedure is technically demanding and requires microsurgical skills. The advantage of this approach is the possibility to expose the MCA at its origin from the internal carotid artery without retracting parts of the brain. Vascular occlusion can thus be performed without the risk of brain trauma. On the other hand, removal of the eyeball is invasive and may evoke functional disturbances which should not be ignored. Surgery may also cause generalized vasospasm which may interfere with the collateral circulation and, hence, induce variations in infarct size. The procedure therefore requires extensive training before reproducible results can be expected.

The occlusion of the MCA at its origin interrupts blood flow to the total vascular territory, including the basal ganglia which are supplied by the lenticulostriate arteries. These MCA branches are end-arteries which in contrast to the cortical branches do not form collaterals with the adjacent vascular territories. As a consequence, the basal ganglia are consistently part of the infarct core whereas the cerebral cortex exhibits a gradient of blood flow which decreases from the peripheral towards the central parts of the vascular territory. Depending on the steepness of this gradient, a cortical core region with the lowest flow values in the lower temporal cortex is surrounded by a variably sized penumbra which may extend up to the parasagittal cortex.

Transcranial occlusion of the middle cerebral artery: post- or retro-orbital transcranial approaches for MCA occlusion are mainly used in rats and mice because in these species the main stem of the artery appears on the cortical surface rather close to its origin from the internal carotid artery [49]. In contrast to transorbital MCA occlusion, transcranial models do not produce ischemic injury in the basal ganglia because the lenticulostriate branches originate proximal to the occlusion site. Infarcts, therefore, are mainly located in the temporo-parietal cortex with a gradient of declining flow values from the peripheral to the central parts of the vascular territory.

Filament occlusion of the middle cerebral artery: the presently most widely used procedure for MCA occlusion in rats and mice is the intraluminal filament occlusion technique, first described by Koizumi *et al.* [50]. A nylon suture with an acryl-thickened tip is inserted into the common carotid artery and orthogradely advanced, until the tip is located at the origin of the MCA. Modifications of the original technique include different thread types for isolated or combined vascular occlusion, adjustments of the tip size to the weight of the animal, poly-L-lysine coating of the tip to prevent incomplete MCA occlusion, or the use of guide-sheaths to allow remote manipulation of the thread for occlusion during polygraphic recordings or magnetic resonance imaging.

The placement of the suture at the origin of the MCA obstructs blood supply to the total MCA supplied territory, including the basal ganglia. It may also reduce blood flow in the anterior and posterior cerebral arteries, particularly when the common carotid artery is ligated to facilitate the insertion of the thread. As this minimizes collateral blood supply from these territories, infarcts are very large and produce massive ischemic brain edema with a high mortality when experiments last for more than a few hours. For this reason, threads are frequently withdrawn 1–2 hours following insertion. The resulting reperfusion salvages the peripheral parts of the MCA territory, and infarcts become smaller [51]. However, the pathophysiology of transient MCA occlusion differs basically from that of the clinically more relevant permanent occlusion models, and neither the mechanisms of infarct evolution nor the pharmacological responsiveness of the resulting lesions replicate that of clinical stroke [52].

Transient filament occlusion is also an inappropriate model for the investigation of spontaneous or thrombolysis-induced reperfusion. Withdrawal of the intraluminal thread induces instantaneous reperfusion whereas spontaneous or thrombolysis-induced recanalization results in slowly progressing recirculation. As post-ischemic recovery is greatly influenced by the dynamics of reperfusion, outcome and pharmacological responsiveness of transient filament occlusion is distinct from most clinical situations of reversible ischemia, where the onset of reperfusion is much less abrupt.

Clot embolism of middle cerebral artery: MCA embolism with autologous blood clots is a clinically highly relevant but also inherently variable stroke model which requires careful preparation and placement of standardized clots to induce reproducible brain infarcts [53]. The most reliable procedure for clot preparation is thrombin-induced clotting of autologous blood within calibrated tubings, which results in cylindrical clots that can be dissected in segments of equal length. Selection of either fibrin-rich (white) or fibrin-poor (red) segments influences the speed of spontaneous reperfusion and results in different outcome. Clots can also be produced *in situ* by microinjection of thrombin [54] or photochemically by ultraviolet illumination of the MCA following injection of rose Bengal [55].

The main application of clot embolism is for the investigation of experimental thrombolysis. The drug most widely used is human recombinant tissue plasminogen activator (rtPA) but the dose required in animals is much higher than in humans, which must be remembered when possible side-effects such as rtPA toxicity are investigated. The hemodynamic effect, in contrast, is similar despite the higher dose and adequately reproduces the slowly progressing recanalization observed under clinical conditions.

A recent development of clinical stroke treatment and possibly the central challenge for future animal research is *interventional thrombectomy* [56]. The animal most widely used for this research is the swine but as in this species the carotid access to the anterior cerebral vasculature is impeded by a rete mirabile, clot embolism and retrieval is carried out via the internal maxillary or lingual artery [57]. Angiographic studies confirm that clot retrieval using either aspiration or removable stent devices results in immediate recanalization but a detailed pathophysiological analysis of post-ischemic reperfusion is not yet available. It is, therefore, premature to speculate whether this treatment and its effect on post-ischemic recovery can also be replicated in smaller animals by technically simpler mechanical occlusion models, such as transient filament occlusion.

> Various procedures for artery occlusion models, mostly middle cerebral artery occlusion models, were developed to study focal ischemia in animals.

Hemodynamics of stroke
Normal regulation of blood flow
In the *intact brain*, CBF is tightly coupled to the metabolic requirements of tissue (metabolic regulation) but the flow rate remains essentially constant over a wide range of blood pressures (autoregulation).

An important requirement for *metabolic regulation* is the responsiveness of blood vessels to carbon dioxide (*CO₂ reactivity*), which can be tested by the application of carbonic anhydrase inhibitors or CO_2 ventilation. Under physiological conditions, blood flow doubles when CO_2 rises by about 30 mmHg, and is reduced by one-third when CO_2 declines by 15 mmHg. The vascular response to CO_2 depends mainly on the changes of extracellular pH but it is also modulated by other factors such as prostanoids, NO, and neurogenic influences.

Autoregulation of CBF is the remarkable capacity of the vascular system to adjust its resistance in such a way that blood flow is kept constant over a wide range of cerebral perfusion pressures (80–150 mmHg). The range of autoregulation is shifted to the right, i.e. to higher values, in patients with hypertension and to the left during hypercarbia.

The mechanism of autoregulation is complex [58]. The dominating factor is a pressure-sensitive direct myogenic response initiated by the activation of stretch-sensitive cation channels of vascular smooth muscle. In addition, a flow-sensitive indirect smooth muscle response is initiated by changes in the shear stress of endothelial cells, which result in activation of various signal transduction pathways. Other influences are mediated by metabolic and neurogenic factors but these may be secondary effects and are of lesser significance.

> Metabolic regulation: cerebral blood flow is coupled to metabolic requirements of tissue by a vascular response to changes in CO_2. Autoregulation: cerebral blood flow is kept constant over a wide range of cerebral perfusion pressures.

Disturbances of flow regulation

Focal cerebral ischemia is associated with tissue acidosis which leads to vasoparalysis and, in consequence, to a severe disturbance of the regulation of blood flow [59]. In the center of the ischemic territory, CO_2 reactivity is abolished or even reversed, i.e. blood flow may decrease with increasing arterial pCO_2. This paradoxical "steal" effect has been attributed to the rerouting of blood to adjacent non-ischemic brain regions in which CO_2 reactivity remains intact.

Stroke also impairs autoregulation but the disturbance is more severe with decreasing rather than with increasing blood pressure. This is explained by the fact that in the ischemic tissue a decrease of local

brain perfusion pressure cannot be compensated by further vasorelaxation whereas an increase may shift the local perfusion pressure into the autoregulatory range and cause vasoconstriction. An alternative explanation is "false autoregulation" due to brain edema which causes an increase in local tissue pressure that precludes a rise of the actual tissue perfusion pressure. Failure of cerebral autoregulation can be demonstrated in such instances by dehydrating the brain in order to reduce brain edema.

After transient ischemia, vasorelaxation persists for some time, which explains the phenomenon of post-ischemic hyperemia or luxury perfusion. During luxury perfusion, oxygen supply exceeds oxygen requirements of the tissue, as reflected by the appearance of red venous blood. With the cessation of tissue acidosis, vascular tone returns, and blood flow declines to or below normal. At longer recirculation times autoregulation – but not CO_2 reactivity – may recover, resulting in persisting failure of metabolic regulation. This is one of the reasons why primary post-ischemic recovery may be followed by delayed post-ischemic hypoxia and secondary metabolic failure [60].

> Disturbances of flow regulation through ischemia: tissue acidosis leads to vasorelaxation, CO_2 reactivity is abolished or even reversed, and autoregulation is impaired.

Disturbances of microcirculation

With the increasing understanding of the pathobiology of the neurovascular unit, microcirculatory disturbances are recognized to contribute to the evolution of ischemic brain injury [61]. Such disturbances develop at the capillary level within the first hour of focal ischemia and may persist even after full reversal of vascular occlusion (incomplete microcirculatory reperfusion). The dominating pathology is the narrowing of the capillary lumen, induced by constriction of pericytes and swelling of pericapillary astrocytic endfeet. The capillaries are filled with aggregated red blood cells, leukocytes, and fibrin/platelet deposits, the high viscosity of which adds to the increased vascular resistance of the reduced capillary lumen.

The mechanism of microcirculatory impairment is multifactorial. Pericytes constrict in response to the generation of reactive oxygen species (ROS), swelling of astrocytic endfeet is due to cytotoxic brain edema, and leukocyte adhesion to the vessel wall is part of the

11

inflammatory response mediated by the generation of chemoattractants, cytokines, and chemokines. Finally, the activation of proteolytic enzymes contributes to the dismantlement of basal lamina and results in damage of the blood–brain barrier, an increase in interstitial tissue pressure, and the risk of hemorrhagic transformation.

The impairment of microcirculation is equivalent to a reduction of nutritional blood flow. During permanent vascular occlusion it aggravates the effect of primary ischemia, particularly in the borderzone of the infarct, and after transient vascular occlusion it prevents adequate reoxygenation despite recanalization of the supplying artery. It is still unresolved to what extent microcirculatory impairment contributes to or originates from ischemic injury but there is general consent that microvascular protection is a requirement for successful stroke treatment [62].

> Focal brain ischemia is aggravated by microcirculatory disturbances which may persist despite recanalization.

Anastomotic steal phenomena

The brain is protected against focal disturbances of blood flow by the collateral circulation, which provides a subsidiary network of vascular channels when principal conduits fail [63]. However, the connection of ischemic and non-ischemic vascular territories by anastomotic channels may divert blood from one brain region to another, depending on the magnitude and direction of the blood pressure gradients across the anastomotic connections (for review see Tode and McGraw [64]). The associated change of regional blood flow is called "steal" if it results in a decrease in flow, or "inverse steal" if it results in an improvement in flow. Inverse steal has also been referred to as the Robin Hood syndrome in analogy to the legendary hero who took from the rich and gave to the poor.

Steals are not limited to a particular vascular territory and may affect both the extra- and intracerebral circulation. Examples of extracerebral steals are the subclavian, the occipital-vertebral, and the ophthalmic steal syndrome. Intracerebral steal occurs across collateral pathways of brain, notably the circle of Willis and Heubner's network of pial anastomoses. The pathophysiological importance of steal has been disputed but as it depends on the individual hemodynamic situation it may explain unintended effects when flow is manipulated by alterations of arterial pCO_2 or vasoactive drugs. Most authors, therefore, do not recommend such manipulations for the treatment of stroke.

> "Steal": decrease in focal blood flow when blood is diverted from one brain region to another by anastomotic channels; "inverse steal" if that results in an improvement in flow.

The concept of ischemic penumbra
Energy requirements of brain tissue

The energy demand of the central nervous tissue is very high and therefore sufficient blood supply to the brain must be maintained constantly. A normal adult male's brain containing about 130 billion neurons (21.5 billion in the neocortex) [65] comprises only 2% of total body mass, yet consumes at rest approximately 20% of the body's total basal oxygen consumption supplied by 16% of the cardiac blood output. The brain's oxygen consumption is almost entirely for the oxidative metabolism of glucose, which in normal physiological conditions is the almost exclusive substrate for the brain's energy metabolism (Table 1.1) [66]. Glucose metabolized in neuronal cell bodies is mainly to support cellular vegetative and housekeeping functions, e.g. axonal transport, biosynthesis of nucleic acids, proteins, and lipids, as well as other energy-consuming processes not related directly to the generation of action potentials. Therefore, the rate of glucose consumption of neuronal cell bodies is essentially unaffected by neuronal functional activation. Increases in glucose consumption (and regional blood flow) evoked by functional activation are confined to synapse-rich regions, i.e. the neuropil, which contains axonal terminals, dendritic processes, and also the astrocytic processes that envelop the synapses. The magnitudes of these increases are linearly related to the frequency of action potentials in

Table 1.1. Cerebral blood flow (CBF), oxygen utilization (CMRO$_2$), and metabolic rates of glucose (CMRGlc) in man (approximated values)

	Cortex	White matter	Global
CBF (ml/100 g/min)	65	21	47
CMRO$_2$ (µmol/100 g/min)	230	80	160
CMRGlc (µmol/100 g/min)	40	20	32

(a)

(b)

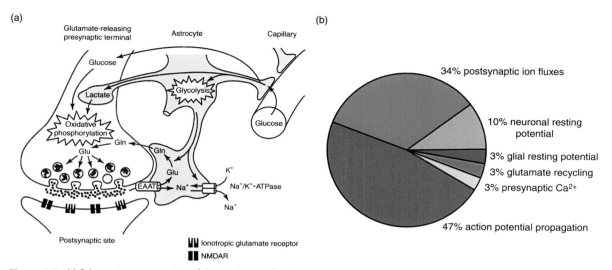

Figure 1.5. (a) Schematic representation of the mechanism for glutamate-induced glycolysis in astrocytes during physiological activation [127]. (b). Distribution of energy expenditure in rat cortex at a mean spike rate of 4 Hz: most energy is required for activity, only 13% is used for maintenance of resting potentials of neurons and glial cells [69,128]. EAAT = excitatory amino-acid transporter; NMDAR = N-methyl-D-aspartate receptor.

the afferent pathways, and increases in the projection zones occur regardless of whether the pathway is excitatory or inhibitory. Energy requirements of functional activation are due mostly to stimulation of the Na$^+$/K$^+$-ATPase activity to restore the ionic gradients across the cell membrane and the membrane potentials following spike activity, and are rather high compared to the basal energy demands of neuronal cell bodies (Figure 1.5) [67].

In excitatory glutamatergic neurons, which account for 80% of the neurons in the mammalian cortex, glucose utilization during activation is mediated by astrocytes which by anaerobic glycolysis provide lactate to the neurons where it is used for oxidative metabolism [68]. Overall, 87% of the total energy consumed is required for signaling, mainly action potential propagation and postsynaptic ion fluxes, and only 13% is expended in maintaining membrane resting potential (Figure 1.5) [69].

The mechanisms by which neurotransmitters other than glutamate influence blood flow and energy metabolism in the brain are still not understood [70].

A normal adult male's brain comprises only 2% of total body mass, yet consumes at rest approximately 20% of the body's total basal oxygen consumption. Glucose is the almost exclusive substrate for the brain's energy metabolism; 87% of the total energy consumed is required for signaling, mainly action potential propagation and postsynaptic ion fluxes.

Viability thresholds of brain ischemia

The different amounts of energy required for the generation of membrane potential and the propagation of electrical activity are reflected by different thresholds of oxygen consumption and blood flow that must be maintained to preserve neuronal function and morphological integrity. Flow values below normal but above the threshold of neuronal function are referred to as "benign oligemia." The flow range between the thresholds of neuronal function and morphological integrity is called the "ischemic penumbra" [71]. It is characterized by the preservation of membrane polarization and the potential of functional recovery without morphological damage, provided that local blood flow can be re-established [72, 73]. The "infarct core" is the area in which blood flow declines below the threshold of morphological integrity and in which tissue necrosis evolves.

According to the classical concept of viability thresholds, functional activity – reflected by the amplitudes of spontaneous and evoked electrical activity – begins to decline at flow values below 50% of control and is completely suppressed at about 30% of control [71]. In awake monkeys these values correspond to the progression of neurological injury from mild paresis at 22 ml/100 g/min to complete paralysis at 8 ml/100 g/min. Morphological damage

13

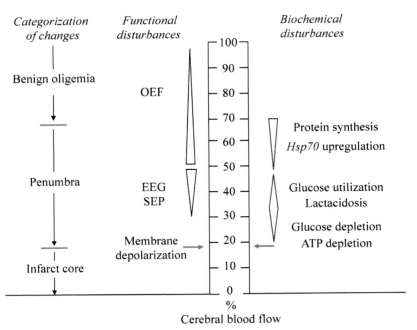

Figure 1.6. Diagrammatic representation of viability thresholds of focal brain ischemia. EEG = electroencephalogram; OEF = oxygen extraction fraction; SEP = somatosensory evoked potential.

evolves as soon as cell membranes depolarize ("terminal" depolarization) and occurs at flow values below 15–20% of control. Biochemically, functional suppression is associated with the inhibition of protein synthesis at about 50% and the development of lactacidosis at 30–40% of control, whereas membrane depolarization and morphological injury correspond to the breakdown of energy metabolism and the loss of adenosine triphosphate (ATP) at about 18% of control (Figure 1.6).

A more detailed picture of the dynamics of injury evolution is obtained by the simultaneous recording of local blood flow and spontaneous unit activity of cortical neurons [74]. According to these measurements, unit activity disappeared at a mean value of 18 ml/100 g/min but the large variability of the functional thresholds of individual neurons (6–22 ml/ 100 g/min) indicates differential vulnerability even within small cortical sectors. This explains the gradual development of neurological deficits, which may be related to differences in single cell activity with regular or irregular discharges at flow levels above the threshold of membrane failure.

Whereas neuronal function is impaired immediately when flow drops below the threshold, the development of irreversible morphological damage is time dependent. Based on recordings from a considerable number of neurons during and after ischemia of varying degree and duration it was possible to construct a discriminant curve representing the worst possible constellation of residual blood flow and duration of ischemia still permitting neuronal recovery (Figure 1.7). These results broaden the concept of the ischemic penumbra: the tissue fate – potential of recovery or irreversible damage – is determined not only by the level of residual flow but also by the duration of the flow disturbance. Each level of decreased flow can, on average, be tolerated for a defined period of time; flow between 17 and 20 ml/ 100 g/min can be tolerated for prolonged but yet undefined periods of time. As a rule used in many experimental models, flow rates of 12 ml/100 g/min lasting for 2–3 hours lead to large infarcts, but individual cells may become necrotic after shorter periods of time and at higher levels of residual flow.

The ischemic penumbra is the range of perfusion between the flow threshold for preservation of function and the flow threshold for preservation of morphological integrity. It is characterized by the potential for functional recovery without morphological damage.

Imaging of penumbra

Based on the threshold concept of brain ischemia, the penumbra can be imaged on quantitative flow maps using empirically established flow thresholds. A more

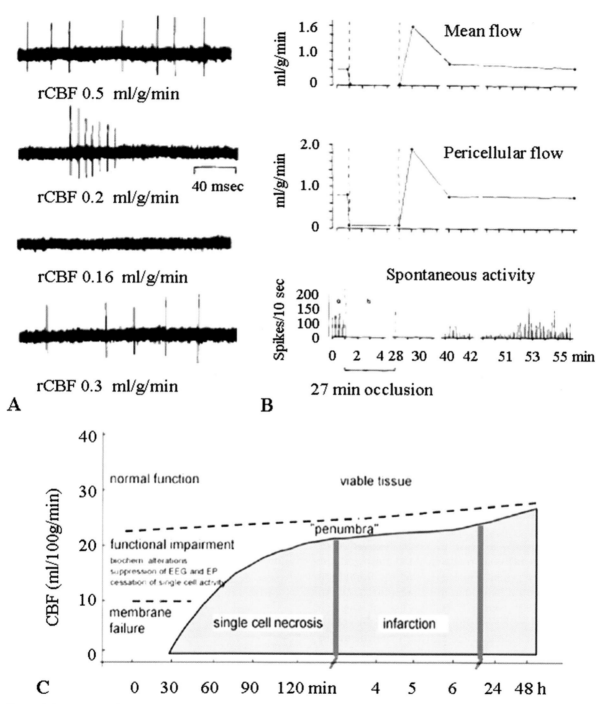

Figure 1.7. (A) Activity of a single neuron during graded ischemia before, during, and after reversible MCA occlusion. (B) Recovery of neuronal function after a limited period of ischemia. (C) Diagram of CBF thresholds required for the preservation of function and morphology of brain tissue. The activity of individual neurons is blocked when flow decreases below a certain threshold (upper dashed line) and returns when flow is raised again above this threshold. The fate of a single cell depends on the duration for which CBF is impaired below a certain level. The solid line separates structurally damaged from functionally impaired, but morphologically intact tissue, the "penumbra." The upper dashed line distinguishes viable from functionally impaired tissue. EP = evoked potentials. (Modified with permission from Heiss and Rosner [129]).

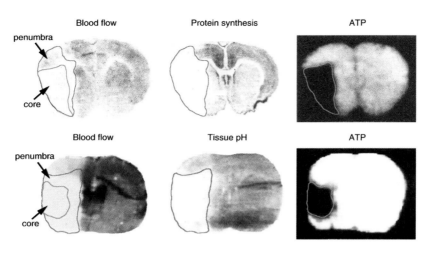

Figure 1.8. Biochemical imaging of infarct core, penumbra, and benign oligemia after experimental middle cerebral artery occlusion. The core is identified by ATP depletion, the penumbra by the mismatch between the suppression of protein synthesis and ATP depletion (top) or by the mismatch between tissue acidosis and ATP (bottom), and benign oligemia by the reduction of blood flow in the absence of biochemical alterations. (Modified with permission from Hossman and Mies [130]).

precise approach is the imaging of threshold-dependent biochemical disturbances to demarcate the mismatch between disturbances which occur only in the infarct core and others which also affect the penumbra (Figure 1.8) [75]. Under experimental conditions the most reliable way to localize the infarct core is the loss of ATP on bioluminescent images of tissue ATP content. A biochemical marker of core plus penumbra is tissue acidosis or the inhibition of protein synthesis. The penumbra is the difference between the respective lesion areas. The reliability of this approach is supported by the precise colocalization of gene transcripts that are selectively expressed in the penumbra, such as the stress protein hsp70, or the documentation of the gradual disappearance of the penumbra with increasing ischemia time [76].

Non-invasive imaging of the penumbra is possible using positron emission tomography (PET) or magnetic resonance imaging (MRI). Widely used PET parameters are the increase in oxygen extraction or the mismatch between reduced blood flow and the preservation of vitality markers, such as flumazenil binding to central benzodiazepine receptors [77]. An alternative PET approach is the use of hypoxia markers such as ^{18}F-misonidazole (F-MISO), which is trapped in viable hypoxic but not in normoxic or necrotic tissue [78].

The best-established MRI approach for penumbra imaging is the calculation of mismatch maps between the signal intensities of perfusion (PWI) and diffusion-weighted images (DWI), but its reliability has been questioned [79]. An alternative method is quantitative mapping of the apparent diffusion coefficient (ADC) of water, which reveals a robust correlation with the biochemically characterized penumbra for ADC values between 90% and 77% of control [80]. Recently MR stroke imaging has been performed by combining PWI, DWI, and pH-weighted imaging (pHWI) [81]. The mismatch between DWI and pHWI detects the penumbra, and that between PWI and pHWI the area of benign oligemia, i.e. a region in which flow reduction is not severe enough to cause metabolic disturbances. Diffusion kurtosis imaging (DKI), an extension of diffusion imaging, demarcates the regions with structural damage that cannot be salvaged upon reperfusion [82].

Finally, new developments in MR molecular imaging are of increasing interest for stroke research [83]. These methods make use of contrast-enhanced probes that trace gene transcription or of intracellular conjugates that reflect the metabolic status and/or bind to stroke markers. The number of molecules that can be identified by these methods rapidly expands and greatly facilitates the regional analysis of stroke injury.

> Non-invasive imaging of the penumbra is possible using positron emission tomography (PET) or magnetic resonance imaging (MRI).

Mechanisms of infarct expansion

With the advent of non-invasive imaging evidence has been provided that brain infarcts grow (Figure 1.9). This growth is not due to the progression of ischemia because the activation of collateral blood supply and spontaneous thrombolysis tend to improve blood flow over time. Infarct progression can be differentiated into three phases. During the acute phase tissue

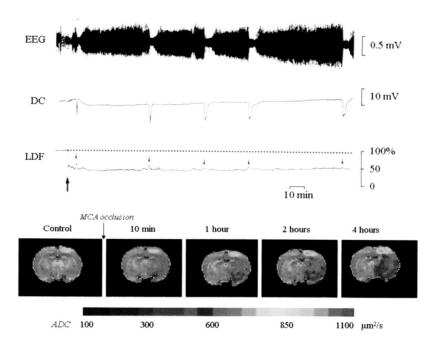

Figure 1.9. Relationship between peri-infarct spreading depressions (above) and infarct growth (below) during permanent focal brain ischemia induced by occlusion of the middle cerebral artery in rat. The effect of spreading depressions on electrical brain activity (EEG) and blood flow (LDF) are monitored by DC recording of the cortical steady potential, and infarct growth by MR imaging of the apparent diffusion coefficient (ADC) of brain water. (Modified with permission from Hossmann [131,132]).

injury is the direct consequence of the ischemia-induced energy failure and the resulting terminal depolarization of cell membranes. At flow values below the threshold of energy metabolism this injury is established within a few minutes after the onset of ischemia. During the subsequent subacute phase, the infarct core expands into the peri-infarct penumbra until, after 4–6 hours, core and penumbra merge. The reasons for this expansion are peri-infarct spreading depressions and a multitude of cell biological disturbances, collectively referred to as molecular cell injury. Moreover, a delayed phase of injury evolves which may last for several days or even weeks. During this phase secondary phenomena such as vasogenic edema, inflammation, and possibly programmed cell death may contribute to a further progression of injury.

The largest increment of infarct volume occurs during the subacute phase in which the infarct core expands into the penumbra. Using multiparametric imaging techniques for the differentiation between core and penumbra, evidence could be provided that in small rodents submitted to permanent occlusion of the MCA at its origin, the penumbra equals the volume of the infarct core at 1 hour, but after 3 hours more than 50% and between 6 and 8 hours almost all of the penumbra has disappeared and is now part of the irreversibly damaged infarct core [76]. In larger

animals the infarct core may be heterogeneous with multiple mini-cores surrounded by multiple mini-penumbras but these lesions also expand and eventually progress to a homogeneous defect with a similar time course [84].

Brain infarcts evolve in three phases:

- acute phase, within a few minutes after the onset of ischemia; terminal depolarization of cell membranes;
- subacute phase, within 4–6 hours; spreading depression and molecular cell injury, the infarct core expands into the peri-infarct penumbra;
- delayed phase, several days to weeks; vasogenic edema, inflammation, and possibly programmed cell death.

In the following, the most important mediators of infarct progression will be discussed.

Peri-infarct spreading depression

A functional disturbance contributing to the growth of the infarct core into the penumbra zone is the generation of peri-infarct spreading depression-like depolarizations (Figure 1.9) [85]. These depolarizations are initiated at the border of the infarct core and spread over the entire ipsilateral hemisphere. During spreading depression the metabolic rate of the tissue markedly increases in response to the

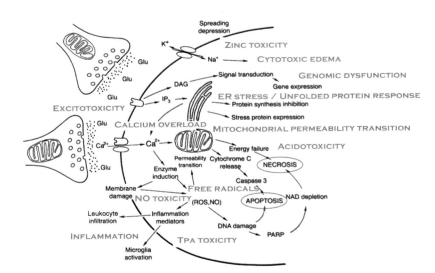

Figure 1.10. Schematic representation of molecular injury pathways leading to necrotic or apoptotic brain injury after focal brain ischemia. Injury pathways can be blocked at numerous sites, providing multiple approaches for the amelioration of both necrotic and apoptotic cell death. DAG = diacylglycerol; IP_3 = inositol 1, 4, 5-trisphosphate; PARP = poly (ADP-ribose) polymerase; TPA = tissue plasminogen activator.

greatly enhanced energy demands of the activated ion exchange pumps. In the healthy brain the associated increase of glucose and oxygen demands are coupled to a parallel increase of blood flow but in the peri-infarct penumbra this flow response is suppressed or even reversed [86]. As a result, a misrelationship arises between the increased metabolic workload and the low oxygen supply, leading to transient episodes of hypoxia and the stepwise increase in lactate during the passage of each depolarization.

The pathogenic importance of peri-infarct depolarizations for the progression of ischemic injury is supported by the linear relationship between the number of depolarizations and infarct volume. Correlation analysis of this relationship suggests that during the initial 3 hours of vascular occlusion each depolarization increases the infarct volume by more than 20%. This is probably one of the reasons that glutamate antagonists, which are potent inhibitors of spreading depression, reduce the volume of brain infarcts [87].

> Peri-infarct spreading depressions are depolarizations initiated at the border of the infarct core and may contribute to progression of ischemic injury.

Molecular mechanisms of injury progression

In the borderzone of permanent focal ischemia or in the core of the ischemic territory after transient vascular occlusion, cellular disturbances may evolve that cannot be explained by a lasting impairment of blood flow or energy metabolism. These disturbances are referred to as molecular injury, where the term "molecular" does not anticipate any particular injury pathway (for reviews see [88], [89]). The molecular injury cascades (Figure 1.10) are interconnected in complex ways, which makes it difficult to predict their relative pathogenic importance in different ischemia models. In particular, molecular injury induced by transient focal ischemia is not equivalent to the alterations that occur in the penumbra of permanent ischemia. Therefore, the relative contribution of the following injury mechanisms differs in different types of ischemia.

Acidotoxicity: during ischemia oxygen depletion and the associated activation of anaerobic glycolysis cause an accumulation of lactic acid which, depending on the severity of ischemia, blood glucose levels, and the degree of ATP hydrolysis, results in a decline of intracellular pH to between 6.5 and below 6.0. As the severity of acidosis correlates with the severity of ischemic injury, it has been postulated that acidosis is neurotoxic. Recently, evidence has been provided that ASICs (acid-sensing ion channels) are glutamate-independent vehicles of calcium flux, and that blockade of ASICs attenuates stroke injury. This suggests that acidosis may induce calcium toxicity, and that this effect is the actual mechanism of acidotoxicity [90].

Excitotoxicity: shortly after the onset of ischemia, excitatory and inhibitory neurotransmitters are released, resulting in the activation of their specific receptors. Among these neurotransmitters, particular attention has been attributed to glutamate, which under certain experimental conditions may produce excitotoxic cell death [91]. The activation of ionotropic glutamate receptors results in the inflow of calcium from the extracellular into the intracellular compartment, leading to mitochondrial calcium overload and the activation of calcium-dependent catabolic enzymes. The activation of metabotropic glutamate receptors induces the inositol 1,4,5-trisphosphate (IP$_3$)-dependent signal transduction pathway, leading among others to the stress response of ER, and by induction of immediate-early genes (IEGs) to adaptive genomic expressions. At very high concentration, glutamate results in primary neuronal necrosis. However, following pharmacological inhibition of ionotropic glutamate receptors, an apoptotic injury mechanism evolves that may prevail under certain pathophysiological conditions. The importance of excitotoxicity for ischemic cell injury has been debated, but this does not invalidate the beneficial effect of glutamate antagonists for the treatment of focal ischemia. An explanation for this incongruity is the above-described pathogenic role of peri-infarct depolarizations in infarct expansion. As glutamate antagonists inhibit the spread of these depolarizations, the resulting injury is also reduced.

Calcium toxicity: in the intact cell, highly efficient calcium transport systems assure the maintenance of a steep calcium concentration gradient of approximately 1:10 000 between the extra- and the intracellular compartment on the one hand, and between the cytosol and the ER on the other. During ischemia anoxic depolarization in combination with the activation of ionotropic glutamate and acid-sensing ion channels causes a sharp rise of cytosolic calcium [92]. At the onset of ischemia this rise is further enhanced by activation of metabotropic glutamate receptors which mediate the release of calcium from ER, and after recovery from ischemia by activation of transient receptor potential (TRP) channels which perpetuate intracellular calcium overload despite the restoration of ion gradients (Ca^{2+} paradox) [93]. The changes in intracellular calcium activity are highly pathogenic. Prolonged elevation of cytosolic calcium causes mitochondrial dysfunction and induces catabolic changes, notably by activation of Ca^{2+}-dependent effector proteins and enzymes such as endonucleases, phospholipases, protein kinases, and proteases that damage DNA, lipids, and proteins. The release of calcium from the ER evokes an ER stress response, which mediates a great number of ER-dependent secondary disturbances, notably inhibition of protein synthesis. Calcium-dependent pathological events are therefore complex and contribute to a multitude of secondary molecular injury pathways.

Free radicals: in brain regions with low or intermittent blood perfusion, reactive oxygen species (ROS) are formed which produce peroxidative injury of plasma membranes and intracellular organelles [94]. The reaction with NO leads to the formation of peroxynitrite, which also causes violent biochemical reactions. Secondary consequences of free radical reactions are the release of biologically active free fatty acids such as arachidonic acid, the induction of ER stress and mitochondrial disturbances, the initiation of an inflammatory response, breakdown of the blood–brain barrier, and fragmentation of DNA. The last may induce apoptosis and thus enhance molecular injury pathways related to mitochondrial dysfunction. The therapeutic benefit of free radial scavengers, however, is limited, as documented by the therapeutic failure of the free-radical-trapping agent NXY-059 [95].

Nitric oxide toxicity: NO is a product of NO synthase (NOS) acting on arginine. There are at least three isoforms of NOS: eNOS is constitutively expressed in endothelial cells, nNOS in neurons, and the inducible isoform iNOS mainly in macrophages. Pathophysiologically, NO has two opposing effects [96]. In endothelial cells the generation of NO leads to vascular dilatation, an improvement of blood flow and the alleviation of hypoxic injury, whereas in neurons it contributes to glutamate excitotoxicity and – by formation of peroxynitrite – to free-radical-induced injury. The net effect of NO thus depends on the individual pathophysiological situation and is difficult to predict.

Zinc toxicity: zinc is an essential catalytic and structural element of numerous proteins and a secondary messenger which is released from excitatory synapses during neuronal activation. Cytosolic zinc overload may promote mitochondrial dysfunction and generation of ROS, activate signal transduction pathways such as mitogen-activated protein kinase (MAPK), enhance calcium toxicity, and promote apoptosis [97]. However, at low concentration zinc may also exhibit neuroprotective properties, indicating that cells may possess a specific zinc set-point by which too little or too much zinc can promote ischemic injury [98].

ER stress and inhibition of protein synthesis: a robust molecular marker for the evolution of ischemic injury is inhibition of protein synthesis, which persists throughout the interval from the onset of ischemia until the manifestation of cell death [45]. It is initiated by a disturbance of the calcium homoeostasis of the ER, which results in ER stress and various cell biological abnormalities such as un- or misfolding of proteins, expression of stress proteins, and a global inhibition of the protein synthesizing machinery. The last is due to the activation of protein kinase R (PKR), which causes phosphorylation and inactivation of the alpha subunit of eukaryotic initiation factor eIF_2. This again leads to selective inhibition of polypeptide chain initiation, disaggregation of ribosomes, and inhibition of protein synthesis at the level of translation.

To restore ER function un- or misfolded proteins must be refolded (by activation of the unfolded protein response, UPR) or degraded (by ER-associated degradation, ERAD). Cells in which UPR and ERAD fail to restore ER function die by apoptosis [99].

Obviously, persistent inhibition of protein synthesis is incompatible with cell survival but as the manifestation of cell death greatly varies in different cell populations, other factors must also be involved.

Mitochondrial disturbances: to mitigate metabolic or environmental stress, functional mitochondria are maintained by fission and fusion [100]. However, the concurrence of an increased cytosolic calcium activity with the generation of ROS may lead to an increase in permeability of the inner mitochondrial membrane (mitochondrial permeability transition, MPT), which has been associated with the formation of a permeability transition pore (PTP). The PTP is a Ca^{2+}-, ROS- and voltage-dependent, cyclosporine A-sensitive high-conductance channel, located in the inner mitochondrial membrane. It is also a reversible fast Ca^{2+} release channel, facilitated by the mitochondrial matrix protein cyclophilin D [101]. The increase in permeability of the inner mitochondrial membrane has two pathophysiologically important consequences. The breakdown of the electrochemical gradient interferes with mitochondrial oxidative phosphorylation and, in consequence, with aerobic energy production. Furthermore, the equilibration of mitochondrial ion gradients causes swelling of the mitochondrial matrix, which eventually will cause disruption of the outer mitochondrial membrane and the release of pro-apoptotic mitochondrial proteins (see below). Ischemia-induced mitochondrial disturbances thus contribute to delayed cell death both by impairment of the energy state and the activation of apoptotic injury pathways [102].

> A large number of molecular disturbances are involved in the progression of ischemic damage.

Inflammation

Brain infarcts evoke a strong inflammatory response which is thought to contribute to the progression of ischemic brain injury. Gene expressions related to this response have, therefore, been extensively investigated to search for possible pharmacological targets (for review see Rothwell and Luheshi [103]). The inflammatory response of the ischemic tissue has been associated, among others, with the generation of free radicals in reperfused or critically hypoperfused brain tissue. The prostaglandin synthesizing enzyme cyclo-oxygenase-2 (COX-2) and nuclear factor-kappa B (NF-kappa B), a transcription factor that responds to oxidative stress, are strongly upregulated and may be neurotoxic, as suggested by the beneficial effect of COX-2 inhibitors. Infarct reduction was also observed after genetic or pharmacological inhibition of matrix metalloproteinase (MMP)-9 but this effect has been disputed.

A key player in the intracellular response to cytokines is the JAK (janus kinase)/STAT (signal transducer and activator of transcription) pathway, which induces alterations in the pattern of gene transcription. These changes are associated with either cell death or survival and suggest that inflammation may be both neurotoxic and neuroprotective [104]. Inflammatory reactions and the associated free-radical-mediated processes are, therefore, important modulators of ischemic injury but the influence on the final outcome is difficult to predict.

> Inflammatory reactions are important modulators of ischemic injury.

Brain edema

Ischemic brain edema can be differentiated into two pathophysiologically different types: an early cytotoxic type, followed after some delay by a late vasogenic type of edema. The cytotoxic type of edema is threshold dependent. It is initiated at flow values of similar to 30% of control when stimulation of anaerobic metabolism causes an increase of brain tissue osmolality and, hence, an osmotically obliged cell swelling. At flow values below 20% of control, anoxic depolarization and equilibration of ion gradients across the cell membranes further enhance intracellular osmolality and the associated cell swelling. The intracellular uptake of sodium is also associated with a coupled movement of water that is independent of an osmotic gradient and which is referred to as "anomalous osmosis."

In the absence of blood flow, cell swelling occurs at the expense of the extracellular fluid volume, leading to the shrinkage of the extracellular compartment, but not to a change in the net water content. The shift of fluid is reflected by a decrease of the ADC of water, which is the reason for the increase of signal intensity in diffusion-weighted MR imaging [80]. However, if some residual blood flow persists, water is taken up from the blood, and the net tissue water content increases. After vascular occlusion this increase starts within a few minutes after the onset of ischemia and causes a gradual increase in brain volume.

With the evolution of tissue necrosis and the degradation of basal lamina, the blood–brain barrier breaks down [105], and after 4–6 hours serum proteins begin to leak from the blood into the brain. This disturbance initiates a vasogenic type of edema, which further enhances the water content of the tissue. Vasogenic edema reaches its peak at 1–2 days after the onset of ischemia and may cause an increase of tissue water by more than 100%. If brain infarcts are large, the volume increase of the edematous brain tissue may be so pronounced that transtentorial herniation results in compression of the midbrain. Under clinical conditions, this "malignant" form of brain infarction is by far the most dangerous complication of stroke and an indication for decompressive craniectomy [106].

Vasogenic edema, in contrast to the early cytotoxic type of edema, is isoosmotic and accumulates mainly in the extracellular compartment. This reverses the cytotoxic narrowing of the extracellular space and explains the "pseudonormalization" of the signal intensity observed in diffusion-weighted MR imaging [107]. However, as the total tissue water content is increased at this time, the high signal intensity in T_2-weighted images clearly differentiates this situation from a "real" recovery to normal.

The formation of cytotoxic and, to a lesser extent, also vasogenic edema requires the passage of water through aquaporin channels located in the plasma membrane [108]. Inhibition of aquaporin water conductance may, therefore, reduce the severity of ischemic brain edema. Similarly, the inhibition of sodium transport across sodium channels has been suggested to reduce edema formation. However, as the driving force for the generation of edema is the gradient of osmotic and ionic concentration differences built up during ischemia, aquaporin and sodium channels may modulate the speed of edema generation but not the final extent of tissue water accumulation. Their pathophysiological importance is, therefore, limited.

> Early cytotoxic edema is caused by osmotically induced cell swelling; the later vasogenic edema is isoosmotic, caused by breakdown of the blood–brain barrier, and accumulates in the extracellular compartment.

Apoptosis

Apoptosis is an evolutionary conserved form of programmed cell death that in multicellular organisms matches cell proliferation to preserve tissue homoeostasis [109]. It is an active process that requires intact energy metabolism and protein synthesis, and it is initiated essentially by two pathways: an extrinsic death receptor-dependent route, and an intrinsic pathway which depends on the mitochondrial release of pro-apoptotic molecules such as apoptosis-inducing factor (AIF) and cytochrome C. In focal ischemia pro-apoptotic pathways are also initiated by activation of toll-like receptors 2 and 4, the NOTCH-1 receptor, and the adiponectin receptor 1. Apoptotic pathways involve a series of enzymatic reactions and converge in the activation of caspase-3, a cystine protease, which contributes to the execution of cell death. An end stage of this process is the ordered disassembly of the genome, resulting in a laddered pattern of oligonucleosomal fragments as detected by electrophoresis or TUNEL.

Although apoptosis is mainly involved in physiological cell death, it is widely assumed to contribute to the pathogenesis of diseases, including cerebral ischemia [110]. In the context of stroke this is difficult to understand because in areas with primary cell death the obvious cause is energy failure, and in regions with delayed injury the dominating biochemical disturbance is the irreversible suppression of protein synthesis. However, ischemia induces a multitude of biochemical reactions that are reminiscent of apoptosis, such as the expression of p53, JNK, c-jun, p38, cyclin-dependent kinase 5, or caspase 3, all of which correlate to some degree with the severity of injury.

Moreover, inhibition of these reactions by gene manipulation or pharmacological interventions reduces the volume of brain infarcts. It has, therefore, been suggested that ischemic cell death is a hybrid of necrosis and apoptosis, appearing on a continuum with the two forms of cell death at its poles [111].

> Apoptosis, an active form of programmed cell death, may contribute to a certain extent to ischemic cell death.

Pre- and postconditioning of ischemic injury

The molecular signaling cascades initiated by brain ischemia are not solely destructive but may also exert a neuroprotective effect. In fact, most of the above-described injury pathways including ischemia itself induce a transient state of increased ischemic tolerance, provided the initial injury remains subliminal for tissue destruction. This effect is called "ischemic preconditioning" and can be differentiated into three phases: during the induction phase molecular sensors which respond to the preconditioning stimulus are activated by transcription factors; the transduction phase results in the amplification of the signal; and during the effector phase proteins with a protective impact are switched on [112]. The increase in ischemia tolerance appears 2 to 3 days after the preconditioning stimulus, and it slowly disappears after 1 week.

An important preconditioning pathway is the upregulation of the hypoxia-inducible factor 1 (HIF-1) in astrocytes. HIF-1 is a transcription factor that among others induces the expression of erythropoietin (EPO) which binds to the neuronal EPO receptor and which exhibits potent neuroprotective effects. Another putative mechanism is the ER stress response. Depletion of ER calcium stores causes accumulation of unfolded proteins in the ER lumen and induces the activation of two highly conserved stress responses, the ER overload response (EOR) and the unfolded protein response (UPR). EOR triggers activation of the transcription factor NF-kappa B, and UPR causes a suppression of the initiation of protein synthesis. As the latter contributes to delayed ischemic injury (see above) its reduction may have a neuroprotective effect.

Evidence has also been provided that ischemic injury can be alleviated by repeated mechanical interruptions of blood reperfusion after a period of transient focal ischemia [113]. This phenomenon, termed "ischemic postconditioning," has been associated with the phosphorylation of several prosurvival protein kinases, such as extracellular signal-regulated kinase (ERK), p38 MAPK, and Akt. The possibility to influence ischemic injury after the primary impact is challenging but it remains to be shown for which kind of clinical situation this finding is of practical relevance.

> Short episodes of ischemia can improve the tolerance of brain tissue for subsequent blood flow disturbance.

Regeneration and cell therapy

Brain infarcts produced by focal ischemia are seemingly irresolvable in agreement with Cajal's classical statement that in the adult brain "everything may die, nothing may be regenerated." This dogma was reversed by the discovery of three permanently neurogenic regions, i.e. the subventricular zone (SVZ), the subgranular zone (SGZ), and the posterior perireticular (PPr) area, which provide lifelong supply of newly generated neurons to the hippocampus and olfactory bulb. After stroke, neurogenesis increases in these areas, and some of the newly formed cells migrate into the infarct penumbra, differentiate into glia and mature neurons, and survive for at least several weeks [114]. Neurogenesis may also occur through the neurovascular unit. After ischemia pericytes strongly migrate into the peri-infarct surrounding and contribute to tissue repair by controlling neurogenesis, angiogenesis, and blood–brain barrier function [115].

Ischemia-induced neurogenesis is enhanced by growth factors, NO, inflammation, and various hormones and neurotransmitters, notably estradiol and dopamine, but it is repressed by activation of the N-methyl-D-aspartate (NMDA) subtype of glutamate receptors. The functional consequences of spontaneous or drug-enhanced neurogenesis are modest but optimism is building up for targeted interventions. Similarly, considerable expectations are placed on the transplantation of neural progenitor cells, particularly in combination with growth factors and/or strategies that permit recruitment of transplanted cells to the site of injury [116]. However, cell therapy carries the risk of tumorigenesis, and as major breakthroughs have not yet been achieved, further research is necessary to explore the actual potentials of stroke regenerative medicine.

> Several brain regions may provide lifelong supply of newly generated neurons.

Translation of experimental concepts to clinical stroke

Experimental research has advanced our knowledge about the pathophysiology of brain disorders, but the transfer of this knowledge into clinical application is difficult and often lacks behind. One of the reasons are differences between the brain of experimental animals and humans with respect to evolutionary state (non-gyrencephalic vs. gyrencephalic anatomy (amount of gray vs. white matter), relative size, cellular density, blood supply, and metabolism). Additionally, experimental models in animals cannot be easily compared to complex human diseases often based on a different pathophysiology and affecting multimorbid patients. The other problem arises from the investigative procedures, which cannot be equally applied in animals and patients. This is especially true when pathophysiological changes obtained by invasive procedures in animals, e.g. by analysis of tissue samples, by autoradiography, or by histology, should be related to the course of a disease, but cannot be assessed repeatedly and regionally. To facilitate the transfer of knowledge from experimental neuroscience to clinical neurology, it is necessary to develop methods which can be equally applied in patients and animal models, and which are not invasive and can be performed repeatedly without affecting or harming the object. To this task of transferring experimental results into clinical application functional imaging modalities are successfully applied.

Detection of the penumbra by PET

PET is still the only method allowing quantitative determination of various physiological variables in the brain and was applied extensively for studies in patients with acute, subacute, or chronic stages of ischemic stroke (review in Heiss [77]). The introduction of scanners with high resolution (2.5–5 mm for human, 1 mm for animal application) made PET a tool for studying animal models and to compare repeat examinations of various variables from experiments to the course of disease in humans. The regional decrease of CBF can be directly observed in PET as in other studies (single-photon emission computed tomography [SPECT], PWI-MRI, perfusion computed tomography [PCT]). However, already in early PET studies [117] preserved glucose consumption

was observed in regions with decreased flow in the first hours after the ictus. Since the 1980s, PET with oxygen-15 tracers became the gold standard for the evaluation of pathophysiological changes in early ischemic stroke [118]. The quantitative measurement of CBF, oxygen utilization ($CMRO_2$), oxygen extraction fraction (OEF), and cerebral blood volume (CBV) permitted the independent assessment of perfusion and energy metabolism, and demonstrated the uncoupling of these usually closely related variables. These studies provided data on flow and metabolic variables predicting final infarction on late CTs (rCBF less than 12 ml/100 g/min, $CMRO_2$ less than 65 μmol/100 g/min). Relatively preserved $CMRO_2$ indicated maintained neuronal function in regions with severely reduced CBF; this pattern was coined "misery perfusion" and served as a definition for the penumbra, which is characterized by increased oxygen extraction fraction (up to more than 80% from the normal 40–50%). Late CT or MRI often showed these regions as morphologically intact.

Sequential PET studies of CBF, $CMRO_2$, and metabolic rate of glucose (CMRGlc) before and repeatedly up to 24 hours after MCA occlusion in cats could demonstrate the development and growth of irreversible ischemic damage. Immediately after MCA occlusion CBF within the supplied territory dropped, but $CMRO_2$ was less diminished and was preserved at an intermediate level. As a consequence, OEF was increased, indicating misery perfusion, i.e. penumbra tissue. However, as OEF is also increased in benign oligemia, demarcation of the penumbra from normal tissue is not possible. With time, OEF was decreased, a process which started in the center and developed centrifugally to the borderline of the ischemic territory, indicating the conversion into irreversible damage and the growth of the MCA infarct. In experiments with transient MCA occlusion it could be demonstrated that an infarct did not develop when reperfusion was initiated to tissue with increased OEF. Comparable to patients with early thrombolysis, reperfusion could salvage ischemic tissue in the condition of "penumbra" (Figure 1.11). Similar results were obtained in ischemia models of baboons. PET thus permits the differentiation of various tissue compartments within an ischemic territory: irreversible damage by decreased flow and oxygen consumption below critical thresholds; misery perfusion, i.e. penumbra, by decreased flow, but preserved oxygen utilization above a critical threshold, expressed by

23

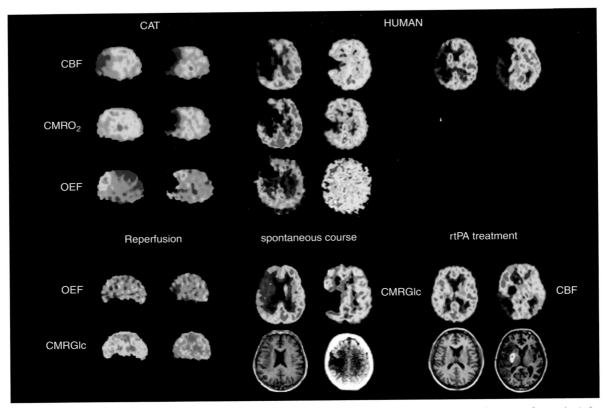

Figure 1.11 Sequential PET images of CBF, CMRO₂, and OEF of MCA occlusion in cats compared to images of patients after stroke: Left columns: In the right cat, the progressive decrease of CMRO₂ and the reduction of OEF predict infarction that cannot benefit from reperfusion. Only if OEF is increased until the start of reperfusion can the infarct be salvaged (left cat). Middle columns: In the patient the areas with preserved OEF are not infarcted and can survive in spontaneous course (posterior part of ischemic cortex in left, anterior part in right patient, as indicated on late MRI and CT). Right columns: In patients receiving rtPA treatment measurements of CMRO₂ and OEF are not feasible, but flow determinations show the effect. If reperfusion occurs early enough and before tissue damage, tissue can be salvaged (left patient). If reperfusion is achieved too late, tissue cannot be salvaged despite hyperperfusion in some parts (right patient).

increased OEF; luxury perfusion by flow increased above the metabolic demand; anaerobic glycolysis by a change in the ratio between glucose metabolism and oxygen utilization. However, PET has severe disadvantages limiting its routine application in patients with stroke: it is a complex methodology, requires multitracer application, and quantitative analysis necessitates arterial blood sampling.

> Positron emission tomography (PET) is the most reliable non-invasive method to identify irreversible tissue damage and penumbra.

Prediction of irreversible tissue damage

The prediction of the portion of irreversibly damaged tissue within the ischemic area early after the stroke

is of utmost importance for the efficiency of treatment. Meticulous analyses of CBF and CMRO₂ data indicated that CMRO₂ below 65 μmol/100 g/min predicted finally infarcted tissue, but also large portions with flow and oxygen utilization in the penumbra range were included in the final cortical–subcortical infarcts. Determination of oxygen utilization additionally requires arterial blood sampling, which limits clinical applicability. These facts stress the need for a marker of neuronal integrity that can identify irreversibly damaged tissue irrespective of the time elapsed since the vascular attack, and irrespective of the variations in blood flow over time.

Central benzodiazepine receptor (BZR) ligands can be used as markers of neuronal integrity as they bind to the gamma-aminobutyric acid (GABA) receptors abundant in cerebral cortex that are sensitive to ischemic damage. After successful testing in the cat MCA occlusion model, cortical binding of flumazenil (FMZ) was investigated in patients with acute ischemic stroke [119]. In all patients, defects in FMZ binding were closely related to areas with severely depressed oxygen consumption and predicted the size of the final infarcts, whereas preserved FMZ binding indicated intact cortex. Additionally, FMZ distribution within 2 minutes after tracer injection was highly correlated with CBF measured by

H_2O and therefore can be used as a relative flow tracer yielding reliable perfusion images. PET with FMZ therefore can be used as a non-invasive procedure to image irreversible damage and critically reduced perfusion (i.e. penumbra) in early ischemic stroke.

> Special tracers, e.g. ligands to benzodiazepine receptors, can be used as early markers of irreversible neuronal damage, since they bind to GABA receptors of cortical neurons, which are very sensitive to ischemic damage.

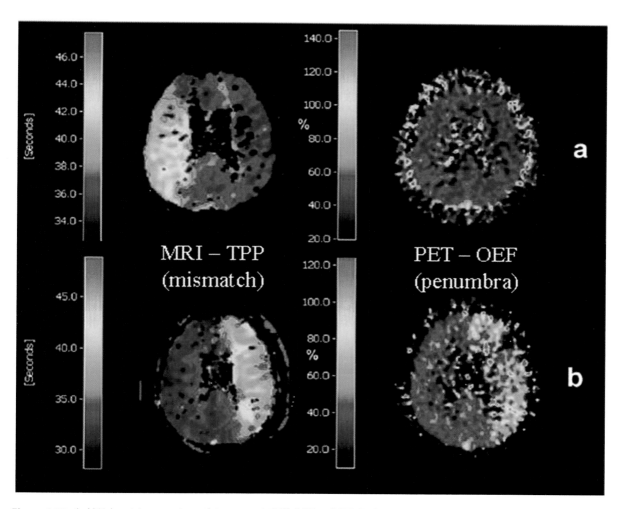

Figure 1.12. (a, b) Volumetric comparison of time to peak (TTP) (MRI) and OEF (PET) images in two patients measured in the chronic phase of stroke. In both patients a TTP delay of >4 seconds indicates a considerable mismatch volume (red contour on TTP images). The mismatch volumes were 473 cm^3 for patient a and 199.7 cm^3 for patient b. However, only patient b had a corresponding volume of penumbra (260 cm^3). (c) Volumes of penumbra defined by increased OEF (black) and mismatch defined by TTP > 4 (gray) in 13 patients: all 13 patients showed mismatch, only 8 patients showed penumbra, which comprised 1–75% of the mismatch volume. (Modified with permission from Sobesky et al. [124].)

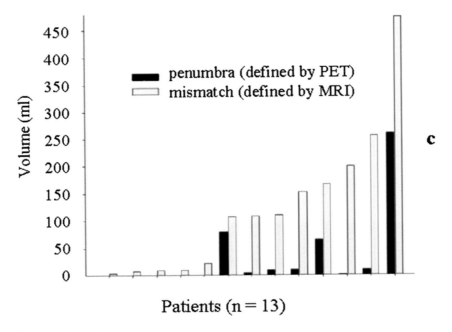

Figure 1.12. (*cont.*)

Surrogate markers for penumbra and irreversible damage

Although PET remains the imaging gold standard for identification of the penumbra in stroke patients, MR studies using DWI and perfusion-weighted imaging (PWI) might provide a differentiation between the core and the penumbra: the early DWI lesion might define the ischemic core and adjacent critically hypoperfused tissue might be identified with PWI [120]. Therefore, brain regions with hypoperfusion assessed by PWI but without restricted diffusion (PWI/DWI mismatch) were assumed to represent the penumbra. This surrogate definition of the penumbra has several uncertainties [121]: the initial diffusion lesion does not only consist of irreversibly infarcted tissue; diffusion lesions may be reversed if blood flow is restored at an early time point; critically perfused tissue (i.e. penumbra) cannot be clearly differentiated from tissue experiencing benign oligemia; the PWI abnormality often overestimates the amount of tissue at risk. These facts are further accentuated by methodological limitations, because perfusion techniques and data evaluation are not quantitative and vary among centers. Despite the attempts to correct the mismatch area by subtracting the region of benign oligemia and

adding the portion of reversible diffusion abnormality [121] the definition of the penumbra remains controversial and suffers from lack of standardization of methodological approaches to imaging, post processing, and analysis, which restricts pooling of data and cross-comparison of results across studies.

A validation of PWI/DWI results with quantitative measurements of flow values and oxygen consumption or FMZ uptake in the same patients early after stroke is necessary for the assessment of the accuracy of the applied signatures for predicting tissue outcome. Several studies were performed in order to validate mismatch as a surrogate of penumbra on PET-derived discrimination of irreversibly damaged, critically perfused "at risk," and oligemic "not at risk" tissue. The studies demonstrated that the DWI lesion predicts more or less the finally infarcted tissue [122], but contains up to 25% false positive, i.e. surviving tissue.

The inaccuracy in defining the penumbra with PWI/DWI mismatch is thought to be mainly related to PW data acquisition, since the parameters used to estimate perfusion are variable and somewhat arbitrary. As a consequence, perfusion lesion size differs markedly depending on the parameters calculated [123] and usually is overestimated and extends into considerable areas with non-critical oligemia especially when short delays are used. Overall, PWI is unable to provide a reliable quantitative estimation of cerebal perfusion when compared to gold-standards such as PET, SPECT, or Xe-CT and overestimated the size of the critically perfused tissue and therefore also the volume of critically perfused but salvageable tissue, i.e. the penumbra (Figure 1.12) [124]. Of 13 patients showing considerable PWI/DWI mismatch only 8 had areas with elevated OEF typical for penumbra tissue, and these areas were always smaller than MR mismatch. Overall, the mismatch volume in PWI/DWI as conventionally calculated does not reliably reflect misery perfusion, i.e. the penumbra as defined by PET. Recently, several methods have been proposed to improve the reliability of assessment of perfusion using MR methods [125], but they all need to be validated by quantitative measures.

> The mismatch between perfusion-weighted and diffusion-weighted MRI can be used as a surrogate marker of the penumbra, but the applied parameters need to be validated.

Chapter summary

Atherosclerosis is the most widespread disorder leading to death and serious morbidity including stroke. It develops over years from initial fatty streaks to atheromatous plaques with the risk of plaque disruption and formation of thrombus, from which emboli might originate. Lipohyalinosis affects small vessels, leading to lacunar stroke. The vascular lesions and emboli from the heart cause territorial infarcts, whereas borderzone infarcts are due to low perfusion in the peripheral parts of the vascular territories (last meadows). Ischemic infarcts may be converted into hemorrhagic infarctions by leakage of vessels, whereas intracerebral hemorrhages (5–15% of all strokes) result from rupture of arteries typically in deep portions of the hemispheres. Venous infarcts usually result from thrombosis of sinuses or veins and are often accompanied by edema, hemorrhagic transformation, and bleeding. Primary ischemic cell death is the result of severe ischemia; early signs are potentially reversible swelling or shrinkage; irreversible necrotic neurons have condensed acidophilic cytoplasm and pyknotic nuclei. Delayed neuronal death can occur after moderate or short-term ischemia; it goes along with nuclear fragmentation and development of apoptotic bodies. The pathophysiology of ischemic cell damage in animal models reflects only certain aspects of ischemia and cannot give a complete picture of ischemic stroke in humans. However, from these experimental models principles of regulation of cerebral blood flow and flow thresholds for maintenance of function and morphology can be deduced. As the energy requirement of the brain is very high, already mild decreases of blood supply lead to potentially reversible disturbance of function and, if the shortage is more severe and persists for certain periods, to irreversible morphological damage. Tissue perfused in the range between the thresholds of functional and morphological injury has been called the penumbra, a concept which has great importance for treatment. The ischemia-induced energy failure triggers a complex cascade of electrophysiological disturbances, biochemical changes, and molecular dysfunction, which lead to progressive cell death and growth of infarction. The progression of ischemic injury is further boosted by inflammatory reactions and the development of early cytotoxic and later vasogenic brain edema. The translation of these experimental concepts into clinical application and management of stroke patients, however, is difficult. It can be achieved in some instances by special functional imaging techniques, such as positron emission tomography, but requires further refinements to predict the outcome of neuroprotective interventions. Solid understanding of experimental and clinical stroke pathophysiology is, therefore, needed to improve the reliability of translational research.

References

1. Sanz J, Moreno PR, Fuster V. The year in atherothrombosis. *J Am Coll Cardiol* 2012; **60**:932–42.

2. Rajamani K, Fisher M, Fisher M. Atherosclerosis – pathogenesis and pathophysiology. In: Ginsberg MD, Bogousslavsky J, eds. *Cerebrovascular Disease: Pathophysiology, Diagnosis and Management.* London: Blackwell Science; 1998: 308–18.

3. Willeit J, Kiechl S. Biology of arterial atheroma. *Cerebrovas Dis* 2000; **10**(Suppl 5):1–8.

4. Ross R. Atherosclerosis–an inflammatory disease. *N Engl J Med* 1999; **340**:115–26.

5. Faxon DP, Fuster V, Libby P, *et al.* Atherosclerotic Vascular Disease Conference: Writing Group III: pathophysiology. *Circulation* 2004; **109**:2617–25.

6. Aikawa M, Libby P. The vulnerable atherosclerotic plaque: pathogenesis and therapeutic approach. *Cardiovasc Pathol* 2004; **13**:125–38.

7. Koga J, Aikawa M. Crosstalk between macrophages and smooth muscle cells in atherosclerotic vascular diseases. *Vascul Pharmacol* 2012; **57**:24–8.

8. Dzau VJ, Braun-Dullaeus RC, Sedding DG. Vascular proliferation and atherosclerosis: new perspectives and therapeutic strategies. *Nat Med* 2002; **8**:1249–56.

9. Madden JA. Role of the vascular endothelium and plaque in acute ischemic stroke. *Neurology* 2012; **79**:S58–62.

10. Glagov S, Weisenberg E, Zarins CK, Stankunavicius R, Kolettis GJ. Compensatory enlargement of human atherosclerotic coronary arteries. *N Engl J Med* 1987; **316**:1371–5.

11. Rauch U, Osende JI, Fuster V, *et al.* Thrombus formation on atherosclerotic plaques: pathogenesis and clinical consequences. *Ann Intern Med* 2001; **134**:224–38.

12. Lubos E, Handy DE, Loscalzo J. Role of oxidative stress and nitric oxide in atherothrombosis. *Front Biosci* 2008; **13**:5323–44.

13. Fisher CM. Cerebral miliary aneurysms in hypertension. *Am J Pathol* 1972; **66**:313–30.

14. Zülch K-J. *The Cerebral Infarct. Pathology, Pathogenesis, and Computed Tomography*. Berlin, Heidelberg, New York, Tokyo: Springer-Verlag; 1985.

15. Russell RWR. Observations on intracerebral aneurysms. *Brain* 1963; **86**:425–42.

16. Zülch K-J. Über die Entstehung und Lokalisation der Hirninfarkte. *Zentralbl Neurochir* 1961; **21**:158–78.

17. Dichgans M. Genetics of ischaemic stroke. *Lancet Neurol* 2007; **6**:149–61.

18. Mohr JP, Choi DW, Grotta JC, Weir B, Wolf PA (eds.). *Stroke – Pathophysiology, Diagnosis, and Management*, 4th edn. Philadelphia: Churchill Livingstone; 2004.

19. Pantoni L. Cerebral small vessel disease: from pathogenesis and clinical characteristics to therapeutic challenges. *Lancet Neurol* 2010; **9**:689–701.

20. Ringelstein EB, Nabavi DG. Cerebral small vessel diseases: cerebral microangiopathies. *Curr Opin Neurol* 2005; **18**:179–88.

21. Wolf PA. Epidemiology of stroke. In: Mohr JP, Choi DW, Grotta JC, Weir B, Wolf PA, eds. *Stroke – Pathophysiology, Diagnosis, and Management*, 4th edn. Philadelphia: Churchill Livingstone; 2004: 13–34.

22. Stochdorph O. Der Mythos der letzten Wiese. *Zentralbl Allg Pathol Path Anat* 1977; **121**:554.

23. Ringelstein EB, Zunker P. Low-flow infarction. In: Ginsberg MD, Bogousslavsky J, eds. *Cerebrovascular Disease: Pathophysiology, Diagnosis, and Management*. London: Blackwell Science; 1998: 1075–89.

24. Fisher CM. Lacunes: small, deep cerebral infarcts. *Neurology* 1965; **15**:774–84.

25. Amarenco P, Bogousslavsky J, Caplan LR, Donnan GA, Hennerici MG. New approach to stroke subtyping: the A-S-C-O (phenotypic) classification of stroke. *Cerebrovasc Dis* 2009; **27**:502–8.

26. Beghi E, Bogliun G, Cavaletti G, *et al.* Hemorrhagic infarction: risk factors, clinical and tomographic features, and outcome. A case-control study. *Acta Neurol Scand* 1989; **80**:226–31.

27. Lodder J, Krijne-Kubat B, Broekman J. Cerebral hemorrhagic infarction at autopsy: cardiac embolic cause and the relationship to the cause of death. *Stroke* 1986; **17**:626–9.

28. Fisher M, Adams RD. Observations on brain embolism with special reference to the mechanism of hemorrhagic infarction. *J Neuropathol Exp Neurol* 1951; **10**:92–4.

29. Mohr JP, Caplan LR, Melski JW, *et al.* The Harvard Cooperative Stroke Registry: a prospective registry. *Neurology* 1978; **28**:754–62.

30. Sacco RL, Wolf PA, Bharucha NE, *et al.* Subarachnoid and intracerebral hemorrhage: natural history, prognosis, and precursive factors in the Framingham Study. *Neurology* 1984; **34**:847–54.

31. Feldman E. *Intracerebral Hemorrhage*. Armonk, New York: Futura; 1994.

32. Schütz H. *Spontane intrazerebrale Hämatome. Pathophysiologie, Klinik und Therapie*. Berlin, Heidelberg, New York: Springer-Verlag; 1988.

33. Qureshi AI, Tuhrim S, Broderick JP, *et al.* Spontaneous intracerebral hemorrhage. *N Engl J Med* 2001; **344**:1450–60.

34. Kase CS, Mohr JP, Caplan LR. Intracerebral hemorrhage. In: Mohr JP, Choi DW, Grotta JC, Weir B, Wolf PA, eds. *Stroke – Pathophysiology, Diagnosis, and Management*, 4th edn. Philadelphia: Churchill Livingstone; 2004: 327–76.

35. Fisher CM. Pathological observations in hypertensive cerebral hemorrhage. *J Neuropathol Exp Neurol* 1971; **30**:536–50.

36. Brott T, Broderick J, Kothari R, *et al.* Early hemorrhage growth in patients with intracerebral hemorrhage. *Stroke* 1997; **28**:1–5.

37. Gonzalez-Duarte A, Cantu C, Ruiz-Sandoval JL,

Barinagarrementeria F. Recurrent primary cerebral hemorrhage: frequency, mechanisms, and prognosis. *Stroke* 1998; **29**: 1802–5.

38. Bousser MG, Barnett HJM. Cerebral venous thrombosis. In: Mohr JP, Choi DW, Grotta JC, Weir B, Wolf PA, eds. *Stroke – Pathophysiology, Diagnosis, and Management*, 4th edn. Philadelphia: Churchill Livingstone; 2004: 301–25.

39. Petito CK. *The Neuropathology of Focal Brain Ischemia*. Basel: ISN Neuropath; 2005.

40. Brown AW, Brierley JB. Anoxic-ischaemic cell change in rat brain light microscopic and fine-structural observations. *J Neurol Sci* 1972; **16**:59–84.

41. Jortner BS. The return of the dark neuron. A histological artifact complicating contemporary neurotoxicologic evaluation. *Neurotoxicology* 2006; **27**:628–34.

42. Kirino T, Sano K. Selective vulnerability in the gerbil hippocampus following transient ischemia. *Acta Neuropathol* 1984; **62**:201–8.

43. Martin LJ. Neuronal cell death in nervous system development, disease, and injury (Review). *Int J Mol Med* 2001; **7**:455–78.

44. Charriaut-Marlangue C, Ben-Ari Y. A cautionary note on the use of the TUNEL stain to determine apoptosis. *Neuroreport* 1995; **7**:61–4.

45. Hossmann KA. Disturbances of cerebral protein synthesis and ischemic cell death. *Prog Brain Res* 1993; **96**:161–77.

46. DeGracia DJ, Jamison JT, Szymanski JJ, Lewis MK. Translation arrest and ribonomics in post-ischemic brain: layers and layers of players. *J Neurochem* 2008; **106**:2288–301.

47. Stanimirovic DB, Friedman A. Pathophysiology of the neurovascular unit: disease cause

or consequence? *J Cereb Blood Flow Metab* 2012; **32**:1207–21.

48. Hudgins WR, Garcia JH. Transorbital approach to the middle cerebral artery of the squirrel monkey: a technique for experimental cerebral infarction applicable to ultrastructural studies. *Stroke* 1970; **1**:107–11.

49. Tamura A, Graham DI, McCulloch J, Teasdale GM. Focal cerebral ischaemia in the rat: 1. Description of technique and early neuropathological consequences following middle cerebral artery occlusion. *J Cereb Blood Flow Metab* 1981; **1**:53–60.

50. Koizumi J, Yoshida Y, Nakazawa T, Ooneda G. Experimental studies of ischemic brain edema. 1. A new experimental model of cerebral embolism in rats in which recirculation can be introduced in the ischemic area. *Jpn J Stroke* 1986; **8**:1–8.

51. Rogers DC, Campbell CA, Stretton JL, Mackay KB. Correlation between motor impairment and infarct volume after permanent and transient middle cerebral artery occlusion in the rat. *Stroke* 1997; **28**:2060–5; discussion 2066.

52. Hossmann KA. The two pathophysiologies of focal brain ischemia: implications for translational stroke research. *J Cereb Blood Flow Metab* 2012; **32**:1310–16.

53. DiNapoli VA, Rosen CL, Nagamine T, Crocco T. Selective MCA occlusion: a precise embolic stroke model. *J Neurosci Methods* 2006; **154**:233–8.

54. Orset C, Macrez R, Young AR, *et al.* Mouse model of in situ thromboembolic stroke and reperfusion. *Stroke* 2007; **38**:2771–8.

55. Chen F, Suzuki Y, Nagai N, *et al.* Rodent stroke induced by photochemical occlusion of proximal middle cerebral artery: evolution monitored with MR

imaging and histopathology. *Eur J Radiol* 2007; **63**:68–75.

56. Mehra M, Henninger N, Hirsch JA, *et al.* Preclinical acute ischemic stroke modeling. *J Neurointerv Surg* 2012; **4**:307–13.

57. Mordasini P, Frabetti N, Gralla J, *et al.* In vivo evaluation of the first dedicated combined flow-restoration and mechanical thrombectomy device in a swine model of acute vessel occlusion. *AJNR Am J Neuroradiol* 2011; **32**:294–300.

58. Koller A, Toth P. Contribution of flow-dependent vasomotor mechanisms to the autoregulation of cerebral blood flow. *J Vasc Res* 2012; **49**:375–89.

59. Symon L. Regional vascular reactivity in the middle cerebral arterial distribution. An experimental study in baboons. *J Neurosurg* 1970; **33**:532–41.

60. Hata R, Maeda K, Hermann D, Mies G, Hossmann KA. Evolution of brain infarction after transient focal cerebral ischemia in mice. *J Cereb Blood Flow Metab* 2000; **20**:937–46.

61. del Zoppo GJ. The neurovascular unit in the setting of stroke. *J Intern Med* 2010; **267**:156–71.

62. Gursoy-Ozdemir Y, Yemisci M, Dalkara T. Microvascular protection is essential for successful neuroprotection in stroke. *J Neurochem* 2012; **123** (Suppl 2):2–11.

63. Liebeskind DS. Collateral circulation. *Stroke* 2003; **34**:2279–84.

64. Toole JF, McGraw CP. The steal syndromes. *Annu Rev Med* 1975; **26**:321–9.

65. Pakkenberg B, Gundersen HJ. Neocortical neuron number in humans: effect of sex and age. *J Comp Neurol* 1997; **384**:312–20.

66. Clarke DD, Sokoloff L. Circulation and energy metabolism of the brain. In: Siegel G, Agranoff B, Albers RW, Fisher

29

S, eds. *Basic Neurochemistry: Molecular, Cellular, and Medical Aspects*, 6th edn. Philadelphia: Lippincott-Raven; 1999: 637–69.

67. Sokoloff L. Energetics of functional activation in neural tissues. *Neurochem Res* 1999; **24**:321–9.

68. Magistretti PJ, Pellerin L. Astrocytes couple synaptic activity to glucose utilization in the brain. *News Physiol Sci* 1999; **14**:177–82.

69. Laughlin SB, Attwell D. The metabolic cost of neural information: from fly eye to mammalian cortex. In: Frackowiak RSJ, Magistretti PJ, Shulman RG, Altman JS, Adams M, eds. *Neuroenergetics: Relevance for Functional Brain Imaging.* Strasbourg: HFSP Workshop XI; 2001: 54–64.

70. Frackowiak RSJ, Magistretti PJ, Shulman RG, Altman JS, Adams M (eds.). *Neuroenergetics: Relevance for Functional Brain Imaging.* Strasbourg: HFSP Workshop XI; 2001.

71. Astrup J, Siesjö BK, Symon L. Thresholds in cerebral ischemia – the ischemic penumbra. *Stroke* 1981; **12**:723–5.

72. Heiss WD. Experimental evidence of ischemic thresholds and functional recovery. *Stroke* 1992; **23**:1668–72.

73. Hossmann KA. Viability thresholds and the penumbra of focal ischemia. *Ann Neurol* 1994; **36**:557–65.

74. Heiss W-D, Hayakawa T, Waltz AG. Cortical neuronal function during ischemia. Effects of occlusion of one middle cerebral artery on single-unit activity in cats. *Arch Neurol* 1976; **33**:813–20.

75. Hossmann KA. Cerebral ischemia: models, methods and outcomes. *Neuropharmacology* 2008; **55**:257–70.

76. Hata R, Maeda K, Hermann D, Mies G, Hossmann KA. Dynamics of regional brain metabolism and gene expression after middle cerebral artery occlusion in mice. *J Cereb Blood Flow Metab* 2000; **20**:306–15.

77. Heiss WD. Ischemic penumbra: evidence from functional imaging in man. *J Cereb Blood Flow Metab* 2000; **20**:1276–93.

78. Takasawa M, Beech JS, Fryer TD, *et al.* Imaging of brain hypoxia in permanent and temporary middle cerebral artery occlusion in the rat using 18F-fluoromisonidazole and positron emission tomography: a pilot study. *J Cereb Blood Flow Metab* 2007; **27**:679–89.

79. Kane I, Sandercock P, Wardlaw J. Magnetic resonance perfusion diffusion mismatch and thrombolysis in acute ischaemic stroke: a systematic review of the evidence to date. *J Neurol Neurosurg Psychiatry* 2007; **78**:485–91.

80. Hoehn-Berlage M, Norris DG, Kohno K, *et al.* Evolution of regional changes in apparent diffusion-coefficient during focal ischemia of rat brain: the relationship of quantitative diffusion NMR imaging to reduction in cerebral blood flow and metabolic disturbances. *J Cereb Blood Flow Metab* 1995; **15**:1002–11.

81. Sun PZ, Zhou J, Sun W, Huang J, van Zijl PC. Detection of the ischemic penumbra using pH-weighted MRI. *J Cereb Blood Flow Metab* 2007; **27**:1129–36.

82. Cheung JS, Wang E, Lo EH, Sun PZ. Stratification of heterogeneous diffusion MRI ischemic lesion with kurtosis imaging: evaluation of mean diffusion and kurtosis MRI mismatch in an animal model of transient focal ischemia. *Stroke* 2012; **43**:2252–4.

83. Kidwell CS, Heiss WD. Advances in stroke: imaging. *Stroke* 2012; **43**:302–4.

84. del Zoppo GJ, Sharp FR, Heiss WD, Albers GW. Heterogeneity in the penumbra. *J Cereb Blood Flow Metab* 2011; **31**:1836–51.

85. Dreier JP. The role of spreading depression, spreading depolarization and spreading ischemia in neurological disease. *Nat Med* 2011; **17**: 439–47.

86. Strong AJ, Anderson PJ, Watts HR, *et al.* Peri-infarct depolarizations lead to loss of perfusion in ischaemic gyrencephalic cerebral cortex. *Brain* 2007; **130**:995–1008.

87. Mies G, Iijima T, Hossmann K-A. Correlation between periinfarct DC shifts and ischemic neuronal damage in rat. *Neuroreport* 1993; **4**:709–11.

88. Moskowitz MA, Lo EH, Iadecola C. The science of stroke: mechanisms in search of treatments. *Neuron* 2010; **67**:181–98.

89. Tymianski M. Emerging mechanisms of disrupted cellular signaling in brain ischemia. *Nat Neurosci* 2011; **14**:1369–73.

90. Simon R, Xiong Z. Acidotoxicity in brain ischaemia. *Biochem Soc Trans* 2006; **34**:1356–61.

91. Choi DW. Excitotoxicity, apoptosis and ischemic stroke. *J Biochem Mol Biol* 2001; **34**:8–14.

92. Szydlowska K, Tymianski M. Calcium, ischemia and excitotoxicity. *Cell Calcium* 2010; **47**:122–9.

93. MacDonald JF, Xiong ZG, Jackson MF. Paradox of Ca^{2+} signaling, cell death and stroke. *Trends Neurosci* 2006; **29**:75–81.

94. Chan PH. Reactive oxygen radicals in signaling and damage in the ischemic brain. *J Cereb Blood Flow Metab* 2001; **21**:2–14.

95. Shuaib A, Lees KR, Lyden P, *et al.* NXY-059 for the treatment of acute ischemic stroke. *N Engl J Med* 2007; **357**:562–71.

96. Dalkara T, Moskowitz MA. The complex role of nitric oxide in the pathophysiology of focal cerebral ischemia. *Brain Pathol* 1994; **4**:49–57.

97. Shuttleworth CW, Weiss JH. Zinc: new clues to diverse roles in brain ischemia. *Trends Pharmacol Sci* 2011; **32**:480–6.

98. Sensi SL, Jeng JM. Rethinking the excitotoxic ionic milieu: the emerging role of Zn(2+) in ischemic neuronal injury. *Curr Mol Med* 2004; **4**:87–111.

99. Paschen W. Endoplasmic reticulum dysfunction in brain pathology: critical role of protein synthesis. *Curr Neurovasc Res* 2004; **1**:173–81.

100. Youle RJ, van der Bliek AM. Mitochondrial fission, fusion, and stress. *Science* 2012; **337**:1062–5.

101. Gouriou Y, Demaurex N, Bijlenga P, De Marchi U. Mitochondrial calcium handling during ischemia-induced cell death in neurons. *Biochimie* 2011; **93**:2060–7.

102. Norenberg MD, Rao KV. The mitochondrial permeability transition in neurologic disease. *Neurochem Int* 2007; **50**:983–97.

103. Rothwell NJ, Luheshi GN. Interleukin 1 in the brain: biology, pathology and therapeutic target. *Trends Neurosci* 2000; **23**:618–25.

104. Planas AM, Gorina R, Chamorro A. Signalling pathways mediating inflammatory responses in brain ischaemia. *Biochem Soc Trans* 2006; **34**:1267–70.

105. Wang CX, Shuaib A. Critical role of microvasculature basal lamina in ischemic brain injury. *Prog Neurobiol* 2007; **83**:140–8.

106. Walz B, Zimmermann C, Bottger S, Haberl RL. Prognosis of patients after hemicraniectomy in malignant middle cerebral artery infarction. *J Neurol* 2002; **249**:1183–90.

107. Lansberg MG, Thijs VN, O'Brien MW, *et al.* Evolution of apparent diffusion coefficient, diffusion-weighted, and T2-weighted signal intensity of acute stroke. *AJNR Am J Neuroradiol* 2001; **22**:637–44.

108. Badaut J, Lasbennes F, Magistretti PJ, Regli L. Aquaporins in brain: distribution, physiology, and pathophysiology. *J Cereb Blood Flow Metab* 2002; **22**:367–78.

109. Kerr JF, Wyllie AH, Currie AR. Apoptosis: a basic biological phenomenon with wide-ranging implications in tissue kinetics. *Br J Cancer* 1972; **26**:239–57.

110. Niizuma K, Yoshioka H, Chen H, *et al.* Mitochondrial and apoptotic neuronal death signaling pathways in cerebral ischemia. *Biochim Biophys Acta* 2010; **1802**:92–9.

111. MacManus JP, Buchan AM. Apoptosis after experimental stroke: fact or fashion? *J Neurotrauma* 2000; **17**:899–914.

112. Dirnagl U, Simon RP, Hallenbeck JM. Ischemic tolerance and endogenous neuroprotection. *Trends Neurosci* 2003; **26**:248–54.

113. Zhao H, Sapolsky RM, Steinberg GK. Interrupting reperfusion as a stroke therapy: ischemic postconditioning reduces infarct size after focal ischemia in rats. *J Cereb Blood Flow Metab* 2006; **26**:1114–21.

114. Wiltrout C, Lang B, Yan Y, Dempsey RJ, Vemuganti R. Repairing brain after stroke: a review on post-ischemic neurogenesis. *Neurochem Int* 2007; **50**:1028–41.

115. Kamouchi M, Ago T, Kuroda J, Kitazono T. The possible roles of brain pericytes in brain ischemia and stroke. *Cell Mol Neurobiol* 2012; **32**:159–65.

116. Abe K, Yamashita T, Takizawa S, *et al.* Stem cell therapy for cerebral ischemia: from basic science to clinical applications. *J Cereb Blood Flow Metab* 2012; **32**:1317–31.

117. Kuhl DE, Phelps ME, Kowell AP, *et al.* Effects of stroke on local cerebral metabolism and perfusion: mapping by emission computed tomography of ^{18}FDG and ^{13}NH$_3$. *Ann Neurol* 1980; **8**:47–60.

118. Baron JC, Frackowiak RS, Herholz K, *et al.* Use of PET methods for measurement of cerebral energy metabolism and hemodynamics in cerebrovascular disease. *J Cereb Blood Flow Metab* 1989; **9**:723–42.

119. Heiss WD, Grond M, Thiel A, *et al.* Permanent cortical damage detected by flumazenil positron emission tomography in acute stroke. *Stroke* 1998; **29**:454–61.

120. Baird AE, Benfield A, Schlaug G, *et al.* Enlargement of human cerebral ischemic lesion volumes measured by diffusion-weighted magnetic resonance imaging. *Ann Neurol* 1997; **41**:581–9.

121. Kidwell CS, Alger JR, Saver JL. Beyond mismatch: evolving paradigms in imaging the ischemic penumbra with multimodal magnetic resonance imaging. *Stroke* 2003; **34**:2729–35.

122. Heiss WD, Sobesky J, Smekal U, *et al.* Probability of cortical infarction predicted by flumazenil binding and diffusion-weighted imaging signal intensity: a comparative positron emission tomography/magnetic resonance imaging study in early ischemic stroke. *Stroke* 2004; **35**:1892–8.

123. Kane I, Carpenter T, Chappell F, *et al.* Comparison of 10 different magnetic resonance perfusion imaging processing methods in acute ischemic stroke: effect on lesion size, proportion of patients with diffusion/perfusion mismatch, clinical scores, and radiologic outcomes. *Stroke* 2007; **38**:3158–64.

124. Sobesky J, Weber OZ, Lehnhardt FG, *et al.* Does the mismatch match the penumbra? Magnetic resonance imaging and positron emission tomography in early ischemic stroke. *Stroke* 2005; **36**:980–5.

125. Olivot JM, Albers GW. Diffusion-perfusion MRI for triaging transient ischemic attack and

acute cerebrovascular syndromes. *Curr Opin Neurol* 2011; **24**:44–9.

126. Garcia JH, Liu KF, Ho KL. Neuronal necrosis after middle cerebral artery occlusion in Wistar rats progresses at different time intervals in the caudoputamen and the cortex. *Stroke* 1995; **26**:636–42.

127. Magistretti PJ. Coupling synaptic activity to glucose metabolism. In: Frackowiak RSJ, Magistretti PJ, Shulman RG, Altman JS, Adams M, eds. *Neuroenergetics: Relevance for Functional Brain Imaging.* Strasbourg: HFSP Workshop XI; 2001: 133–42.

128. Attwell D, Laughlin SB. An energy budget for signaling in the grey matter of the brain. *J Cereb Blood Flow Metab* 2001; **21**:1133–45.

129. Heiss WD, Rosner G. Functional recovery of cortical neurons as related to degree and duration of ischemia. *Ann Neurol* 1983; **14**:294–301.

130. Hossmann KA, Mies G. *Multimodal Mapping of the Ischemic Penumbra in Animal Models.* New York: Marcel Dekker, Inc.; 2007.

131. Hossmann KA. Periinfarct depolarizations. *Cerebrovasc Brain Metab Rev* 1996; **8**: 195–208.

132. Hossmann KA. Pathophysiology and therapy of experimental stroke. *Cell Mol Neurobiol* 2006; **26**:1057–83.

Chapter

2

Common causes of ischemic stroke

Bo Norrving

Introduction

This chapter focuses on the major causes of ischemic stroke. Common and less common stroke syndromes are described in Chapters 9 and 10.

Ischemic stroke is not a single disease but a heterogeneous condition with several very different pathophysiological mechanisms. Identification of the underlying cause is important for several reasons. It helps to group patients into specific subtypes for the study of different aspects of prognosis, which may be used for planning and information purposes. It also helps for selecting patients for some specific therapies, which are among the most effective secondary preventive measures currently available. Identification of the mechanism of ischemic stroke should therefore be part of the routine diagnostic workup in clinical practice.

Ischemic stroke is generally caused by one of three pathogenic mechanisms:

- large artery atherosclerosis in extracranial and large intracranial arteries
- embolism from the heart
- intracranial small-vessel disease (lacunar infarcts).

These three types account for about 75% of all ischemic strokes (Figure 2.1). In about 20% of patients no clear cause of ischemic stroke can be identified despite appropriate investigations; this is labeled cryptogenic stroke. About 5% of all ischemic strokes result from more uncommon causes. These frequencies relate to ischemic stroke aggregating all age groups: in younger patients with stroke the pathogenic spectrum is much different, with arterial dissection as the most common single cause in patients <45 years of age (Chapter 10, Less common stroke syndromes).

As described in Chapter 9 (Common stroke syndromes), there are several classification schemes for ischemic stroke based on the underlying pathophysiology. The most widely used is the Trial of Org 10172 in Acute Stroke Treatment (TOAST) classification, which divides ischemic stroke into atherothrombotic, cardioembolic, small-vessel occlusion, other determined cause, and undetermined cause [1]. The last category comprises both truly cryptogenic strokes, ischemic strokes that are "undetermined" because of incomplete investigation, and strokes that are "undetermined" because multiple possible causes coexist in the same patient. In a further development of the TOAST classification the "undetermined cause" category has been subdivided, and definitions of subtypes have been further refined, taking more recent advances in diagnostic tools into account [2, 3]. A computerized algorithm of this classification has been developed, and further defines categories into evident, probable, and possible based on the level of diagnostic support (Table 2.1). Although these classification schemes were developed for use in clinical trials, they also form a useful framework for identifying causes of stroke in clinical practice.

> The TOAST classification divides ischemic stroke into atherothrombotic, cardioembolic, small-vessel occlusion, other determined cause, and undetermined cause.

Large artery atherosclerosis

Atherosclerosis of the major vessels supplying the brain is an important mechanism in ischemic stroke. Although the common occurrence of atherosclerosis in the region of the carotid bifurcation was observed early in the twentieth century, and the mechanism of

---

Table 2.1. Causative Classification System for Ischemic Stroke (CCS)

Large artery atherosclerosis	Evident – probable – possible
Cardio-aortic embolism	Evident – probable – possible
Small artery occlusion	Evident – probable – possible
Other causes	Evident – probable – possible
Undetermined causes	

unknown – cryptogenic embolism

unknown – other cryptogenic

unknown – incomplete evaluation

unclassified

Source: Adapted from Ay *et al.* [2].

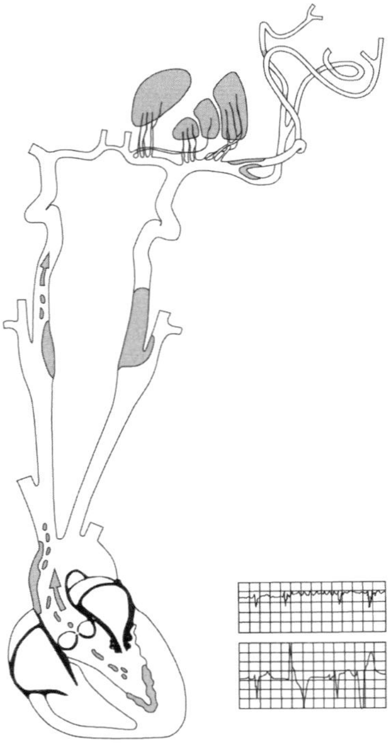

Figure 2.1. Graphic illustration of the major causes of ischemic stroke.

distal embolization in causing strokes was proposed, it was widely assumed that most cerebral ischemic strokes were caused by *in situ* middle cerebral artery (MCA) thrombosis. The full implications of extracranial atherosclerosis for ischemic stroke were not recognized until the mid-twentieth century with the advent of the diagnostic techniques of catheter angiography and later ultrasound, the links with clinical syndromes, and the therapeutic implications of carotid surgery for carotid bifurcation disease.

Large-vessel disease may cause ischemia through embolism (artery-to-artery embolism) or reduction of blood flow (hemodynamic causes). Emboli from large-vessel disease are usually platelet aggregates or thrombus formed on atherosclerotic plaques. Atherosclerotic debris and cholesterol crystals may also contribute. In many patients carotid or vertebral artery occlusion occurs without symptoms because good collateral supply is provided through the circle of Willis, the external carotid artery, and cortical pial anastomoses.

Patients with stroke often have generalized atherosclerosis in other vascular beds. About one-quarter of patients with transient ischemic attach (TIA) or stroke have a history of a symptomatic coronary event, and an additional 25–50% have asymptomatic coronary plaques, stenoses, or silent myocardial infarcts [4, 5]. Although coronary heart disease is somewhat more prevalent in patients with large atherosclerosis of the cervical arteries, it is commonly present also in patients with other stroke subtypes.

> Large-vessel disease may cause ischemia through embolism or reduction of blood flow.

Prevalence of large atherosclerosis: extra- and intracranial

Symptomatic atherosclerosis is most common at the bifurcation of the common carotid artery into the external and internal carotid arteries (Figure 2.2). Other common extracranial sites are the aortic arch, the proximal subclavian arteries, and the vertebral artery origins. Severe carotid stenosis (50–99%) is present in 10–15% of patients with anterior circulation ischemic strokes, with proportions increasing with age. The proportions are similar in patients with TIAs. Intracranial atherosclerosis, in white populations less common than extracranial, most often affects the carotid siphon, the intracranial vertebral arteries as they penetrate the dura, and the basilar artery. Severe atherosclerosis in the proximal MCA is rarer; in whites MCA occlusion is usually the result of embolism from the heart or a proximal arterial site. Overall, large artery atherosclerosis is estimated to account for about 30% of all ischemic strokes.

However, the pattern of atherosclerosis is widely different in other populations. Intracranial

atherosclerosis appears to be much more common in the Asian and African-American population (Figure 2.3). Intracranial large artery disease has long been a relatively neglected disorder because of a research focus on the more accessible extracranial carotid artery occlusive disease lesions. However, intracranial large artery disease appears to be the most common stroke subtype worldwide [6, 7]. In Chinese and Japanese populations intracranial atherosclerosis accounts for up to half of all strokes, and in Korean studies up to a quarter. The underlying causes of racial differences in the distribution of extracranial and intracranial occlusive disease are not fully understood: they are presumably related to differences in risk-factor patterns but findings from different regions do not show a consistent pattern.

> Intracranial atherosclerosis is in white populations less common than extracranial but appears to be the most common stroke subtype worldwide.

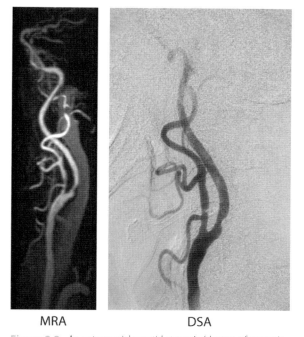

MRA   DSA

Figure 2.2. An extracranial carotid stenosis (degree of stenosis 67%) as visualized by MR angiography (left) and digital subtraction angiography (right). (Courtesy of Dr. Mats Cronqvist.)

Large artery atherosclerosis in the aortic arch

The link between atherosclerosis of the aortic arch and ischemic stroke was not clearly recognized until the early 1990s when autopsy studies revealed a high prevalence of such lesions in particular in patients with cryptogenic strokes [8]. At that time examination of the aortic arch was not part of the routine echocardiographic examination. Protruding aortic atheromas (>4–5 mm) have been found to be 3–9 times more common in stroke patients than in healthy controls. Later studies have established that aortic arch atheroma is clearly associated with ischemic stroke, possibly both by serving as a source of

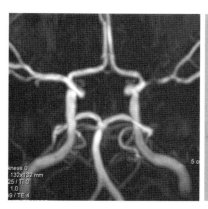

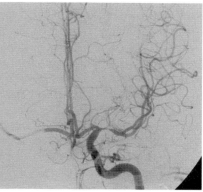

Figure 2.3. Stenosis of the middle cerebral artery visualized by MR angiography (left) and digital subtraction angiography (right). (Courtesy of Dr. Mats Cronqvist.)

emboli and by being a marker of generalized large artery atherosclerosis including cerebral vessels. In stroke patients thick or complex aortic atheromas are associated with advanced age, carotid stenosis, coronary heart disease, atrial fibrillation (AF), diabetes, and smoking. For the long-term prognosis, the characteristics of thickness over 4–5 mm, ulceration, noncalcified plaque, and presence of mobile components are associated with a 1.6–4.3 times increased risk of recurrent stroke.

> Protruding aortic atheromas are frequently found in stroke patients.

Mechanisms of cerebral ischemia resulting from extracranial and intracranial large artery atherosclerosis

Artery-to-artery embolism is considered the most common mechanism of TIA and ischemic stroke due to large artery atherosclerosis. Thrombosis at the site of an atherosclerotic lesion is due to interplay between the vessel wall lesion, blood cells, and plasma factors. Severe stenosis alters blood flow characteristics, and turbulence replaces laminar flow when the degree of stenosis exceeds about 70%. Platelets are activated when exposed to abnormal or denuded endothelium in the region of an atheromatous plaque. Plaque hemorrhage may contribute to thrombus formation, similar to the mechanisms in coronary artery disease. Plaque instability appears to be a dynamic phenomenon [9], and may explain the observation that the risk of recurrent ischemic events is highest early after a TIA and is much lower from 1 to 3 months and onwards [10, 11]. Plaque instability is characterized by a thin fibrous cap, large lipid core, reduced smooth muscle content, and a high macrophage density. Complicating thrombosis occurs mainly when the thrombogenic center of the plaque is exposed to flowing blood.

> Artery-to-artery embolism is considered the most common mechanism of TIA and ischemic stroke due to large artery atherosclerosis.

Reduction of blood flow in the carotid artery is not affected until the degree of stenosis approaches 70%, corresponding to a luminal diameter of less than 1.5 mm. However, the degree of carotid stenosis correlates poorly with intracranial hemodynamic alterations because of the variability of the collateral circulation. Embolic and hemodynamic causes of ischemic stroke and TIA are not mutually exclusive mechanisms. Ultrasound studies with transcranial Doppler have documented the frequent occurrence of microembolic signals not associated with apparent clinical symptoms in patients with symptomatic ischemic vascular disease of the brain. Hemodynamically compromised brain regions appear to have a diminished capacity for wash-out or clearance of small emboli which are more likely to cause infarcts in low-flow areas [12].

> Blood flow in the carotid artery is reduced if stenosis is more than 70%.

Clinical features of large artery atherosclerosis

Large artery atherosclerosis is a prototype of stroke mechanism that may cause almost any clinical stroke syndrome. Furthermore, some degree of atherosclerosis in brain-supplying arteries is present in most patients with ischemic stroke, raising the issue of determining the likely cause if multiple potential causes are identified. The clinical spectrum of large artery atherosclerosis ranges from asymptomatic arterial disease, TIA affecting the eye or the brain, and ischemic stroke of any severity in the anterior and posterior circulation. Less common clinical syndromes due to large artery atherosclerosis, e.g. those due to hemodynamic causes, are detailed in Chapter 10.

Cardioembolic stroke

Cardioembolic stroke accounts for 25–35% of all ischemic strokes, making cardiac disease the most common major cause of stroke overall – a practical point often forgotten. Non-valvular AF is the commonest cause of cardioembolic stroke. The heart is of particular importance in ischemic stroke for other reasons also: cardiac disorders (in particular coronary heart disease) frequently coexist in patients with stroke and are important long-term prognostic determinants. Whereas recurrent stroke is the most common vascular event during the first few years after a first stroke, with time an increasing proportion of new vascular events are due to coronary heart disease.

> Cardiac disease is the most common cause of stroke overall.

Proportion of all strokes due to cardioembolic stroke

The proportion of strokes associated with cardioembolic strokes increases sharply with age, mainly because of the epidemiological characteristics in the population of AF, the single most common major cardioembolic source.

In some cases of cardioembolic stroke the association may be coincidental. This is certainly true for several of the minor cardioembolic sources (see below), for which findings from case–control studies show divergent results. As technology advances further more cardiac conditions that may constitute potential causes of stroke are detected. It is also true for AF, which is associated with several other stroke risk factors, and is very common in the general population. However, the finding that anticoagulant therapy reduces the risk of ischemic stroke by about 60% in patients with AF suggests that the majority of strokes associated with AF are the result of cardiac embolism. An autopsy study of patients with stroke dying within 30 days showed that 70% of patients with a diagnosis of cardioembolic stroke in this study (based on cardiac conditions that may produce emboli in the heart or through the heart) were found to have intracardiac thrombi, which were of similar composition to persistent emboli detected in the major intracerebral arteries [13].

Cardioembolic sources: major and minor

There are several cardiac disorders that may constitute a source of embolus, but not all sources pose equal threats. They are commonly divided by origin in the heart (atrial, valvular, ventricular) and potential for embolism (high risk versus low or uncertain risk, or major versus minor) (Table 2.2). The clinically most important cardioembolic sources are nonrheumatic AF, infective endocarditis, prosthetic heart valve, recent myocardial infarction, dilated cardiomyopathy, intracardiac tumors, and rheumatic mitral valve stenosis.

Atrial fibrillation

Non-valvular AF is by far the commonest major cardioembolic source, and an arrhythmia of considerable importance for ischemic stroke due to its prevalence in the population and the substantial increase in stroke risk. In the general population 5–6% of persons

Table 2.2. Cardioembolic sources and risk of embolism

High risk	Low/uncertain risk
I Atrial	
Atrial fibrillation	Patent foramen ovale
Sustained atrial flutter	Atrial septal aneurysm
Sick sinus syndrome	Atrial auto-contrast
Left atrial/atrial appendage thrombus	
Left atrial myxoma	
II Valvular	
Mitral stenosis	Mitral annulus calcification
Prosthetic valve	Mitral valve prolapse
Infective endocarditis	Fibroelastoma
Non-infective endocarditis	Giant Lambl's excrescences
III Ventricular	
Left ventricular thrombus	Akinetic/dyskinetic ventricular wall segment
Left ventricular myxoma	Subaortic hypertrophic cardiomyopathy
Recent anterior myocardial infarct	Congestive heart failure
Dilated cardiomyopathy	

Source: Modified from Ferro [21].

>65 years and 12% of persons >75 years have AF. Fifty-six percent of people with AF are over 75 years of age. Epidemiological studies have shown that non-valvular AF is associated with at least a 5-fold increased risk of stroke. However, the individual risk of embolism in AF varies 20-fold among AF patients, depending on age and other associated risk factors. To predict the future risk for embolism in AF risk stratification schemes (such as $CHADS_2$ and CHADS-VASC) have been developed (see Chapter 22, Secondary prevention).

The proportion of ischemic strokes associated with AF increases with age, and in the highest age group >80 years about 40% of all strokes occur in patients with this arrhythmia [14]. The mean age of patients with stroke associated with AF is 79 years in European stroke registries, about 4 years higher than the average age of stroke in general. The importance of AF for ischemic stroke is likely to increase even further in the future because the prevalence of AF in the population is increasing (because persons with AF tend to live longer, and a larger proportion of people are reaching a higher age).

Paroxysmal AF carries a risk for embolism similar to the average risk for chronic AF, which is of importance for therapeutic purposes. Paroxysmal AF after ischemic stroke appears to be undetected in a substantial proportion of patients. By subsequent use of Holter monitoring and other monitoring techniques new AF is detected in at least 5% of all patients with ischemic stroke who are initially in sinus rhythm [15]. Detection has been shown to improve with prolonged monitoring.

> Cardioembolic stroke accounts for 25–35% of all ischemic strokes. Non-valvular atrial fibrillation is the commonest cause of cardioembolic stroke and carries at least a 5-fold increased risk of stroke.

Prosthetic heart valves

Mechanical prosthetic heart valves are well recognized for their propensity to produce thrombosis and embolism, whereas tissue prostheses appear to have a much lower risk. Long-term anticoagulant therapy is standard practice for patients with mechanical prosthetic heart valves, but despite therapy embolism occurs at a rate of about 2% per year. Any type of prosthetic valve may be complicated by infective endocarditis, which should be considered in patients who experience embolic events.

Endocarditis

Infectious and non-infectious endocarditis is covered in Chapter 10 (Less common stroke syndromes).

Recent anterior myocardial infarct

Ischemic stroke may occur in close temporal proximity (hours, days, weeks) to an acute myocardial infarct, suggesting a cause-and-effect relationship due to embolism. Left ventricular mural thrombi have been diagnosed by echocardiography in up to 20% of patients with large anterior infarcts, but the frequency has not been well determined in the current era of much more active antithrombotic drug treatments and endovascular procedures in the acute phase of coronary heart disease. Studies have reported a frequency of about 5% for ischemic stroke during the first few weeks after myocardial infarction. After this

period the stroke risk appears to be much lower, and is probably related to the presence of shared risk factors for coronary heart disease and ischemic stroke in the vast majority of these patients.

> Five percent of ischemic strokes are related to a myocardial infarct.

Dilated cardiomyopathy

Dilated cardiomyopathies are a well-recognized cause of embolism, which may be due to the formation of intracardiac thrombus from severe ventricular dysfunction, AF, or endocarditis. In contrast, hypertrophic cardiomyopathies appear not to be associated with an increased risk of stroke per se.

Patent foramen ovale (PFO) and atrial septal aneurysm (ASA)

Patent foramen ovale (PFO) has been linked to ischemic stroke mainly in young adults, in whom frequencies for this cardiac finding of up to 40% are detected, about twice the rate in the general population [16, 17]. PFO is more commonly observed in patients with cryptogenic stroke than in those with a known cause, and this association appears to hold also for elderly patients [18]. PFO may cause stroke through paradoxical embolism, which requires the coexistence of thrombosis in lower limb, pelvic, or visceral veins or pulmonary embolism, a cardiac right-to-left shunt, or cough or other Valsalva maneuver immediately preceding stroke onset. However, the exact mechanism by which PFO may cause stroke is still not clear, and evidence mainly comes indirectly from statistical associations. Concurrent venous thrombosis or pulmonary embolism is rarely detected even in patients with a high suspicion of paradoxical embolism. Besides paradoxical embolism PFO may be linked to stroke through causing a propensity for supraventricular arrhythmias, and through thrombus from a coexisting ASA. The long-term risk of recurrent stroke from PFO has not been precisely determined; it appears that mainly the coexistence of PFO and ASA is associated with a clearly increased risk of recurrence. PFO has also been linked to migraine (which increases the risk of stroke in young adults), but recent studies have not confirmed this association [19].

> Patent foramen ovale may cause strokes through paradoxical embolism.

Mitral valve prolapse

Early studies proposed mitral valve prolapse to be the major cause of unexplained stroke in particular in young persons. However, revised diagnostic criteria and subsequent observational and case–control studies have questioned the overall role of mitral valve prolapse as a cardioembolic source.

Clinical and neuroimaging features of cardioembolic ischemic strokes

Although cardioembolism may cause almost any clinical stroke syndrome, some features are statistically linked to this cause and are therefore characteristic (Table 2.3). However, it should be borne in mind that the positive predictive value of clinical features suggesting cardioembolism is very modest, at only about 50% [20, 21]. Conversely, some clinical and neuroimaging syndromes, such as a lacunar syndrome found on diffusion-weighted magnetic resonance imaging (DWI) to be due to a single small infarct, are very unlikely to be due to cardioembolism.

Traditionally it was thought that cardioembolic strokes almost always had a sudden onset of symptoms that were maximal from the beginning, but this doctrine has not stood the test of time. Exceptions with gradual and stuttering progressive courses are not rare, and may be due to distal migration of an embolus or early recurrence of embolism in the same vascular territory [22]. Strokes due to cardioembolism are usually more severe than average, probably because emboli from the heart tend to be larger than emboli from arterial sources. However, cardioembolism may well cause TIAs, and the proportion of cardioembolic strokes preceded by TIA is similar to findings in other stroke subtypes.

The risk of early hemorrhagic transformation (multifocal or in the form of secondary hematoma) is about twice as high in cardiac embolism compared to other stroke subtypes [23]. Hemorrhagic transformation has been thought to be due to leakage of blood through a vessel wall with ischemia-induced increased permeability, but the process is likely to be much more complex. In patients with cardioembolism predictive factors of hemorrhagic transformation are decreased level of consciousness, high stroke severity, proximal occlusion, extensive early infarct signs in the MCA territory, and delayed recanalization [24].

> Strokes due to cardioembolism are usually more severe than those from other causes and the risk of early hemorrhagic is about twice as high in cardiac embolism compared to other stroke subtypes.

Some patients with a major cerebral hemispheric stroke syndrome due to distal internal carotid artery or proximal MCA occlusion may have rapid spontaneous improvement of neurological deficits, a phenomenon that has been labeled "spectacular shrinking deficit" [25]. This clinical syndrome is usually, but not exclusively, caused by cardioembolism. The rapid improvement is due to distal propagation, fragmentation, and subsequent spontaneous lysis of the embolus.

Emboli from the heart may occlude the internal artery in the neck, but more commonly they occlude one of the main intracranial vessels. In the anterior circulation cardioembolism and artery-to-artery embolism are the two major causes of full MCA infarcts due to proximal MCA occlusion as well as partial (pial territorial) MCA infarcts due to more distal occlusions. Large artery disease tends to be somewhat more common for anterior MCA infarcts, whereas cardioembolism is more common in posterior MCA lesions. Cardioembolism is also a recognized cause of the restricted cortical MCA syndrome of acute ischemic distal arm paresis, which may mimic peripheral radial or ulnar nerve lesion [26].

In the posterior circulation cardioembolism is no less frequent and tends to occur at characteristic "embolic" sites, common for embolism from cardiac and arterial sources. Cardioembolism is the cause of about a quarter of all lateral medullary infarcts, and

Table 2.3. Features suggestive of cardioembolic stroke

Sudden onset of maximal deficit

Decreased level of consciousness

Rapid regression of initially massive symptoms ("spectacular shrinking deficit")

Supratentorial stroke syndromes of isolated motor or sensory dysphasia, or visual field defects

Infratentorial ischemic stroke involving the cerebellum (posterior inferior cerebellar artery [PICA] or superior cerebellar artery [SCA] territories), top of the basilar

Hemorrhagic transformation

Neuroimaging finding of acute infarcts involving multiple vascular territories in the brain, or multiple levels of the posterior circulation about three-quarters of cerebellar infarcts in the posterior inferior cerebellar artery (PICA) and superior cerebellar artery (SCA) territories, and distal basilar artery occlusions. Basilar artery occlusion presenting with sudden onset of severe brainstem symptoms is often due to cardioembolism [27].

Studies with DWI in patients with acute ischemic stroke have demonstrated that acute ischemic abnormalities involving multiple territories are much more common than previously thought; about 40% of all patients have scattered lesions in one vascular territory or multiple lesions in multiple vascular territories. As should be logically plausible, these ischemic lesion patterns have been associated with embolism from cardiac or large artery sources [28].

Small-vessel disease

Infarcts due to small-vessel disease of the brain were first recognized by French neurologists and neuropathologists in the nineteenth century, who also coined the term "lacune" from the autopsy finding of a small cavitation. However, the importance of lacunar infarcts as one of the main ischemic stroke subtypes was not clearly recognized until the investigations of C. Miller Fisher in the 1960s, who on the basis of careful clinicopathological observations laid the foundation for our pathological understanding of lacunar infarction.

Lacunar infarcts are small (<15 mm diameter) subcortical infarcts that result from occlusion of a single penetrating artery (Figure 2.4). Lacunar infarcts are usually located in the basal ganglia, thalamus, internal capsule, corona radiate, and the brainstem. The arterial pathology is characterized by intrinsic disease of small arterioles (40–200 µm) attributed to microatheroma or segmental arterial disorganization. Lacunar infarcts may also be caused by intracranial atherosclerosis (*in situ* atheroma at the mouth of the penetrating vessel). However, the detailed microvascular characteristics of lacunar infarcts are based on quite few observations, partly due to the difficulties in obtaining adequate and timely autopsy specimens. Lacunar infarcts are part of the spectrum of cerebral small-vessel disease, and more recently generalized endothelial failure has been increasingly recognized as a common underlying factor [29].

Lacunar infarcts usually result from occlusion of single penetrating arteries.

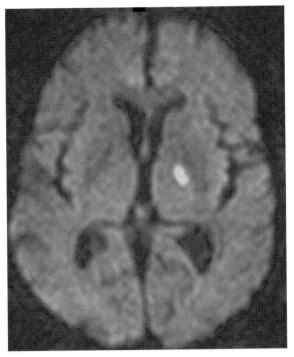

Figure 2.4. Diffusion-weighted MRI of a lacunar infarct in the internal capsule. (Courtesy of Professor Stig Holtås.)

Prevalence and risk factors

In most series lacunar infarcts are thought to account for about one-quarter of all ischemic strokes, a proportion similar to cardioembolic stroke and infarcts due to large-vessel atherosclerosis. Patients with lacunar infarcts are on average a few years younger than patients with ischemic stroke in general. This is likely to be indirectly linked to the fact that cardioembolic sources become more prevalent with age and consequently patients with cardiac embolism tend to be older.

Lacunar infarcts are formed on a risk-factor profile that comprises age, gender, hypertension, diabetes, smoking, previous TIA, and possibly ischemic heart disease. In particular, hypertension was initially thought to be a prerequisite for the development of small-vessel occlusion. However, later studies have demonstrated that the vascular risk-factor profile is not specific for lacunar infarction, but is largely similar to other stroke types [30]. Genetic factors may also play an important role in the development of lacunar infarcts and other types of cerebral small-vessel disease. Lacunar infarcts are part of the clinical spectrum of cerebral autosomal dominant arteriopathy with subcortical infarcts and leukencephalopathy (CADA-SIL), a genetic disease affecting the small arteries of the brain (see Chapter 10).

Clinical features

Lacunar infarcts cause stroke, i.e. give rise to acute stroke symptoms, when they occur at strategic sites where descending and ascending long tracts are concentrated in their course subcortically or in the brainstem.

Classic lacunar syndromes

When symptomatic, lacunar infarcts are associated with clinical "lacunar" syndromes, five of which are well recognized: pure motor hemiparesis, pure sensory stroke, sensorimotor stroke, dysarthria–clumsy hand syndrome, and ataxic hemiparesis. Face, arm, and leg involvement are characteristic of the first three syndromes. The most important clinical feature is the absence of cognitive symptoms or signs and visual field defects. Preceding TIAs occur in about 25% of all cases, usually only shortly before the infarct occurs. Sometimes patients present with a burst of dramatic TIAs with dense hemiparesis for 5–15 minutes alternating with normal function – the "capsular warning syndrome." About half of these patients go on to develop a lacunar infarct within the first 1–2 days, despite routine antiplatelet and even heparin therapies. Initial progression of the neurological deficit is observed in up to 40% of all cases, making lacunar infarct the most common subtype of progressive stroke. The exact mechanisms of the progression is still not well understood [31].

The classic lacunar syndromes are further detailed in Chapter 9.

Other clinical presentations of lacunar infarcts

Several other more rare clinical syndromes may also be caused by occlusion of single penetrating arteries, but the clinicopathological evidence for this is more limited. Descriptions include movement disorders such as chorea, dystonia, hemibalismus, and asterixis. Brainstem syndromes (such as internuclear ophthalmoplegia, horizontal gaze palsy, Bendikt's syndrome, Claude's syndrome, pure motor hemiplegia plus sixth nerve palsies) and isolated cranial nerve palsies (most often third nerve palsies) may be caused by a micro infarct in the brainstem (visualized only by MRI), presumably most often due to occlusion of a small penetrating artery, though the mechanism is likely to vary. The old doctrine that isolated vascular cranial nerve syndromes were usually caused by affection of vasa vasorum to the peripheral nerve outside the brainstem is probably incorrect [32].

Silent lacunar infarcts

Lacunar infarcts cause clinical symptoms when they affect the long motor and sensory tracts in the subcortical areas, linked to their clinical presentation. However, MRI studies of the general population have disclosed that most lacunar infarcts do not produce acute stroke symptoms but are clinically unrecognized or "silent" [33]. Silent cerebral infarcts (95% of which are "lacunar") are at least five times as common as symptomatic ones, and have been shown to increase the risk of vascular events (including stroke), cognitive decline, and dementia.

Imaging criteria for silent lacunar infarcts have been imprecise. A recent consensus statement defines a lacune of presumed vascular origin as a round or ovoid, subcortical, fluid-filled (similar signal as cerebrospinal fluid) cavity, of between 3 mm and about 15 mm in diameter, consistent with a previous acute small deep brain infarct or hemorrhage in the territory of one perforating arteriole [34]. Longitudinal imaging studies have shown that acute lacunar infarcts often cavitate with time, but this is not always the case: acute lacunar infarcts may disappear, or have a similar appearence as white matter hyperintensities in the chronic phase (Figure 2.5) [29, 34].

> Silent lacunar infarcts are five times more frequent than symptomatic ones.

Specificity of the clinical lacunar syndromes

Studies have shown that the majority of patients with lacunar syndromes have DWI findings suggestive of lacunar infarcts, i.e. that the imaged ischemic abnormality is compatible with the territory of a single perforating artery. In the acute stage the diameter should be less than 15 mm, but may extend up to 20 mm in some cases. The infarct size shrinks by at least half from the acute to the chronic stage, and most late lacunar infarcts are less than 5 mm in diameter [29, 34]. However, with DWI in no less than one-third of patients lesion patterns of multiple ischemic areas in the cortex or subcortex are seen, suggesting embolism as the underlying cause. Because multiple small embolic infarcts are present in a

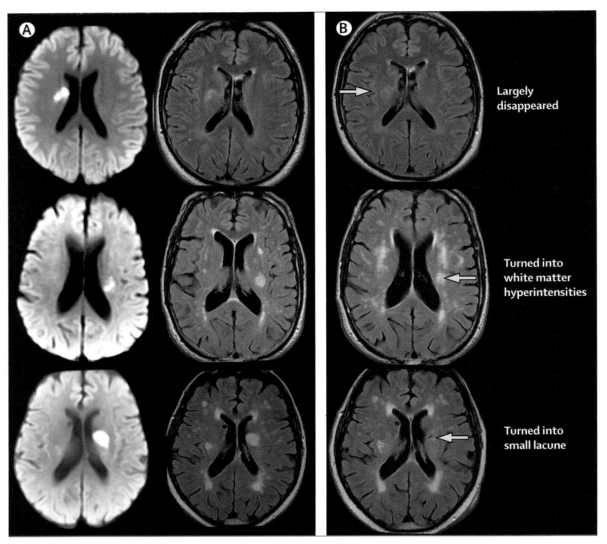

Figure 2.5. Common late sequelae of acute small deep (lacunar) infarcts. (A) Acute stage diffusion-weighted imaging (left column), FLAIR (right column). (B) About 1 year later FLAIR. These infarcts can: disappear (top), look like white matter hyperintensities indefinitely (middle), or cavitate to create a lacune (bottom). FLAIR = fluid-attenuated inversion recovery. From Wardlaw *et al.* [29] with permission from the publisher.

proportion of all patients presenting with a lacunar syndrome, carotid artery ultrasound, ECG, and cardiac monitoring to detect AF should also be part of clinical routine in such patients.

Multiple overlapping causes of ischemic stroke

In some patients multiple overlapping causes of ischemic stroke are identified. In such cases, whether these findings are purely coincidental or represent the cause of the infarct is not clear. For example, patients with clinical and neuroimaging features that are compatible with lacunar infarction may have associated findings of large artery atherosclerosis or a cardioembolic source (most commonly AF). The cause of stroke in such patients is difficult to establish on an individual basis, but large artery or cardiac causes of stroke are not always coincidental.

Cryptogenic ischemic stroke

Patients experiencing a TIA/stroke frequently have no determined etiology after standard diagnostic evaluation. Previous reports show that 20–25% of stroke survivors are classified as cryptogenic stroke, but it is a matter of debate which strokes should be labeled cryptogenic – what level of evidence is needed for accepting a finding or risk factor as the "cause?" Such debate has surrounded PFO, which can be an incidental finding or possibly an underlying mechanism: methods for distinguishing incidental PFOs from pathogenic ones in cryptogenic stroke patients and for identifying patients at high risk of recurrence would be clinically most useful but are currently not available.

A proportion of such "cryptogenic" strokes may stem from unrecognized cardiac embolism (paroxysmal AF), subclinical aortic, and large artery atherothrombotic embolism, in particular among elderly patients. The spectrum of potential causes of cryptogenic ischemic stroke in the young may be different. In a recent large study of causes of stroke in patients <55 years of age, no less than 33% were found to be cryptogenic despite a comprehensive diagnostic protocol including monogenetic causes of ischemic stroke [35].

Chapter summary

> The Trial of Org 10172 in Acute Stroke Treatment (TOAST) classification divides ischemic stroke into
>
> - atherothrombotic (30% of ischemic strokes, mostly emboli from the bifurcation of the carotid artery)
> - cardioembolic (25–35% of ischemic strokes, mostly due to atrial fibrillation [AF])

- small-vessel occlusion (25% of ischemic strokes, leading to lacunar infarcts)
- other determined cause
- and undetermined cause.

Sometimes, overlapping causes can be identified.

Large artery atherosclerosis is estimated to account for about 30% of all ischemic strokes. Large-vessel disease may cause ischemia through embolism (artery-to-artery embolism) or reduction of blood flow (hemodynamic causes) or both (hemodynamically compromised brain regions appear to have a diminished capacity for wash-out or clearance of small emboli). The clinical spectrum of large artery atherosclerosis ranges from asymptomatic arterial disease, TIA affecting the eye or the brain, and ischemic stroke of any severity in the anterior and posterior circulation.

Cardioembolic stroke accounts for 25–35% of all ischemic strokes. The clinically most important cardioembolic source of cardioembolic stroke is nonvalvular AF followed by infective endocarditis, prosthetic heart valve, recent myocardial infarction, dilated cardiomyopathy, intracardiac tumors, and rheumatic mitral valve stenosis. Paroxysmal AF carries a risk for embolism similar to the average risk for chronic AF. Strokes due to cardioembolism are usually more severe than average and the risk of early hemorrhagic embolism is about twice as high in cardiac embolism compared to other stroke subtypes.

In most series lacunar infarcts are thought to account for about one-quarter of all ischemic strokes. Lacunar infarcts are small (<15 mm diameter) subcortical infarcts that result from occlusion of a single penetrating artery. Lacunar infarcts are associated with clinical lacunar syndromes, but the specificity of the syndromes is only moderate: lacunar syndromes may be caused by other mechanisms than small artery disease in one-third of all cases.

References

1. Adams HP, Bendixen BH, Kappelle LJ, et al. Classification of subtype of acute ischemic stroke. Definitions for use in a multicenter clinical trial. Stroke 1993; 24:35–41.

2. Ay H, Benner T, Arsava EM, Furie KL, et al. A computerized algorithm for etiologic classification of ischemic stroke: the Causative Classification of Stroke System. Stroke 2007; 38:2979–84.

3. Arsava EM, Ballabio E, Benner T, et al. The Causative Classification of Stroke system: an international reliability and optimization study. Neurology 2010; 75:1277–84.

4. Adams RJ, Chimowitz MI, Alpert JS, et al. Coronary risk evaluation in patients with transient ischemic attack and ischemic stroke: a scientific statement for healthcare professionals from the Stroke Council and the Council on Clinical Cardiology of the American Heart Association/American Stroke Association. Stroke 2003; 34:2310–22.

5. Gongora-Rivera F, Labreuche J, Jaramillo A, et al. Autopsy prevalence of coronary atherosclerosis in patients with fatal stroke. Stroke 2007; 38:1203–10.

6. Gorelick PB, Wong KS, Hee-Joon Bae, Pandey DK. Large artery intracranial occlusive disease. A large worldwide burden but a relatively neglected frontier. *Stroke* 2008; **39**:2396–9.

7. Pu Y, Liu L, Wang Y, *et al.* Geographic and sex difference in the distribution of intracranial atherosclerosis in China. *Stroke* 2013; **44**:2109–14.

8. Amarenco P, Cohen A, Tzuorio C, *et al.* Atherosclerotic disease of the aortic arch and the risk of ischemic stroke. *N Engl J Med* 1994; **331**:1474–9.

9. Rothwell PM. Atherothrombosis and ischaemic stroke. *BMJ* 2007; **334**:379–80.

10. Giles MF, Rothwell PM. Risk of stroke early after transient ischaemic attack: a systematic review and meta-analysis. *Lancet Neurol* 2007; **6**:1063–72.

11. Wu CM, McLaughlin K, Lorenzetti DL, *et al.* Early risk of stroke after transient ischemic attack. A systematic review and meta-analysis. *Arch Intern Med* 2007; **167**:2417–22.

12. Caplan LR, Wong KS, Gao S, Hennerici MH. Is hypoperfusion an important cause of strokes? If so, how? *Cerebrovasc Dis* 2006; **21**(3):145–53.

13. Ogata J, Yutani C, Otsubo R, *et al.* Heart and vessel pathology underlying brain infarction in 142 stroke patients. *Ann Neurol* 2008; **63**:770–81.

14. Marini C, De Santis F, Sacco S, *et al.* Contribution of atrial fibrillation to incidence and outcome of ischemic stroke: results from a population-based study. *Stroke* 2005; **36**:1115–19.

15. Liao J, Khalid Z, Scallan C, Morillo C, O'Donnell M. Noninvasive cardiac monitoring for detecting paroxysmal atrial fibrillation or flutter after acute ischemic stroke: a systematic review. *Stroke* 2007; **38**:2935–40.

16. Mas JL, Arquizan C, Lamy C, *et al.* Recurrent cerebrovascular events associated with patent foramen ovale, atrial septal aneurysm, or both. *N Engl J Med* 2001; **345**:1740–6.

17. Lamy C, Giannesini C, Zuber M, *et al.* Clinical and imaging findings in cryptogenetic stroke patients with and without patent foramen ovale: the PFO-ASA Study. *Stroke* 2002; **33**:706–11.

18. Handke M, Harloff A, Olschewski M, Hetzel A, Geibel A. Patent foramen ovale and cryptogenic stroke in older patients. *N Engl J Med* 2007; **357**:2262–8.

19. Rundek T, Elkind MS, Di Tullio MR, *et al.* Patent foramen ovale and migraine: a cross-sectional study from the Northern Manhattan Study (NOMAS). *Circulation* 2008; **118**:1419–24.

20. Palacio S, Hart RG. Neurologic manifestations of cardiogenic embolism: an update. *Neurol Clin* 2002; **20**:179–93.

21. Ferro JM. Cardioembolic stroke: an update. *Lancet Neurol* 2003; **2**:177–88.

22. Kang DW, Latour LL, Chalela JA, Dambrosia J, Warach S. Early ischemic lesion recurrence within a week after acute ischemic stroke. *Ann Neurol* 2003; **54**:66–74.

23. Paciaroni M, Agnelli G, Corea F, *et al.* Early hemorrhagic transformation of brain infarction: rate, predictive factors, and influence on clinical outcome: results of a prospective multicenter study. *Stroke* 2008; **39**:2249–56.

24. Molina CA, Montaner J, Abilleira S, *et al.* Timing of spontaneous recanalization and risk of hemorrhagic transformation in acute cardioembolic stroke. *Stroke* 2001; **32**:1079–84.

25. Minematsu K, Yamaguchi T, Omae T. Spectacular shrinking deficit: rapid recovery from a major hemispheric syndrome by migration of an embolus. *Neurology* 1992; **42**:17–62.

26. Gass A, Szabo K, Behrens S, Rossmanith C, Hennerici M. A diffusion-weighted MRI study of acute ischemic distal arm paresis. *Neurology* 2001; **57**:1589–94.

27. Caplan LR. *Posterior Circulation Disease. Clinical Findings, Diagnosis and Management.* Cambridge MA: Blackwell Science; 1996.

28. Kang DW, Chalela JA, Ezzeddine MA, *et al.* Association of ischaemic lesion patterns on early diffusion-weighted imaging with TOAST stroke subtypes. *Arch Neurol* 2003; **60**:1730–4.

29. Wardlaw JM, Smith C, Dichgans M. Mechanisms of sporadic cerebral small vessel disease: insights from neuroimaging. *Lancet Neurol* 2013; **12**:483–97.

30. Jackson C, Sudlow C. Are lacunar strokes really different? A systematic review of differences in risk factor profiles beween lacuna and nonlacunar infarcts. *Stroke* 2005; **36**:891–901.

31. Steinke W, Ley SC. Lacunar stroke is the major cause of progressive motor deficits. *Stroke* 2002; **33**:1510–16.

32. Thömke F, Gutmann L, Stoeter P, Hopf HC. Cerebrovascular brainstem diseases with isolated cranial nerve palsies. *Cerebrovasc Dis* 2002; **13**:147–55.

33. Vermeer S, Longstreth WT Jr, Koudstaal PJ. Silent brain infarcts: a systematic review. *Lancet Neurol* 2007; **6**:611–19.

34. Wardlaw JM, Smith EE, Biessels GJ, *et al.* Neuroimaging standards for research into small vessel disease and its contribution to ageing and neurodegeneration. *Lancet Neurol* 2013; **12**:822–38.

35. Rolfs A, Fazekas F, Grittner U, *et al.* Acute cerebrovascular disease in the young: the Stroke in Young Fabry Patients Study. *Stroke* 2013; **44**:340–9.

Neuroradiology

PART A: IMAGING OF ACUTE ISCHEMIC AND HEMORRHAGIC STROKE: CT, PERFUSION CT, CT ANGIOGRAPHY

Patrik Michel

Practical aspects of acute stroke CT

Plain CT has a long track record of a safe exam that is feasible in most patients. An occasional patient will need sedation or anesthesia for cerebrovascular images after sedation. Two or three injections of contrast are needed to obtain sufficient CT angiography (CTA) images of head and neck vessels (starting at the aortic arch) and perfusion CT (PCT) from supratentorial structures. Contrast nephrotoxicity or allergic contrast reactions are a rare occurrence [1], especially if contrast is not administered to patients with a pre-existing history of renal failure and metformin medication. In our institution, contrast is injected for CTA and PCT before knowledge of the creatinine clearance in hyperacute patients who are potential candidates for revascularization treatment. Several precautions may be applied [2] to help limit nephrotoxicity. Other than a creatinine clearance <30 ml/min/m^2 are early pregnancy, thyroid disorders and known contrast allergy.

Non-contrast CT (NCCT)

NCCT can be performed in less than a minute with a helical CT scanner, and is considered sufficient to select patients for intravenous thrombolysis with intravenous recombinant tissue plasminogen activator (RTPA) within 4.5 hours, or endovascular treatment within 6 hours. It is a highly accurate method for identifying acute intracerebral hemorrhage (ICH)

and subarachnoid hemorrhage, but quite insensitive for detecting acute ischemia. The approximate sensitivity of CT and PCT in different ischemic stroke subtypes is depicted in Figure 3.A.1. The "fogging effect" on NCCT relates to the potential disappearance of hypoattenuation from approximately day 7 for up to 2 months after the acute stroke. It may result in false-negative NCCT in the subacute stage of ischemic stroke.

Focal hypoattenuation (hypodensity) is very specific and predictive for irreversible ischemia, whereas early edema without hypoattenuation indicates low perfusion pressure with increased cerebral blood volume (CBV) and therefore represents potentially salvageable tissue [3]. In addition to hypoattenuation, loss of gray–white matter differentiation including in the insular cortex ("insular ribbon sign") and isodense basal ganglia constitute the four early ischemic changes (EIC) that are mostly irreversible and are used to calculate the Alberta Stroke Program Early CT Score (ASPECTS) [4, 5]. Using this score, detection of EIC is better. It remains uncertain, however, whether the ASPECTS improves the prediction of clinical outcome independently of demographic and clinical variables.

> Non-contrast CT (NCCT) is considered sufficient to select patients for intravenous thrombolysis with intravenous RTPA within 4.5 hours, or endovascular treatment within 6 hours.

Regarding treatment response, ASPECTS based on NCCT does not add substantially to prediction of response to intravenous thrombolysis [6, 7], but lower ASPECTS scores are related to a poorer response to endovascular recanalization treatment [6]. EIC on NCCT predict post-thrombolysis symptomatic ICH independently of other factors [8, 9]. On the other

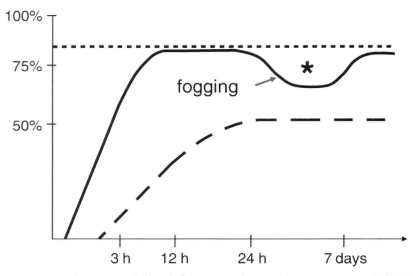

Figure 3.A.1. Approximate likelihood of detecting ischemic stroke on non-contrast CT (NCCT) in territorial (continuous line) and lacunar (dashed line) infarcts. * indicates the fogging effect observed in the subacute phase on NCCT. The dotted line indicates approximate sensitivity of perfusion CT in non-lacunar supratentorial strokes. PCT data are from the ASTRAL registry.

hand, extent of EIC on very early NCCT has not been shown to predict mass effect after acute ischemic stroke.

Perfusion CT (PCT)

PCT with iodinated contrast may be used in two ways:

- as a slow-infusion/whole-brain technique
- as dynamic PCT with first-pass bolus-tracking methodology.

The latter is preferable as it is quantitative and allows accurate identification of the ischemic penumbra [10].

In a patient with suspected acute ischemic stroke, a non-contrast baseline cerebral CT is immediately followed by PCT. Then, a CTA of the head and neck, and a contrast-enhanced CT of the brain are performed, with a total of about 15 minutes from the start to the end of the examination. If the patient fulfills criteria for intravenous thrombolysis based on the NCCT, treatment may be started in the scanner while the patient is undergoing PCT and CTA. Similarly, image acquisition and processing usually overlap.

PCT examinations usually consist of two 40-second series separated by 5 minutes. For each series, CT scanning is initiated 7 seconds after injection of 50 ml of iso osmolar iodinated contrast material into an antecubital vein using a power injector. Multidetector-array technology currently allows the

acquisition of data from four adjacent 5–10 mm sections for each series. The lowest of these eight cerebral CT sections usually cuts through the midbrain and hippocampi; the other slices cover most of the supratentorial brain.

The PCT data are analyzed according to the central volume principle to create parametric maps of regional cerebral blood volume (rCBV), mean transit time (MTT), and regional cerebral blood flow (rCBF). The rCBV map is calculated from a quantitative estimation of the partial size averaging effect, which is completely absent in a reference pixel at the center of the large superior sagittal venous sinus. The MTT maps result from a deconvolution of the parenchymal time–concentration curves by a reference arterial curve. Finally, the rCBF values can be calculated from the rCBV and MTT values for each pixel using the following equation: rCBF = rCBV/MTT. The maps can then be displayed graphically (Figure 3.A.2.).

Table 3.A.1. Alterations of MTT, rCBF, and rCBV in case of ischemia (comparison with contralateral homologous region)

	MTT	rCBF	rCBV
Healthy parenchyma	=	=	=
Penumbra	↑↑	↓	= or ↑
Infarct	↑↑↑	↓↓	↓

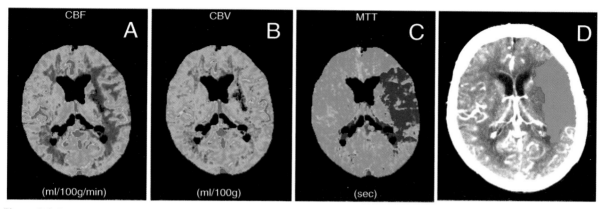

Figure 3.A.2. A 77-year-old patient, found on awakening with aphasia and right hemiparesis, NIHSS = 20. Perfusion CT maps depicting (A) regional cerebral blood flow, (B) regional cerebral blood volume, (C) mean transit time, and (D) core infarct maps according to a threshold model [14]. In (D), green: reversible ischemia (penumbra), and red: low likelihood of survival (infarct).

Raw maps of PCT images may be interpreted in a non-quantitative way by comparing the different parameters given in Table 3.A.1.

MTT is the most sensitive measure for decreased blood flow but overestimates ischemia. rCBF is more specific in identifying salvageable tissue, and rCBV is the most specific parameter for irreversibly damaged tissue [11, 12], also in white matter [13]. Threshold maps separate reversible from irreversible ischemia [14, 15] and result in high interobserver agreement [15].

The 64-slice CT scanners allowing for eight or more brain slices have increased the detection rate for acute ischemic stroke [16], but diffusion-weighted MRI (DWI) remains more sensitive for small and infratentorial lesions. PCT has an overall sensitivity of about 75% for ischemic stroke, above 85% for non-lacunar supratentorial infarcts (Figure 3.A.1), and a high specificity for ischemia [11, 15].

Several PCT-based threshold models to differentiate ischemic, non-viable tissue ("core"), viable tissue ("penumbra"), and non-threatened tissue ("benign oligemia") have been developed. According to calculations by Wintermark's group [17], the ischemic area (penumbra and infarct) is defined by pixels with a greater than 145% prolongation of MTT compared with the corresponding region in the contralateral cerebral hemisphere [17]. Within this selected area, 2.0 ml/100 g represents the rCBV threshold: pixels belong to the infarct core if the rCBV value is inferior to the threshold, and to the penumbra if the rCBV value is superior to the threshold. Salvageable penumbra is displayed in green, and tissue with low likelihood of survival (infarct core) is displayed in red (Figure 3.A.2). According to Parsons' group, penumbra is present if the relative delay time is >2 seconds [18], and infarct if the mean CBF is <31% of the contralateral side [19]. Determination of PCT-based thresholds using positron emission tomography (PET) is currently ongoing.

PCT also shows brain perfusion alterations in about 25% of patients with transient ischemic attacks, which are sometimes still present after the resolution of the patients' symptoms [20]. Focal hyperperfusion in relationship with epileptic seizures has been described, and focal hypoperfusion is rare [21, 22]. During the migrainous aura, poorly delimited hypoperfusion contralateral to the aura symptoms is found occasionally [23] and may be mistaken as ischemic stroke.

Overall, in the absence of an abnormality on PCT in a patient with stroke symptoms, one might suspect a posterior fossa stroke, a lacunar stroke, small cortical stroke [16], or a stroke-imitating condition (migraine, Todd's paralysis, venous thrombosis, encephalitis, conversion syndrome). Acute recanalization treatments might be inappropriate in some of these patients.

Baseline PCT volumes correlate with stroke severity in the acute stage, and do so better in left-sided infarctions [24]. Although several PCT parameters have been associated with clinical outcome, few of them were tested in combination with well-established clinical variables, such as age or initial stroke severity. Initial penumbra volume seems to be an independent predictor depending on recanalization: if recanalization occurs, large initial penumbra is an indicator of favorable prognosis and vice versa [25, 26].

PCT predictors of treatment response are partially established; it has been shown that thrombolysis saves salvageable tissue as identified by PCT [27], and the presence of large penumbra volumes is associated with better clinical outcome if recanalization is achieved [26]. In patients undergoing endovascular treatment, smaller CBVs were associated with better outcomes [28]. These results points to similar principles as found in multimodal MRI-based prediction of treatment response.

PCT-based predictors of post-thrombolytic symptomatic ICH are only partially known. Severity and volume of hypoperfusion on PCT seems to play a role [29, 30], but independence of such variables from EIC on NCCT, stroke severity, or glucose sugar need to be demonstrated. Similarly, PCT has the potential to predict mass effect after middle cerebral artery (MCA) stroke. No consensus has been found of the

most promising marker, however; volumes of decreases CBF or CBV [31, 32] and blood–brain barrier permeability [33] have been proposed.

Perfusion CT (PCT) has an overall sensitivity of about 75% for ischemic stroke, above 85% for non-lacunar supratentorial infarcts (Figure 3.A.1), and a high specificity for ischemia, but diffusion-weighted MRI (DWI) remains more sensitive for small and infratentorial lesions. Still, in the absence of an abnormality on PCT in a patient with stroke symptoms, acute recanalization treatments might be inappropriate.

CT angiography

Cerebral and cervical CTA is performed using intravenous administration of 50 ml of iodinated contrast material at a rate of 3 ml per second, and an acquisition delay of about 15 seconds. Data acquisition is performed from the origin of the aortic arch branch vessels to the circle of Willis and reconstructed as maximum-intensity projections (MIP) and three-dimensional reconstructions (Figure 3.A.3).

CTA has been shown to identify the site of arterial occlusion in acute ischemic stroke patients, with

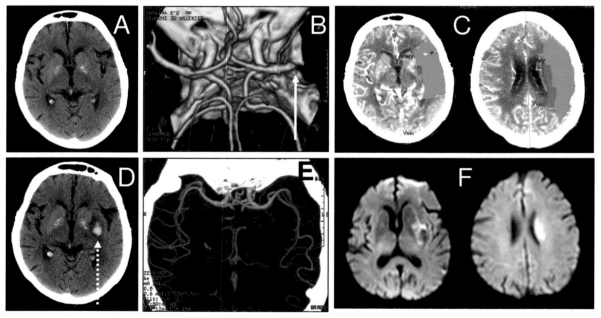

Figure 3.A.3. Same patient as Figure 3.A.2. **Upper row:** imaging at 12 hours after going to bed: (A) plain CT, (B) CT angiography with occlusion of the middle cerebral artery (white arrow), and (C) perfusion CT with threshold maps. The patient was then given intravenous thrombolysis with rtPA at 13 hours after going to bed and 2.5 hours after awaking (approved study protocol with informed consent from family). **Lower row:** (D) plain CT at 24 hours with a small left basal ganglion bleed (dotted arrow). (E) CT angiography with repermeabilization, and (F) diffusion-weighted MRI at 5 days, showing a small, partially hemorrhagic lesion.

similar accuracy as digital subtractive angiography (DSA) and probably better than MR angiography (MRA) [34, 35]. Clot length can be assessed by thin-sliced NCCT [36] and CTA, although the latter may overestimate unless late images with collateral filling are considered [37]. Similar to clot length, a clot burden score can be calculated and correlates with stroke severity [38]. Clot presence, localization, length, and burden seem to predict clinical outcome [38–41], but it is not known whether they do it independently of known clinical and demographic outcome predictors. Clot length and site do seem to predict recanalization after intravenous thrombolysis, however [36, 42, 43].

Good collateral circulation is associated with smaller early infarct volume and National Institutes of Health Stroke Scale (NIHSS) scores [42, 44, 45]. Correlation with better clinical outcome has been shown [42, 44, 46, 47] but as with clot length, its added value to other predictors needs to be confirmed.

CTA source images (CTA-SI) have been used to estimate infarct core and penumbra in anterior [48, 49] and posterior circulation [50]. The value of this method to predict tissue fate, clinical outcome, and treatment response still requires more work [51].

> CT angiography (CTA) has been shown to identify the site of arterial occlusion in acute ischemic stroke patients, with similar accuracy as DSA and probably better than MRA. Clot length can be assessed by thin-sliced NCCT and CTA. Clot presence, localization, length, and burden seem to predict clinical outcome and clot length and site do seem to predict recanalization after intravenous thrombolysis.

CT and intracranial hemorrhage

Hyperintensity in acute intracranial hemorrhage (ICH) is present on NCCT from its onset in virtually all patients. Intraparenchymal calcifications or melanin-containing metastases may sometimes give false-positive results. Adding CTA is debated, but is probably useful in patients with higher risk of vascular malformations underlying the ICH, such as patients with superficial (lobar) ICH, without hypertension, and of younger age. One main advantage of adding iodinated contrast in ICH is that contrast extravasation ("leakage") is an independent predictor of hematoma growth and poorer clinical outcome [52]. It is now a target for immediate hemostatic therapy in randomized trials. Various radiological methods, including PCT [53], indicate that there is no significant ischemia around the hematoma.

PART B: IMAGING OF ACUTE ISCHEMIC AND HEMORRHAGIC STROKE: MRI AND MR ANGIOGRAPHY

Jochen B. Fiebach, Patrik Michel, and Jens Fiehler

Practical aspects of acute stroke MRI

Magnetic resonance imaging (MRI) can be used as the first and sole modality for the emergency imaging of patients with suspected acute stroke. An acute multi-parametric stroke imaging should combine diffusion-weighted (DWI), fluid attenuated inversion recovery (FLAIR), T2*-weighted imaging, and MR angiography (MRA; usually using magnetic contrast agent, but time-of-flight MRA is also possible) of head and neck arteries. Total acquisition time with 1.5T or 3T systems is about 10 minutes and enables examinations of acute stroke patients with moderate cooperation. Once contraindications are excluded, medication can be administered and additional sequences can be acquired. This may include perfusion-weighted imaging (PWI; usually using contrast agent), T2 sequences, and T1 imaging following injection of contrast. Fast image reconstruction makes the results of MRA or PWI available within a few minutes.

Such a comprehensive set of acute examinations not only identifies ischemia in most patients, but provides valuable information on potential stroke imitators, high bleeding risk with thrombolysis, prognostic information, and pathogenetic mechanisms of the current stroke.

Contraindications to acute stroke MRI are most implantable electronic devices (such as cardiac pacemakers) and other metallic elements in the head region (such as first-generation aneurysm clips or foreign bodies in the eye). Agitated and claustrophobic patients will usually not tolerate this exam well enough to obtain high-quality images. In pregnant women, the potential effects on the fetus are poorly known, particularly in the first trimester. Magnetic contrast agent should not be injected in patients with a creatinine clearance <30 ml/min because of the risk of systemic nephrogenic fibrosis.

49

Multiparametric MRI can be used as the first and sole imaging modality in suspected acute stroke. It provides valuable information on potential stroke imitators, high bleeding risk with thrombolysis, prognostic information, and pathogenetic mechanisms of the current stroke, but contraindications have to be considered.

Diffusion images, FLAIR

The invention of echo-planar imaging in the mid 1990s made DWI available for examinations in acute stroke patients. Water molecules show random motion in brain tissue which is limited by intracellular organelles, increased along white matter tracts, and reduced perpendicular to tracts and bundles. This anisotropy of diffusion caused by white matter tracts is technically compensated by diffusion measurements in three orthogonal directions and calculation of mean diffusion (trace) images (Figure 3.B.1).

Sensitivity of DWI at standard slice thickness of 5–6 mm is 80–90% [54, 55], which is about twice the sensitivity of acute non-contrast CT examinations (30–60%) [55, 56]. DWI lesions represent infarction in the majority of stroke patients but are not completely specific for infarction. Transient global amnesia is associated with hippocampal DWI positive spots [57] and DWI hyperintensities have been reported after seizures [58], and in multiple sclerosis (MS) plaques [59]. DWI hyperintensity is also seen along the margins of acute intracerebral hemorrhage and in brain abscesses.

Stroke symptoms with initially negative DWI can be explained by symptomatic hypoperfusion above 12 ml/100 g/min, by a very small lesion below the resolution of the MRI, or are initially considered negative due to noise or motion artifacts. A normal DWI exam in a patient with suspected stroke may also indicate a stroke imitator such as epileptic seizures, hypoglycemia, and migraine with aura. Such patients presenting with stroke-like symptoms but showing neither infarction/ischemia nor vessel obstruction are unlikely to benefit from thrombolysis [60].

Lesions on DWI are also a good marker for the core volume in acute ischemic stroke, because only about 10% of it is reversible [61]. This percentage may be higher in very early imaging such as within 3 hours [62]. Several studies have identified an acute DWI lesion volume above 70–100 ml to be a critical size beyond which favorable outcome is highly unlikely [63–65].

At first sight, FLAIR imaging does not seem to be of particular value in acute ischemic stroke, given its lower sensitivity and less contrast between affected healthy tissue compared to DWI. On DWI, there is a much stronger contrast between affected and healthy tissue compared to conventional FLAIR images. As opposed to DWI, FLAIR abnormalities develop more slowly over several hours in acute stroke. Using this knowledge, attempts have been made to employ MRI patterns for identifying strokes within the 4.5-hour time window. In the PRE-FLAIR study, a multinational team assessed FLAIR signal intensity of acute DWI lesions [66]. In 543 patients examined within 12 hours of ictus DWI indicated infarction in 95% and 50% of those lesions were visible on FLAIR. The so-called DWI-FLAIR mismatch with FLAIR negative DWI lesions identified patients within 4.5 hours of symptom onset with 62% sensitivity and 83% positive predictive value. About 14% of acute stroke symptoms are diagnosed at awakening [67]. Those patients cannot be treated with thrombolysis as the actual time of symptom onset is unclear. Safety and efficacy of thrombolysis in wake-up stroke patients presenting with DWI-FLAIR mismatch within 4.5 hours after awakening is currently being investigated in randomized trials and cannot be recommended in clinical routine [68]. Further use of FLAIR is discussed in the MRA section below.

A typical sequence of multimodal imaging including DWI, FLAIR, PWI, and susceptibility-weighted imaging (SWI) in an acute stroke patient is shown in Figure 3.B.2.

In summary, the advantages of acute DWI MRI lie in its high sensitivity, and the characterization of the lesion extent and potentially of the stroke mechanism, thus providing a pathophysiological basis for rational decision-making. FLAIR imaging may be used as a substitute for the time clock in patients with unknown stroke onset as it seems to separate with reasonable accuracy the patient within and outside the 4.5-hour (thrombolysis) window.

Magnetic resonance angiography (MRA)

MRA directly reveals the location of the vessel occlusion. The size of the thrombus – related to the site of vessel occlusion in MRA – is an important determinant of vessel recanalization rates. It may be overestimated with MRA because stasis around a thrombus appears as occlusion.

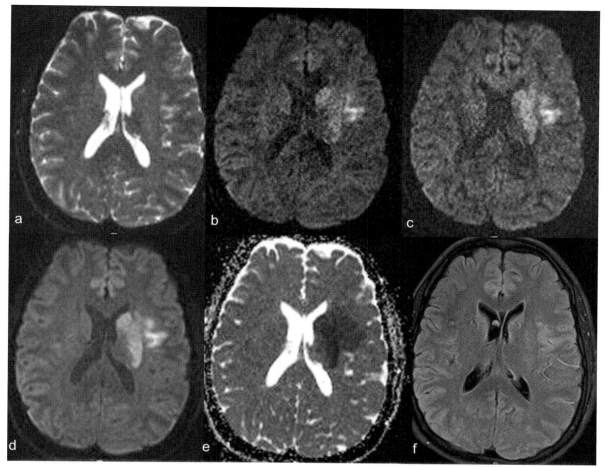

Figure 3.B.1. Technical aspects of DWI. Two diffusion sensitizing magnetic field gradients are added to a T2-weighted echo-planar imaging sequence (a). On DWI source images the signal is reduced if diffusion is measured in the direction of a tract (corpus callosum; b) and increased if measured perpendicular (c). On postprocessed isotropic DWI (d), healthy tissue such as the right hemisphere shows low contrast between gray and white matter. Acute infarction is hyperintense on DWI (d; left caudate and lentiform nucleus and the insular cortex). The apparent diffusion coefficient (ADC) is reduced in the infarcted tissue (e). On DWI there is a much stronger contrast between affected and healthy tissue compared to conventional FLAIR images (f).

Patients presenting with a major vessel occlusion or severe stenosis seem more likely to benefit from thrombolytic treatment [60, 69]. Still, many patients with more proximal occlusions on MRA reveal a considerable lesion growth and a poor outcome [70], especially if not rapidly revascularized.

Without MRA, signal intensity changes within vessels ("vessel signs") in FLAIR images can be helpful in diagnosing the site of vessel occlusion (Figure 3.B.3). However, the hypointense vessel sign in T2*- weighted MRI and the hyperintense vessel sign in FLAIR does not independently predict recanalization, risk for secondary intracerebral hemorrhage, or clinical outcome [71].

MRA directly reveals the location of the vessel occlusion. Patients presenting with a major vessel occlusion or severe stenosis seem more likely to benefit from thrombolytic treatment.

Perfusion imaging (PWI) and the mismatch concept

PWI maps are derived from the signal intensity change caused by the passage of contrast agent through the capillary bed and reflect several aspects of cerebral perfusion. Dynamic susceptibility contrast (DSC)-PWI is based on repetitive T2*-weighted acquisitions typically performed every 1.5 seconds.

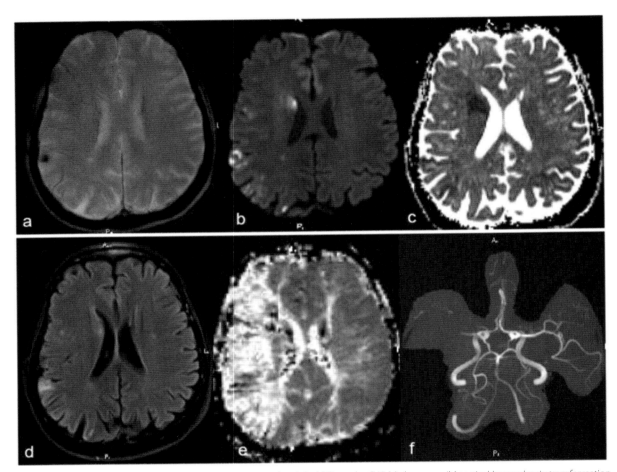

Figure 3.B.2. Multimodal MR-based imaging in a patient with a right MCA stroke. SWI (a) shows a mild cortical hemorrhagic transformation which is a contraindication for intravenous thrombolysis. A typical mismatch pattern can be seen with scattered DWI lesions on DWI (b) and ADC (c) and perfusion deficit on MTT map (e). MRA (f) shows MCA occlusion on the right. Thrombolysis was withheld with respect to the hemorrhagic transformation of one cortical infarction (a) and the different ADC values (c) and FLAIR (d) signal intensities indicating a timely distribution.

The signal drop during contrast passage can be post-processed to maps of cerebral blood flow (CBF), cerebral blood volume (CBV), mean transit time (MTT), time to bolus arrival or bolus peak, Tmax using delay corrected or uncorrected algorithms. Results can be expressed as relative (to unaffected hemisphere) or absolute values and different software provide different results for the same parameter maps [72]. Both the volume and the severity of the initial perfusion deficit are associated with the growth of the initial DWI lesion at follow-up imaging.

The penumbra in acute stroke patients has been defined as brain tissue with loss of electric activity and potential recovery after timely recanalization of the occluded artery. It is widely accepted that extension of hypoperfusion on PWI beyond the corresponding DWI boundary represents penumbra [73, 74]. This PWI > DWI mismatch has been used, validated, and refined in several studies [74–76]. Such baseline MRI findings can identify patients that are likely to benefit from reperfusion therapies and can potentially identify subgroups that are unlikely to benefit or may be harmed [77, 78]. This concept is now being used for patient selection into clinical trials, both within and beyond established time windows.

Systematic analysis of DWI and PWI patterns in the non-randomized DEFUSE study [77] and post-hoc analyses [65] have allowed the identification of patients presenting at high risk for bleeding and poor outcome despite thrombolysis ("malignant" profile): presence of

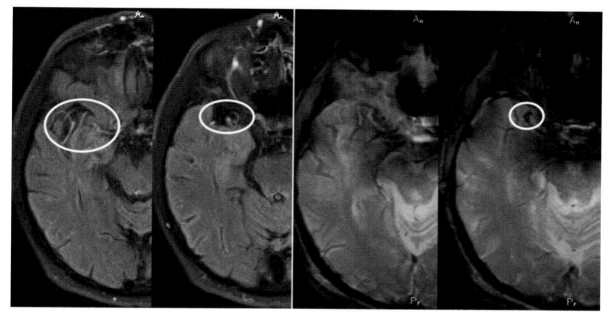

Figure 3.B.3. Value of FLAIR and T2* images in vessel pathology. In a patient with distal MCA occlusion there is a hyperintense vessel sign of the MCA and its branches on FLAIR (white circles on two left images) indicating slow flow. There is a hypointense thrombus sign on a T2*-weighted image in the distal MCA. The thrombus causes a blooming artifact that is larger than the diameter of the affected vessel (white circle on the right).

>100 ml DWI lesion and/or Tmax 8 seconds delay perfusion. Similarly, the initial mismatch definition of a perfusion deficit of 10 ml or more and 120% or more of the DWI lesion was then refined to "target mismatch," i.e. a core <70 ml, a significant hypoperfusion of <100 ml, and a mismatch ratio of ≥1.8. In patients who had reperfusion after thrombolysis, only the ones with an initial "target mismatch" had a more favorable clinical outcome.

In the post-hoc analysis of the randomized EPITHET thrombolysis trial, target mismatch patients who were thrombolyzed had less infarct growth [79]. In a similar post-hoc analysis of the phase II and III trials with the fibrinolytic substance desmoteplase a perfusion deficit exceeding DWI lesion of at least 60 ml identified treatment responders [80]. Furthermore, fully automated assessments of perfusion deficits failed to reliably differentiate between critical ischemia and oligemia [81]. The RAPID software used in DEFUSE 2 enabled investigators to identify those patients who responded to early endovascular recanalization therapy [82].

The PWI > DWI mismatch concept has also been challenged [62, 83] on the grounds that the PWI lesion cannot discriminate reliably between benign oligemia and true penumbra, and because of noted overestimation of the extent of infarction seen at follow-up [84].

Arterial spin labeling (ASL) has recently been introduced as new perfusion imaging technology not requiring contrast agent. Blood labeled with a radiofrequency pulse can be used as an endogenous contrast agent. Zaharchuk *et al.* [85] and Bokkers *et al.* [86] compared ASL-DWI mismatch to DSL perfusion-DWI mismatch. They found moderate agreement between the two methods, and called for further studies. Niibo *et al.* [87] found good correlations of ASL values with traditional MRI core and penumbra thresholds.

Based on these very recently published studies, ASL should be focused on patients with contraindications to gadolinium contrast agents. Ongoing clinical development of ASL technology and further improvement concerning robustness and accuracy in stroke imaging can be anticipated.

The extension of hypoperfusion on perfusion imaging (PWI) beyond the corresponding DWI boundary represents penumbra. This PWI>DWI mismatch has been used to identify patients that are likely to benefit from reperfusion therapies.

Arterial spin labeling (ASL) enables imaging of perfusion without contrast agent. Blood labeled with a radiofrequency pulse can be used as an endogenous contrast agent. ASL should be focused on patients with contraindications to gadolinium contrast agents.

Susceptibility weighted imaging (SWI) and intracerebral hemorrhage

For the evaluation of intracerebral hemorrhage, clinicians have traditionally relied on CT, in fear of missing or misdiagnosing an intracerebral hemorrhage by utilizing MRI only. Thrombolysis as the most effective treatment of ischemic stroke requires a rapid and reliable imaging assessment to exclude hemorrhage. Systematic studies suggest that MRI identifies intracranial hemorrhages rapidly and reliably, in particular if appropriate sequences are performed such as SWI (or gradient echo [GRE] or T2*) for intracerebral hemorrhage [88] and FLAIR for subdural hematomas (SDHs) and subarachnoid hemorrhage (SAH).

MRI in fact may be superior to CT, especially for the detection of small chronic hemorrhages, the cerebral microbleeds (CMBs). CMBs in the brain parenchyma diagnosed in T2*-weighted MRI should be interpreted in the light of the patient's history as well as the location, number, and distribution of the lesions and associated imaging findings. The retrospective BRASIL study does not support the hypothesis that CMBs are associated with a higher risk for a clinically relevant intracerebral hemorrhage after anticoagulation/antiaggregation therapy or after thrombolytic therapy in stroke patients, and thus does not support the general exclusion of patients from therapy based on the presence of CMBs [89, 90].

SDHs can also be identified reliably with MRI. In the hyperacute setting, SDHs are best demonstrated on FLAIR sequences since FLAIR imaging nulls the effect of cerebrospinal fluid. On DWI, SDHs appear hyperintense and on T2*-weighted images they tend to be hypointense. The presence of mixed signal intensity within the SDH may indicate the presence of blood with different ages and MRI may emerge as a tool in selecting the therapeutic approach to SDHs [91]. Proton density-weighted images may add further value to the diagnosis of SDH [92].

For SAH detection, the best imaging sequences on MRI are FLAIR and proton density-weighted images.

> MRI identifies intracranial hemorrhages rapidly and reliably, in particular if appropriate sequences are performed.

PART C: MULTIMODAL IMAGING-GUIDED ACUTE STROKE TREATMENT BASED ON CT AND MR IMAGING

Patrik Michel

Comparison of MR- and CT-based acute stroke imaging

The original PWI/DWI mismatch concept is based on MR imaging and postulates that critical hypoperfusion on PWI exceeding the borders of the DWI lesion indicates salvageable tissue which may justify reperfusion treatment [93]. This concept has now been refined as described below, and CT-based perfusion imaging has become an important focus of research to determine core and salvageable tissue, given its wide availability.

With regard to information about brain perfusion, PCT appears at least equivalent to MRI [12, 48, 94–96]. Significant correlation has been demonstrated between PCT-CBV and DWI, between PCT-MTT and PWI-TTP, and between CTA source images and DWI [12, 48]. If threshold models are used, the PCT core correlates well with DWI and PCT total ischemia with PWI-MTT [14, 94]. It has to be cautioned, however, that both imaging methods still need better standardization of terminology, better knowledge about thresholds, further validation of their independent prediction of clinical outcome, and testing in phase III clinical studies [97].

DWI as a marker of early infarct has the advantage of widespread availability and relative robustness. On the other hand, the linear relationship between contrast concentration and signal intensity may be an advantage of CT perfusion imaging over gadolinium-based MR perfusion imaging, allowing a more quantitative estimation of cerebral blood flow [98].

Both CTA and MRA detect significant stenosis and vascular malformations quite reliably [35, 99]. Whereas CTA better quantifies the degree of stenosis and identifies arterial calcifications, MRA is probably more specific in diagnosing cervical artery dissections [100].

Valid criticisms of MR imaging include its cost, limited availability, more difficult patient monitoring, pace maker incompatibility, and the longer time required for scanning [101]. Although exposure to radiation seems acceptable [102], it prohibits frequent use of PCT and CTA because of a probable risk of inducing cancer by radiation, particularly in younger subjects and with multiple exposures [103]. There are reports of radiation overdosing from wrongly calibrated scanners. Iodinated contrast can occasionally be associated with allergy, hyperthyroidism, or renal failure, although the last seems to occur rarely [104]. These drawbacks are counterbalanced by the availability of CT in most emergency rooms, its easy accessibility, and the easy monitoring of patients. Patients with known severe renal failure (creatinine clearance <30 ml/min) should probably receive neither iodinated contrast agents nor gadolinium [105].

Both CT- and MR-based perfusion and arterial imaging are feasible in the emergency setting. Both detect intracranial hemorrhage with high accuracy, and exclude the major contraindications for thrombolysis. Decisions for endovascular therapy based on non-invasive arterial imaging can be obtained by both methods with a sufficient degree of confidence. Advantages of MRI of a higher sensitivity to detect acute ischemic stroke (DWI) have to be balanced with the somewhat easier accessibility of CT. Both methods have certain limitations in patients with agitation and renal failure, as described below. Ideally, a stroke-receiving hospital offers both CT- and MRI-based imaging on an emergency basis, allowing physicians to choose the most appropriate one for a clinical question and situation. More realistically, most hospitals will chose one method as their first-line imaging, where indications and contraindications to multimodal sequences should be integrated in standard operating procedures of hyperacute stroke care.

With regard to information about brain perfusion, PCT appears at least equivalent to MRI, but both imaging methods still need better standardization. DWI has the advantage of widespread availability and relative robustness. On the other hand, the linear relationship between contrast concentration and signal intensity may be an advantage of CT perfusion imaging over gadolinium-based MR perfusion imaging.

Advantages of CT: available in most emergency rooms, easily accessible, and the monitoring of patients is easy. Disadvantages: iodinated contrast can be associated with allergy, hyperthyroidism, or renal failure.

Advantages of MRI: higher sensitivity to detect acute ischemic stroke (DWI). Disadvantages: higher costs, limited availability, more difficult patient monitoring, pacemaker incompatibility, and the longer time required for scanning.

Treatment decisions based on multimodal imaging

The concept of using advanced imaging for treatment decisions is similar for MR- and CT-based imaging. Through the above-mentioned systematic work, several important markers for benefit from acute revascularization treatment have been identified: low core volumes, large penumbra volumes accompanied by reperfusion, reperfusion (mostly through recanalization of large arteries), good collateral blood flow. In general, there are important relationships and codependence between such multimodal imaging parameters [51], and the most reliable and simple combination of variables for each clinical question still needs to be determined. In addition, generally applied thresholds in perfusion imaging might be inappropriate because the same degree of perfusion impairment might have a different impact on the tissue depending on patient age, the anatomic location, and time from stroke onset.

Analysis of multimodal MR-based treatment trials assessing the predictive value of multimodal imaging has shown its added value in some [77, 82], but not in others [78, 106], or only after reanalysis [69, 107]. The combination on MRI-based imaging of a core <70 ml, a significant hypoperfusion of <100 ml, and a mismatch ratio of ≥1.8 has been labeled "target mismatch" by the DEFUSE group in order to describe the patient with an increased benefit from acute revascularization [65].

Some [108, 109] but not all [69, 106, 110] retrospective analyses of recanalization treatments incorporating multimodal CT show a potential benefit.

Given the proven benefits in the first 2–3 hours after stroke onset and the high likelihood of substantial penumbra and limited infarct size very early on, intravenous thrombolytics should probably be given immediately after exclusion of major contraindications. Multimodal imaging may then be added during thrombolysis and guide further treatment decisions such as:

- adding or not mechanical revascularization treatment
- treating patients arriving late or with unknown stroke onset

- selecting the best treatment modality to achieve rapid reperfusion
- avoiding overtreatment that is likely futile or harmful.

Several important markers for benefit from acute revascularization treatment can be identified by **multimodal CT and MRI investigations**: low core volumes, large penumbra volumes accompanied by reperfusion, reperfusion (mostly through recanalization of large arteries), and good collateral blood flow.

Patient selection for clinical trials based on multimodal imaging

Several important markers for benefit from acute revascularization treatment can be identified by multimodal CT and MRI investigations, as described above. Such knowledge was gained in randomized and non-randomized trials applying multimodal imaging systematically before revascularization trials, with various results:

- DEFUSE-1: non-randomized trial of intravenous rtPA at 0–6 hours. Finding: if mismatch pattern was present and reperfusion was achieved, clinical outcome was improved [77]
- EPITHET: randomized trial using intravenous rtPA vs. placebo at 3–6 hours. Findings: initial analysis negative [78]. Post-hoc analysis of target mismatch patients, using coregistration techniques: less infarct growth was observed with rtPA [79].
- DEFUSE-2: non-randomized trial of standard treatment vs. endovascular reperfusion treatment. Findings: if mismatch pattern was present and reperfusion was achieved, clinical outcome was improved [82]
- MR RESCUE: randomized trial using standard treatment (including intravenous rtPA) vs. endovascular recanalization up to 8 hours. Findings: mismatch pattern was not associated with outcome [106].

Several randomized revascularization trials using advanced neuroimaging for treatment selection have been completed:

- DIAS-2: intravenous desmoteplase vs. placebo in the 3–9-hour window if ≥20% mismatch on PWI or PCT

  - Overall result negative regarding 3 months handicap
  - Subgroup of occlusion patients had benefit [69]
  - Subgroup of patients with ≥60% mismatch had benefit [80]
  - Intravenous tenecteplase vs. rtPA in the 0–6-hour window if ≥20% mismatch on PCT → tenecteplase was superior to rtPA regarding 3 months handicap
- Wake-up pilot trial: n = 12 based on PCT mismatch
  - PCT-based wake-up study is feasible
  - Number of patients too small to make conclusions on efficacy.

Knowledge from such trials can be combined with insight obtained from case series and randomized recanalization trials that did not use multimodal imaging, such as PROACT-2 [111], IMS-3 [112], and SYNTHESIS [113]. Such lessons include:

- Presence of initial arterial occlusion matters: if there is visible occlusion, revascularization treatments are more likely to work
- Time is brain also for endovascular treatment [114]
- Completeness of recanalization matters, in addition to speed.

Reperfusion trials using multimodal imaging are now under way, selecting patients based on tissue viability, occlusion patterns, or both (see Table 3.C.1). All these trials are using non-invasive arterial information for patient selection, and all CT-based trials set an upper limit for the volume of early ischemic changes.

Automated mismatch analyzer software in acute ischemic stroke is part of some of these trials and needs further validation; at this stage, such programs cannot be recommended for routine clinical use because of limited knowledge about their limitations and accuracy. Further work on methodological standardization and thresholds is needed for a practical and operation core/penumbra definition [115]. Other acute imaging parameters such as site of arterial occlusion, thrombus length or load, and degree of collateralization also need to be integrated in patient selection models.

Reperfusion trials using multimodal imaging are now under way, selecting patients based on tissue viability, occlusion patterns, or both.

Table 3.C.1. Ongoing randomized phase IIB or III acute stroke revascularization trials

Name	Arterial criteria	Tissue viability	Treatment tested
DIAS-3/4	√	CT : EIC	IV desmoteplase (3–9 h)
BASICS	√	CT : EIC	IV rtPA vs. bridging (0–6 h)
THRACE	√	CT : EIC	Endovascular vs. IV rtPA
PISTE	√	CT : EIC	IV rtPA vs. bridging
MR CLEAN	√	CT : EIC	Endovascular vs. standard
THERAPY	√	CT : EIC	IV rtPA vs. bridging (<8 h)
POSITIVE	√	CT : EIC	Endovascular vs. standard for IV thrombolysis ineligible (<12 h)
°* WAKE-UP	–	DWI/FLAIR	IV rt-PA vs. placebo for wake-up
° DAWN	√	DWI or PCT (max. core)	Endovascular vs. standard for wake-up or late (<24 h)
° REVASCAT	√	DWI or PCT (max. core)	Endovascular vs. standard (<8 h)
° ESCAPE	√	CT or PCT (max. core)	Endovascular vs. standard (<12 h)
°* EXTEND/ ECASS-4	–	PWI (or PCT)	IV rtPA vs. placebo (4.5–9 h)
°* DEFUSE-3	√	PWI/DWI	Endovascular vs. standard (<15 h)
°* SWIFT-PRIME	√	PWI/DWI or PCT	IV rtPA vs. bridging (0–4.5 h)
°* EXTEND-IA	√	PWI/DWI or PCT	IV rtPA vs. bridging (0–4.5 h)

° indicates that multimodal imaging core information based on advanced imaging is required as a selection criterion for the trial.
* indicates that some form of radiological mismatch information is required.
EIC = early ischemic changes on non-contrast CT; IV = intravenous; Bridging = IV rtPA followed rapidly by an endovascular revascularization procedure.

Chapter summary

CT, perfusion CT, CT angiography

Non-contrast CT (NCCT) is considered sufficient to select patients for intravenous thrombolysis with intravenous RTPA within 4.5 hours, or endovascular treatment within 6 hours. It is a highly accurate method for identifying acute intracerebral hemorrhage and subarachnoid hemorrhage, but quite insensitive for detecting acute ischemia. Early ischemic changes (EIC) on NCCT predict post-thrombolysis symptomatic ICH independently of other factors.

Perfusion CT (PCT) with iodinated contrast can be used to create parametric maps of regional cerebral blood volume, mean transit time, and regional cerebral blood flow. PCT has an overall sensitivity of about 75% for ischemic stroke, above 85% for non-lacunar supratentorial infarcts, and a high specificity for ischemia, but diffusion-weighted MRI (DWI) remains more sensitive for small and infratentorial lesions. Still, in the absence of an abnormality on PCT in a patient with stroke symptoms, acute recanalization treatments might be inappropriate.

CT angiography (CTA) has been shown to identify the site of arterial occlusion in acute ischemic stroke patients, with similar accuracy as DSA and probably better than MRA. Clot length can be assessed by thin-sliced NCCT and CTA. Clot presence, localization, length, and burden seem to predict clinical outcome and clot length and site seem to predict recanalization after intravenous thrombolysis.

Hyperintensity in acute intracranial hemorrhage (ICH) is present on NCCT from its onset in virtually all patients, but one main advantage of adding iodinated contrast in ICH is that contrast extravasation ("leakage") is an independent predictor of hematoma growth and poorer clinical outcome.

MRI and MR angiography

Sensitivity of diffusion-weighted imaging (DWI) at standard slice thickness of 5–6 mm is 80–90%, which is about twice the sensitivity of acute non-contrast CT examinations. DWI lesions represent infarction in the majority of stroke patients but are not completely specific for infarction – hyperintensities have also been reported after seizures and in multiple sclerosis plaques. A normal DWI exam in a patient with suspected stroke may also indicate a stroke imitator such as epileptic seizures, hypoglycemia, and migraine with aura. Such patients presenting with stroke-like symptoms but showing neither infarction/ischemia nor vessel obstruction are unlikely to benefit from thrombolysis.

The so-called DWI-FLAIR mismatch with FLAIR (fluid attenuated inversion recovery) negative DWI lesions identified patients within 4.5 hours of symptom onset with 62% sensitivity and 83% positive predictive value. FLAIR imaging may be used as a substitute for the time clock in patients with unknown stroke onset as it seems to separate with reasonable accuracy the patient within and outside the 4.5-hour (thrombolysis) window.

MRA directly reveals the location of the vessel occlusion. Patients presenting with a major vessel occlusion or severe stenosis seem more likely to benefit from thrombolytic treatment.

The extension of hypoperfusion on perfusion imaging (PWI) beyond the corresponding DWI boundary represents penumbra. This PWI > DWI mismatch has been used to identify patients that are likely to benefit from reperfusion therapies.

Arterial spin labeling (ASL) enables imaging of perfusion without contrast agent. Blood labeled with a radiofrequency pulse can be used as an endogenous contrast agent. ASL should be focused on patients with contraindications to gadolinium contrast agents.

MRI identifies intracranial hemorrhages rapidly and reliably, in particular if appropriate sequences are performed. MRI in fact may be superior to CT for the detection of small chronic hemorrhages, the cerebral microbleeds. Subdural hematomas can also be identified reliably with MRI and are best demonstrated on FLAIR sequences. For subarachnoidal hemorrhage detection, the best imaging sequences on MRI are FLAIR and proton density-weighted images.

Comparison of MR- and CT-based acute stroke imaging

With regard to information about brain perfusion, PCT appears at least equivalent to MRI, but both imaging methods still need better standardization. DWI has the advantage of widespread availability and relative robustness. On the other hand, the linear relationship between contrast concentration and signal intensity may be an advantage of CT perfusion imaging over gadolinium-based MR perfusion imaging.

Iodinated contrast can occasionally be associated with allergy, hyperthyroidism, or renal failure. On the other hand, CT is available in most emergency rooms, is easily accessible, and the monitoring of patients is easy.

Advantages of MRI of a higher sensitivity to detect acute ischemic stroke (DWI) have to be balanced with its cost, limited availability, more difficult patient monitoring, pacemaker incompatibility, and the longer time required for scanning.

Several important markers for benefit from acute revascularization treatment can be identified by **multimodal CT and MRI investigations**: low core volumes, large penumbra volumes accompanied by reperfusion, reperfusion (mostly through recanalization of large arteries), and good collateral blood flow. Reperfusion trials using multimodal imaging are now under way, selecting patients based on tissue viability, occlusion patterns, or both.

References

1. Krol AL, Dzialowski I, Roy J, *et al.* Incidence of radiocontrast nephropathy in patients undergoing acute stroke computed tomography angiography. *Stroke* 2007; **38**:2364–6.

2. Michel P, Odier C, Rutgers M, *et al.* The Acute STroke Registry and Analysis of Lausanne (ASTRAL): design and baseline analysis of an ischemic stroke registry including acute multimodal imaging. *Stroke* 2010; **41**:2491–8.

3. Na DG, Kim EY, Ryoo JW, *et al.* CT sign of brain swelling without concomitant parenchymal hypoattenuation: comparison with diffusion- and perfusion-weighted MR imaging. *Radiology* 2005; **235**:992–48.

4. Barber PA, Demchuk AM, Zhang J, Buchan AM. Validity and reliability of a quantitative computed tomography score in predicting outcome of hyperacute stroke before thrombolytic therapy. ASPECTS Study Group.

Alberta Stroke Programme Early CT Score. *Lancet* 2000; **355**:1670–4.

5. Puetz V, Dzialowski I, Hill MD, Demchuk AM. The Alberta Stroke Program Early CT Score in clinical practice: what have we learned? *Int J Stroke* 2009; **4**:354–64.

6. Hill MD, Rowley HA, Adler F, *et al.* Selection of acute ischemic stroke patients for intra-arterial thrombolysis with pro-urokinase by using ASPECTS. *Stroke* 2003; **34**:1925–31.

7. Demchuk AM, Hill MD, Barber PA, *et al.* Importance of early ischemic computed tomography changes using ASPECTS in NINDS rtPA Stroke Study. *Stroke* 2005; **36**:2110–15.

8. Strbian D, Engelter S, Michel P, *et al.* Symptomatic intracranial hemorrhage after stroke thrombolysis: the SEDAN score. *Ann Neurol* 2012; **71**:634–41.

9. Nezu T, Koga M, Nakagawara J, *et al.* Early ischemic change on CT versus diffusion-weighted imaging for patients with stroke receiving intravenous recombinant tissue-type plasminogen activator therapy: stroke acute management with urgent risk-factor assessment and improvement (SAMURAI) rt-PA registry. *Stroke* 2011; **42**:2196–200.

10. Latchaw RE, Yonas H, Hunter GJ, *et al.* Guidelines and recommendations for perfusion imaging in cerebral ischemia: a scientific statement for healthcare professionals by the writing group on perfusion imaging, from the Council on Cardiovascular Radiology of the American Heart Association. *Stroke* 2003; **34**:1084–104.

11. Koenig M, Kraus M, Theek C, *et al.* Quantitative assessment of the ischemic brain by means of perfusion-related parameters derived from perfusion CT. *Stroke* 2001; **32**:431–7.

12. Eastwood JD, Lev MH, Azhari T, *et al.* CT perfusion scanning with deconvolution analysis: pilot study in patients with acute middle cerebral artery stroke. *Radiology* 2002; **222**:227–36.

13. Murphy BD, Fox AJ, Lee DH, *et al.* White matter thresholds for ischemic penumbra and infarct core in patients with acute stroke: CT perfusion study. *Radiology* 2008; **247**:818–25.

14. Wintermark M, Reichhart M, Thiran JP, *et al.* Prognostic accuracy of cerebral blood flow measurement by perfusion computed tomography, at the time of emergency room admission, in acute stroke patients. *Ann Neurol* 2002; **51**:417–32.

15. Wintermark M, Fischbein NJ, Smith WS, *et al.* Accuracy of dynamic perfusion CT with deconvolution in detecting acute hemispheric stroke. *AJNR Am J Neuroradiol* 2005; **26**:104–12.

16. Youn SW, Kim JH, Weon YC, *et al.* Perfusion CT of the brain using 40-mm-wide detector and toggling table technique for initial imaging of acute stroke. *AJR Am J Roentgenol* 2008; **191**:W120–6.

17. Wintermark M, Flanders AE, Velthuis B, *et al.* Perfusion-CT assessment of infarct core and penumbra: receiver operating characteristic curve analysis in 130 patients suspected of acute hemispheric stroke. *Stroke* 2006; **37**:979–85.

18. Bivard A, Spratt N, Levi C, Parsons M. Perfusion computer tomography: imaging and clinical validation in acute ischaemic stroke. *Brain* 2011; **134**:3408–16.

19. Campbell BC, Christensen S, Levi CR, *et al.* Cerebral blood flow is the optimal CT perfusion parameter for assessing infarct core. *Stroke* 2011; **42**:3435–40.

20. Michel P, Reichhart M, Wintermark M, Maeder Ph, Bogousslavsky R. Perfusion-CT in transient ischemic attacks (abstract). *Stroke* 2005; **36**:484.

21. Gelfand JM, Wintermark M, Josephson SA. Cerebral perfusion-CT patterns following seizure. *Eur J Neurol* 2010; **17**:594–601.

22. Bezerra DC, Michel P, Reichhart M, *et al.* Perfusion-CT guided acute thrombolysis in patients with seizures at stroke onset (abstract). *Stroke* 2005; **36**:484.

23. Gonzalez-Delgado M, Michel P, Reichhart M, *et al.* The significance of focal hypoperfusion during migraine with aura (abstract). *Stroke* 2005; **36**:444.

24 Furtado AD, Smith WS, Koroshetz W, *et al.* Perfusion CT imaging follows clinical severity in left hemispheric strokes. *Eur Neurol* 2008; **60**:244–52.

25. Zhu G, Michel P, Aghaebrahim A, *et al.* Computed tomography workup of patients suspected of acute ischemic stroke: perfusion computed tomography adds value compared with clinical evaluation, noncontrast computed tomography, and computed tomography angiogram in terms of predicting outcome. *Stroke* 2013; **44**:1049–55.

26. Zhu G, Michel P, Aghaebrahim A, *et al.* Prediction of recanalization trumps prediction of tissue fate: the penumbra: a dual-edged sword. *Stroke* 2013; **44**:1014–19.

27. Silvennoinen HM, Hamberg LM, Lindsberg PJ, Valanne L, Hunter GJ. CT perfusion identifies increased salvage of tissue in patients receiving intravenous recombinant tissue plasminogen activator within 3 hours of stroke onset. *AJNR Am J Neuroradiol* 2008; **29**:1118–23.

28. Psychogios MN, Schramm P, Frölich AM, *et al.* Early CT scale evaluation of multimodal computed tomography in predicting clinical outcomes of

stroke patients treated with aspiration thrombectomy. *Stroke* 2013; **44**:2188–93.

29. Souza LC, Payabvash S, Wang Y, *et al.* Admission CT perfusion is an independent predictor of hemorrhagic transformation in acute stroke with similar accuracy to DWI. *Cerebrovasc Dis* 2012; **33**:8–15.

30. Hermitte L, Cho TH, Ozenne B, *et al.* Very low cerebral blood volume predicts parenchymal hematoma in acute ischemic stroke. *Stroke* 2013; **44**:2318–20.

31. Dittrich R, Kloska SP, Fischer T, *et al.* Accuracy of perfusion-CT in predicting malignant middle cerebral artery brain infarction. *J Neurol* 2008; **255**:896–902.

32. Minnerup J, Wersching H, Ringelstein EB, *et al.* Prediction of malignant middle cerebral artery infarction using computed tomography-based intracranial volume reserve measurements. *Stroke* 2011; **42**:3403–9.

33. Bektas H, Wu TC, Kasam M, *et al.* Increased blood-brain barrier permeability on perfusion CT might predict malignant middle cerebral artery infarction. *Stroke* 2010; **41**:2539–44.

34. Bash S, Villablanca JP, Jahan R, *et al.* Intracranial vascular stenosis and occlusive disease: evaluation with CT angiography, MR angiography, and digital subtraction angiography. *AJNR Am J Neuroradiol* 2005; **26**:1012–21.

35. Knauth M, von Kummer R, Jansen O, *et al.* Potential of CT angiography in acute ischemic stroke. *AJNR Am J Neuroradiol* 1997; **18**:1001–10.

36. Riedel CH, Zimmermann P, Jensen-Kondering U, *et al.* The importance of size: successful recanalization by intravenous thrombolysis in acute anterior stroke depends on thrombus length. *Stroke* 2011; **42**:1775–7.

37. Riedel CH, Yoo AJ. Clot characterization by noncontrast CT to predict IV tPA failure. *AJNR Am J Neuroradiol* 2012; **33**:E63.

38. Puetz V, Dzialowski I, Hill MD, *et al.* Intracranial thrombus extent predicts clinical outcome, final infarct size and hemorrhagic transformation in ischemic stroke: the clot burden score. *Int J Stroke* 2008; **3**:230–6.

39. Sylaja PN, Dzialowski I, Puetz V, *et al.* Does intravenous rtPA benefit patients in the absence of CT angiographically visible intracranial occlusion? *Neurol India* 2009; **57**:739–43.

40. Smith WS, Schwab S. Advances in stroke: critical care and emergency medicine. *Stroke* 2012; **43**:308–9.

41. González RG, Lev MH, Goldmacher GV, *et al.* Improved outcome prediction using CT angiography in addition to standard ischemic stroke assessment: results from the STOPStroke study. *PLoS One* 2012; **7**:e30352.

42. Tan IY, Demchuk AM, Hopyan J, *et al.* CT angiography clot burden score and collateral score: correlation with clinical and radiologic outcomes in acute middle cerebral artery infarct. *AJNR Am J Neuroradiol* 2009; **30**:525–31.

43. Saarinen JT, Sillanpää N, Rusanen H, *et al.* The mid-M1 segment of the middle cerebral artery is a cutoff clot location for good outcome in intravenous thrombolysis. *Eur J Neurol* 2012; **19**:1121–7.

44. Menon BK, Smith EE, Modi J, *et al.* Regional leptomeningeal score on CT angiography predicts clinical and imaging outcomes in patients with acute anterior circulation occlusions. *AJNR Am J Neuroradiol* 2011; **32**:1640–5.

45. Tan JC, Dillon WP, Liu S, *et al.* Systematic comparison of perfusion-CT and CT-angiography in acute stroke patients. *Ann Neurol* 2007; **61**:533–43.

46. Miteff F, Levi CR, Bateman GA, *et al.* The independent predictive utility of computed tomography angiographic collateral status in acute ischaemic stroke. *Brain* 2009; **132**:2231–8.

47. Angermaier A, Langner S, Kirsch M, *et al.* CT-angiographic collateralization predicts final infarct volume after intra-arterial thrombolysis for acute anterior circulation ischemic stroke. *Cerebrovasc Dis* 2011; **31**:177–84.

48. Schramm P, Schellinger PD, Fiebach JB, *et al.* Comparison of CT and CT angiography source images with diffusion-weighted imaging in patients with acute stroke within 6 hours after onset. *Stroke* 2002; **33**:2426–32.

49. Lev MH, Segal AZ, Farkas J, *et al.* Utility of perfusion-weighted CT imaging in acute middle cerebral artery stroke treated with intra-arterial thrombolysis: prediction of final infarct volume and clinical outcome. *Stroke* 2001; **32**:2021–8.

50. Puetz V, Sylaja PN, Hill MD, *et al.* CT angiography source images predict final infarct extent in patients with basilar artery occlusion. *AJNR Am J Neuroradiol* 2009; **30**:1877–83.

51. Mortimer AM, Simpson E, Bradley MD, Renowden SA. Computed tomography angiography in hyperacute ischemic stroke: prognostic implications and role in decision-making. *Stroke* 2013; **44**:1480–8.

52. Demchuk AM, Dowlatshahi D, Rodriguez-Luna D, *et al.* Prediction of haematoma growth and outcome in patients with intracerebral haemorrhage using the CT-angiography spot sign (PREDICT): a prospective observational study. *Lancet Neurol* 2012; **11**:307–14.

53. Fainardi E, Borrelli M, Saletti A, *et al.* CT perfusion mapping of hemodynamic disturbances associated to acute spontaneous intracerebral hemorrhage. *Neuroradiology* 2008; **50**:729–40.

54. Fiebach J, Schellinger P, Jansen O, *et al.* CT and diffusion-weighted MR imaging (DWI) in randomized order: DWI results in higher accuracy and lower interrater variability in the diagnosis of hyperacute ischemic stroke. *Stroke* 2002; **33**:2206–10.

55. Chalela JA, Kidwell CS, Nentwich LM, *et al.* Magnetic resonance imaging and computed tomography in emergency assessment of patients with suspected acute stroke: a prospective comparison. *Lancet* 2007; **369**:293–8.

56. von Kummer R, Bourquain H, Bastianello S, *et al.* Early prediction of irreversible brain damage after ischemic stroke at CT. *Radiology* 2001; **219**:95–100.

57. Sedlaczek O, Hirsch JG, Grips E, *et al.* Detection of delayed focal MR changes in the lateral hippocampus in transient global amnesia. *Neurology* 2004; **62**:2165–70.

58. Chatzikonstantinou A, Gass A, Förster A, Hennerici MG, Szabo K. Features of acute DWI abnormalities related to status epilepticus. *Epilepsy Res* 2011; **97**:45–51.

59. Eisele P, Szabo K, Griebe M, *et al.* Reduced diffusion in a subset of acute MS lesions: a serial multiparametric MRI study. *AJNR Am J Neuroradiol* 2012; **33**:1369–73.

60. Ma L, Gao PY, Lin Y, *et al.* Can baseline magnetic resonance angiography (MRA) status become a foremost factor in selecting optimal acute stroke patients for recombinant tissue plasminogen activator (rt-PA) thrombolysis beyond 3 hours? *Neurol Res* 2009; **31**:355–61.

61. Chemmanam T, Campbell BC, Christensen S, *et al.* Ischemic diffusion lesion reversal is uncommon and rarely alters perfusion-diffusion mismatch. *Neurology* 2010; **75**:1040–7.

62. Fiehler J, Knudsen K, Kucinski T, *et al.* Predictors of apparent diffusion coefficient normalization in stroke patients. *Stroke* 2004; **35**:514–19.

63. Yoo AJ, Barak ER, Copen WA, *et al.* Combining acute diffusion-weighted imaging and mean transmit time lesion volumes with National Institutes of Health Stroke Scale Score improves the prediction of acute stroke outcome. *Stroke* 2010; **41**:1728–35.

64. Parsons MW, Christensen S, McElduff P, *et al.* Pretreatment diffusion- and perfusion-MR lesion volumes have a crucial influence on clinical response to stroke thrombolysis. *J Cereb Blood Flow Metab* 2010; **30**:1214–25.

65. Mlynash M, Lansberg MG, De Silva DA, *et al.* Refining the definition of the malignant profile: insights from the DEFUSE-EPITHET pooled data set. *Stroke* 2011; **42**:1270–5.

66. Thomalla G, Cheng B, Ebinger M, *et al.* DWI-FLAIR mismatch for the identification of patients with acute ischaemic stroke within 4.5 h of symptom onset (PRE-FLAIR): a multicentre observational study. *Lancet Neurol* 2011; **10**:978–86.

67. Mackey J, Kleindorfer D, Sucharew H, *et al.* Population-based study of wake-up strokes. *Neurology* 2011; **76**:1662–7.

68. Thomalla G, Fiebach JB, Ostergaard L, *et al.* A multicenter, randomized, double-blind, placebo-controlled trial to test efficacy and safety of magnetic resonance imaging-based thrombolysis in wake-up stroke (WAKE-UP). *Int J Stroke* 2013 Mar 12, doi: 10.1111/ijs.12011.

69. Fiebach JB, Al-Rawi Y, Wintermark M, *et al.* Vascular occlusion enables selecting acute ischemic stroke patients for treatment with desmoteplase. *Stroke* 2012; **43**:1561–6.

70. Fiehler J, Knudsen K, Thomalla G, *et al.* Vascular occlusion sites determine differences in lesion growth from early apparent diffusion coefficient lesion to final infarct. *AJNR Am J Neuroradiol* 2005; **26**:1056–61.

71. Schellinger PD, Chalela JA, Kang DW, Latour LL, Warach S. Diagnostic and prognostic value of early MR imaging vessel signs in hyperacute stroke patients imaged <3 hours and treated with recombinant tissue plasminogen activator. *AJNR Am J Neuroradiol* 2005; **26**:618–24.

72. Galinovic I, Ostwaldt AC, Soemmer C, *et al.* Search for a map and threshold in perfusion MRI to accurately predict tissue fate: a protocol for assessing lesion growth in patients with persistent vessel occlusion. *Cerebrovasc Dis* 2011; **32**:186–93.

73. Rovira A, Orellana P, Alvarez-Sabin J, *et al.* Hyperacute ischemic stroke: middle cerebral artery susceptibility sign at echo-planar gradient-echo MR imaging. *Radiology* 2004; **232**:466–73.

74. Thomalla G, Schwark C, Sobesky J, *et al.* Outcome and symptomatic bleeding complications of intravenous thrombolysis within 6 hours in MRI-selected stroke patients: comparison of a German multicenter study with the pooled data of ATLANTIS, ECASS, and NINDS tPA trials. *Stroke* 2006; **37**:852–8.

75. Hacke W, Albers G, Al-Rawi Y, *et al.* The Desmoteplase in Acute Ischemic Stroke Trial (DIAS): a phase II MRI-based 9-hour window acute stroke thrombolysis trial with intravenous

61

desmoteplase. *Stroke* 2005; **36**:66–73.

76. Butcher K, Parsons M, Allport L, *et al.* Rapid assessment of perfusion-diffusion mismatch. *Stroke* 2008; **39**:75–81.

77. Albers GW, Thijs VN, Wechsler L, *et al.* Magnetic resonance imaging profiles predict clinical response to early reperfusion: the diffusion and perfusion imaging evaluation for understanding stroke evolution (DEFUSE) study. *Ann Neurol* 2006; **60**:508–17.

78. Davis SM, Donnan GA, Parsons MW, *et al.* Effects of alteplase beyond 3 h after stroke in the Echoplanar Imaging Thrombolytic Evaluation Trial (EPITHET): a placebo-controlled randomised trial. *Lancet Neurol* 2008; **7**:299–309.

79. Nagakane Y, Christensen S, Brekenfeld C, *et al.* EPITHET: positive result after reanalysis using baseline diffusion-weighted imaging/perfusion-weighted imaging co-registration. *Stroke* 2011; **42**:59–64.

80. Warach S, Al-Rawi Y, Furlan AJ, *et al.* Refinement of the magnetic resonance diffusion-perfusion mismatch concept for thrombolytic patient selection: insights from the desmoteplase in acute stroke trials. *Stroke* 2012; **43**:2313–18.

81. Galinovic I, Brunecker P, Ostwaldt AC, *et al.* Fully automated postprocessing carries a risk of substantial overestimation of perfusion deficits in acute stroke magnetic resonance imaging. *Cerebrovasc Dis* 2011; **31**:408–13.

82. Lansberg MG, Straka M, Kemp S, *et al.* MRI profile and response to endovascular reperfusion after stroke (DEFUSE 2): a prospective cohort study. *Lancet Neurol* 2012; **11**:860–7.

83. Kidwell CS, Alger JR, Saver JL. Beyond mismatch: evolving paradigms in imaging the ischemic penumbra with multimodal magnetic resonance imaging. *Stroke* 2003; **34**:2729–35.

84. Kucinski T, Naumann D, Knab R, *et al.* Tissue at risk is overestimated in perfusion-weighted imaging: MR imaging in acute stroke patients without vessel recanalization. *AJNR Am J Neuroradiol* 2005; **26**:815–19.

85. Zaharchuk G, El Mogy IS, Fischbein NJ, Albers GW. Comparison of arterial spin labeling and bolus perfusion-weighted imaging for detecting mismatch in acute stroke. *Stroke* 2012; **43**:1843–8.

86. Bokkers RP, Hernandez DA, Merino JG, *et al.* Whole-brain arterial spin labeling perfusion MRI in patients with acute stroke. *Stroke* 2012; **43**:1290–4.

87. Niibo T, Ohta H, Yonenaga K, *et al.* Arterial spin-labeled perfusion imaging to predict mismatch in acute ischemic stroke. *Stroke* 2013; **44**:2601–3.

88. Kidwell CS, Chalela JA, Saver JL, *et al.* Comparison of MRI and CT for detection of acute intracerebral hemorrhage. *JAMA* 2004; **292**:1823–30.

89. Fiehler J. Cerebral microbleeds: old leaks and new haemorrhages. *Int J Stroke* 2006; **1**:122–30.

90. Fiehler J, Albers GW, Boulanger JM, *et al.* Bleeding risk analysis in stroke imaging before thromboLysis (BRASIL): pooled analysis of T2*-weighted magnetic resonance imaging data from 570 patients. *Stroke* 2007; **38**:2738–44.

91. Tanikawa M, Mase M, Yamada K, *et al.* Surgical treatment of chronic subdural hematoma based on intrahematomal membrane structure on MRI. *Acta Neurochir (Wien)* 2001; **143**:613–19.

92. Wiesmann M, Mayer TE, Yousry I, *et al.* Detection of hyperacute subarachnoid hemorrhage of the brain by using magnetic resonance imaging. *J Neurosurg* 2002; **96**:684–9.

93. Baird AE, Benfield A, Schlaug G, *et al.* Enlargement of human cerebral ischemic lesion volumes measured by diffusion-weighted magnetic resonance imaging. *Ann Neurol* 1997; **41**:581–9.

94. Schaefer PW, Barak ER, Kamalian S, *et al.* Quantitative assessment of core/penumbra mismatch in acute stroke: CT and MR perfusion imaging are strongly correlated when sufficient brain volume is imaged. *Stroke* 2008; **39**:2986–92.

95. Wintermark M, Reichhart M, Cuisenaire O, *et al.* Comparison of admission perfusion computed tomography and qualitative diffusion- and perfusion-weighted magnetic resonance imaging in acute stroke patients. *Stroke* 2002; **33**:2025–31.

96. Wintermark M, Meuli R, Browaeys P, *et al.* Comparison of CT perfusion and angiography and MRI in selecting stroke patients for acute treatment. *Neurology* 2007; **68**:694–7.

97. Dani KA, Thomas RG, Chappell FM, *et al.* Computed tomography and magnetic resonance perfusion imaging in ischemic stroke: definitions and thresholds. *Ann Neurol* 2011; **70**:384–401.

98. Wintermark M, Maeder P, Thiran JP, Schnyder P, Meuli R. Quantitative assessment of regional cerebral blood flows by perfusion CT studies at low injection rates: a critical review of the underlying theoretical models. *Eur Radiol* 2001; **11**:1220–30.

99. Liu Y, Karonen JO, Vanninen RL, *et al.* Acute ischemic stroke: predictive value of 2D phase-contrast MR angiography–serial study with combined diffusion and perfusion MR imaging. *Radiology* 2004; **231**:517–27.

100. Schievink WI. Spontaneous dissection of the carotid and vertebral arteries. *N Engl J Med* 2001; **344**:898–906.

101. Lev MH, Koroshetz WJ, Schwamm LH, Gonzalez RG. CT or MRI for imaging patients with acute stroke: visualization of "tissue at risk"? *Stroke* 2002; **33**:2736–7.

102. Mnyusiwalla A, Aviv RI, Symons SP. Radiation dose from multidetector row CT imaging for acute stroke. *Neuroradiology* 2009; **51**:635–40.

103. Smith-Bindman R, Lipson J, Marcus R, *et al*. Radiation dose associated with common computed tomography examinations and the associated lifetime attributable risk of cancer. *Arch Intern Med* 2009; **169**:2078–86.

104. Aulicky P, Mikulík R, Goldemund D, *et al*. Safety of performing CT angiography in stroke patients treated with intravenous thrombolysis. *J Neurol Neurosurg Psychiatry* 2010; **81**:783–7.

105. Thomsen HS. ESUR guideline: gadolinium-based contrast media and nephrogenic systemic fibrosis. *Eur Radiol* 2007; **17**:2692–6.

106. Kidwell CS, Jahan R, Gornbein J, *et al*. A trial of imaging selection and endovascular treatment for ischemic stroke. *N Engl J Med* 2013; **368**:914–23.

107. Ogata T, Christensen S, Nagakane Y, *et al*. The effects of alteplase 3 to 6 hours after stroke in the EPITHET-DEFUSE combined dataset: post hoc case-control study. *Stroke* 2013; **44**:87–93.

108. Sztriha LK, Manawadu D, Jarosz J, Keep J, Kalra L. Safety and clinical outcome of thrombolysis in ischaemic stroke using a perfusion CT mismatch between 3 and 6 hours. *PLoS One* 2011; **10**:e25796.

109. Obach V, Oleaga L, Urra X, *et al*. Multimodal CT-assisted thrombolysis in patients with acute stroke: a cohort study. *Stroke* 2011; **42**:1129–31.

110. Hassan AE, Zacharatos H, Rodriguez GJ, *et al*. A comparison of computed tomography perfusion-guided and time-guided endovascular treatments for patients with acute ischemic stroke. *Stroke* 2010; **41**:1673–8.

111. Furlan A, Higashida R, Wechsler L, *et al*. Intra-arterial prourokinase for acute ischemic stroke. The PROACT II study: a randomized controlled trial. Prolyse in Acute Cerebral Thromboembolism. *JAMA* 1999; **282**:2003–11.

112. Broderick JP, Palesch YY, Demchuk AM, *et al*. Endovascular therapy after intravenous t-PA versus t-PA alone for stroke. *N Engl J Med* 2013; **368**:893–903.

113. Ciccone A, Valvassori L, Nichelatti M, *et al*. Endovascular treatment for acute ischemic stroke. *N Engl J Med* 2013; **368**:904–13.

114. Mazighi M, Chaudhry SA, Ribo M, *et al*. Impact of onset-to-reperfusion time on stroke mortality: a collaborative pooled analysis. *Circulation* 2013; **127**:1980–5.

115. Wintermark M, Albers GW, Broderick JP, *et al*. Acute Stroke Imaging Research Roadmap II. *Stroke* 2013; **44**:2628–39.

Imaging for prediction of functional outcome and for assessment of recovery

Wolf-Dieter Heiss

Introduction

Stroke is the third most frequent cause of acquired adult disability [1]. Stroke recovery is heterogeneous: it is estimated that 25–74% of the 50 million stroke survivors require assistance or are dependent for activities of daily living (ADL) after stroke [2]: approximately 14% of the stroke survivors achieve full recovery of ADL, between 25% and 50% require some assistance, and approximately half experience long-term dependency [3]. Prediction of outcome after ischemic stroke therefore is important for setting realistic and attainable treatment goals, informing clients and their relatives properly, facilitating discharge planning, and anticipating possible consequences for home adjustments and community support [4]. The knowledge of the expected recovery pattern is also necessary to assess the effectiveness of new therapeutic interventions and their contribution to recovery and should be applied to select comparable patient populations for treatment trials [5]. ADL, most importantly concerning dressing, mobility, and bathing, are assessed most frequently by the Barthel Index (BI) [6], and by the modified Rankin Scale (mRS) [7], but the Glasgow Outcome Scale [8], the Functional Independence Measure [9], or other ADL assessment tools [10] can also be used. In some instances the National Institute of Health Stroke Scale (NIHSS) [11], which is the standard to assess deficits in the acute state and during follow-up, is applied to measure outcome. A considerable number of prognostic stroke studies used the BI and the mRS as outcome measure reached after 3–6 months and found that scores on scales assessing severity of neurological deficits, such as the NIHSS [12–15], and the Canadian Neurological Scale [16] assessed in acute stroke (i.e. within 72 hours) are strongly associated with outcome

beyond 3 months [4, 17]. A systemic review of prognostic studies [10] indicated that gender and presence of risk factors did not significantly affect the prediction of outcome; only age emerged as a highly significant inverse predictor of good functional outcome [18]. With the applied simple models a large percentage of patients could be correctly classified with respect to survival and functional recovery (70.4% and 72.9% [14]) and to the severity of impairment on the BI (severe vs. mild neurological deficits, area under curve [AuC] 0.789 to 0.808 depending on time of assessment, 2 days to 5 days [19]). Addition of more clinical variables and application of more complex models improved prediction accuracy only slightly (83.9%, [15]). In a similar way measurement of the BI within 72 hours after stroke showed good discriminative properties for final outcome of BI at 6 months (AuC 0.837) and may be used for initiating early rehabilitation management [4] whereas the added value of imaging data for the prediction of ADL outcome is limited when compared to the contribution of clinical variables alone [20, 21]. Neuroimaging modalities are able to measure the extent of damage to brain tissue and to indicate alternative functional networks and thereby may help to assess functional outcome and to predict the efficacy of rehabilitation in individual patients.

> Neuroimaging modalities may help to assess functional outcome and to predict the efficacy of rehabilitation in individual patients additionally to functional assessment scales such as the NIHSS and others.

Structural imaging

Computed tomography

Computed tomography (CT) and magnetic resonance imaging (MRI) are the most important procedures for

Textbook of Stroke Medicine, Second Edition, ed. Michael Brainin and Wolf-Dieter Heiss. Published by Cambridge University Press. © Michael Brainin and Wolf-Dieter Heiss 2014.

diagnosis and management of acute stroke (Chapter 3). The most widely used imaging procedure in acute stroke is CT, especially for differentiation between hemorrhagic and ischemic stroke, for localization of the lesion, and for decision-making regarding administration of potentially risky stroke therapies as thrombolysis. As a measure for quantifying ischemic changes on CT the Alberta Stroke Program Early Computed Tomography Score (ASPECTS) was developed which evaluates the extent and location of ischemic changes in 10 regions within the territory of the middle cerebral artery (MCA) [22]. ASPECTS has been found to be better reproducible than the one-third MCA rule and can help to predict functional outcome on the mRS at 3 months post-stroke and to

select patients for acute intravascular treatment [23]. In combination with age and the severity of neurological deficits a subacute ASPECTS of greater than 5 had a significant predictive value of greater functional independence at 3 months ($R^2 = 0.701$) and 1 year post-stroke ($R^2 = 0.528$) [24]. In another large study initial lesion volume was found to be a strong and independent predictor of stroke outcome in a statistical regression model that also accounts for age and NIHSS. By including the lesion volume as an additive predictive factor the fraction of unexplained variability could be reduced by 15% [25] (Figure 4.1). As a consequence, the inclusion of lesion size in predictive models of outcome will improve stratification of samples and increase power for effect detection in

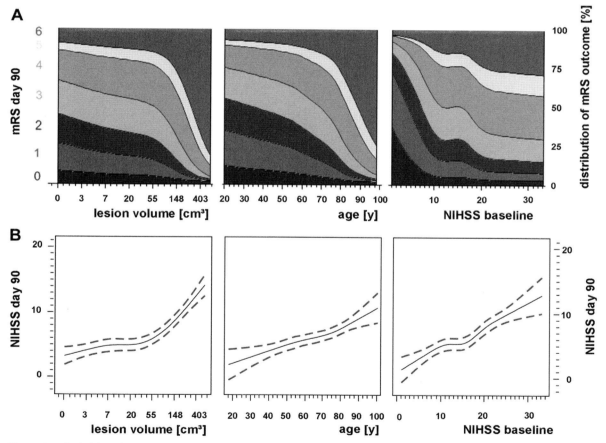

Figure 4.1. Probability of outcome (mRS and NIHSS) dependent on baseline parameters in patients with ischemic stroke. (A) Probability of mRS outcome dependent on baseline parameters in patients with ischemic stroke. mRS is modeled as an ordinal variable using logistic regression analysis. The 7 points on the mRS scale are color-coded. The height of each color segment corresponds to the probability of mRS outcome at the x-axis values. (B) Probability of outcome on the NIHSS at day 90. NIHSS, age, and lesion volume (log-transformed) are modeled using knotted splines. The x-axis of lesion volume is a log-scale, but nontransformed values (cm³) are given as labels. Dashed lines in B indicate the 95% CI. mRS indicates modified Rankin Scale; NIHSS, National Institutes of Health Stroke Scale. Used with permission from Vogt et al. [25].

trials of acute therapy and of rehabilitative strategies in ischemic stroke.

ASPECTS (the Alberta Stroke Program Early Computed Tomography Score) is a measure to quantify ischemic changes on CT within the territory of the middle cerebral artery (MCA) and can help select patients for acute intravascular treatment.

Magnetic resonance imaging

High-resolution MRI reproducibly identifies even small stroke lesions, but relating the size of lesions to clinical impairment and functional outcome is difficult since small lesions of the subcortical white matter or the brainstem especially can produce disproportionate clinical disturbances [26]. The effect on the corticospinal tract by the ischemic lesion is a particularly important factor limiting motoric recovery [27]. The size of the lesion can be outlined early by diffusion-weighted imaging (DWI), which is sensitive to the movement of water molecules within the tissue and reduced by cytotoxic edema in early ischemia. In patients with non-lacunar strokes in the anterior circulation, lesion volume assessed by DWI in addition to age and NIHSS score was an independent predictor of outcome separating patients with a final BI above or below 85 [28]. DWI lesion volume significantly increased the power of prediction models, but this effect was not large enough to be clinically important in another analysis [29]. However, the likelihood of achieving excellent neurological outcome diminishes substantially with growth in DWI infarct volume in the first 5 days after ischemic stroke of mild to moderate severity [30].

Diffusion tensor imaging (DTI) permits the visualization of white matter pathways in the brain and was used especially to demonstrate damage to the corticospinal tract which is associated with motoric impairment in chronic stroke patients [31]. DTI measures may also be used to predict outcome: extent of damage to the corticospinal tract following a corona radiata infarct assessed 7–30 days after a stroke was related to motor function of the affected hand 6 months later (Figure 4.2) [32, 33]. Progressive damage to the pyramidal tract was observed as assessed by fractional anisotropy (FA) in DTI, which progressively decreased in the medulla as well as in proximal portions 1–12 weeks after pontine infarction; these anterograde and retrograde degenerations were accompanied by deterioration in the clinical

scales [34]. The prediction of motor impairment and recovery was improved if not merely the pyramidal tract but also alternative motor fibers were included in the classification of damage [27]. Efficiency of rehabilitative therapy was related to DTI parameters of individual tracts and tract combinations and may indicate a patient's individual recovery potential and the optimal rehabilitative intervention [35]. Additionally, gains from treatment were related to the degree of injury to specific motor tracts (descending from primary motor cortex, supplementary motor area, dorsal premotor cortex, and ventral premotor cortex, respectively), and the damage to these tracts had a greater impact on the therapeutic effect than infarct volume or baseline clinical status [36]. Damage to the posterior limb of the internal capsule within 12 hours of symptoms onset correlated well with motor impairment at 30 and 90 days; the sensitivity and specificity of the DTI parameters were superior to lesion volume in the corona radiata or the cortex and to baseline clinical scores [37].

Nonmotor pathways can also be studied and their damage related to higher brain function, e.g. language performance [38]. Lower FA values in the superior longitudinal and arcuate fasciculi of the left hemisphere were correlated with decreased ability to repeat spoken language, lower FA values in the arcuate fasciculus were associated with comprehension deficits; these relationships were independent of the degree of damage to cortical areas [39].

All these data stress that the connectivity in networks as assessed by DTI is more important for outcome and recovery than the extent of the primary structural lesion. However, despite all these promising results, structural neuroimaging neither provides information on the cause of the ischemic lesion and compensatory mechanisms, nor on whether or how surviving tissues are working [40]. The functional connectivity between cortical and subcortical components of neural networks determines the capacity for reorganization and recovery. The studies of these measures require modalities for physiological, molecular, and functional imaging.

With diffusion-weighted imaging (DWI), the size of the lesion can be outlined early and DWI lesion volume significantly increased the power of prediction models.

Diffusion tensor imaging (DTI) measures may also be used to predict outcome: the connectivity in networks as assessed by DTI is more important for outcome and recovery than the extent of the primary structural lesion.

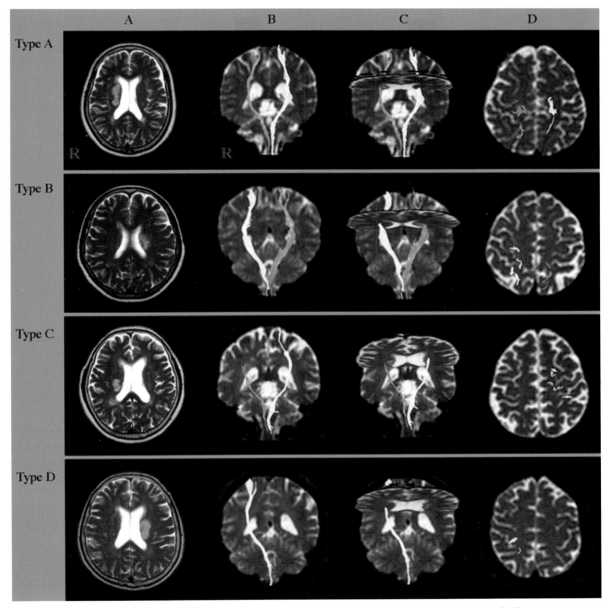

Figure 4.2. Diffusion tensor imaging: Prediction of motor outcome by corticospinal tract integrity. Classification of diffusion tensor tractography: (A) T2-weighted MR images, (B) Coronal images of diffusion tensor tractography (DTT), (C) combined axial (at the infarct level) and coronal images of DTT and (D) axial images (at the primary motor cortex level) of DTT. Motricity index (MI) for hand distribution at 6 months from the time of stroke onset. The MI distribution was significantly uneven (Pearson's chi-squared test; p = 0.003) and was significantly influenced by the diffusion tensor tractography type (Kruskal–Wallis test, p = 0.0002). MBC = modified Brunnstrom classification. Used with permission from Cho *et al.* [32].

Assessment of brain blood supply and cerebral perfusion

The cause of ischemic stroke is the reduction of tissue blood flow below a critical threshold for a critical period of time (Chapter 1). Usually this shortage in blood supply is due to the occlusion of the feeding vessel and the insufficiency of collateral perfusion. Occlusion of a large intracranial vessel, such as basilar, internal carotid, and middle cerebral artery, is

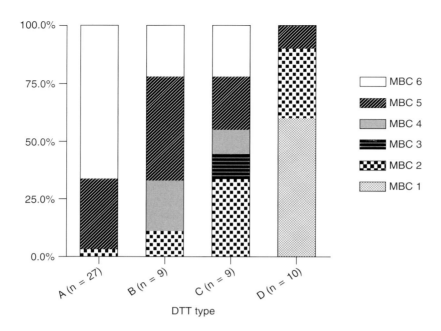

Figure 4.2. (*cont.*)

associated with higher mortality and more severe permanent deficits and therefore the pathological vascular state can be expected to contribute predictive value to models of stroke outcome. Retrospective studies of patients undergoing conventional angiography found that basilar and internal carotid artery occlusions had the highest NIHSS scores [41] whereas normal angiograms predict a good prognosis. In a prospective study results from CT angiography performed within 24 hours of symptoms onset were related to outcome after 6 months (Figure 4.3) [42]. Larger-vessel occlusion significantly increased 6 months mortality (4.5-fold increase) and was negatively correlated to good outcome (mRS ≤ 2 threefold reduction). In a multivariate analysis the presence of basilar and internal carotid occlusions independently predicted outcome in addition to age and NIHSS. Inclusion of information from CT angiography contributed significantly more to outcome prediction than the ASPECTS score [43, 44]. Evidence of large-vessel occlusion, therefore, is crucial for improving outcome by early endovascular interventions.

The vascular occlusion and its eventual recanalization are decisive for the evolution of tissue damage and for the clinical deficits, but the final size of an infarct is also influenced by the extent and quality of collateral circulation to the affected brain area. The presence of robust collateral flow is best visualized by conventional angiography and has been linked to improved clinical outcomes and reduced infarct volumes; in cases receiving thrombolysis collateralization was a significant univariate predictor in addition to occlusion type and recanalization [45, 46]. CT angiography as a non-invasive alternative has better spatial resolution than transcranial Doppler or MR angiography and can depict leptomeningeal collaterals. Rapid recruitment of sufficient collaterals was related to favorable outcome, whereas patients with diminished sylvian and leptomeningeal collaterals had a greater risk of worsening [47]. Univariate analysis identified the grade of leptomeningeal vascularity as an independent predictor of good outcome [48].

The validity of perfusion parameters obtained by CT or MRI for prediction of long-term outcome has not been accurately established, but some data indicate a weak relationship of perfusion-weighted imaging (PWI) lesion size early after the ictus [49] as well as perfusion CT mismatch [50] and mRS 3 months after the stroke, confirming early results of the relationship between cerebral blood flow (CBF) measured with 133 xenon [51] or with 99m technetium-labeled hexamethylpropyleneamine [52] and final outcome.

CT angiography contributes to outcome prediction, can provide evidence of large-vessel occlusion for early endovascular interventions, and visualizes collateral circulation to the affected brain area.

A

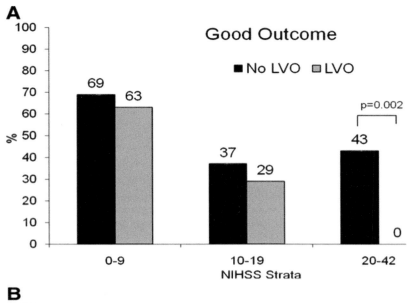

B

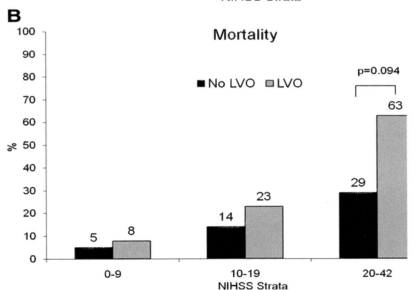

Figure 4.3. Large vessel occlusion (LVO) within NIHSS strata and probability of good outcome (A) and mortality (B): Influence of LVO within NIHSS strata on probability of good outcome (A) and mortality (B). Used with permission from Smith *et al.* [42].

Role of functional imaging in stroke patients

The functional deficit after a focal brain lesion is determined by the localization and the extent of the tissue damage; recovery depends on the adaptive plasticity of the undamaged brain, especially the cerebral cortex, and of the non-affected elements of the functional network. Since destroyed tissue usually cannot be replaced in the adult human brain, improvement or recovery of neurological deficits can be achieved only by reactivation of functionally disturbed but morphologically preserved areas or by recruitment of alternative pathways within the functional network. This activation of alternative pathways may be accompanied by the development of different strategies to deal with the new functional-anatomical situation at the behavioral level. Additionally, the sprouting of fibers from surviving neurons and the formation of new synapses could play a role in long-term recovery. These compensatory mechanisms are expressed in altered patterns of blood flow or metabolism at rest and during activation within the functional network involved in a special task, and

69

therefore functional imaging tools can be applied successfully for studying physiological correlates of plasticity and recovery non-invasively after localized brain damage. The observed patterns depend on the site, the extent, and also the type and the dynamics of the development of the lesion; they change over time and thereby are related to the course and the recovery of a deficit. The visualization of disturbed interaction in functional networks and of their reorganization in the recovery after focal brain damage is the domain of functional imaging modalities such as positron emission tomography (PET) and functional magnetic resonance imaging (fMRI).

For the analysis of the relationship between disturbed function and altered brain activity, studies can be designed in several ways: measurement at rest, comparing location and extent to deficit and outcome (eventually with follow-up); measurement during activation tasks, comparing changes in activation patterns to functional performance; and measurement at rest and during activation tasks early and later in the course of disease (e.g. after stroke) to demonstrate recruiting and compensatory mechanisms in the functional network responsible for complete or partial recovery of disturbed functions. Only a few studies have been performed applying this last and most complete design together with extensive testing for the evaluation of the quality of performance finally achieved.

A large amount of data has been collected over the past years with functional imaging of changes in activation patterns related to recovery of disturbed function after stroke [53–59].

> The visualization of disturbed interaction in functional networks and of their reorganization in the recovery after focal brain damage is the domain of functional imaging modalities such as PET and functional resonance imaging (fMRI).

The principle of functional and activation studies using positron emission tomography (PET)

The energy demand of the brain is very high and relies almost entirely on the oxidative metabolism of glucose (see Chapter 1). Mapping of neuronal activity in the brain can be primarily achieved by quantitation of the regional cerebral metabolic rate for glucose (rCMRGlc), as introduced for autoradiographic experimental studies by Sokoloff et al. [60] and

adapted for PET in humans by Reivich et al. [61]. The cerebral metabolic rate for glucose (CMRGlc) can be quantified with PET using 2-[^{18}F]fluoro-2-deoxyglucose (FDG) and a modification of the three-compartment model equation developed for autoradiography by Sokoloff et al. [60]. Like glucose, FDG is transported across the blood–brain barrier and into brain cells, where it is phosphorylated by hexokinase. However, FDG-6-phosphate cannot be metabolized to its respective fructose-6-phosphate analog, and does not diffuse out of the cells in significant amounts. The distribution of the radioactivity accumulated in the brain remains quite stable between 30 and 50 minutes after intravenous tracer injection, thus permitting multiple intercalated scans. Using (i) the local radioactivity concentration measured with PET during this steady-state period, (ii) the concentration–time course of tracer in arterial plasma, (iii) plasma glucose concentration, and (iv) a lumped constant correcting for the differing behavior in brain of FDG and glucose, CMRGlc can be computed pixel by pixel according to an optimized operational equation [62]. The resulting pseudocolor-coded images reflect all effects on cerebral glucose metabolism. Because of its robustness with regard to procedure and model assumptions, the FDG method has been employed in many PET studies, including prediction of recovery after stroke [63].

Almost all commonly applied methods for the quantitative imaging of CBF are based on the principle of diffusible tracer exchange. Using ^{15}O-labeled water administered either directly by intravenous bolus injection or by the inhalation of ^{15}O-labeled carbon dioxide, which is converted into water by carbonic anhydrase in the lungs, CBF can be estimated from steady-state distribution or from the radioactivity concentration–time curves in arterial plasma and brain. Typical measuring times range between 40 seconds and 2 minutes, and, because of the short biological half-life of the radiotracers, repeat studies can be performed [64, 65].

Various PET methods have been developed for determining the cerebral metabolic rate for oxygen (CMRO$_2$), using continuous [65] or single-breath inhalation [66] of air containing trace amounts of ^{15}O-labeled molecular oxygen. All require the concurrent estimation or paired measurement of CBF in order to convert the measured oxygen extraction fractions (OEFs) into images of CMRO$_2$ as given by the product of arterial oxygen concentration, local

OEF, and local CBF. Because ^{15}O has a short half-life (123 seconds), an on-site cyclotron is necessary; this and other methodological complexities limit the use of $CMRO_2$ as a measure of brain function. Application of this method for detection of penumbra tissue is described in Chapter 1.

Functional activation studies as they are used now rely primarily on the hemodynamic response, assuming a close association between energy metabolism and blood flow. Whereas it is well documented that increases in blood flow and glucose consumption are closely coupled during neuronal activation, the increase in oxygen consumption is considerably delayed, leading to a decreased OEF during activation [67]. PET detects and, if required, can quantify changes in CBF and CMRGlc accompanying different activation states of brain tissue. The regional values of CBF or CMRGlc represent the brain activity due to a specific state, task, or stimulus in comparison to the resting condition, and color-coded maps can be analyzed or correlated to morphological images. Due to the radioactivity of the necessary tracers, activation studies with PET are limited to a maximum of 12 doses of ^{15}O-labeled tracers, e.g. 12 flow scans, or two doses of ^{18}F-labeled tracers, e.g. two metabolic scans. Especially for studies of glucose consumption, the time to metabolic equilibrium (20–40 minutes) must be taken into consideration, as well as the time interval between measurements required for isotope decay (half-life for ^{18}F 108 minutes, for ^{15}O 2 minutes).

PET used to quantify the regional concentration of these tracers relies on the labeling of the compounds with short-lived cyclotron-produced radioisotopes (e.g. ^{15}O, ^{11}C, ^{13}N, ^{18}F) which are characterized by a unique decay scheme. A positron, i.e. a positively charged particle of the mass of an electron, is emitted from a labeled probe molecule (Figure 4.4). Following emission from the atomic nucleus, the positron takes a path marked by multiple collisions with ambient electrons. Approximately 1–3 mm from its origin, it has lost so much energy that it combines with an electron, resulting in the annihilation of the two oppositely charged particles by the emission at an angle of $180° \pm 0.5°$ of two 511 keV (kilo electron volt) gamma rays that are recorded as coincident events, using pairs of uncollimated (convergent) detectors facing each other. Therefore, the origin of the gamma rays can be localized directly to the straight line between these coincidence detectors. State-of-the-art PET scanners are equipped with thousands of detectors arranged in up to 24 rings, simultaneously scanning 47 slices of <5 mm thickness. Pseudocolor-coded tomographic images of the radioactivity distribution are then reconstructed from the many projected coincidence counts by a computer, using CT-like algorithms and reliable scatter and attenuation corrections. Typical in-plane resolution (full width at half-maximum) is <5 mm; 3D data accumulation and reconstruction permits imaging of the brain in any selected plane or view.

> In PET, radioactive tracers can be used to detect and quantify changes in cerebral blood flow (CBF) and cerebral metabolic rate of glucose (CMRGlc). Color-coded maps of different activation states of brain tissue can be analyzed or coregistered to morphological images.

Functional magnetic resonance imaging (fMRI)

fMRI measures signals that depend on the differential magnetic properties of oxygenated and deoxygenated hemoglobin, termed the blood-oxygen-level-dependent (BOLD) signal, which gives an estimate of changes in oxygen availability [68]. This means that mainly the amount of deoxyhemoglobin in small blood vessels is recorded, which depends on the flow of well-oxygenated arterial blood (CBF), on the outflow of oxygen to the tissue ($CMRO_2$) and on the cerebral blood volume (CBV) [69]. The magnitude of these changes in signal intensity relative to the resting conditions is color-coded to produce fMRI images that map changes in brain function, which can be superimposed on the anatomical image. This results in a spatial resolution of fMRI of 1–3 mm with a temporal resolution of approx. 10 seconds. As fMRI does not involve ionizing radiation and thus is also used without limitation in healthy subjects, and allows more rapid signal acquisition and more flexible experimental set-ups, it has become the dominant technique for functional imaging. There are some advantages of PET, however – physiologically specific measures, better quantitation, better signal-to-noise ratio, fewer artifacts, actual activated and reference values – which support its continued use especially in complex clinical situations and in combination with special stimulating techniques, such as transcranial magnetic stimulation (TMS).

71

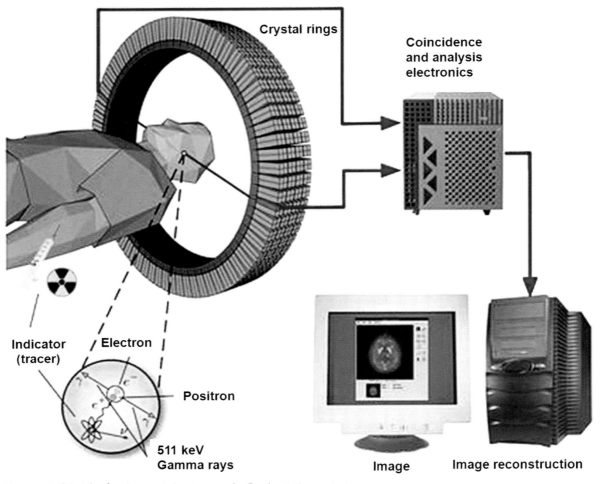

Figure 4.4. Principle of positron emission tomography. For description see text.

Functional MRI (fMRI) detects changes in brain function by measuring differences in magnetic properties of hemoglobin depending on the blood oxygen level.

Motor and somatosensory deficits

Motor function may be impaired by damage to a widely distributed network, involving multiple cortical representations and complex fiber tracts. The degree of motor impairment and the potential for recovery depends on the site of the lesion, the combination of lesions in cortical areas and in fiber tracts, and the involvement of deep gray structures, e.g. the basal ganglia, thalamus, and brainstem. The patterns of altered metabolism and blood flow and the patterns of activation after stimuli or during motor tasks are manifold and reflect the site and extent of the lesion,

but they are also dependent on the paradigm of stimulus or task. With severe motor impairment, patients cannot carry out complex or even simple motor tasks, and the activation paradigm must be restricted to passive movement or imagination of motor performance. The diverging experimental conditions make the interpretation and comparison of different studies extremely difficult, and might help explain the lack of a clear concept of "neuronal plasticity" applicable to recovery from motor stroke (reviews in [54, 56, 57, 70, 71]). A recent review concluded that "motor recovery after stroke depends on a variety of mechanisms including perilesional motor reorganization, use of motor pathways in subcortical structures, use of collateral pathways in the ipsilateral hemisphere, or use of collateral pathways in the contralateral hemisphere, or possibly the development of entirely new motor

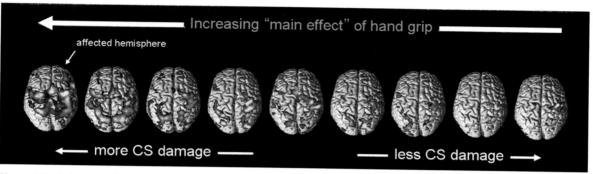

Figure 4.5. Brain activity for hand grip compared to rest for individual subjects with corticospinal (CS) damage. These fMRI studies demonstrate that increasing corticospinal damage leads to a shift in the pattern of activation from the primary to the secondary motor system. Modified from Ward [56].

networks" [54]. In most fMRI or PET studies involving active or passive movements, a widespread network of neurons was activated in both hemispheres. The areas included frontal and parietal cortices, and sometimes the basal ganglia and cerebellum. In particular, (ipsilateral) premotor cortex, supplementary motor area (SMA), anterior parts of the insula/frontal operculum, and bilateral inferior parietal cortices are often activated (Figure 4.5). These results suggest that sensorimotor functions are represented in extended, variable, probably parallel processing, bilateral networks [58, 72]. Whereas changes in both the damaged and the undamaged hemisphere can be observed, ipsilateral activation of motor cortex is consistently found to be stronger for movement of the paretic fingers after recovery from stroke, whereas movements of the unaffected hand (as in normal subjects) are accompanied mainly by activation of the contralateral cerebral cortex. In addition to stronger intensity, the spatial extent of activation in motor cortex was enlarged, and activation on the ipsilateral side was also seen in premotor and insular cortex. These results indicate that recruitment of ipsilateral cortices plays a role in recovery: the higher the activation in the ipsilesional M1(BA4p), S1, and insula, the better the recovery 1 year after stroke [73]; patients who activated the posterior primary motor cortex early after stroke had a better recovery of hand function (Figure 4.6).

Task-oriented arm training increased activation bilaterally in the inferior parietal area, in premotor areas, and in the contralateral sensorimotor cortex, suggesting an improved functional brain reorganization in the bilateral sensory and motor systems [74]. Similar results were obtained by fMRI, by which an evolution of the activation in the sensorimotor cortex

from early contralesional activity to late ipsilateral activity was found [75], suggesting a dynamic bihemispheric reorganization of motor networks during recovery from hemiparesis. It was also shown that the over-activation observed a few weeks after a stroke diminishes over time, suggesting compensatory mechanisms appearing even late in the course [76]. Ipsilateral cortical recruitment seems to be a compensatory cortical process related to the lesion of the contralateral primary motor cortex; this process of compensatory recruitment will persist if the primary motor cortex is permanently damaged. Newly learned movements after focal cortical injury are represented over larger cortical territories, an effect which is dependent on the intensity of rehabilitative training. It is of importance that the unaffected hemisphere actually inhibits the generation of a voluntary movement by the paretic hand [77]. This effect of transcallosal inhibition can be reduced by repetitive transcranial magnetic stimulation (rTMS) [78, 79]. Recovery from infarction is also accompanied by substantial changes in the activity of the proprioceptive systems of the paretic and non-paretic limb, reflecting an interhemispheric shift of attention to proprioceptive stimuli associated with recovery [80].

> During recovery from hemiparesis, a dynamic bihemispheric reorganization of motor networks takes place. fMRI and PET studies can display the compensatory cortical processes and show the importance of transcallosal inhibition.

Post-stroke aphasia

Studies of glucose metabolism in aphasia after stroke have shown metabolic disturbances in the ipsilateral

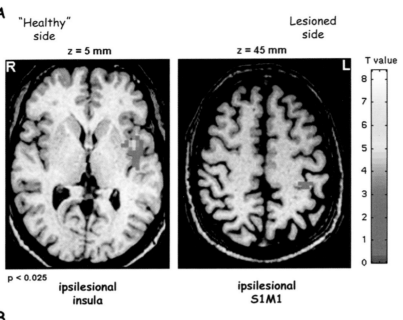

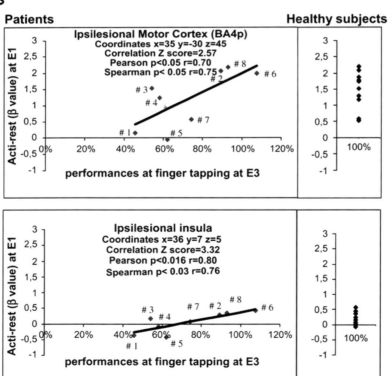

Figure 4.6. Prognostic value of MRI in recovery of hand function: (A) Areas where the intensity of activation 20 days after stroke (E1) correlates with finger-tapping motor performance at E3 (1 year after stroke). Activations are overlaid on a healthy brain. The lesioned side is on the left of the image (radiological convention). (B) Corresponding plots of the positive correlations between the individual β values and finger-tapping performance. The β values of the 10 healthy subjects at E1 are also given for the same coordinates. Used with permission from Loubinoux *et al.* [73].

hemisphere caused by the lesion and in the contra-lateral hemisphere caused by functional deactivation (diaschisis) (review in Heiss *et al.* [71]). In right-handed individuals with language dominance in the left hemisphere, the left temporo-parietal region, in particular the angular gyrus, supramarginal gyrus, and lateral and transverse superior temporal gyrus (STG) are the most frequently and consistently impaired, and the degree of impairment is related to the severity of aphasia. The functional disturbance as measured by rCMRGlc in speech-relevant brain regions early after stroke is predictive of the eventual outcome of aphasia but the metabolism in the hemisphere outside the infarct was also significantly related to outcome of post-stroke aphasia, a finding supporting previous results of a significant correlation of CMRGlc outside the infarct with functional recovery [63]. Additionally, the functionality of the bihemispheric network has a significant impact on outcome: although the brain recruits right-hemispheric regions for speech-processing when the left-hemispheric centers are impaired, outcome studies reveal that this strategy is significantly less effective than repair of the speech-relevant network in adults. That the quality of recovery is mainly dependent on undamaged portions of the language network in the left hemisphere and to a lesser extent on homologous right hemisphere areas can be deduced from activation studies in the course after post-stroke aphasia [81]. The differences in improvement of speech deficits were reflected in different patterns of activation in the course after stroke (Figure 4.7): the subcortical and frontal groups improved substantially and activated the right inferior frontal gyrus and the right STG at baseline and regained regional left STG activation at follow-up. The temporal group improved only in word comprehension; it activated the left

Broca area and SMAs at baseline and the precentral gyrus bilaterally as well as the right STG at follow-up, but could not reactivate the left STG. These results were confirmed in comparable studies [82–84].

> Studies of glucose metabolism in aphasia after stroke have shown metabolic disturbances in the ipsilateral hemisphere caused by the lesion and contralateral hemisphere caused by functional deactivation (diaschisis).

Combination of repetitive transcranial magnetic stimulation (rTMS) with activated imaging

rTMS is a non-invasive procedure to create electric currents in discrete brain areas which, depending on frequency, intensity, and duration, can lead to transient increases and decreases in excitability of the affected cortex. Low frequencies of rTMS (below 5 Hz) can suppress excitability of the cortex, while higher-frequency stimulation (5–20 Hz) leads to an increase in cortical excitability [85]. Increases in relative CBV in contralateral homologous language regions during overt propositional speech fMRI in chronic, non-fluent aphasia patients indicated over-activation of right language homologs. This right hemisphere over-activation may represent a maladaptive strategy and can be interpreted as a result of

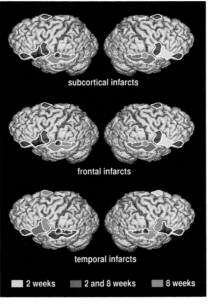

subcortical infarcts

frontal infarcts

temporal infarcts

2 weeks   2 and 8 weeks   8 weeks

Reactivation of left temporal gyrus

Only activation of left frontal and homologous language areas

Figure 4.7. Activation patterns in patients with left hemispheric stroke 2 and 8 weeks after stroke. In the case of subcortical and frontal infarction, the left temporal areas are reactivated correlating to better recovery of language function. Used with permission from Heiss *et al.* [81].

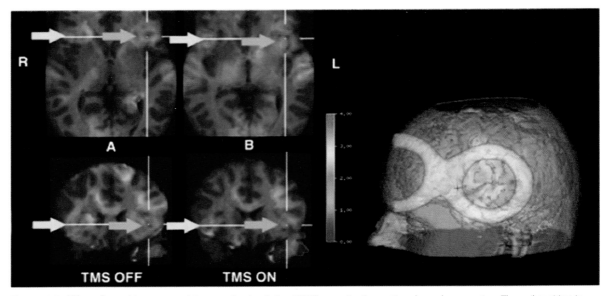

Figure 4.8. Effect of repetitive transcranial magnetic stimulation (rTMS) on activation pattern by verb generation. The coil position is shown in the 3D rendering. (A) shows inferior frontal gyrus activation during simple verb generation. (B) clearly shows the decreased activation on the left (blue arrow) and increased activity on the right side (yellow arrow) during rTMS interference. Modified from Thiel *et al.* [87].

decreased transcallosal inhibition due to damage of the specialized and lateralized speech areas. TMS studies with blockade of this contralateral over-activation by a series of 1 Hz rTMS [86] have improved picture-naming ability in chronic non-fluent aphasia patients. Collateral ipsilateral as well as transcallosal contralateral inhibition can be demonstrated by simultaneous rTMS and PET activation studies [87]: at rest, rTMS decreased blood flow ipsilaterally and contralaterally. During verb generation, regional CBF was decreased ipsilaterally under the coil during rTMS, but increased ipsilaterally outside the coil and in the contralateral homologous area (Figure 4.8). The effect of rTMS was accompanied by a prolongation of reaction time latencies to verbal stimuli.

The role of activation in the right hemisphere for residual language performance can be investigated by combining rTMS with functional imaging, e.g. PET. In patients in whom verb generation activated predominantly the right inferior frontal gyrus, this response could be blocked by rTMS over this region. These patients had lower performance in verbal fluency tasks than patients with effects of rTMS only over the left inferior frontal gyrus, suggesting a less effective compensatory potential of right-sided network areas. These results indicate a

potential for rTMS in the treatment of post-stroke aphasia [88].

The activation studies in the course of recovery of post-stroke aphasia suggest various mechanisms for the compensation of the lesion within the functional network. Despite differences among the activation and stimulation paradigms and the heterogeneity of patients included in different imaging studies, a hierarchy for effective recovery might be deduced:

- Best, even complete, recovery can only be achieved by restoration of the original activation pattern after small brain damage outside primary centers.
- If primary functional centers are damaged, reduction of collateral inhibition leads to activation of areas around the lesion (intrahemispheric compensation).
- If the ipsilateral network is severely damaged, reduction of transcallosal inhibition causes activation of contralateral homotopic areas, which is usually not as efficient as intrahemispheric compensation. In some patients with slowly developing brain damage the language function can be completely shifted to the right hemisphere.

In most instances the disinhibition of homotopic areas contralateral to the lesion impairs the capacity for recovery – a mechanism which might be counteracted by rTMS of these contralateral active areas. This approach might open a new therapeutic strategy for post-stroke aphasia.

The role of activation in the right hemisphere for residual language performance can be investigated by combining rTMS with functional imaging, e.g. PET. Counteraction by rTMS of contralateral active areas might open a new therapeutic strategy for post-stroke aphasia.

Chapter summary

Neuroimaging modalities may help to assess functional outcome and to predict the efficacy of rehabilitation in individual patients additionally to functional assessment scales such as NIHSS and others.

CT: the most widely used imaging procedure in acute stroke is CT, especially for differentiation between hemorrhagic and ischemic stroke, for localization of the lesion, and for decision-making regarding administration of potentially risky stroke therapies as thrombolysis. ASPECTS (the Alberta Stroke Program Early Computed Tomography Score) is a measure to quantify ischemic changes on CT within the territory of the middle cerebral artery (MCA) and can help select patients for acute intravascular treatment.

MRI: with diffusion-weighted imaging (DWI), the size of the lesion can be outlined early and DWI lesion volume significantly increased the power of prediction models. Diffusion tensor imaging (DTI) measures may also be used to predict outcome. The connectivity in networks as assessed by DTI is more important for outcome and recovery than the extent of the primary structural lesion.

Assessment of brain blood supply and cerebral perfusion

Inclusion of information from CT angiography contributed significantly more to outcome prediction than the ASPECTS score. Evidence of large-vessel occlusion is crucial for improving outcome by early endovascular interventions.

The final size of an infarct is also influenced by the extent and quality of collateral circulation to the affected brain area. The presence of robust collateral flow is best visualized by conventional angiography, but CT angiography as a non-invasive alternative has better spatial resolution than transcranial Doppler or MR angiography and can depict leptomeningeal collaterals.

The visualization of disturbed interaction in functional networks and of their reorganization in the recovery after focal brain damage is the domain of functional imaging modalities such as PET and fMRI.

PET: mapping of neuronal activity in the brain can be primarily achieved by quantitation of the regional **cerebral metabolic rate for glucose** (CMRGlc). Quantitative imaging of **cerebral blood flow** (CBF) is based on the principle of diffusible tracer exchange, using ^{15}O-labeled water.

PET detects and, if required, can quantify changes in CBF and CMRGlc accompanying different activation states of brain tissue. The regional values of CBF or CMRGlc represent the brain activity due to a specific state, task, or stimulus in comparison with the resting condition, and color-coded maps can be analyzed or correlated to morphological images.

fMRI measures signals that depend on the differential magnetic properties of oxygenated and deoxygenated hemoglobin, termed the blood-oxygen-level-dependent (BOLD) signal, which gives an estimate of changes in oxygen availability. The amount of deoxyhemoglobin in small blood vessels depends on the flow of well-oxygenated arterial blood (CBF), on the outflow of oxygen to the tissue (CMRO$_2$), and on the cerebral blood volume (CBV). fMRI images map changes in brain function and can be superimposed on the anatomical image.

Motor and somatosensory deficits

In most fMRI or PET studies involving active or passive movements, a widespread network of neurons was activated in both hemispheres. During recovery from hemiparesis, a dynamic bihemispheric reorganization of motor networks takes place. Ipsilateral cortical recruitment seems to be a compensatory cortical process related to the lesion of the contralateral primary motor cortex. The unaffected hemisphere actually inhibits the generation of a voluntary movement by the paretic hand. This effect of transcallosal inhibition can be reduced by repetitive transcranial magnetic stimulation (rTMS).

Post-stroke aphasia

Studies of glucose metabolism in aphasia after stroke have shown metabolic disturbances in the ipsilateral hemisphere caused by the lesion and contralateral hemisphere caused by functional deactivation (diaschisis). Patients with an eventual good recovery predominantly activated structures in the ipsilateral hemisphere.

Combination of repetitive transcranial magnetic stimulation (rTMS) with activated imaging

Activation studies in the course of recovery of post-stroke aphasia suggest various mechanisms for the compensation of the lesion within the functional network: restoration of the original activation pattern, activation of areas around the lesion (intra-hemispheric compensation), and reduction of trans-callosal inhibition causing activation of contralateral homotopic areas. rTMS is a non-invasive procedure for creating electric currents in discrete brain areas which, depending on frequency, intensity, and duration, can lead to transient increases (with higher frequencies) and decreases (with lower frequencies) in excitability of the affected cortex. The role of activation in the right hemisphere for residual language performance can be investigated by combining rTMS with functional imaging, e.g. PET. Counteraction by rTMS of contralateral active areas might open a new therapeutic strategy for post-stroke aphasia.

References

1. WHO. *Shaping the Future*. Geneva: World Health Organization; 2003.

2. Miller EL, Murray L, Richards L, *et al*. Comprehensive overview of nursing and interdisciplinary rehabilitation care of the stroke patient: a scientific statement from the American Heart Association. *Stroke* 2010; 41(10):2402–48.

3. Gordon NF, Gulanick M, Costa F, *et al*. Physical activity and exercise recommendations for stroke survivors: an American Heart Association scientific statement from the Council on Clinical Cardiology, Subcommittee on Exercise, Cardiac Rehabilitation, and Prevention; the Council on Cardiovascular Nursing; the Council on Nutrition, Physical Activity, and Metabolism; and the Stroke Council. *Stroke* 2004; 35(5):1230–40.

4. Kwakkel G, Veerbeek JM, Harmeling-van der Wel BC, van Wegen E, Kollen BJ, Early Prediction of functional Outcome after Stroke (EPOS) Investigators Diagnostic accuracy of the Barthel Index for measuring activities of daily living outcome after ischemic hemispheric stroke: does early post-stroke timing of assessment matter? *Stroke* 2011; 42(2): 342–6.

5. Young FB, Lees KR, Weir CJ, Committee GITS, Investigators. Improving trial power through use of prognosis-adjusted end points. *Stroke* 2005; 36(3): 597–601.

6. Granger CV, Dewis LS, Peters NC, Sherwood CC, Barrett JE. Stroke rehabilitation: analysis of repeated Barthel index measures. *Arch Phys Med Rehabil* 1979; 60(1):14–17.

7. Sulter G, Steen C, De Keyser J. Use of the Barthel index and modified Rankin scale in acute stroke trials. *Stroke* 1999; 30(8):1538–41.

8. Johnston KC, Connors AF Jr, Wagner DP, *et al*. A predictive risk model for outcomes of ischemic stroke. *Stroke* 2000; 31(2):448–55.

9. Alexander MP. Stroke rehabilitation outcome. A potential use of predictive variables to establish levels of care. *Stroke* 1994; 25(1):128–34.

10. Veerbeek JM, Kwakkel G, van Wegen EE, Ket JC, Heymans MW. Early prediction of outcome of activities of daily living after stroke: a systematic review. *Stroke* 2011; 42(5):1482–8.

11. Brott T, Adams HP Jr, Olinger CP, *et al*. Measurements of acute cerebral infarction: a clinical examination scale. *Stroke* 1989; 20(7):864–70.

12. Adams HP Jr, Davis PH, Leira EC, *et al*. Baseline NIH Stroke Scale score strongly predicts outcome after stroke: a report of the Trial of Org 10172 in Acute Stroke Treatment (TOAST). *Neurology* 1999; 53(1):126–31.

13. Meyer BC, Hemmen TM, Jackson CM, Lyden PD. Modified National Institutes of Health

Stroke Scale for use in stroke clinical trials: prospective reliability and validity. *Stroke* 2002; **33**(5):1261–6.

14. Konig IR, Ziegler A, Bluhmki E, *et al*. Predicting long-term outcome after acute ischemic stroke: a simple index works in patients from controlled clinical trials. *Stroke* 2008; **39**(6):1821–6.

15. Muscari A, Puddu GM, Santoro N, Zoli M. A simple scoring system for outcome prediction of ischemic stroke. *Acta Neurol Scand* 2011; **124**(5):334–42.

16. Fiorelli M, Alperovitch A, Argentino C, *et al*. Prediction of long-term outcome in the early hours following acute ischemic stroke. Italian Acute Stroke Study Group. *Arch Neurol* 1995; **52**(3):250–5.

17. Heuschmann PU, Wiedmann S, Wellwood I, *et al*. Three-month stroke outcome: the European Registers of Stroke (EROS) investigators. *Neurology* 2011; **76**(2):159–65.

18. Knoflach M, Matosevic B, Rucker M, *et al*. Functional recovery after ischemic stroke–a matter of age: data from the Austrian Stroke Unit Registry. *Neurology* 2012; **78**(4):279–85.

19. Kwakkel G, Veerbeek JM, van Wegen EE, *et al*. Predictive value of the NIHSS for ADL outcome after ischemic hemispheric stroke: does timing of early assessment matter? *J Neurol Sci* 2010; **294**(1–2):57–61.

20. Reid JM, Gubitz GJ, Dai D, *et al*. Predicting functional outcome after stroke by modelling baseline clinical and CT variables. *Age Ageing* 2010; **39**(3):360–6.

21. Schiemanck SK, Kwakkel G, Post MW, Kappelle LJ, Prevo AJ. Predicting long-term independency in activities of daily living after middle cerebral artery stroke: does information from

22. Barber PA, Demchuk AM, Zhang J, Buchan AM, Group AS. Validity and reliability of a quantitative computed tomography score in predicting outcome of hyperacute stroke before thrombolytic therapy. *Lancet* 2000; 355:1670–4.

23. Hill MD, Rowley HA, Adler F, *et al*. Selection of acute ischemic stroke patients for intra-arterial thrombolysis with pro-urokinase by using ASPECTS. *Stroke* 2003; **34**(8):1925–31.

24. Alexander LD, Pettersen JA, Hopyan JJ, Sahlas DJ, Black SE. Long-term prediction of functional outcome after stroke using the Alberta stroke program early computed tomography score in the subacute stage. *J Stroke Cerebrovasc Dis* 2012; **21**(8):737–44.

25. Vogt G, Laage R, Shuaib A, Schneider A, VISTA Collaboration. Initial lesion volume is an independent predictor of clinical stroke outcome at day 90: an analysis of the Virtual International Stroke Trials Archive (VISTA) database. *Stroke* 2012; **43**(5):1266–72.

26. Schiemanck SK, Kwakkel G, Post MW, Prevo AJ. Predictive value of ischemic lesion volume assessed with magnetic resonance imaging for neurological deficits and functional outcome post-stroke: a critical review of the literature. *Neurorehabil Neural Repair* 2006; **20**(4):492–502.

27. Lindenberg R, Renga V, Zhu LL, *et al*. Structural integrity of corticospinal motor fibers predicts motor impairment in chronic stroke. *Neurology* 2010; **74**(4):280–7.

28. Thijs VN, Lansberg MG, Beaulieu C, *et al*. Is early ischemic lesion volume on diffusion-weighted

imaging an independent predictor of stroke outcome? A multivariable analysis. *Stroke* 2000; **31**(11):2597–602.

29. Johnston KC, Wagner DP, Wang XQ, *et al*. Validation of an acute ischemic stroke model: does diffusion-weighted imaging lesion volume offer a clinically significant improvement in prediction of outcome? *Stroke* 2007; **38**(6):1820–5.

30. Barrett KM, Ding YH, Wagner DP, *et al*. Change in diffusion-weighted imaging infarct volume predicts neurological outcome at 90 days: results of the Acute Stroke Accurate Prediction (ASAP) trial serial imaging substudy. *Stroke* 2009; **40**(7):2422–7.

31. Jang SH. Prediction of motor outcome for hemiparetic stroke patients using diffusion tensor imaging: a review. *NeuroRehabilitation* 2010; **27**(4):367–72.

32. Cho SH, Kim DG, Kim DS, *et al*. Motor outcome according to the integrity of the corticospinal tract determined by diffusion tensor tractography in the early stage of corona radiata infarct. *Neurosci Lett* 2007; **426**(2):123–7.

33. Radlinska B, Ghinani S, Leppert IR, *et al*. Diffusion tensor imaging, permanent pyramidal tract damage, and outcome in subcortical stroke. *Neurology* 2010; **75**(12):1048–54.

34. Liang Z, Zeng J, Zhang C, *et al*. Longitudinal investigations on the anterograde and retrograde degeneration in the pyramidal tract following pontine infarction with diffusion tensor imaging. *Cerebrovascu Dis* 2008; **25**(3):209–16.

35. Lindenberg R, Zhu LL, Ruber T, Schlaug G. Predicting functional motor potential in chronic stroke patients using diffusion tensor

imaging. *Hum Brain Mapp* 2012; **33**(5):1040–51.

36. Riley JD, Le V, Der-Yeghiaian L, *et al.* Anatomy of stroke injury predicts gains from therapy. *Stroke* 2011; **42**(2):421–6.

37. Puig J, Pedraza S, Blasco G, *et al.* Acute damage to the posterior limb of the internal capsule on diffusion tensor tractography as an early imaging predictor of motor outcome after stroke. *AJNR Am J Neuroradiol* 2011; **32**(5):857–63.

38. Kim SH, Lee DG, You H, *et al.* The clinical application of the arcuate fasciculus for stroke patients with aphasia: a diffusion tensor tractography study. *NeuroRehabilitation* 2011; **29**(3):305–10.

39. Breier JI, Hasan KM, Zhang W, Men D, Papanicolaou AC. Language dysfunction after stroke and damage to white matter tracts evaluated using diffusion tensor imaging. *AJNR Am J Neuroradiol* 2008; **29**(3):483–7.

40. Stinear CM, Ward NS. How useful is imaging in predicting outcomes in stroke rehabilitation? *Int J Stroke* 2013; **8**(1):33–7.

41. Fischer U, Arnold M, Nedeltchev K, *et al.* NIHSS score and arteriographic findings in acute ischemic stroke. *Stroke* 2005; **36**(10):2121–5.

42. Smith WS, Lev MH, English JD, *et al.* Significance of large vessel intracranial occlusion causing acute ischemic stroke and TIA. *Stroke* 2009; **40**(12):3834–40.

43. Gonzalez RG, Lev MH, Goldmacher GV, *et al.* Improved outcome prediction using CT angiography in addition to standard ischemic stroke assessment: results from the STOPStroke study. *PLoS One* 2012; **7**(1):e30352.

44. Mortimer AM, Simpson E, Bradley MD, Renowden SA.

Computed tomography angiography in hyperacute ischemic stroke: prognostic implications and role in decision-making. *Stroke* 2013; **44**(5): 1480–8.

45. Kucinski T, Koch C, Eckert B, *et al.* Collateral circulation is an independent radiological predictor of outcome after thrombolysis in acute ischaemic stroke. *Neuroradiology* 2003; **45**(1):11–18.

46. Bang OY, Saver JL, Kim SJ, *et al.* Collateral flow predicts response to endovascular therapy for acute ischemic stroke. *Stroke* 2011; **42**(3):693–9.

47. Maas MB, Lev MH, Ay H, *et al.* Collateral vessels on CT angiography predict outcome in acute ischemic stroke. *Stroke* 2009; **40**(9):3001–5.

48. Lima FO, Furie KL, Silva GS, *et al.* The pattern of leptomeningeal collaterals on CT angiography is a strong predictor of long-term functional outcome in stroke patients with large vessel intracranial occlusion. *Stroke* 2010; **41**(10):2316–22.

49. Kane I, Carpenter T, Chappell F, *et al.* Comparison of 10 different magnetic resonance perfusion imaging processing methods in acute ischemic stroke: effect on lesion size, proportion of patients with diffusion/perfusion mismatch, clinical scores, and radiologic outcomes. *Stroke* 2007; **38**(12):3158–64.

50. Bivard A, Spratt N, Levi C, Parsons M. Perfusion computer tomography: imaging and clinical validation in acute ischaemic stroke. *Brain* 2011; **134**(Pt 11): 3408–16.

51. Heiss WD, Zeiler K, Havelec L. Hirndurchblutung und soziale Prognose nach ischämischem zerebralem Insult. *Dtsch Med Wschr* 1978; **103**:597–602.

52. Giubilei F, Lenzi GL, Di Piero V, *et al.* Predictive value of brain

perfusion single-photon emission computed tomography in acute ischemic stroke. *Stroke* 1990; **21**(6):895–900.

53. Rijntjes M, Weiller C. Recovery of motor and language abilities after stroke: the contribution of functional imaging. *Prog Neurobiol* 2002; **66**(2):109–22.

54. Thirumala P, Hier DB, Patel P. Motor recovery after stroke: Lessons from functional brain imaging. *Neurol Res* 2002; **24**:453–8.

55. Herholz K, Heiss WD. Functional imaging correlates of recovery after stroke in humans. *J Cereb Blood Flow Metab* 2000; **20**:1619–31.

56. Ward NS. Future perspectives in functional neuroimaging in stroke recovery. *Eura Medicophys.* 2007; **43**(2):285–94.

57. Cramer SC. Repairing the human brain after stroke: I. Mechanisms of spontaneous recovery. *Ann Neurol* 2008; **63**(3):272–87.

58. Rossini PM, Calautti C, Pauri F, Baron JC. Post-stroke plastic reorganisation in the adult brain. *Lancet Neurol* 2003; **2**:493–502.

59. Eliassen JC, Boespflug EL, Lamy M, *et al.* Brain-mapping techniques for evaluating post-stroke recovery and rehabilitation: a review. *Top Stroke Rehabil* 2008; **15**(5):427–50.

60. Sokoloff L, Reivich M, Kennedy C, *et al.* The (14 C)-deoxyglucose method for the measurement of local cerebral glucose utilization: theory, procedure, and normal values in the conscious and anesthetized albino rat. *J Neurochem* 1977; **28**:897–916.

61. Reivich M, Kuhl D, Wolf A, *et al.* The (18 F)fluorodeoxyglucose method for the measurement of local cerebral glucose utilization in man. *Circ Res* 1979; **44**:127–37.

62. Wienhard K, Pawlik G, Herholz K, Wagner R, Heiss WD.

Estimation of local cerebral glucose utilization by positron emission tomography of [18F]2-fluoro-2-deoxy-D-glucose: a critical appraisal of optimization procedures. *J Cereb Blood Flow Metab* 1985; **5**(1):115–25.

63. Heiss WD, Emunds HG, Herholz K. Cerebral glucose metabolism as a predictor of rehabilitation after ischemic stroke. *Stroke* 1993; **24**(12):1784–8.

64. Herscovitch P, Martin WRW, Raichle ME. The autoradiographic measurement of regional cerebral blood flow (CBF) with positron emission tomography: validation studies. *J Nucl Med* 1983; **24**:P62–3.

65. Frackowiak RSJ, Lenzi GL, Jones T, Heather JD. Quantitative measurement of regional cerebral blood flow and oxygen metabolism in man using ^{15}O and positron emission tomography: theory, procedure, and normal values. *J Comput Assist Tomogr* 1980; **4**:727–36.

66. Mintun MA, Raichle ME, Martin WRW, Herscovitch P. Brain oxygen utilization measured with O-15 radiotracers and positron emission tomography. *J Nucl Med* 1984; **25**:177–87.

67. Mintun MA, Lundstrom BN, Snyder AZ, *et al.* Blood flow and oxygen delivery to human brain during functional activity: theoretical modeling and experimental data. *Proc Natl Acad Sci U S A* 2001; **98**(12):6859–64.

68. Ogawa S, Lee TM, Kay AR, Tank DW. Brain magnetic resonance imaging with contrast dependent on blood oxygenation. *Proc Natl Acad Sci U S A* 1990; **87**(24):9868–72.

69. Turner R, Howseman A, Rees G, Josephs O. Functional imaging with magnetic resonance. In: Frackowiak RSJ, Friston KJ, Frith CD, Dolan RJ, Mazziotta JC, eds. *Human Brain Function*. San Diego: Academic Press; 1997: 467–86.

70. Weiller C. Recovery from motor stroke: human positron emission tomography studies. *Cerebrovasc Dis* 1995; **5**:282–91.

71. Heiss WD, Thiel A, Winhuisen L, *et al.* Functional imaging in the assessment of capability for recovery after stroke. *J Rehab Med* 2003; **41**:27–33.

72. Rizzolatti G, Luppino G, Matelli M. The organization of the cortical motor system: new concepts. *Electroencephalogr Clin Neurophysiol* 1998; **106**(4):283–96.

73. Loubinoux I, Dechaumont-Palacin S, Castel-Lacanal E, *et al.* Prognostic value of FMRI in recovery of hand function in subcortical stroke patients. *Cereb Cortex* 2007; **17**(12):2980–7.

74. Nelles G, Jentzen W, Jueptner M, Müller S, Diener HC. Arm training induced brain plasticity in stroke studied with serial positron emission tomography. *Neuroimage* 2001; **13**(6):1146–54.

75. Marshall RS, Perera GM, Lazar RM, *et al.* Evolution of cortical activation during recovery from corticospinal tract infarction. *Stroke* 2000; **31**(3):656–61.

76. Calautti C, Leroy F, Guincestre JY, Baron JC. Dynamics of motor network overactivation after striatocapsular stroke: a longitudinal PET study using a fixed-performance paradigm. *Stroke* 2001; **32**(11):2534–42.

77. Murase N, Duque J, Mazzocchio R, Cohen LG. Influence of interhemispheric interactions on motor function in chronic stroke. *Ann Neurol* 2004; **55**(3):400–9.

78. Shimizu T, Hosaki A, Hino T, *et al.* Motor cortical disinhibition in the unaffected hemisphere after unilateral cortical stroke. *Brain* 2002; **125**(Pt 8):1896–907.

79. Hsu WY, Cheng CH, Liao KK, Lee IH, Lin YY. Effects of repetitive transcranial magnetic stimulation on motor functions in patients with stroke: a meta-analysis. *Stroke* 2012; **43**(7):1849–57.

80. Thiel A, Aleksic B, Klein JC, Rudolf J, Heiss W-D. Changes in proprioceptive systems activity during recovery from post-stroke hemiparesis. *J Rehabil Med* 2007; **39**(7):520–5.

81. Heiss WD, Kessler J, Thiel A, Ghaemi M, Karbe H. Differential capacity of left and right hemispheric areas for compensation of post-stroke aphasia. *Ann Neurol* 1999; **45**(4):430–8.

82. Cao Y, Vikingstad EM, George KP, Johnson AF, Welch KMA. Cortical language activation in stroke patients recovering from aphasia with functional MRI. *Stroke* 1999; **30**(11):2331–40.

83. Warburton E, Price CJ, Swinburn K, Wise RJS. Mechanisms of recovery from aphasia: evidence from positron emission tomography studies. *J Neurol Neurosurg Psychiatry* 1999; **66**(2):155–61.

84. Saur D, Lange R, Baumgaertner A, *et al.* Dynamics of language reorganization after stroke. *Brain* 2006; **129**(6):1371–84.

85. Kobayashi M, Pascual-Leone A. Transcranial magnetic stimulation in neurology. *Lancet Neurol* 2003; **2**:145–56.

86. Naeser MA, Martin PI, Nicholas M, *et al.* Improved picture naming in chronic aphasia after TMS to part of right Broca's area: an open-protocol study. *Brain Lang* 2005; **93**(1):95–105.

87. Thiel A, Schumacher B, Wienhard K, *et al.* Direct demonstration of transcallosal disinhibition in language networks. *J Cereb Blood Flow Metab* 2006; **26**(9):1122–7.

88. Thiel A, Hartmann A, Rubi-Fessen I, *et al.* Effects of non-invasive brain stimulation

Ultrasound in acute ischemic stroke

László Csiba

Introduction

The results of non-invasive tests (e.g. ultrasound) can be highly variable, often providing ambiguous results. Although other parameters can be reviewed, calculation of overall accuracy, sensitivity, and specificity as well as positive and negative predictive values are useful to the clinician who is managing the patient.

To calculate these statistics, ultrasound results must be compared with the established gold standards, usually angiography, surgery, or autopsy findings. The simplest statistic compares the outcome of each test as either positive or negative. A true-positive result indicates that both tests are positive. A true-negative result indicates that both tests are negative. A false-positive result means that the gold standard is negative, indicating the absence of disease, while the non-invasive study is positive, indicating the presence of disease. A false-negative result occurs when the non-invasive test indicates the absence of disease but the gold standard is positive. True-positive and true-negative results can be used to calculate sensitivity and specificity. Sensitivity is the ability of a test to correctly diagnose disease. It can be calculated by dividing the number of true-positive tests by the total number of positive results obtained by the gold standard.

Specificity is the ability to diagnose the absence of disease and is calculated by dividing the true negative by the total number of negative results obtained by the gold standard. The positive predictive value (PPV) or likelihood means that disease is present and negative predictive values (NPV) means that disease is not present. Overall accuracy can be calculated by dividing the number of true negatives and true positives by the total number of tests performed. These results are not very specific and can be highly variable, based on

the incidence of disease in the patient population. Because the patient population referred to the ultrasound lab is diverse, high levels of sensitivity and specificity help to make the diagnosis optimal.

$$Sensitivity(\%) = \frac{true\ positives}{true\ positives + false\ negatives} \times 100$$

$$Specificity(\%) = \frac{true\ negatives}{true\ negatives + false\ positives} \times 100$$

Positive predictive value(%)
$$= \frac{true\ positives}{true\ positives + false\ positives} \times 100$$

Negative predictive value(%)
$$= \frac{true\ negatives}{true\ negatives + false\ negatives} \times 100$$

Extracranial ultrasound in acute stroke

The most important diagnostic question in ultrasonography is which extra- and intracranial vessel(s) is/are stenotic or occluded and can it/they be responsible for the clinical symptoms. Note that clinically silent stenotic processes might also influence the cerebral circulation.

Because of the interactions between extra- and intracranial hemodynamics, both extracranial and intracranial ultrasound techniques should be performed in acute stroke. Similarly, clinically silent stenoses should be detected by careful investigation of anterior, posterior, or ipsi- and contralateral vasculature.

Doppler ultrasonography is the primary non-invasive test for evaluating carotid stenosis.

Carotid ultrasonography consists of two steps, imaging and spectral analysis. Images are produced with the brightness-mode (B-mode) technique and

Textbook of Stroke Medicine, Second Edition, ed. Michael Brainin and Wolf-Dieter Heiss. Published by Cambridge University Press. © Michael Brainin and Wolf-Dieter Heiss 2014.

sometimes color flow information is superimposed on the grayscale image. By convention, the color of the pulsating artery is red. The echogenicity of an object on the image determines its brightness. An object that rebounds very little of the pulse is hypoechoic. An object that reflects much of the signal, such as calcified plaque, is hyperechoic. Plaques with irregular surface and/or heterogeneous echogenicity are more likely to embolize. Soft plaques present a higher embolic risk than hard plaques. The sonographic characteristics of symptomatic and asymptomatic carotid plaques are different. Symptomatic plaques are more likely to be hypoechoic and highly stenotic while asymptomatic plaques are hyperechoic and moderately stenotic. Evaluation of the surface of the plaque has not been demonstrated to be a satisfactory index of plaque instability.

The degree of stenosis is better measured on the basis of the waveform and spectral analysis of the common carotid artery (CCA) and its major branches, especially the internal carotid artery (ICA). Spectral (velocity) analysis is essential to identify stenosis or occlusion. An important general rule for ultrasound is the greater the degree of stenosis, the higher the velocity. Power Doppler provides color imaging that is independent of direction or velocity of flow and gives an angiographic-like picture of an artery.

Blood flow can be laminar, disturbed, or turbulent. When no stenosis is present, blood flow is laminar. Flow of blood is even, with the fastest flow in the middle and the slowest at the edges of the vessel. When a small degree of stenosis is present, the blood flow becomes disturbed and loses its laminar quality. Even in normal conditions, such flow can be seen around the carotid bulb. With even greater stenosis, the flow can become turbulent [1].

In normal hemodynamics, as vessel length increases so does resistance. With increasing radius, the resistance decreases significantly.

As vessel diameter (and area) decreases, blood velocity increases to maintain volume flow.

The extracranial ultrasound procedure starts with the CCA, ICA and external carotid artery (ECA); at least two or three spectral analyses of each vessel should be obtained. Color imaging and power Doppler may be used but may not necessarily provide additional information.

Note the carotid bifurcation, look for plaques, attempt to characterize the nature of the plaque, and color may be used at this point to identify flow within the artery and potential areas of high velocity.

The CCA can be identified by pulsatile walls, smaller caliber than the jugular vein, and systolic peak and diastolic endpoints in between those of external and internal carotid arteries on spectral analysis. The ECA has a smaller caliber, while the ICA is often posterolateral to the ECA and the ECA may have a superior thyroid artery branch coming off. The ECA has virtually no diastolic flow (i.e. high-resistance vessel) on spectral analysis. The ECA shows positive "temporal tap" (i.e. undulations in waveform with tapping of the temporal artery). Perform spectral analysis and find the highest velocity or frequency. After assessment of the anterior circulation, the sonographer should assess the vertebral circulation. Usually, the C4–C6 segment is accessible. Vertebral arteries can be identified with a probe parallel to the carotid: angle the probe laterally and inferiorly. The vertebral body processes appear as hypoechoic transverse bars. The vertebral artery (VA) runs perpendicular to vertebral processes.

Use of color flow Doppler enables the more rapid identification of vessels (especially the VA) and often helps identify the area of highest velocity, reduces scan time, and may help in diagnosis of arterial occlusion [1].

> Doppler ultrasonography is the primary non-invasive test for evaluating carotid stenosis.
> Symptomatic and asymptomatic carotid plaques and the degree of stenosis can be analyzed with ultrasonography by examining the echogenicity of the structures and the velocity of the blood flow.

Identification and classification of ICA stenosis

Mild stenoses (<50%) can be estimated by measurement of area and/or diameter in the cross-sectional and longitudinal image using the B- and color-mode of the ultrasound system. Area measurements in high-grade stenosis are difficult. Diagnosis of severe stenosis is based on hemodynamic parameters (measured by pre-, intra-, and post-stenotic Doppler spectrum analysis).

Investigation of flow direction in the ophthalmic artery is a simple, bedside, ancillary method in suspected ICA stenosis or occlusion (equally severe upper and lower extremity paresis). In a case of hemodynamically significant ICA stenosis or occlusion (proximal to the origin of the ophthalmic artery) a reversed (extra → intracranial) flow could be detected in the ophthalmic artery.

Using duplex ultrasound a proximal ICA occlusion (proximal to the origin of the ophthalmic artery, no color-mode signal, and no Doppler flow) can be distinguished from the ICA occlusion distal to the ophthalmic origin (ICA has low flow velocities and a higher pulsatility but preserved diastolic velocity).

Occlusion results in a complete absence of color-flow signal in ICA, and the diagnosis can be confirmed by ultrasound contrast agents.

Some sonographers characterize the degree of stenosis based on diameter or area reduction but estimation of stenosis solely based on this criterion is not reliable. Commonly used methods are:

- peak systolic velocities (PSV) and end-diastolic velocities
- ratios of ICA/CCA maximal systolic flow velocity within the ICA stenosis
- maximal systolic flow velocity within the non-affected CCA
- ICA/ICA
- maximal systolic flow velocity within the ICA stenosis
- maximal systolic flow velocity of the non-affected ICA.

The stroke risk depends on more than the degree of carotid artery narrowing (cardiac diseases, age, sex, hypertension, smoking, and plaque structure). Most studies consider carotid stenosis of 60% or greater to be clinically important. In a case of a suspected stenosis not only the intrastenotic but also the flow from vessel segments proximal and distal to a stenosis have to be analyzed. If normal flow signals are present before and behind the suspected lesion significant stenosis can be excluded. The stenosis ranges vary from laboratory to laboratory. When possible, laboratories should perform their own correlations with angiographic measurements for quality control. A consensus statement of the Society of Radiologists in Ultrasound recommended the following criteria for estimating stenosis [2]:

- Normal: ICA PSV <125 cm/s, no plaque or intimal thickening.
- <50% stenosis: ICA PSV <125 cm/s and plaque or intimal thickening.
- 50–69% stenosis: ICA PSV is 125–230 cm/s and plaque is visible.
- >70% stenosis to near occlusion: ICA PSV >230 cm/s and visible plaque and lumen narrowing.

- Near occlusion: a markedly narrowed lumen on color Doppler ultrasound.
- Total occlusion: no detectable patent lumen is seen on grayscale ultrasound, and no flow is seen on spectral, power, and color Doppler ultrasound.

With stenosis over 90% (near occlusion), velocities may actually drop as mechanisms that maintain flow fail. Ratios may be particularly helpful in situations in which cardiovascular factors (e.g. poor ejection fraction) limit the increase in velocity [1].

<50% stenoses ICA/CCA: <2.0.

50–69% stenoses ICA/CCA: 2.0–4.0.

70% stenoses ICA/CCA: >4.0.

Doppler ultrasonography associated with stenosis might result in false-positive/negative results:

- Ipsilateral CCA-to-ICA flow ratios may not be valid in the setting of contralateral ICA occlusion.
- CCA waveforms may have a high-resistance configuration in ipsilateral ICA lesions.
- ICA waveforms may have a high-resistance configuration in ipsilateral distal ICA lesions.
- ICA waveforms may be dampened in ipsilateral CCA lesions.
- Long-segment ICA stenosis may not have high end-diastolic velocity.
- Velocities supersede imaging in grading stenosis.
- Imaging can be used to downgrade stenosis in the setting of turbulence caused by kinking [3].

A recent consensus paper of Neurosonology Research Group of the World Federation of Neurology suggests the use of NASCET method of measuring a stenosis (local diameter narrowing with the diameter distal to the bulb as denominator). Estimation of carotid stenosis should be primarily based on morphological information (B-mode, color flow, or B-flow imaging) in low to moderate degrees of stenosis. In addition to degree of narrowing, plaque thickness, plaque length, and residual lumen should also be reported. The simply velocity measurement (PSV and carotid ratio) in the stenotic area is not sufficient to differentiate a moderate from a severe (≥70% NASCET) stenosis. The reversed flow in the ophthalmic artery (from extracranial to intracranial direction) should also be investigated. The post-stenotic flow velocity distal to flow disturbances is an important diagnostic value, in which a reduction of velocities (comparison with the unaffected contralateral side or absolute reduction) allows additional grading within the category of severe stenosis. Hemodynamic criteria are appropriate for grading moderate to severe stenoses. Established collateral flow is the most powerful criterion, excluding a less than severe stenosis irrespective of PSV. Special care is recommended for converting Doppler frequencies into velocity by measuring the angle of incidence (Doppler angle). Measurements should be taken using the lowest possible angle of insonation and made in relation to the direction of the jet visualized by color velocity flow and not the vessel course [4].

A carotid occlusion is shown in Figure 5.1.

Morphological measurements (B-mode images and color flow imaging) are the main criteria for low and moderate degrees of stenosis. Most studies consider carotid stenosis of 60% or greater to be clinically important. This equals a peak systolic velocity greater than 125 cm/s. With stenosis greater than 90% (near occlusion), velocities may actually drop as mechanisms that maintain flow fail.

Ratios (maximal systolic flow velocity within the ICA stenosis/maximal systolic flow velocity within the non-affected CCA) may be helpful in situations in which cardiovascular factors (e.g. poor ejection fraction) limit the increase in velocity. Velocity measurements in a stenosis (PSV and carotid ratio) alone are not sufficient to differentiate a moderate from a severe ($\geq$70% NASCET) stenosis.

Additional criteria refer to the effect of a stenosis on pre-stenotic flow (CCA), the extent of post-stenotic flow disturbances, and derived velocity criteria (diastolic peak velocity and the carotid ratio).

The recent American Heart Association /American Stroke Association (AHA/ASA) guideline also recommends that each laboratory should validate its own Doppler criteria for clinically relevant stenosis [5].

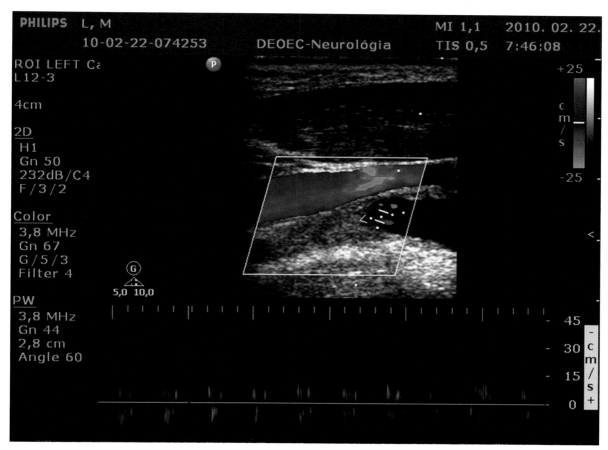

Figure 5.1. A carotid occlusion.

IMT measurement

In the Cardiovascular Health Study, increases in the intimal-medial thickness (IMT) of the carotid artery were associated with an increased risk of myocardial infarction and stroke in older adults without a history of cardiovascular disease [6]. CCA IMT greater than 0.87 mm and ICA IMT greater than 0.90 mm were associated with a progressively increased risk of cardiovascular events. For each 0.20 mm increase in CCA IMT, the risk increased by approximately 27%. For each 0.55 mm increase in ICA IMT, the risk increased approximately 30%.

The following method is suggested by the American Society of Echocardiography and the Society for Vascular Medicine for measuring IMT [7]: (1) use end-diastolic images for IMT measurements; (2) categorization of plaque presence and IMT; (3) avoid use of a single upper limit of normal for IMT because the measure varies with age, sex, and race; and (4) incorporate lumen measurement, particularly when serial measurements are performed, to account for changes in distending pressure.

Treatment with lipid-lowering drugs has been shown to decrease the intimal thickness of the carotid artery. Decrease in the thickness of the intima of the CCA has been correlated directly with successful treatment with drugs that lower serum low-density lipoprotein levels.

A recent consensus paper defines the plaque as a focal structure that encroaches into the arterial lumen of at least 0.5 mm or 50% of the surrounding IMT value or demonstrates a thickness 1–1.5 mm as measured from the media–adventitia interface to the intima–lumen interface. Carotid IMT and plaques are different phenotypes indicating increased vascular risk. Plaque presence demonstrates a higher risk and therefore overrides IMT predictive values. However, IMT without plaque remains a significant marker of an increased risk of vascular events and significantly predicts plaque occurrence [8]. A recent, prospective study on more than 600 patients and 2 years follow-up suggests that the progression of stenosis is also a strong risk factor for cerebrovascular events. The IMT was confirmed as a crucial additional measure, with an increased risk by 25% for each 0.1 mm IMT increase [9].

> With ultrasound, the intimal-medial thickness [IMT] of the carotid artery can be measured. Increases in the IMT of the carotid artery are associated with an increased risk of myocardial infarction and stroke.

> The presence of plaque demonstrates a higher risk and overrides IMT predictive values.

Extracranial vertebral and subclavian arteries

The origin of the VA is one of the most common locations of atherosclerotic stenosis, which is difficult to investigate, especially its origin. Raised flow velocities and spectral broadening can be seen in over 50% of stenoses. A distal extracranial VA occlusion may cause a stump signal or a high pulsatile flow signal with almost absent end-diastolic flow component.

A high grade of subclavian stenosis (>50%) results in increased flow velocities and a turbulent flow. In high-grade subclavian stenosis an alternating flow, or even a retrograde flow, can be detected within the ipsilateral VA. The levels of evidence of the European Federation of Neurological Societies are shown in Table 5.1 [10].

Ultrasound diagnosis of intracranial stenosis and occlusion

Intracranial disease corresponds to approximately 8–10% of acute ischemic stroke, depending on sex and race. Diagnosis is frequently reached through arteriography.

A recent review summarized the existing clinical conditions and standards for which a variety of transcranial Doppler (TCD) tests and monitoring are performed in clinical practice.

TCD has been shown to provide diagnostic and prognostic information that determines patient management decisions in multiple cerebrovascular conditions and periprocedural/surgical monitoring [11, 12].

The consensus confirms the importance of standardized investigation and emphasizes the following aspects:

1. The examiner should follow the course of blood flow in each major branch of the circle of Willis.
2. Identify spectral waveforms at least at two key points per artery.
3. Middle cerebral artery (MCA) signals should be stored as proximal, mid, and distal.
4. VA signals may be stored at 40–50 and 60–70 mm.
5. Basilar artery (BA) signals can be stored as proximal, mid, and distal given the length and variability of velocities in these segments.

Table 5.1. Highlights of the guidelines of the European Federation of Neurological Societies

Domains	Class and level
Ultrasonography is the non-invasive screening technique indicated for the study of vessels involved in causing symptoms of carotid stenosis	Class IV, GCPP
Transcranial Doppler (TCD) is useful for screening for intracranial stenosis and occlusion in patients with cerebrovascular disease	Class II, level B
Transcranial Doppler is very useful for monitoring arterial reperfusion after thrombolysis of acute middle cerebral artery (MCA) occlusions	Class II, level B
Clinical studies have suggested that continuous TCD monitoring in patients with acute MCA occlusion treated with intravenous thrombolysis may improve both early recanalization and clinical outcome	Class II, level A
The presence of embolic signals with carotid stenosis predicts early recurrent stroke risk	Class II, level A
Even in asymptomatic patients, TCD is the only imaging technique that allows detection of circulating emboli	Class II, level A
Asymptomatic embolization is common in acute stroke, particularly in patients with carotid artery disease. In this group the presence of embolic signals has been shown to predict the combined stroke and transient ischemic attack (TIA) risk and more recently the risk of stroke alone	Class II, level A

Source: Masdeu et al. [10]

6. Measure the highest velocity signals at each key point.

General characteristics of the investigation are as follows [13–17]:

- About 15% of patients cannot be examined by transcranial color-coded duplex Doppler (TCCD) because of the insufficient acoustic window. Identification rates decline with advancing age.
- The mean velocity analysis is not enough to identify intracranial vessel abnormalities. It must be combined with other parameters such as asymmetry, segmental elevations, spectral analysis, and knowledge of extracranial circulation.
- Either flow velocities (frequency-based TCCD) or the integrated power of the reflected signal (power TCCD) can be coded. The power TCCD does not display information on the flow direction.
- Flow velocities are determined by spectral Doppler sonography using the color Doppler image as a guide to the correct positioning of the Doppler sample volume.
- The angle correction should only be applied to velocity measurements when the sample volume can be located in a straight vessel segment of at least 2 cm length.
- Flow velocities in the arterial as well as in the venous system are higher in women than in men, and decrease with age, whereas the pulsatility index increases.
- Intracranial stenosis: local increase in the peak systolic flow velocities, post-stenotic flow disturbances with low frequency and high-intensity Doppler signals.
- The intracranial vessel is occluded if the color signal is absent in one segment, while other vessels and parenchymal structures can be correctly visualized.
- The accuracy of ultrasound for detecting intracranial stenosis is summarized in Table 5.2.
- The use of contrast material increases the sensitivity and specificity and only 4% of examinations are inconclusive because of insufficient bone windows.
- After application of echo-contrast enhancing agents (ECE) the diagnostic confidence of TCCD for intracranial vessel occlusion is similar to that of magnetic resonance angiography.
- In an acute stroke study the ability of duplex ultrasound to diagnose main stem arterial occlusions within the anterior circulation was between 50% and 60% of studied vessels in unenhanced TCCD but reached 80–90% after intravenous contrast administration.
- The diagnostic strength of contrast-enhanced TCCD can be the highly specific identification of a normal intracranial arterial status. Therefore, if an experienced sonographer detects no abnormalities by using TCCD in a patient with sufficient bone windows, no more imaging is needed.

Table 5.2. Highlights of the American Academy of Neurology recommendations

		Sensitivity (%)	Specificity (%)
Intracranial steno-occlusive disease	• Anterior circulation	70–90	90–95
	• Posterior circulation occlusion	50–80	80–96
	• MCA	85–95	90–98
	• ICA, VA, BA	55–81	96
	TCD is probably useful **(Type B, Class II–III)** for the evaluation of occlusive lesions of intracranial arteries in the basal cisterns (especially the ICA siphon and MCA) The relative value of TCD compared with MR angiography or CT angiography remains to be determined **(Type U)** Data are insufficient to recommend replacement of conventional angiography with TCD **(Type U)**		
Cerebral thrombolysis	• Complete occlusion	50	100
	• Partial occlusion	100	76
	• Recanalization	91	93
	TCD is probably useful for monitoring thrombolysis of acute MCA occlusions **(Type B, Class II–III)**. More data are needed to assess the frequency of monitoring for clot dissolution and enhanced recanalization and to influence therapy **(Type U)**		
Cerebral microemboli detection	TCD monitoring is probably useful for the detection of cerebral microembolic signals in a variety of cardiovascular/cerebrovascular disorders/procedures **(Type B, Class II–IV)**. Data do not support the use of this TCD technique for diagnosis or monitoring response to antithrombotic therapy in ischemic cerebrovascular disease **(Type U)**		
TCCS	TCCS is possibly useful **(Type C, Class III)** for the evaluation and monitoring of space-occupying ischemic MCA infarctions. More data are needed to show if it has value vs. CT and MRI scanning and if its use affects clinical outcomes **(Type U)**		
Contrast-enhanced TCCS	(CE)-TCCS may provide information in patients with ischemic cerebrovascular disease and aneurysmal subarachnoid hemorrhage (SAH) **(Type B, Class II–IV)**		
	Its clinical utility vs. CT scanning, conventional angiography, or non-imaging TCD is unclear **(Type U)**		

Type A: established as useful/predictive or not useful/predictive for the given condition in the specified population.
Type B: probably useful/predictive or not useful/predictive for the given condition in the specified population.
Type C: possibly useful/predictive or not useful/predictive for the given condition in the specified population.
Type U: data inadequate or conflicting; given current knowledge, test/predictor unproven.
Class I: evidence provided by prospective study in broad spectrum of persons with suspected condition, using a "gold standard" to define cases, where test is applied in blinded evaluation, and enabling assessment of appropriate tests of diagnostic accuracy.
Class II: evidence provided by prospective study in narrow spectrum of persons with suspected condition or well-designed retrospective study of broad spectrum of persons with suspected condition (by "gold standard") compared to broad spectrum of controls where test is applied in blinded evaluation and enabling assessment of appropriate tests of diagnostic accuracy.
Class III: evidence provided by retrospective study where either persons with established condition or controls are of narrow spectrum, and where test is applied in blinded evaluation.
Class IV: any design where test is not applied in blinded fashion OR evidence provided by expert opinion or descriptive case series.
Source: Sloan *et al.* [14].

• A correctly performed TCD investigation also provides valuable information about the vascular status of the ICA. The presence of collaterals and delayed flow acceleration on TCD usually indicates a hemodynamically significant lesion (>80% ICA stenosis or occlusion).
• The investigation should start on the presumably non-affected side (road map! clinical symptoms).

Table 5.3. Velocity values for ultrasound grading of intracranial stenosis

Stenosis	≥50%	50–80%	≥80%
Middle cerebral artery	≥155 cm/s	≥220	Distal M1/M2-MCA post-stenotic fp A1-ACA and/or P1/P2-PCA↑
Anterior cerebral artery	≥120	≥155	A2-ACA post-stenotic fp ipsilateral M1-MCA and/or contralat. A1↑
Posterior cerebral artery	≥100	≥145	Distal PCA post-stenotic fp ipsilateral M1-MCA↑
Basilar artery	≥100	≥140	Distal BA/PCA post-stenotic fp VA/proximal BA pre-stenotic fp
Vertebral artery	≥90	≥120	Distal VA/BA post-stenotic fp VA extracranial pre-stenotic fp

Fp: flow pattern, ↑ increased velocity as collateral sign.
Source: Modified from Baumgartner [15] and Valdueza *et al.* [16].

- The sonographer looks for a focal velocity rise in a circumscribed vessel segment, and differences between the affected and non-affected sides, extending more than 30 cm/s.
- If a pathological finding is present, the proximal and distal vessel segments should also be evaluated.
- Occlusions are characterized by missing color and Doppler flow signals at the site of the occlusion or reduced flow signals in vessel segments proximal to the occlusion.

MCA stenosis

Stenoses of the M1-MCA can be graded according to flow velocity, turbulence, and asymmetry into mild, moderate, and high-grade stenoses and all detectable MCA segments should be insonated [14–16].

MCA occlusion

Depending on the location of the occlusion, the Doppler spectrum may be completely absent or reduced. If there is a proximal M1-MCA occlusion no flow signal is seen. In occlusions of the middle part of the MCA, a small orthograde flow with increased pulsatility may be present. In distal M1-MCA occlusion a reduced flow velocity is present with variable pulsatility depending on the presence of a temporal branch.

Distal MCA occlusion, e.g. of a relevant M2-MCA branch or more than one M2 branch, will result in a reduced flow with low velocities and a marked bilateral asymmetry.

Stenosis and occlusion in posterior circulation

Again the typical clinical symptoms of vertebrobasilar insufficiency should orient the sonographer. Alteration of flow velocities and turbulence, at least 30 cm/s flow velocity difference between the right and left sides, may also be useful. A proximal posterior cerebral artery (PCA) occlusion can be diagnosed by absent flow signal. Vertebral stenoses can be diagnosed by flow velocity, profile disturbances, and pre- and post-stenotic flow patterns. Velocity values for mild and severe stenosis are given in Table 5.3. Flow signals in VA occlusion strongly depend on the site of the occlusion, mainly on their relation to the origin of the posterior inferior cerebellar artery (PICA) (proximal or distal). Occlusions distal to the PICA origin will result in mild to moderate flow alterations of the extracranial VA, mainly depending on its diameter and its former relevance in the posterior circulation [16].

Basilar artery stenosis and occlusion

Transforaminal and transtemporal insonation allows the investigation of the total length of the BA. The most distal segment of the BA may be better insonated transtemporally, but the visualization of the distal part of the BA appears to be difficult even using ECE.

Occlusions are difficult to assess and diagnostic certainty depends on the site of the occlusion. A proximal BA occlusion will always result in pre-stenotic flow alterations of both extracranial VAs [16]. Therefore, apparently normal VA and proximal BA velocities are not sufficient to exclude top of the basilar occlusion.

However, as this cannot exclude the presence of, for example, a fragmented thrombus, ultrasound should always be used together with other diagnostic tools such as CTA, MRA, or DSA in presumed BA pathology.

The highlights of the recommendation of the American Academy of Neurology [14] summarize the accuracy of TCD in intracranial steno-occlusive disorders (Table 5.2).

With transcranial color-coded duplex sonography (TCCD), using low frequencies to penetrate the skull, most intracranial stenoses and occlusions can be detected by combining velocity analysis with other parameters. With the use of echo-contrast enhancing agents (ECE), the sensitivity and specificity can be increased and the diagnostic confidence of contrast-enhanced TCCD for intracranial vessel occlusion can reach that of magnetic resonance angiography.

Fast-track neurovascular ultrasound examination

Recently, a practical algorithm has been published for urgent bedside neurovascular ultrasound examination with carotid/vertebral duplex and TCD in patients with acute stroke [18].

Using such a protocol, urgent TCD studies can be completed and interpreted quickly at the bedside. The expanded fast-track protocol for combined carotid and transcranial ultrasound testing in acute cerebral ischemia is shown in Table 5.4. Below, we highlight the most important details of the algorithm.

The choice of fast-track insonation steps is determined by the clinical localization of ischemic arterial territory. For example, if patients present with MCA symptoms, the insonation begins with the non-affected side. This is followed by locating the MCA on the affected side, with insonation starting at the mid-M1-MCA depth range, usually 50–58 mm. The waveforms and systolic flow acceleration are compared to the non-affected side. If a normal MCA flow is found, the distal MCA segments are insonated (range 40–50 mm); this is followed by proximal MCA and ICA bifurcation assessment (range 60–70 mm) [18]. The non-invasive vascular ultrasound evaluation (NVUE) in patients with acute ischemic stroke has a high yield and accuracy in diagnosing lesions amenable to interventional treatment (LAIT). The ultrasound screening criteria for LAIT are shown in Table 5.5.

TCD has the highest sensitivity (>90%) for acute arterial obstructions located in the proximal MCA and ICAs. TCD has modest sensitivity for posterior circulation lesions if performed without TCCD or contrast enhancement (Table 5.2). However, with a completely normal spectral TCD, there is less than 5% chance that an urgent angiogram will show any acute obstruction [19].

While TCD demonstration of an arterial occlusion helps to determine the ischemic nature of acute focal neurological deficits, a normal TCD result would support a lacunar mechanism.

In summary, bedside ultrasound in acute stroke may identify thrombus presence, determine thrombus location(s), assess collateral supply, find the worst residual flow signal, and monitor recanalization and re-occlusion.

A practical algorithm has been elaborated for urgent bedside neurovascular ultrasound examination with carotid/vertebral duplex and transcranial Doppler in patients with acute stroke.

Emboli monitoring and acute stroke

TCD identifies microembolic signs (MES) in intracranial circulation. The ultrasound distinguishes signal characteristics through embolic materials – solid or gaseous – from erythrocyte flow velocity. Microembolic signals appear as signals of high intensity and short duration within the Doppler spectrum as a result of their different acoustic properties compared to the circulating blood.

A microembolus signal is visible on TCD registration of ACA (Figure 5.2).

MES have been proven to represent solid or gaseous particles within the blood flow. They occur at random within the cardiac cycle and they can be acoustically identified by a characteristic "chirp" sound. Detection of MES can identify patients with stroke or TIA likely to be due to embolism. Potential applications of MES detection include determining the pathophysiology of cerebral ischemia, identifying patients at increased risk for stroke who may benefit from surgical and pharmacological intervention, assessing the effectiveness of novel antiplatelet therapies, and perioperative monitoring to prevent intra- and postoperative stroke.

The methodology includes simultaneous monitoring of both MCAs for at least 30 minutes, with fixed transducers in order to reduce movement artifacts. With two possible embolic sources – cardiogenic and carotid plaque – the identification of MES contributes higher diagnosis accuracy and support for therapy decision-making. MES detection, in addition, acts as a predictor for new cerebral ischemic event recurrence [19–23].

Table 5.4. Fast-track neurovascular ultrasound examination

Use portable devices with bright display overcoming room light. Stand behind patient headrest. Start with TCD because acute occlusion responsible for the neurological deficit is likely to be located intracranially. Extracranial carotid/vertebral duplex may reveal an additional lesion often responsible for intracranial flow disturbance. Fast-track insonation steps follow clinical localization of patient symptoms.

A. Clinical diagnosis of cerebral ischemia in the anterior circulation

    STEP 1: Transcranial Doppler
1. If time permits, begin insonation on the non-affected side to establish the temporal window, normal MCA waveform (M1 depth 45–65 mm, M2 30–45 mm) and velocity for comparison with the affected side.
2. If short on time, start on the affected side: first assess MCA at 50 mm. If no signals detected, increase the depth to 62 mm. If an anterograde flow signal is found, reduce the depth to trace the MCA stem or identify the worst residual flow signal. Search for possible flow diversion to the ACA, PCA, or M2 MCA. Evaluate and compare waveform shapes and systolic flow acceleration.
3. Continue on the affected side (transorbital window). Check flow direction and pulsatility in the OA at depths 40–50 mm followed by ICA siphon at depths 55–65 mm.
4. If time permits or in patients with pure motor or sensory deficits, evaluate BA (depth 80–100 mm) and terminal VA (40–80 mm).

    STEP 2: Carotid/vertebral duplex
1. Start on the affected side in transverse B-mode planes followed by color or power-mode sweep from proximal to distal carotid segments. Identify CCA and its bifurcation on B-mode and flow-carrying lumens.
2. Document if ICA (or CCA) has a lesion on B-mode and corresponding disturbances on flow images. In patients with concomitant chest pain, evaluate CCA as close to the origin as possible.
3. Perform angle-corrected spectral velocity measurements in the mid-to-distal CCA, ICA and external carotid artery.
4. If time permits or in patients with pure motor or sensory deficits, examine cervical portion of the vertebral arteries (longitudinal B-mode, color or power mode, spectral Doppler) on the affected side.
5. If time permits, perform transverse and longitudinal scanning of the arteries on the non-affected side.

B. Clinical diagnosis of cerebral ischemia in the posterior circulation

    STEP 1: Transcranial Doppler
1. Start suboccipital insonation at 75 mm (VA junction) and identify BA flow at 80–100 mm.
2. If abnormal signals present at 75–100 mm, find the terminal VA (40–80 mm) on the non-affected side for comparison and evaluate the terminal VA on the affected side at similar depths.
3. Continue with transtemporal examination to identify PCA (55–75 mm) and possible collateral flow through the posterior communicating artery (check both sides).
4. If time permits, evaluate both MCAs and ACAs (60–75 mm) for possible compensatory velocity increase as an indirect sign of basilar artery obstruction.

    STEP 2: Vertebral/carotid duplex ultrasound
1. Start on the affected side by locating CCA using longitudinal B-mode plane, and turn transducer downward to visualize shadows from transverse processes of midcervical vertebrae.
2. Apply color or power modes and spectral Doppler to identify flow in intratransverse VA segments.
3. Follow VA course to its origin and obtain Doppler spectra. Perform similar examination on other side.
4. If time permits, perform bilateral duplex examination of the CCA, ICA and external carotid artery as described above.

OA = ophthalmic artery.
Source: Reproduced with permission from Chernyshev *et al.* [17].

At present, monitoring of microembolisms is useful for patients with non-defined acute ischemic stroke, and for determining which is of probable cardio- or carotid-embolic etiology.

Simultaneous monitoring for MES in different vessels may help identify the active embolic source (cardiac? carotid?). Simultaneous monitoring above (i.e. MCA) and below (i.e. CCA) an ICA stenosis is

Table 5.5. Ultrasound screening criteria for lesions amenable for intervention

Lesion location	TCD criteria (at least one present)	CD criteria
M1/M2 MCA	*Primary:* TIBI grades 0–4 (absent, minimal, blunted, dampened, or stenotic) at depths <45 mm (M2) and 45–65 mm (M1) *Secondary:* Flow diversion to ACA, PCA, or M2 Increased resistance in ipsilateral TICA Embolic signals in MCA Turbulence, disturbed flow at stenosis Nonharmonic and harmonic covibrations (bruit or pure musical tones)	Extracranial findings may be normal or may show decreased ICA velocity on the side of the lesion
TICA	*Primary:* TIBI grades 0–4 at 60–70 mm Increased velocities suggest anterior cross-filling or collateral flow in posterior communicating artery *Secondary:* Embolic signals in unilateral MCA Blunted unilateral MCA, MFV >20 cm/s	Decreased ICA velocity unilateral to lesion or normal extracranial findings
Proximal ICA	*Primary:* Increased flow velocities suggest anterior cross-filling through ACommA or collateral flow through PCommA Reversed OA Delayed systolic flow acceleration in or blunted ipsilateral MCA, MFV >20 cm/s *Secondary:* Embolic signals in unilateral MCA Normal OA direction due to retrograde filling of siphon	B-mode evidence of a lesion in ICA ± CCA; Flow imaging evidence of no flow or residual lumen ICA >50% stenosis PSV >125 cm/s EDV >40 cm/s ICA/CCA PSV ratio >2 ICA near-occlusion or occlusion Blunted, minimal, reverberating, or absent spectral Doppler waveforms in ICA
Tandem ICA/ MCA stenosis/ occlusion	*Primary:* TIBI grades 0–4 and: Increased velocities in contralateral ACA, MCA, or unilateral PCommA or: Reversed unilateral OA	B-mode evidence of a lesion in ICA ± CCA; or: Flow imaging evidence of residual lumen or no flow ICA >50% stenosis PSV >125 cm/s EDV >40 cm/s ICA/CCA PSV ratio >2

Table 5.5. *(cont.)*

Lesion location	TCD criteria (at least one present)	CD criteria
	Secondary: Delayed systolic flow acceleration in proximal MCA or TICA Embolic signals in proximal MCA or TICA	ICA near-occlusion or occlusion Blunted, minimal, reverberating, or absent spectral Doppler waveforms in ICA
Basilar artery	*Primary:* TIBI flow grades 0–4 at 75–100 mm *Secondary:* Flow velocity increase in terminal VA and branches, MCAs, or PcommAs High resistance flow signals in VA(s) Reversed flow direction in distal basilar artery (85 mm)	Extracranial findings may be normal or showing decreased VA velocities or VA occlusion
Vertebral artery	*Primary (intracranial VA occlusion):* TIBI flow grades 0–4 at 40–75 mm *Primary (extracranial VA occlusion)* Absent, minimal, or reversed high resistance flow signals in unilateral terminal VA *Secondary:* Embolic signals increased velocities or low pulsatility in contralateral VA	Extracranial findings may be normal (intracranial VA lesion) or showing decreased VA velocities or VA occlusion

TICA = terminal internal carotid artery; TIBI = thrombolysis in brain infarction; MFV = mean flow velocity; ACommA = anterior communicating artery; PCommA = posterior communicating artery; OA = ophthalmic artery; EDV = end-diastolic velocity; CD = cervical duplex.
Source: Reproduced with permission from Chernyshev *et al.* [18].

another possible way of differentiating between artery-to-artery and cardiogenic embolism.

The frequency of MES in acute stroke shows a wide range, from 10% to 70%, probably due to different therapies, different criteria for MES detection, or different elapsed times after stroke. Some investigators used single registration, others serial measurements. The incidence of MES is maximal in the first week after stroke. The occurrence of MES showed more prevalence in completed stroke than in patients with TIA, and in symptomatic than asymptomatic hemispheres and a discrete subcortical or cortical pattern of infarction on computed tomography (CT) compared with a hemodynamic or small-vessel pattern.

Some authors have demonstrated that MES occur predominantly in patients with large-vessel territory stroke patterns and cases of artery-to-artery or cardiogenic embolism with persisting deficit. In contrast, MES are only occasionally detected in patients with small-vessel infarctions.

In addition, TCD monitoring may help to discriminate between different potential sources of embolism (i.e. artery-to-artery or cardioembolic strokes). Different types of emboli (i.e. cardiac or carotid) have different acoustic properties and ultrasonic characteristics, based on composition and size, which could permit differentiation.

MES detection by TCD in carotid endarterectomy (CEA) candidates may allow identification of a particularly high-risk group of patients who merit an early intervention or, if this is not possible, more aggressive antithrombotic therapy. The Clopidogrel and Aspirin for Reduction of Emboli in Symptomatic Carotid Stenosis Study (CARESS) also revealed that the combination of clopidogrel and aspirin was associated with a marked reduction in MES, compared with aspirin alone (e.g. clopidogrel + aspirin versus aspirin) [24].

A recent meta-analysis confirmed the usefulness of MES detection by TCD sonography. MES are a frequent finding in varying sources of arterial brain

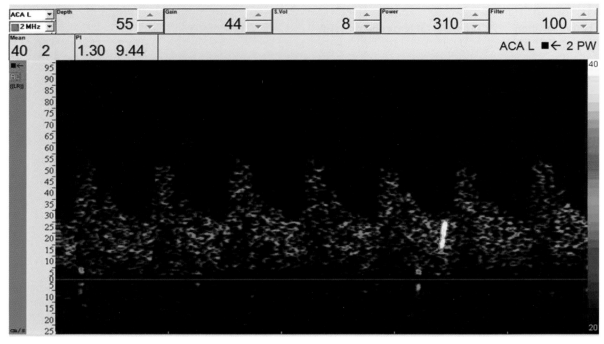

Figure 5.2. A microembolus signal visible on transcranial Doppler registration of anterior cerebral artery.

embolism and MES detection is useful for risk stratification in patients with carotid stenosis [25].

Numerous studies, including a prospective observational one (asymptomatic carotid emboli study
[ACES]), proved that TCD can be used to identify
patients who are at a higher risk of stroke and TIA.
The meta-analyses of ACES with previous studies
confirmed the association of embolic signals with
future risk of ipsilateral stroke and TIA [26].

> TCD identifies MES (microembolic signs) in
> intracranial circulation. Detection of MES can identify
> patients with stroke or TIA likely to be due to
> embolism, acts as a predictor for new cerebral
> ischemic event recurrence, and can influence therapy
> decision-making.

Diagnostic brain perfusion imaging in stroke patients

The availability of new ultrasound contrast agents
(UCAs) and the development of contrast-specific
imaging modalities have established the application
of ultrasound in stroke patients for visualization of
brain perfusion deficits. The UCAs consist of microbubbles composed of a gas that is associated with

various types of shells for stabilization. Because
of their small size, they can pass through the microcirculation. There are interactions between ultrasound and microbubbles: at low ultrasound energies
UCA microbubbles produce resonance, emitting
ultrasound waves at multiples of the insonated fundamental frequency.

The new microbubbles (e.g. SonoVue) generate a
nonlinear response at low acoustic power without
destruction, thus being particularly suitable for real-
time imaging. Harmonic imaging differentiates
echoes from microbubbles from those coming from
tissue. The insonated tissue responds at the fundamental frequency, while resonating microbubbles
cause scattering of multiples of the fundamental frequency – the harmonic frequencies.

Real-time visualization of middle cerebral artery infarction

Perfusion harmonic imaging after SonoVue bolus
injection can be used in patients with acute stroke.
In the early phase of acute ischemic stroke, bolus
imaging after SonoVue injection is useful for analyz-
ing cerebral perfusion deficits at the patient's bedside.

The ultrasound imaging data correlate well with the definite area of infarction and outcome after ischemic stroke. Ultrasound perfusion imaging (UPI) with SonoVue has allowed measurements not only in ischemic stroke but also in intracerebral hemorrhages, due to a characteristic reduction of contrast reaching the lesion.

The real-time UPI can detect hemodynamic impairment in acute MCA occlusion and subsequent improvement following arterial recanalization. This offers the chance for bedside monitoring of the hemodynamic compromise (e.g. during therapeutic interventions such as systemic thrombolysis [27]). In spite of continuous effort, perfusion imaging in acute stroke is still in the experimental phase [28–31].

> New ultrasound contrast agents (UCAs) that can pass through the microcirculation and the development of contrast-specific imaging modalities make it possible to use ultrasound for the visualization of brain perfusion deficits.

Prognostic value of ultrasound in acute stroke

During recent years, ultrasound has become an important non-invasive imaging technique for bedside monitoring of acute stroke therapy and prognosis. By providing valuable information on temporal patterns of recanalization, ultrasound monitoring may assist in the selection of patients for additional pharmacological or interventional treatment. Ultrasound also has an important prognostic role in acute stroke. A prospective, multicenter, randomized study confirmed that a normal MCA finding is predictive of a good functional outcome in more than two-thirds of subjects. After adjustment for age, neurological deficit on admission, CT scan results, and pre-existing risk factors, ultrasound findings remained the only independent predictor of outcomes [32].

The analysis of flow signal changes during thrombolysis acquired by TCD further confirmed the prognostic value of transcranial ultrasound. Acute arterial occlusion is a dynamic process since a thrombus can propagate and break up, thereby changing the degree of arterial obstruction and affecting the correlation between TCD and angiography.

A complete occlusion should not produce any detectable flow signals. However, in reality, some residual flow around the thrombus is often present. The Thrombolysis in Brain Ischemia (TIBI)

flow-grading system was developed to evaluate residual flow non-invasively and monitor thrombus dissolution in real time [33]:

- Grade 0: absent flow.
- Grade 1: minimal flow.
- Grade 2: blunted flow.
- Grade 3: dampened flow.
- Grade 4: stenotic flow.
- Grade 5: normal flow.

(TIBI 0 and 1 refer to proximal occlusion, TIBI 2 and 3 to distal occlusion, and TIBI 4 to recanalization.)

Applying these criteria in acute stroke the TIBI classification correlates with initial stroke severity, clinical recovery, and mortality in patients treated with recombinant tissue plasminogen activator (rtPA). The grading system can be used also to analyze recanalization patterns.

The waveform changes ($0 \rightarrow 5$) correlate well with clinical improvement and a rapid arterial recanalization is associated with better short-term improvement, whereas slow flow improvement and dampened flow signals are less favorable prognostic signs [33].

Even incomplete or minimal recanalization determined 24 hours after stroke onset results in more favorable outcome compared with persistent occlusion [34].

Reperfusion is important for prognosis. Both partial and full early reperfusion led to a lesser extent of neurological deficits irrespective of whether this occurred early or in the 6- to 24-hour interval.

Progressive deterioration after stroke due to cerebral edema, thrombus propagation, or hemodynamic impairment is closely linked to extra- and intracranial occlusive disease. TCCD is also useful for the evaluation of combined intravenous (i.v.)–intra-arterial (i.a.) thrombolysis. Patients receiving combined i.v.–i.a. thrombolysis show greater improvement in flow signal and higher incidence of complete MCA recanalization compared with those receiving i.v. thrombolysis, especially when the MCA was occluded or had only minimal flow [35].

Patients with distal MCA occlusion are twice as likely to have a good long-term outcome as patients with proximal MCA occlusion. Patients with no detectable residual flow signals as well as those with terminal ICA occlusions are least likely to respond early or long term. The distal MCA occlusions are more likely to recanalize with i.v. rtPA therapy; terminal ICA occlusions were the least likely to recanalize or have clinical recovery with i.v. rtPA compared with other occlusion locations [36].

Alexandrov et al. [37] described the patterns of the speed of clot dissolution during continuous TCD monitoring: sudden recanalization (abrupt normalization of flow velocity in a few seconds), stepwise recanalization as a progressive improvement in flow velocity lasting less than 30 minutes, and slow recanalization as a progressive improvement in flow velocity lasting more than 30 minutes. Sudden recanalization reflects rapid and complete restoration of flow, while stepwise and slow recanalization indicate proximal clot fragmentation, downstream embolization, and continued clot migration. Sudden recanalization was associated with a higher degree of neurological improvement and better long-term outcome than stepwise or slow recanalization.

A tandem ICA/MCA occlusion independently predicted a poor response to thrombolysis in patients with a proximal MCA clot, but not in those with a distal MCA clot [38].

> Ultrasound has an important prognostic role in acute stroke and can be used to monitor thrombus dissolution during thrombolysis.

Ultrasound accelerated thrombolysis and microbubbles

TCD can be used not only for diagnostic and prognostic purposes, but also for therapy. The ultrasound enhances the enzymatic thrombolysis, increasing the transport of rtPA into the thrombus and improving the binding affinity, and provides a unique opportunity to detect the recanalization during and after rtPA administration.

Continuous monitoring with 2 MHz TCD in combination with standard i.v. rtPA therapy results in significantly higher recanalization rate or dramatic recovery than i.v. rtPA therapy without TCD monitoring. In the CLOTBUST trial, 126 patients were randomly assigned to receive continuous TCD monitoring or placebo in addition to i.v. rtPA. Complete recanalization or dramatic clinical recovery within 2 hours after the administration of a rtPA bolus occurred in 49% of the target group as compared to 30% in the control group (P = 0.03). Only 4.8% of patients developed symptomatic intracerebral hemorrhage. These results showed the positive effects of 2 MHz continuous TCD monitoring in acute stroke, with no increase in the rate of intracerebral hemorrhage [39].

Recently, combining rtPA, ultrasound, and gaseous microbubbles showed signs of further enhancing arterial recanalization. Although these microbubbles, previously known as diagnostic microbubbles or gaseous microspheres, were originally designed to improve conventional ultrasound images, facilitation of thrombolysis is now emerging as a new treatment application for this technology. Newer-generation bubbles use specific phospholipid molecules that, when exposed to mechanical agitation, arrange themselves in nanobubbles with a consistent 1–2 μm (or even less) diameter. When injected intravenously, nanobubbles carry gas through the circulation. As the bubbles approach and permeate through the thrombus, they can be detected and activated by the ultrasound energy. Upon encountering an ultrasound pressure wave, the phospholipid shell breaks up and releases gas. The result is bubble-induced cavitation with fluid jets that erode the thrombus surface. In the presence of rtPA, this erosion increases the surface area for thrombolytic action and accelerates lysis of clots [40]. Recent studies evaluated the effects of administration of microbubbles on the initial MCA recanalization during systemic thrombolysis and continuous 2 MHz pulsed-wave TCD monitoring. The complete recanalization rate was significantly higher in the rtPA + ultrasound + microbubbles group (55%) than in the rtPA/ultrasound (41%) and rtPA (24%) groups [40] with no increase in symptomatic intracranial hemorrhage after systemic thrombolysis.

A Cochrane analysis indicated that sonothrombolysis produces a significant increase of recanalization rate associated with a non-significant increase of hemorrhagic transformation of the cerebral infarction [41]. There was also a statistically significant clinical improvement at the three-month follow-up in terms of death plus disability rate.

The concomitant use of microbubbles and ultrasound may increase the frequency of asymptomatic and symptomatic cerebral hemorrhage, but the small size of the evaluated population means that these conclusions are not reliable.

The use of any sonothrombolysis plus rtPA versus rtPA alone allowed a statistically significant reduction of death plus disability rate at 3 months in the sonothrombolysis group in comparison to rtPA alone, but with a wide confidence interval.

A significant improvement in the recanalization rate (any degree) was also attained. However, the incidence of cerebral hemorrhage increased, although this result was not statistically significant [40]. The Cochrane analysis [41] urges further investigations with sonothrombolysis, similarly to the statement of the 2013 American Heart Association/American Stroke Association (AHA/ASA) guideline "the effectiveness of sonothrombolysis for treatment of patients with acute stroke is not well established (*Class IIb; Level of Evidence B*)" [5]

> Arterial recanalization can be enhanced by combining rtPA with ultrasound, and even further with gaseous microbubbles, which increase the surface area for the thrombolytic action of rtPA, but further investigations are necessary.

Vasomotor reactivity

Vasomotor reactivity or cerebrovascular reactivity (CVR) describes the ability of the cerebral circulation to respond to vasomotor stimuli; the changes in cerebral blood flow (velocity in TCD studies) in response to such stimuli can be studied by TCD. CO_2 is a widely used agent to measure cerebral vasomotor reactivity. Another widely used agent is i.v. acetazolamide (0.15 mg/kg).

CO_2 results in vasodilatation and increased cerebral blood flow velocity. Measuring vasomotor reactivity requires standard experimental conditions. Markus *et al.* [42] described a simple measurement of the MCA velocity in response to 30 seconds breath-holding and termed it the breath-holding index (BHI):

$$BHI = \frac{MFV_{end} - MFV_{baseline}}{MFV_{baseline}} \times \frac{100}{\text{seconds of breath-holding}}$$

(MFV: mean flow velocity).

Others [43] evaluated BHI in different studies and showed that impaired vasomotor reactivity can help to identify patients at higher risk of stroke. Decreased vasomotor reactivity suggests failure of collateral flow to adapt to the stenosis. Various studies using different provocative measures for assessing cerebral vasomotor reactivity have demonstrated a remarkable ipsilateral event rate of approx. 30% risk of stroke over 2 years.

A recent international multicenter study did not find any association between impaired CVR and recurrent vascular events. Meta-analysis of available

data suggested an association between impaired CVR and future risk. However, currently there are insufficient data to justify the routine clinical use of CVR [44].

> The changes in cerebral blood flow in response to vasomotor stimuli can be studied by TCD.

Right-to-left shunt detection

Right-to-left shunts, particularly a patent foramen ovale (PFO), are common in the general population, with a prevalence of 10–35% in various echocardiography and autopsy studies for PFO. The prevalence is even higher in cryptogenic stroke or TIA and especially in younger patients without an apparent etiology. Contrast-enhanced TCD can be used for detecting the high-intensity transient signals (HITS) passing through the MCA, thus indicating the presence of a right-to-left shunt. The results of contrast-enhanced TCD have been compared with those of contrast-transesophageal echo and found to have a sensitivity and specificity of 68–100% and 67–100%, respectively [45]. Other studies with TCD and transesophageal echocardiography (TEE) proved the strength of TCD in PFO detection and right-to-left (RLS) quantification [46, 47]. Advantages of TCD include calibrated Valsalva maneuver and the ability to change body positioning during the test. The TCD "bubble" test for right-to-left shunt is superior to transthoracic echocardiography, and possibly TEE.

> Contrast-enhanced TCD can also be used to identify patients with a patent foramen ovale.

Sickle-cell disease (SCD)

Children with SCD have a significant risk of stroke before the age of 20 years from a stenosis or occlusion of the distal ICAs and proximal MCAs. Several studies have demonstrated that children with this disease should be monitored with serial TCD evaluations as TCD can be used to identify children with SCD at an increased risk of stroke. The Stroke Prevention in Sickle Cell Disease (STOP) trial evaluated children who had velocities of >200 cm/s in one or both of the MCAs or terminal ICAs at baseline TCD. They were randomized to either blood transfusion or standard care. Greater than 90% relative risk reduction in stroke incidence could be seen in the treated population [48]. The recent American guideline dealing with the primary stroke prevention recommends the use of TCD for selecting SCD children for transfusion therapy. Children with SCD should be screened with TCD starting at age 2 years (Class I; Level of Evidence B) [49].

Chapter summary

Doppler ultrasonography is the primary non-invasive test for evaluating carotid stenosis.

The sonographic characteristics of symptomatic and asymptomatic carotid plaques are different: symptomatic plaques are more likely to be hypo-echoic and highly stenotic, while asymptomatic plaques are hyperechoic and moderately stenotic. The degree of stenosis is better measured on the basis of the waveform and spectral analysis. When no stenosis is present, blood flow is laminar. With greater stenosis, the flow becomes turbulent. An important general rule for ultrasound is the greater the degree of stenosis, the higher the velocity.

Most studies consider carotid stenosis of 60% or greater to be clinically important.

Commonly used methods to estimate stenosis with ultrasonography are:
- Peak systolic velocities:
    - Normal: ICA PSV <125 cm/s, no plaque or intimal thickening.
    - <50% stenosis: ICA PSV <125 cm/s and plaque or intimal thickening.
    - 50–69% stenosis: ICA PSV is 125–230 cm/s and plaque is visible.
    - >70% stenosis to near occlusion: ICA PSV >230 cm/s and visible lumen narrowing.
    - Near occlusion: a markedly narrowed lumen on color Doppler ultrasound.
    - Total occlusion: no detectable patent lumen is seen on grayscale ultrasound, and no flow is seen on spectral, power, and color Doppler ultrasound.
- Ratios of the maximal systolic flow velocity within the ICA stenosis to the maximal systolic flow velocity within the non-affected CCA:
    - <50% stenoses ICA/CCA: <2.0.
    - 50–69% stenoses ICA/CCA: 2.0–4.0.
    - ≥70% stenoses ICA/CCA: >4.0.

Ratios may be particularly helpful in situations in which cardiovascular factors (e.g. poor ejection fraction) limit the increase in velocity.

Velocity measurements in a stenosis (PSV and carotid ratio) alone are not sufficient to differentiate a moderate from a severe (≥70% NASCET) stenosis.

Additional criteria refer to the effect of a stenosis on pre-stenotic flow (common carotid artery), the extent of post-stenotic flow disturbances, and derived velocity criteria (diastolic peak velocity and the carotid ratio).

With ultrasound, the intimal-medial thickness (IMT) of the carotid artery can be measured. Increases in the IMT of the carotid artery are associated with an increased risk of myocardial infarction and stroke.

In case of hemodynamically significant ICA stenosis or occlusion (proximal to the origin of the ophthalmic artery) a reversed (extra → intracranial) flow can be detected in the ophthalmic artery. Occlusion results in a complete absence of color-flow signal in ICA, and the diagnosis can be confirmed by ultrasound contrast agents (UCAs).

Intracranial stenosis and occlusion corresponds to approximately 8–10% of acute ischemic stroke.

Transcranial color-coded duplex sonography (TCCD) combines the imaging of intracranial vessels and parenchymal structures. To penetrate the skull, TCCD uses low frequencies (1.75–3.5 MHz), which limit the spatial resolution. Some patients cannot be examined because of an insufficient acoustic window. The duplex mode of TCCD enables sampling of vessels and Doppler measurements of angle-corrected blood-flow velocities. Mean velocity analysis is not enough to identify intracranial vessel abnormalities. It must be combined with other parameters such as asymmetry, segmental elevations, spectral analysis, and knowledge of extracranial circulation. The use of echo-contrast enhancing agents (ECE) increases the sensitivity and specificity and with ECE the diagnostic confidence of TCCD for intracranial vessel occlusion is similar to that of magnetic resonance angiography.

Recently, a practical algorithm has been published for urgent bedside neurovascular ultrasound examination.

Sonography in acute stroke of the anterior cerebral circulation.

- Technical requirements: extracranial and transcranial duplex, supplemented by Doppler if necessary (e.g.supratrochlear artery)
- Course of examination: color-coded visualization of the ipsilateral internal carotid artery and middle cerebral artery (MCA) with Doppler spectrum, supported by signal enhancers if necessary. In case of a suspected proximal

occlusion of the MCA, color-coded visualization of the other ipsilateral and contralateral arteries of the cerebral circle in the same acoustic window. In case of a suspected distal occlusion of the MCA or its branches, angle-oriented determination of the blood-flow velocity in the proximal MCA. In case of unclear situations, also sonographic detection of the supratrochlear artery and the common carotid artery comparing the two sides.

With a completely normal spectral TCD, there is less than 5% chance that an urgent angiogram will show any acute obstruction.

TCD identifies microembolic signs (MES) in the intracranial circulation. Detection of MES can identify patients with stroke or TIA likely to be due to embolism and, in addition, acts as a predictor for new cerebral ischemic event recurrence. TCD monitoring may help to discriminate between different potential sources of embolism (i.e. artery-to-artery or cardio-embolic strokes). Different types of emboli (i.e. cardiac or carotid) have different acoustic properties and ultrasonic characteristics, based on composition and size, which could permit differentiation. MES detection by TCD in carotid endarterectomy (CEA) candidates may allow identification of a particularly high-risk group of patients who merit an early intervention or, if this is not possible, more aggressive antithrombotic therapy.

New UCAs that can pass through the microcirculation and the development of contrast-specific imaging modalities make it possible to use ultrasound for the visualization of brain perfusion deficits. But perfusion imaging in acute stroke is still in the experimental phase.

Ultrasound has an important prognostic role in acute stroke and can be used to monitor thrombus dissolution during thrombolysis. The waveform changes correlate well with clinical improvement and a rapid arterial recanalization is associated with better short-term improvement, whereas slow flow improvement and dampened flow signals are less favorable prognostic signs.

TCD can be used not only for diagnostic and prognostic purposes, but also for therapy. The ultrasound enhances enzymatic thrombolysis, increasing the transport of rtPA into the thrombus and improving the binding affinity, and provides a unique opportunity to detect recanalization during and after rtPA administration. Arterial recanalization can be further enhanced by combining rtPA, ultrasound, and gaseous microbubbles. Newer-generation bubbles permeate through the thrombus and erode the thrombus surface, which increases the surface area for the thrombolytic action of rtPA.

The changes in cerebral blood flow in response to vasomotor stimuli can be studied by TCD. Decreased vasomotor reactivity suggests failure of collateral flow to adapt to a stenosis and can help identify patients at higher risk of stroke.

Contrast-enhanced TCD can also be used to identify patients with a patent foramen ovale.

TCD can further help in clinical decision-making by

- monitoring during CEA and thus reducing perioperative complications due to cerebral hypoperfusion– if flow velocity in the MCA velocity decreases by more than 30% on carotid cross-clamping
- detecting microembolism during release of carotid cross-clamps
- identifying the possibility of cerebral hyperperfusion syndrome if MCA velocities increase by more than 1.5 times pre-cross-clamp values and last more than 30 seconds after release of carotid cross-clamps
- monitoring sickle-cell disease children to determine those suitable for receiving transfusion therapy.

Acknowledgement

The author is very grateful for the help and advice of Professor Manfred Kaps in preparing the manuscript.

References

1. Silver B. Carotid ultrasound. http://emedicine.medscape.com/article/1155193-overview. Updated: 15 Dec 2008.

2. Grant EG, Benson CB, Moneta GL, *et al.* Carotid artery stenosis: grayscale and Doppler ultrasound diagnosis – Society of Radiologists in Ultrasound consensus conference. *Ultrasound Q* 2003; **19**(4):190–8.

3. Nadalo LA, Walters MC. Carotid artery, stenosis: imaging. http://emedicine.medscape.com/article/417524-imaging.

4. von Reutern GM, Goertler MW, Bornstein NM, *et al.* Grading carotid stenosis using ultrasonic methods. *Stroke* 2012; **43**(3):916–21.

5. Jauch EC, Saver JL, Adams HP Jr, *et al.* Guidelines for the early management of patients with acute ischemic stroke: a guideline for healthcare professionals from the American Heart Association/American

Stroke Association. *Stroke* 2013; **44**(3):870–947.

6. Cao JJ, Thach C, Manolio TA, *et al*. C-reactive protein, carotid intima-media thickness, and incidence of ischemic stroke in the elderly: the Cardiovascular Health Study. *Circulation* 2003; **108**(2):166–70.

7. Roman MJ, Naqui TZ, Gardin MJ, *et al*. Clinical application of non-invasive vascular ultrasound in cardiovascular risk stratification: A report from the American Society of Echocardiography and the Society of Vascular Medicine and Biology. *Am Soc Echocardiogr* 2006; **19**:943–54.

8. Touboul PJ, Hennerici MG, Meairs S, *et al*. Mannheim carotid intima-media thickness and plaque consensus (2004–2006–2011). *Cerebrovasc Dis* 2012; **34**:290–6.

9. Silvestrini M, Altamura C, Cerqua R, *et al*. Ultrasonographic markers of vascular risk in patients with asymptomatic carotid stenosis. *J Cereb Blood Flow Metab* 2013; **33**(4):619–24.

10. Masdeu JC, Irimiaa P, Asenbaumb S, *et al*. EFNS guideline on neuroimaging in acute stroke. Report of an EFNS task force. *Eur J Neurol* 2006; **13**:1271–83.

11. Alexandrov AV, Sloan MA, Wong LK, *et al*. American Society of Neuroimaging Practice Guidelines Committee. Practice standards for transcranial Doppler ultrasound: part I–test performance. *J Neuroimaging* 2007; **17**(1):11–18.

12. Alexandrov AV, Sloan MA, Tegeler CH, *et al*. Practice standards for transcranial Doppler (TCD) ultrasound. Part II. Clinical indications and expected outcomes. *J Neuroimaging* 2012; **22**(3):215–24.

13. Zipper SG, Stolz E. Clinical application of transcranial colour-coded duplex sonography–a review. *Eur J Neurol* 2002; **9**:1–8.

14. Sloan MA, Alexandrov AV, Tegeler CH, *et al*. Assessment transcranial Doppler ultrasonography report of the therapeutics and technology assessment subcommittee of the American Academy of Neurology. *Neurology* 2004; **62**:1468–81.

15. Baumgartner RW. Transcranial color-coded duplex sonography. *J Neurol* 1999; **246**(8):637–47.

16. Valdueza JM, Schreiber SJ, Roehl JE, Klingebiel R. *Neurosonology and Neuroimaging of Stroke*. Stuttgart: Thieme; 2008.

17. Gerriets T, Goertler M, Stolz E, *et al*. Feasibility and validity of transcranial duplex sonography in patients with acute stroke. *J Neurol Neurosurg Psychiatry* 2002; **73**:17–20.

18. Chernyshev OY, Garami Z, Calleja S, *et al*. Yield and accuracy of urgent combined carotid-transcranial ultrasound testing in acute cerebral ischemia. *Stroke* 2005; **36**:32–7.

19. Sharma VK, Venketasubramanian N, Khurana DK, Tsivgoulis G, Alexandrov AV. Role of transcranial Doppler ultrasonography in acute stroke. *Ann Indian Acad Neurol* 2008; **11**:39–51.

20. Azarpazhooh MR, Chambers BR. Clinical application of transcranial Doppler monitoring for embolic signals. *J Clin Neurosci* 2006; **13**(8):799–810.

21. Segura T, Serena J, Castellanos M, *et al*. Embolism in acute middle cerebral artery stenosis. *Neurology* 2001; **56**:497–501.

22. Tegos TJ, Sabetai MM, Nicolaides AN, *et al*. Correlates of embolic events detected by means of transcranial Doppler in patients with carotid atheroma. *J Vasc Surg* 2001; **33**:131–8.

23. Del Sette M, Angeli S, Stara I, Finocchi C, Gandolfo C. Microembolic signals with serial transcranial Doppler monitoring

in acute focal ischemic deficit. A local phenomenon? *Stroke* 1997; **28**:1311–13.

24. Markus HS, Droste DW, Kaps M, *et al*. Dual antiplatelet therapy with clopidogrel and aspirin in symptomatic carotid stenosis evaluated using doppler embolic signal detection: the Clopidogrel and Aspirin for Reduction of Emboli in Symptomatic Carotid Stenosis (CARESS) trial. *Circulation* 2005; **111**:2233–40.

25. Ritter MA, Dittrich R, Thoenissen N, Ringelstein EB, Nabavi DG. Prevalence and prognostic impact of microembolic signals in arterial sources of embolism. A systematic review of the literature. *J Neurol* 2008; **255**(7):953–61.

26. Markus HS, King A, Shipley M, *et al*. Asymptomatic embolisation for prediction of stroke in the Asymptomatic Carotid Emboli Study (ACES): a prospective observational study. *Lancet Neurol* 2010; **9**(7):663–71.

27. Bolognese M, Artemis D, Alonso A, *et al*. Real-time ultrasound perfusion imaging in acute stroke: assessment of cerebral perfusion deficits related to arterial recanalization. *Ultrasound Med Biol*. 2013; **39**(5):745–52.

28. Della Martina A, Meyer-Wiethe K, Allemann E, Seidel G. Ultrasound contrast agents for brain perfusion imaging and ischemic stroke therapy. *J Neuroimaging* 2005; **15**:217–32.

29. Seidel G, Meyer-Wiethe K. Acute stroke: perfusion imaging. *Front Neurol Neurosci* 2006; **21**:127–39.

30. Meairs S. Contrast-enhanced ultrasound perfusion imaging in acute stroke patients. *Eur Neurol* 2008; **59**(Suppl 1):17–26.

31. Seidel G, Meyer-Wiethe K, Berdien G, *et al*. Ultrasound perfusion imaging in acute middle

cerebral artery infarction predicts outcome. *Stroke* 2004; **35**:1107–11.

32. Allendoerfer J, Goertler M, Reutern GM. Prognostic relevance of ultra-early doppler sonography in acute ischaemic stroke: a prospective multicentre study. *Lancet Neurol* 2006; **5**:835–40.

33. Demchuk AM, Burgin WS, Christou I, *et al.* Thrombolysis in brain ischemia (TIBI) transcranial Doppler flow grades predict clinical severity, early recovery, and mortality in patients treated with intravenous tissue plasminogen activator. *Stroke* 2001; **32**:89–93.

34. Baracchini C, Manara R, Ermani M, Meneghetti G. The quest for early predictors of stroke evolution: can TCD be a guiding light? *Stroke* 2000; **31**:2942–7.

35. Perren F, Loulidi J, Graves R, *et al.* Combined IV–intraarterial thrombolysis: a color-coded duplex pilot study. *Neurology* 2006; **67**:324–6.

36. Saqqur M, Uchino K, Demchuk AM, *et al.* Site of arterial occlusion identified by transcranial Doppler predicts the response to intravenous thrombolysis for stroke. *Stroke* 2007; **38**(3):948–54.

37. Alexandrov AV, Burgin SW, Demchuk AM, El-Mitwalli A, Grotta JC. Speed of intracranial clot lysis with intravenous tissue plasminogen activator therapy: sonographic classification and short-term improvement. *Circulation* 2001; **103**:2897–902.

38. Rubiera M, Ribo M, Delgado-Mederos R, *et al.* Tandem internal carotid artery/middle cerebral artery occlusion: an independent predictor of poor outcome after systemic thrombolysis. *Stroke* 2006; **37**:2301–5.

39. Alexandrov AV, Molina CA, Grotta JC, *et al.*; CLOTBUST Investigators. Ultrasound-enhanced thrombolysis for acute ischemic stroke. *N Engl J Med* 2004; **351**:2170–8.

40. Molina CA, Ribo M, Rubiera M, *et al.* Microbubbles administration accelerates clot lysis during continuous 2-MHz ultrasound monitoring in stroke patients treated with intravenous rtPA. *Stroke* 2006; **37**:425–9.

41. Ricci S, Dinia L, Del Sette M, *et al.* Sonothrombolysis for acute ischaemic stroke (Review). *The Cochrane Library* 2012, Issue 10. 1–35.

42. Markus HS, Harrison MJ. Estimation of cerebrovascular reactivity using transcranial Doppler, including the use of breath-holding as the vasodilatory stimulus. *Stroke* 1992; **23**:668–73.

43. Silvestrini M, Vernieri F, Pasqualetti P, *et al.* Impaired cerebral vasoreactivity and risk of stroke in patients with asymptomatic carotid stenosis. *JAMA* 2000; **283**:2122–7.

44. King A, Serena J, Bornstein NM, Markus HS; ACES Investigators. Does impaired cerebrovascular reactivity predict stroke risk in asymptomatic carotid stenosis? A prospective substudy of the asymptomatic carotid emboli study. *Stroke* 2011; **42**(6):1550–5.

45. Droste DW, Silling K, Stypmann J, *et al.* Contrast transcranial Doppler ultrasound in the detection of right-to-left shunts: time window and threshold in microbubble numbers. *Stroke* 2000; **31**:1640–5.

46. Belvis R, Leta RG, Marti-Fabregas J, *et al.* Almost perfect concordance between simultaneous transcranial Doppler and transesophageal echocardiography in the quantification of right-to-left shunts. *J Neuroimaging* 2006; **16**:133–8.

47. Jauss M, Zanette E. Detection of right-to-left shunt with ultrasound contrast agent and transcranial Doppler sonography. *Cerebrovasc Dis* 2000; **10**(6):490–6.

48. Adams RJ, McKie VC, Hsu L, *et al.* Prevention of a first stroke by transfusions in children with sickle cell anemia and abnormal results on transcranial Doppler ultrasonography. *N Engl J Med* 1998; **339**(1):5–11.

49. Goldstein LB, Bushnell CD, Adams RJ, *et al.* Guidelines for the primary prevention of stroke: a guideline for healthcare professionals from the American Heart Association/American Stroke Association. *Stroke* 2011; **42**(2):517–84.

Basic epidemiology of stroke and risk assessment

Jaakko Tuomilehto

Definition of stroke

In epidemiological studies, stroke is defined by clinical findings and symptoms [1]: rapidly developed signs of focal (or global) disturbance of cerebral function lasting more than 24 hours (unless interrupted by surgery or death), with no apparent cause other than a vascular origin. This approach is supplemented with neuroimaging but even with advanced imaging techniques the diagnosis is based on clinical signs. Therefore, precise definitions of clinical signs are needed. World Health Organization (WHO) definitions are [1]:

Definite focal signs:

- unilateral or bilateral motor impairment (including dyscoordination)
- unilateral or bilateral sensory impairment
- aphasis/dysphasis (non-fluent speech)
- hemianopia (half-sided impairment of visual fields)
- diplopia
- forced gaze (conjugate deviation)
- dysphagia of acute onset
- apraxia of acute onset
- ataxia of acute onset
- perception deficit of acute onset.

Not acceptable as sole evidence of focal dysfunction:

- dizziness, vertigo
- localized headache
- blurred vision of both eyes
- dysarthria (slurred speech)
- impaired cognitive function (including confusion)
- impaired consciousness
- seizures.

(Although strokes can present in this way, these signs are not specific and cannot therefore be accepted as definite evidence of stroke.)

Neuroimaging studies are needed for classification of stroke by subtypes: subarachnoid hemorrhage (SAH), intracerebral hemorrhage, and brain infarction (necrosis). Although there may be large variations in stroke subtype distributions between populations, thrombotic and embolic strokes are responsible for about 80–85% of all strokes in the Indo-European populations, and as low as 65% in some Asian populations. SAH represents 5–10% of all strokes, and may often occur in middle-aged people [2], while both intracerebral and especially thrombotic and embolic stroke events increase markedly with age.

The scope of the problem

Stroke is the second leading cause of death worldwide in the adult population, the first being coronary heart disease [3]. Of note, stroke is an increasing problem in low- and middle-income countries, where 87% of all stroke deaths occur [2–7]. Stroke is the fourth leading cause of disease burden (as measured in disability-adjusted life years [DALYs]) after heart disease, HIV/AIDS, and unipolar depressive disorders [3, 6]. In the 1990s, it caused about 4.4 million deaths worldwide in 1990, 5.4 million in 1999, and 5.7 million in 2004 [7, 8], with two-thirds of these deaths occurring in less-developed countries [3, 5–8]. While in high-income countries 9.9% of all deaths could be attributed to stroke, in low- and middle-income countries this proportion was 9.5%, almost equal; because the total number of deaths in low- and middle-income countries is much greater than in high-income countries, globally the highest burden of stroke is among people living in low- and middle-income countries.

DALYs due to stroke were 62.67 per million person-years in high-income countries, corresponding to 4.5% of the total DALYs, when the corresponding estimate for low- and middle-income countries was 9.35 per million person-years, and this translated to 6.3% of the total DALYs [7]. The recent estimate indicated that in the USA the cost of stroke (direct and indirect costs together) was $73.7 billion [9] in 2010.

Incidence, mortality, and case fatality

There are several issues related to the occurrence of stroke that are important from an epidemiological (and clinical) perspective. While it would be useful to know the *incidence* (occurrence of first stroke events), in most populations data may be available on *mortality* from stroke only, but not on non-fatal events. The *case fatality* at the stroke event, usually

determined as the proportion of deaths occurring during the first 4 weeks after the onset of stroke event, gives information about the severity of stroke and may also reflect the efficacy of early management of acute stroke. The relative frequency of different subtypes of stroke varies among populations, and in particular among different ethnic groups. This variation may be in part due to genetic differences or due to differences in risk-factor profiles.

A comparison of routinely collected stroke mortality data from many countries shows that, in general, mortality rates have declined over recent decades, most notably in Japan, Australia, North America, and Western Europe (Figure 6.1) [10]. Mortality from stroke was highest in the world in Finland in the 1970s, together with Japan [10–14]. The burden of stroke is particularly high in Eastern Europe, North Asia, Central Africa, and the South Pacific, with a 10-fold difference in stroke mortality and morbidity

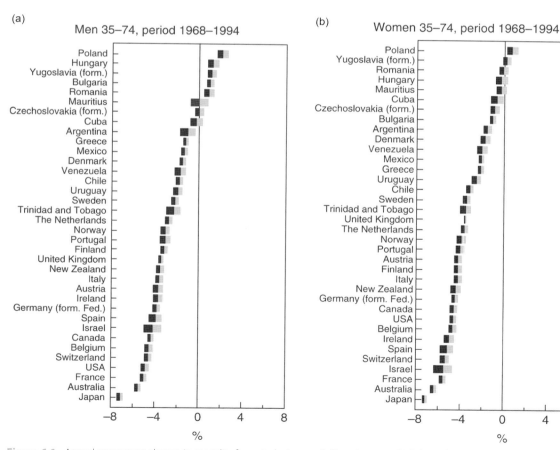

Figure 6.1. Annual percentage change in mortality from stroke in men (left) and women (right) aged 35–74 years in selected countries during the entire study period, 1968–1994. For source and copyright, see Sarti *et al*. [10].

Table 6.1. Top 20 and bottom 20 countries ranked by age-adjusted stroke mortality rates among 192 WHO member countries in 2002

	Country	Mortality (per 100 000)
1	Russia	251
2	Kyrgyzstan	237
3	Saint Kitts and Nevis	216
4	Kazakhstan	200
5	Albania	198
6	Georgia	198
7	Mongolia	195
8	Guyana	187
9	Sierra Leone*	179
10	Tuvalu*	173
11	Latvia	172
12	Haiti	172
13	Moldova	171
14	Angola*	169
15	Marshall Islands*	168
16	Liberia*	168
17	Kiribati	166
18	Macedonia	165
19	Uzbekistan	164
20	Democratic Republic of Congo	162
Median		111
173	El Salvador	42
174	Dominica	41
175	New Zealand	41
176	Netherlands	41
177	Sweden	40
178	Iceland	39
179	Belgium	39
180	Costa Rica	39
181	Spain	38
182	San Marino	36
183	Andorra*	34
184	Australia	33
185	Bahrain	33
186	USA	32
187	France	28
188	Monaco*	28
189	Canada	27
190	Israel	27
191	Switzerland	26
192	Seychelles	24

Rates rounded to nearest whole number.
* Mortality rates estimated from modelling.
Source and copyright, see Feigin et al. [6].

rates between the most affected and least affected countries [7]. For example, Russia's standardized stroke mortality rate is 251 per 100 000 compared with a rate of 32 per 100 000 in the United States [15]. The top 20 and bottom 20 countries ranked by age-adjusted stroke mortality rates among 192 WHO member countries in 2002 are shown in Table 6.1. The highest rate was found in Russia and also several other countries from the previous Soviet Union are among the top 20. There are also countries from Africa, Caribbean region, and Pacific islands. The lowest rate was seen in Seychelles and Switzerland. Most of the low mortality countries were found in Europe, and also in North and Central America, Australia, and New Zealand. In the global analysis, mortality rates were 3.5-fold higher in low-income countries than in middle-income and high-income countries; DALY loss rates were 3.8-fold higher in low-income countries than in middle-income and high-income countries. In the multivariable analysis, the association of stroke mortality rates with gross national income remained significant even after adjustment for national indicators of cardiovascular disease risk, with a 4% reduction in stroke mortality for every additional US$1000 in gross national income per capita (Table 6.2). Furthermore, national income was the strongest predictor in the multivariable model ($p < 0.0001$), others being mean systolic blood pressure ($p = 0.028$), prevalence of tobacco smoking ($p = 0.041$), and low body mass index (BMI) ($p = 0.017$).

There are few studies with validated data from stroke registers or other sources. The incidence of stroke has declined sharply in Finland during the last decades [12], and in 1998 it was 241/100 000, not far

Table 6.2. Univariate and multivariate prediction of age-adjusted stroke mortality in 192 countries

	n	Univariate		Multivariable	
		Relative risk (95% CI)	p	Relative risk (95% CI)	p
National income					
World Bank classification (per category)	188	0.71 (0.68–0.74)	<0.0001	..	..
Gross national income per capita (per US$1000)	164	0.96 (0.95–0.96)	<0.0001	0.96 (0.96–0.97)	<0.0001
Mean systolic blood pressure (per mmHg)	192	1.02 (1.00–1.03)	0.031	1.02 (1.00–1.03)	0.028
Diabetes prevalence (per%)	191	0.92 (0.89–0.95)	<0.0001	0.98 (0.94–1.02)	0.32
Tobacco smoking prevalence (per%)	129	0.99 (0.99–1.00)	0.16	1.01 (1.00–1.02)	0.041
Alcohol					
Per capita consumption (per L/year)	184	0.99 (0.97–1.00)	0.10	1.00 (0.98–1.02)	0.90
Drinking score (per index point)	141	1.34 (1.20–1.50)	<0.0001	1.05 (0.94–1.17)	0.38
Weight					
Mean BMI (per kg/m^3)	192	0.94 (0.92–0.97)	<0.0001	0.95 (0.91–0.99)	0.017
Prevalence of overweight (BMI ≥25, per%)	192	0.99 (0.99–0.99)	<0.0001	..	..
Prevalence of obesity (BMI ≥30, per%)	192	0.99 (0.98–0.99)	0.0004	..	..
Total serum cholesterol (mmol/L)	192	0.67 (0.59–0.76)	<0.0001	0.93 (0.78–1.11)	0.43

Data are based on negative binomial regression with age-adjusted analysis, including all measures for which relative risks are shown. BMI = body mass index. CI = confidence interval. .. = no data available.
Source and copyright, see Johnston *et al.* [7].

from other Western industrialized countries, after a steady fall of about 3% per year throughout the 15 years studied. Mortality from stroke declined even more steeply, around 4% per year, with a standardized mortality rate in 1998 of 50/100 000 among men and 30/100 000 among women [12]. Other countries that already had comparatively lower stroke incidence rates in the 1980s, for example New Zealand [15], the USA [16], or Denmark [17], have reported no fall in stroke incidence, while an increase in the incidence of stroke has been observed in Eastern Europe and Russia [2, 6, 7, 18–20]. In Shanghai, China, almost no decline in incidence of stroke but a clear decline in stroke mortality was reported [21]. The differences observed between countries in mortality rates, and even more in incidence rates, are, however, difficult to interpret, as they largely depend on the study design, the accuracy of the data collection, and the time point when the measurements were made.

The overall case fatality (the proportion of deaths among all strokes) is roughly 20% within the first month, and subsequently increases around 5% per year. There is, however, a large variation in case fatality of stroke among populations; in the WHO Monitoring of Trends and Determinants in Cardiovascular Disease (MONICA) Stroke Study among men, the case fatality of stroke ranged from 12% in northern Sweden to 53% in Moscow in Russia [18]. Overall, the case fatality was high in all eastern European countries. In women, the difference in case fatality of stroke between populations was larger than in men, ranging from 16% in Kuopio, Finland to 57% in Moscow.

In general, stroke mortality rates have declined over recent decades. The overall case fatality (the proportion of deaths among all strokes) is roughly 20% within the first month, and subsequently increases around 5% per year. Mortality rates were 3.5-fold higher in low-income countries than in middle-income and high-income countries.

Trends in stroke event rates, case fatality, and mortality of stroke

Table 6.3 shows the trends, separately for each MONICA population, in stroke event rates, case fatality, and mortality of stroke, both in the register and in routine mortality statistics [22]. Stroke event rates

Table 6.3. Age standardized stroke attack rate, case fatality, and mortality in the WHO MONICA Stroke Study populations

Country	Population	Attack Rate per 100 000		Case Fatality,%		Mortality Rate per 100 000	
		First 3 Years	Last 3 Years	First 3 Years	Last 3 Years	First 3 Years	Last 3 Years
	Men						
China	Beijing	248 (234–264)	241 (226–255)	27 (24–29)	26 (23–29)	67 (59–75)	63 (56–71)
Denmark	Glostrup	218 (197–241)	160 (143–179)	16 (12–20)	20 (15–25)	34 (26–44)	31 (24–40)
Finland	Kuopio	372 (340–407)	310 (292–340)	19 (16–23)	16 (13–20)	72 (58–88)	50 (39–63)
Finland	North Karelia	288 (254–325)	257 (226–290)	22 (17–28)	20 (15–25)	69 (53–89)	51 (38–68)
Finland	Turku/Loimaa	236 (209–267)	228 (201–257)	23 (18–29)	17 (12–21)	54 (41–70)	37 (27–50)
Italy	Friuli	129 (120–139)	121 (112–130)	35 (32–39)	24 (21–27)	46 (41–52)	29 (25–34)
Lithuania	Kaunas	309 (234–335)	347 (322–374)	23 (19–25)	24 (21–27)	69 (58–83)	84 (72–97)
Poland	Warsaw	171 (166–188)	171 (166–187)	52 (47–57)	40 (35–44)	88 (77–101)	69 (59–79)
Russia	Moscow (control)	270 (241–302)	216 (190–245)	32 (26–37)	53 (45–59)	86 (70–105)	111 (93–133)
Russia	Moscow (intervention)	249 (231–269)	237 (220–259)	38 (34–42)	51 (43–55)	96 (84–108)	122 (110–135)
Russia	Novosibirsk (intervention)	438 (382–500)	449 (409–500)	27 (21–33)	35 (30–40)	122 (93–159)	160 (132–192)
Sweden	Gothenburg	129 (115–145)	149 (133–165)	17 (13–21)	18 (14–22)	22 (17–29)	27 (21–34)
Sweden	Northern Sweden	221 (205–230)	219 (203–235)	16 (12–19)	12 (10–15)	35 (29–42)	26 (21–33)
Yugoslavia	Novi Sad	222 (198–248)	211 (190–233)	37 (31–42)	41 (36–47)	82 (68–98)	87 (74–102)
	Women						
China	Beijing	175 (163–188)	182 (160–195)	30 (27–34)	27 (24–31)	54 (47–61)	50 (43–58)
Denmark	Glostrup	99 (85–114)	90 (77–104)	19 (14–25)	22 (15–28)	20 (14–28)	19 (13–26)
Finland	Kuopio	189 (167–213)	130 (113–140)	27 (22–32)	16 (11–21)	48 (38–61)	21 (14–30)
Finland	North Karelia	124 (103–148)	117 (97–140)	23 (16–31)	20 (13–27)	29 (19–41)	23 (15–34)

Table 6.3. (cont.)

Country	Population	Attack Rate per 100 000		Case Fatality,%		Mortality Rate per 100 000	
		First 3 Years	Last 3 Years	First 3 Years	Last 3 Years	First 3 Years	Last 3 Years
Finland	Turku/Loimaa	117 (99–137)	108 (91–128)	24 (17–31)	24 (17–31)	29 (20–39)	27 (18–37)
Italy	Friuli	63 (57–70)	59 (53–65)	42 (37–47)	31 (26–36)	26 (22–30)	18 (15–22)
Lithuania	Kaunas	154 (139–170)	182 (166–199)	24 (19–28)	26 (22–30)	35 (28–44)	46 (38–55)
Poland	Warsaw	90 (79–101)	93 (83–104)	54 (48–60)	44 (38–49)	48 (40–56)	40 (33–47)
Russia	Moscow (control)	146 (129–165)	94 (79–110)	38 (31–44)	47 (30–55)	53 (43–65)	44 (35–56)
Russia	Moscow (intervention)	133 (122–145)	107 (98–118)	30 (35–44)	57 (52–68)	52 (45–60)	61 (54–69)
Russia	Novosibirsk (intervention)	341 (303–383)	391 (352–433)	25 (20–31)	23 (18–27)	87 (68–109)	82 (65–103)
Sweden	Gothenburg	71 (61–82)	72 (62–84)	24 (17–30)	25 (18–32)	17 (12–23)	18 (13–24)
Sweden	Northern Sweden	119 (107–132)	136 (123–150)	21 (17–25)	17 (13–20)	25 (20–31)	23 (18–20)
Yugoslavia	Novi Sad	114 (99–132)	127 (112–144)	49 (40–65)	42 (35–48)	55 (44–67)	53 (43–64)

Note: Values in parentheses are 95% CIs.
Source: Thorvaldsen *et al.* [18].

declined in 9 of 14 populations in men and 8 of 14 populations in women. In men, the case fatality of stroke declined in seven populations, increased in eight, and fluctuated only slightly in two. Among women, a decline in case fatality was seen in eight populations, no obvious change was seen in three, and an increase was observed in three. The trends in case fatality were statistically significant among men in only two populations with declining trends and in two with increasing trends. Among women, there was a significant downward trend in four populations. Within each population, the confidence intervals (CIs) for the case fatality trends were larger than those for the trends in stroke event rates. Of the 14 populations, stroke mortality declined in eight populations among men and 10 populations among women. Stroke mortality increased in all the eastern European populations except in Warsaw, Poland. In Beijing,

China and in the nine western European populations, stroke mortality declined.

Changes in incidence and improved survival on the downward trend in stroke mortality are not easy to quantify, due to the difficulty of measuring accurately the incidence of stroke. The MONICA Stroke Study, for example, compared stroke incidence (or more precisely attack rate, which included various proportions of recurrent strokes), mortality, and case fatality in 14 populations aged 35–64 years (mostly located in Europe except two – one in China and one in Novosibirsk in Asian Russia). The study confirmed the above observed trends in stroke incidence and mortality, and reported a large geographical variation also in case fatality. In most populations, changes in stroke mortality, whether declining or increasing, were principally attributable to changes in case fatality rather than changes in event rates [22]. Since only

107

limited advances in acute stroke care took place during that time, it is likely that the natural history of stroke events has changed and they have become less severe.

Feigin *et al.* carried out a systematic review of published stroke incidence studies from 1970 to 2008 [2]. They found adequate data from 47 centers in 28 countries. Over the four decades, age-adjusted stroke incidence rates in high-income countries decreased by 42% (from 163 per 100 000 person-years in 1970–1979 to 94 per 100 000 person-years in 2000–2008; p = 0.0004), whereas in low- to middle-income countries the stroke incidence rates more than doubled (52 per 100 000 and 117 per 100 000 person-years, respectively; p < 0.0001) and for the first time exceeded the rate observed in high-income countries in the last decade. The pattern of changes in stroke incidence rates in high-income and low-to middle-income countries corresponded to those reported in studies of international mortality trends, suggesting that changes in stroke mortality rates are most likely to be attributable to the corresponding changes in stroke incidence rates. Early stroke case fatality was decreasing in both high-income and low- to middle-income countries but, overall, early stroke case fatality in low- to middle-income countries in the past decade was 25% higher than early stroke case fatality in high-income countries.

Since the MONICA Stroke Study no proper multi-national comparison of stroke incidence has been organized. There are, however, data from a number of countries. The Swedish National Stroke Register, Riks-Stroke, has demonstrated that it is possible to develop a nationwide data collection system for acute stroke events [23]. Riks-Stroke is the world's longest-running national stroke quality register (established in 1994) and includes all 76 hospitals in Sweden admitting acute stroke patients and it covers approximately 85% of all stroke events. In Canada, the Canadian Institute for Health Information's Hospital Morbidity Database that includes International Statistical Classification of Diseases (ICD) codes has been used to assess trends in hospital admissions and in-hospital case fatality for stroke [24]. The age- and sex-standardized rate of hospital admissions decreased 28% for stroke but case fatality decreased only 9% during 1994 to 2004. The average annual rate of decline in stroke mortality was about 3%. In Finland the national Hospital Discharge Register has been used to evaluate the outcome of stroke patients [13].

During 1999 to 2007 stroke outcome in Finland has improved as length-of-stay in hospital decreased for ischemic stroke patients. Acute treatment has become more specialized, which was shown to be associated with improved patient outcome. Nevertheless, a significant portion of Finnish stroke patients still did not receive optimal care. The situation is likely to be similar in other countries. In the USA, stroke mortality fell by 33.5% from 1996 to 2006, with the total number of stroke deaths declining by 18.4% [9]. The previously set goal of a 25% reduction was exceeded in 2008. A study from Dublin, Ireland, in 2005–2006 found the crude incidence of 165 per 100 000 person-years for first-ever stroke and 28 for recurrent stroke, and 45 for first-ever transient ischemic attack (TIA) [25]. Age-adjusted stroke rates in Dublin were higher than those reported earlier in nine other recent population-based samples from high-income countries. Data from Oxfordshire [26] and London, UK [27], and from Beijing, Shanghai, and Changsha, China [28], suggest that the implementation of preventive treatments and decreases in risk factors at the population level have contributed to the significant fall in stroke incidence. On the other hand, the data from Belarus during 2001–2003 confirmed that the stroke incidence in eastern Europe is higher than in western Europe [28].

> The MONICA Stroke Study compared stroke incidence (or more precisely attack rate, which included various proportions of recurrent strokes), mortality, and case fatality in 14 populations aged 35–64 years. After the MONICA Stroke Study no proper multinational comparison of stroke incidence has been organized but various nationwide registers have been established, e.g. in Sweden (Riks-Stroke), Canada, Finland, the USA, and Ireland.

Risk factors for stroke

Stroke has a multifactorial origin and a plethora of putative and confirmed risk factors have been listed and tested in various types of studies. The assessment of the global epidemiology is severely hindered by the lack of any kind of data on stroke occurrence and risk factors in most populations in the world. Although over 65% of all deaths due to stroke occur in developing countries, studies of stroke epidemiology in these populations hardly exist.

The American Heart Association Stroke Council's Scientific Statement Oversight Committee guideline has provided an overview of the evidence on various established and potential stroke risk factors and pro-posed recommendations for the reduction of stroke risk in 2006 [29] with an extensive update in 2011 [9]. The committee used systematic literature reviews published since 2001, reference to previously pub-lished guidelines, personal files, and expert opinions to summarize existing evidence on standard criteria. Risk factors or risk markers for a first stroke were classified according to their potential for modification (non-modifiable, modifiable, or potentially modifi-able) and strength of evidence (well-documented or less well-documented). Non-modifiable risk factors include age, sex, low birth weight, race/ethnicity, and genetic factors. Well-documented and modifiable risk factors include hypertension, exposure to cigar-ette smoke, diabetes, atrial fibrillation and certain other cardiac conditions, dyslipidemia, carotid artery stenosis, excessive alcohol drinking, sickle-cell disease, postmenopausal hormone therapy, poor diet, physical inactivity, and obesity and central body fat distribu-tion. Less well-documented or potentially modifiable risk factors include the metabolic syndrome, drug abuse, oral contraceptive use, sleep-disordered breathing, migraine headache, elevated gamma-glutamyl transferase, hyperhomocysteinemia, ele-vated lipoprotein(a), elevated lipoprotein-associated phospholipase, hypercoagulability, inflammation, and infection. This paper represents probably the most thorough assessment of the prediction and potential for the prevention of stroke.

> Well-documented and modifiable risk factors include hypertension, exposure to cigarette smoke, diabetes, atrial fibrillation and certain other cardiac conditions, dyslipidemia, carotid artery stenosis, excessive alcohol drinking, sickle-cell disease, postmenopausal hormone therapy, poor diet, physical inactivity, and obesity and central body fat distribution.

Non-modifiable risk factors of stroke

Age is probably the most important determinant of stroke; the risk of stroke doubles for each successive decade after age 55 years [30, 31]. This is also true for ischemic stroke, while the age relation of intracerebral hemorrhage is less steep and the peak age of SAH incidence is around 45–55 years. Stroke is a common disease in both men and women, but it is more common in men within the age range of 45–84 years [32–34].

Racial or ethnic specific stroke risk is difficult to interpret. While within a country such as the USA

clear ethnic group differences exist, African Americans [32, 34, 35] and some Hispanic Americans [36, 37] have higher stroke incidence and mortality rates as compared with European Americans, globally stroke mortality does not follow any ethnic patterns [38]. Nevertheless, it is well known that intracerebral bleed-ing is more common in oriental populations, and SAH is most common in Finland and Sweden [10, 39].

Both paternal and maternal history of stroke are associated with an increased stroke risk [9, 40–43]. It is not necessarily "stroke genes" that are behind this familial aggregation, but one or more mechanisms may contribute to it such as (i) familial occurrence of risk factors for stroke, (ii) genetic susceptibility to these risk factors, (iii) familial sharing of environ-mental/lifestyle factors associated with stroke, and (iv) the interaction between genetic and environmen-tal effects [41–43]. Currently, rapid advances in gen-etic research are taking place and have resulted in the identification of genes associated with stroke, and its subtypes. Low birth weight is another risk factor for stroke [44, 45], as it is for cardiovascular disease in general. Although these risk factors themselves cannot be modified, it does not mean that the stroke risk in such individuals could not be modified. In them, it is particularly important to pay attention to the control of modifiable risk factors.

There are several well-documented medical condi-tions and diseases that have importance as risk factors for stroke. These are described in Chapter 7. In this chapter, some general observations are made on life-style factors, and their relative importance for stroke incidence or recurrence is reported.

> Among the non-modifiable risk factors old age, racial or ethnic factors, low birth weight, and sometimes genetic susceptibility play a role. In individuals with non-modifiable risk factors, prevention focused on the modifiable ones is particularly important.

Overall lifestyle patterns and stroke risk

In the analysis of the data from the Health Profes-sionals Follow-up Study and from the Nurses' Health Study the impact on stroke risk of a combination of healthy lifestyle characteristics was evaluated and the burden of stroke that may be attributed to these unhealthy lifestyle choices was calculated [46]. Diet and other lifestyle factors were updated from self-reported questionnaires. A low-risk healthy lifestyle was defined as: (i) not smoking, (ii) a BMI $<25 \text{ kg/m}^2$,

(iii) ≥30 min/day of moderate activity, (iv) modest alcohol consumption (men, 5 to 30 g/day; women, 5 to 15 g/day), and (v) scoring within the top 40% of a healthy diet score. Women with all five low-risk factors had a relative risk of 0.21 for total and 0.19 for ischemic stroke compared with women who had none of these factors. Among men, the corresponding relative risks were 0.31 for total and 0.20 for ischemic stroke. Among women, 47% of total and 54% of ischemic stroke cases were attributable to lack of adherence to a low-risk lifestyle, and among men the corresponding proportions were 35% and 52%, respectively. Low-risk lifestyle was not significantly associated with risk of hemorrhagic stroke, nor was it in the Women's Health Study [47]. Other studies have also evaluated joint effects of multiple lifestyle-related risk profiles on stroke risk. In the German EPIC Potsdam study, almost 60% of ischemic stroke cases could be attributed to hypertension, diabetes, hypercholesterolemia, smoking, and heavy alcohol consumption (>15 g alcohol/day in women, >30 g alcohol/day in men) [48]. Stamler *et al.* found that a low-risk lifestyle, defined as cholesterol <200 mg/dl, blood pressure <120/80 mmHg, and not smoking, was associated with 52–76% lower risk of total stroke mortality [49]. In the Women's Health Study, women with the healthiest lifestyle score, defined as never smoking, having a BMI <22 kg/m^2, exercising ≥4 times a week, consuming 0.5 to 1.5 drinks a day, and following a healthy diet, had 71% lower risk of ischemic stroke compared with women with the least healthy lifestyle [47]. The recent analysis of the Finnish prospective study has confirmed these findings [50]. People who simultaneously practiced several healthy lifestyle habits (no smoking, non-obese, physically active, regular consumption of fruits and vegetables, and moderate alcohol drinking) had significantly reduced risk of stroke. The multivariate adjusted hazard ratios associated with adherence to 0 to 1 (reference group), 2, 3, 4, and 5 healthy lifestyle habits were 1, 0.67, 0.60, 0.50, and 0.30 for ischemic stroke; and 1, 0.63, 0.49, 0.49, and 0.40 for hemorrhagic stroke, respectively (Table 6.4). In addition, compared with hypertensive people who did not use antihypertensive drugs and adhered to ≥3 healthy lifestyle factors, the multivariable-adjusted hazard ratios in hypertensive people who used antihypertensive drugs and adhered to <3 healthy lifestyle factors were associated with 37–42% increased risks of total, ischemic, and hemorrhagic stroke in men and 121–131% increased risks of stroke in women. Thus,

a low-risk healthy lifestyle that is associated with a reduced risk of multiple chronic diseases also seems to be beneficial in the prevention of stroke, even in hypertensive people.

In the WHO MONICA Project, repeated population surveys of cardiovascular risk factors and continuous monitoring of stroke events were conducted in 35–64-year-old people over a 7–13-year period in 15 populations in nine countries. Stroke trends were compared with trends in individual risk factors and their combinations [51]. A 3–4-year time lag between changes in risk factors and change in stroke rates was considered. Population-level trends in systolic blood pressure showed a strong association with stroke event trends in women, but there was no association in men. In women, 38% of the variation in stroke event trends was explained by changes in systolic blood pressure. Combining trends in daily cigarette smoking, serum cholesterol, and BMI with systolic blood pressure into a risk score explained only a small additional fraction of the variation in stroke event trends.

> People who simultaneously practice several healthy lifestyle habits (no smoking, non-obese, physically active, regular consumption of fruits and vegetables, and moderate alcohol drinking) have a significantly reduced risk of stroke.

Prediction of stroke in patients with TIA

Ischemic stroke is often preceded by early symptoms, i.e. a TIA [52]. The risk of stroke after a TIA has been underestimated for many years due to issues in study designs [53, 54]. Hospital-based and population-based cohort studies have reported 7-day risks of stroke of up to 10% [55–60]. Models with predictors for long-term risk of stroke after TIA or minor stroke have been developed [55–58, 60–62]. A substantial international variation exists as to how patients with suspected TIA are managed in the acute phase. TIA carries a high risk of early recurrence especially within the first days. Patients who suffered a TIA lasting longer than 1 hour carry a very high risk of suffering a lasting stroke as opposed to those whose TIA lasted only a few minutes. Simple risk scores to assess high versus low stroke risk in TIA patients are clinically useful.

Rothwell *et al.* have developed and validated a simple risk score to predict stroke during the first 7 days after a TIA [63]. A six-point score derived (age [>60 years = 1], blood pressure [systolic

Table 6.4. Hazard ratios (HRs) of total, ischemic, and hemorrhagic stroke according to number of healthy lifestyle factors restricted to adiposity, smoking, physical activity, vegetable consumption, and alcohol consumption in the middle-aged Finnish population at baseline

Characteristic	Healthy Lifestyle Factors, No.					P Value for Trend
	0–1	2	3	4	5	
Total stroke						
Patients, No.	3976	9161	12 093	8713	2743	
Incidence cases, No.	326	480	449	195	28	
Person-years, No.	52 512	128 505	168 449	117 650	36 119	
Age and study years, adjusted HR (95% CI)	1 [Reference]	0.63 (0.55–0.73)	0.52 (0.45–0.60)	0.42 (0.35–0.50)	0.26 (0.18–0.38)	<.001
Model 1, HR (95% CI)[a]	1 [Reference]	0.65 (0.57–0.75)	0.56 (0.48–0.65)	0.47 (0.39–0.57)	0.30 (0.20–0.45)	<.001
Model 2, HR (95% CI)[b]	1 [Reference]	0.66 (0.58–0.76)	0.57 (0.50–0.66)	0.51 (0.42–0.61)	0.33 (0.23–0.50)	<.001
Ischemic stroke						
Incidence cases, No.	260	384	361	145	18	
Age and study years, adjusted HR (95% CI)	1 [Reference]	0.64 (0.55–0.75)	0.54 (0.46–0.63)	0.42 (0.34–0.51)	0.23 (0.14–0.37)	<.001
Model 1, HR (95% CI)[a]	1 [Reference]	0.66 (0.57–0.78)	0.58 (0.49–0.68)	0.47 (0.38–0.58)	0.27 (0.17–0.44)	<.001
Model 2, HR (95% CI)[b]	1 [Reference]	0.67 (0.57–0.79)	0.60 (0.51–0.70)	0.50 (0.41–0.62)	0.30 (0.18–0.49)	<.001
Hemorrhagic stroke						
Incidence cases, No.	66	97	88	50	10	
Age and study years, adjusted HR (95% CI)	1 [Reference]	0.62 (0.45–0.84)	0.46 (0.34–0.64)	0.44 (0.30–0.64)	0.34 (0.17–0.66)	<.001
Model 1, HR (95% CI)[a]	1 [Reference]	0.62 (0.46–0.85)	0.48 (0.34–0.66)	0.46 (0.31–0.67)	0.36 (0.18–0.71)	<.001
Model 2, HR (95% CI)[b]	1 [Reference]	0.63 (0.46–0.87)	0.49 (0.35–0.68)	0.49 (0.34–0.73)	0.40 (0.20–0.79)	<.001

[a] Model 1: adjusted for age, study year, education, and family history of stroke.
[b] Model 2: adjusted for age, sex, study year, education, family history of stroke, history of diabetes, systolic blood pressure, and total cholesterol.
Each lifestyle factor was dichotomized into unhealthy and healthy categories: smoking (current or ever vs. never), BMI (≥ 25 vs. <25 kg/m^2), physical activity (low vs. moderate or high), vegetable consumption (2 vs. 3 times per week), and alcohol consumption (none or 210 g/week in men and 140 g/week in women vs. 1–209 g/week in men and 1–139 g/week in women).
Source and copyright, see Zhang *et al.* [50].

≥ 140 mmHg and/or diastolic ≥ 90 mmHg $= 1$], clinical features [unilateral weakness $= 2$, speech disturbance without weakness $= 1$, other $= 0$], and duration of symptoms in minutes [$\geq 60 = 2$, $10–59 = 1$, $<10 = 0$]) was highly predictive of 7-day risk of stroke in patients with probable or definite TIA (p < 0.0001), in the Oxford Vascular Study population-based cohort of all referrals with suspected TIA (p < 0.0001), and in the hospital-based weekly TIA clinic-referred cohort (p = 0.006). In the suspected TIA cohort, 95% of strokes occurred in 101 (27%) patients with a score of 5 or greater: 7-day risk was 0.4% in 274 (73%)

patients with a score less than 5, 12.1% in 66 (18%) with a score of 5, and 31.4% in 35 (9%) with a score of 6. In the hospital-referred clinic cohort, 14 (7.5%) patients had a stroke before their scheduled appointment, all with a score of 4 or greater. The authors concluded that the risk of stroke during the 7 days after TIA seems to be highly predictable. While they call for further validations and refinements of this score, it is robust enough to be used in routine clinical practice to identify high-risk individuals in European populations who need emergency investigation and treatment.

Transient ischemic attacks (TIAs) carry a high risk of early recurrence especially within the first days. Patients who suffered a TIA lasting longer than 1 hour carry a very high risk of suffering a lasting stroke as opposed to those whose TIA lasted only a few minutes. Simple risk scores to assess high versus low stroke risk in TIA patients are clinically useful.

Prediction of stroke in the general population

Guidelines state that the level of stroke and cardiovascular risk should inform decision-making about initiating treatments such as aspirin or lipid-lowering agents [29]. These strategies are based on the observation that the respective relative risk reduction of aspirin and statin therapies is similar for most subpopulations, and therefore the absolute benefit of treatment is proportional to the absolute risk of stroke or coronary event. Because clinicians do not accurately estimate cardiovascular risk [64, 65] adhering to these guidelines requires the use of explicit risk calculators. Various multivariable models can be generated to estimate a person's risk for stroke in the populations where prospective studies have been carried out. On the other hand, only a few such attempts exist, while plenty of risk prediction scores for coronary heart disease have been developed. This imbalance is mainly due to the fact that most prospective studies of cardiovascular disease have been carried out in the middle-aged populations (men) in whom coronary heart disease is a more common outcome than stroke.

In addition, many risk prediction models have included mostly biological risk factors. It has been repeatedly pointed out that the major risk factors for coronary heart disease, stroke, peripheral vascular disease, type 2 diabetes, and certain types of cancer all share the same lifestyle background. The reason why one person gets a stroke and another one coronary heart disease or type 2 diabetes, etc. is not clear. Variations in genetic factors or interactions between lifestyle-related factors may provide some answers, but it is certainly not possible to make any use of such information for the individual risk assessment.

At least 110 stroke and cardiovascular disease risk scoring methods exist [66]. For stroke risk-assessment tools, complex interactions of risk factors and the effects of certain risk factors stratified by non-modifiable factors such as age, gender, ethnicity, and geography are incompletely captured by such tools. Some risk-assessment tools are gender-specific and give 1-, 5-, or 10-year stroke risk estimates. The Framingham Stroke Profile (FSP) uses a Cox proportional-hazards model with risk factors as covariates and points calculated according to the weight of the model coefficients [67–69]. Independent stroke predictors are shown in Table 6.5. The FSP is widely used, but its validity among various subgroups other than the Framingham cohort has not been adequately studied. Nevertheless risk-prediction tools based on clinical data have been developed [70, 71]. A comparison between two formats of the Framingham calculator suggests that the multivariate equation is more accurate than the approach based on points [72].

In a clinical setting, simple risk-assessment tools that have been developed for instance for type 2 diabetes [73] might be useful since they do not require any laboratory testing. Similar tools have now been developed for dementia [74], but unfortunately we do not have such a simple risk-assessment tool for stroke. Yet it is not difficult to design such given the large number of prospective studies using stroke as the outcome. In both men and women the FINDRISC predicted the stroke incidence well [75]. This avenue in risk assessment needs to be further pursued in order to identify people at risk of stroke as early as possible.

Electronic health records (EHRs) linked to administrative databases are increasingly used to derive and validate risk-prediction models [76]. For example, the Anticoagulation and Risk Factors in Atrial Fibrillation (ATRIA) study used 13 559 patients included in a clinical database of Kaiser Permanente of Northern California to predict the risk of warfarin-associated hemorrhage [77]. An advantage with EHRs is that they may facilitate a transition to a future in which patient- or clinician-selected risk scores are automatically calculated for clinicians to inform treatment decisions, and used by hospitals, accountable care organizations, and insurers for risk adjustment and the prioritization of high-cost interventions. Various health care systems may develop their own stroke-specific risk scores based on their own unique populations. Eventually EHR-linked databases that currently exist, but are rarely used for risk assessment, could be linked so that every person contributes in real time to the derivation and recalibration of risk calculators. Despite the power and flexibility of EHRs, substantial challenges hinder the translation of

Table 6.5. Framingham stroke risk profile

	Points										
	0	+1	+2	+3	+4	+5	+6	+7	+8	+9	+10
Men											
Age, years	54–56	57–59	60–62	63–65	66–68	69–72	73–75	76–78	79–81	82–84	85
Untreated systolic blood pressure, mmHg	97–105	106–115	116–125	126–135	136–145	146–155	156–165	166–175	176–185	186–195	196–205
Treated systolic blood pressure, mmHg	97–105	106–112	113–117	118–123	124–129	130–135	136–142	143–150	151–161	162–176	177–205
History of diabetes	No		Yes								
Cigarette smoking	No			Yes							
Cardiovascular disease	No				Yes						
Atrial fibrillation	No				Yes						
Left ventricular hypertrophy on electrocardiogram	No					Yes					
Women											
Age, years	54–56	57–59	60–62	63–64	65–67	68–70	71–73	74–76	77–78	79–81	82–84
Untreated systolic blood pressure, mmHg		95–106	107–118	119–130	131–143	144–155	156–167	168–180	181–192	193–204	205–216
Treated systolic blood pressure, mmHg		95–106	107–113	114–119	120–125	126–131	132–139	140–148	149–160	161–204	205–216
History of diabetes	No			Yes							
Cigarette smoking	No			Yes							
Cardiovascular disease	No		Yes								
Atrial fibrillation	No						Yes				
Left ventricular hypertrophy on electrocardiogram	No				Yes						

Modified from D'Agostino et al. [68].

improved predictive accuracy into clinical utility. Several important parameters may not be available in EHRs or they are not well standardized. Concerns on privacy issues exist. Numerical literacy on one's own risk estimate in the general population remains low. The science of clinical risk communication is still in its infancy and the ideal format and clinical setting to display and discuss vascular risk remains poorly understood.

> The use of explicit risk calculators such as the Framingham Stroke Profile (FSP) or FINDRISC help in decision-making about initiating treatments such as aspirin or lipid-lowering agents.

New risk factors for stroke

As many as 60–80% of ischemic stroke events can be attributed to high blood pressure, dyslipidemia, smoking, and diabetes, and also to atrial fibrillation and valvular heart disease (cardiogenic and embolic ischemic stroke) [78]. A review indicated that about 10–20% of atherosclerotic ischemic strokes can probably be attributed to recently established, probably causal risk factors for ischemic heart disease: raised ApoB/ApoA1 ratio, obesity, physical inactivity, psychosocial stress, and low fruit and vegetable intake [79]. However, their causal role remains to be proven. While the importance of genes predisposing to stroke cannot be denied [80, 81], the contribution of any single gene towards ischemic stroke is likely to be modest and to apply in selected patients only and in combination with environmental factors or via other epistatic (gene–gene or gene–environmental) effects.

Hankey proposed, based on the well-known Bradford Hill criteria on causality, a practical way to consider the causal significance of a risk factor for ischemic stroke [79]:

- Is there evidence from experiments in *humans*?
- Is the association between exposure to the risk factor and ischemic stroke shown by means of multiple variable regression analysis to be *independent* of other risk factors that may interact with the risk factor or be a confounding risk factor?
- Is the association *strong*?
- Is the association *consistent* from study to study?
- Is the *temporal relation* correct (exposure to the risk factor occurred before the stroke)?
- Is there a *dose–response relation* (increasing risk or severity of stroke associated with increasing dose or duration of exposure to the risk factor)?

- Is the association *biologically* plausible?
- Is the association *epidemiologically* plausible?
- Is there evidence that *reducing* exposure to the risk factor (e.g. by randomized controlled trials or large observational prospective studies) leads to a reduction in the risk of stroke?

It needs to be pointed out that certain issues such as smoking and alcohol drinking, and many other dietary factors, can never be properly tested in real life using a controlled trial design, and if such experiments would appear, they can only be considered as cross-sectional in a particular population. Therefore, it is very important to understand the inferences that can be drawn from various studies. Techniques such as meta-analysis will help, but only if the original studies were done properly and were comparable. Therefore, resources should not be allocated disproportionately to emerging novel risk factors that may account for up to only 20% of all strokes at the expense of researching the determinants of the relatively few established causal factors that account for up to 80% of all strokes. The evidence is strong to suggest that the control of the established risk factors for stroke will result in prevention of a very large number of stroke events and premature deaths.

Chapter summary

On a global scale, stroke is the second most frequent cause of mortality worldwide and a leading cause of disability. It is especially prevalent in low- and middle-income countries. The WHO Monitoring of Trends and Determinants in Cardiovascular Disease (MONICA) Stroke Study compared the stroke incidence (or more precisely attack rate), mortality, and case fatality in 14 populations aged 35–64 years in the 1980–1990s. The study confirmed the large geographical variation in stroke incidence and mortality, and also in case fatality. More recently, a few countries have systematically collected population-based incidence data for stroke. The relative frequency of different subtypes of stroke varies among populations, and in particular among different ethnic groups. This variation may be in part due to genetic differences or due to differences in risk-factor profiles. In most populations, changes in stroke mortality, whether declining or increasing, have been principally attributable to changes in case fatality rather than changes in event rates. In many epidemiological studies strokes have been defined without confirmation by neuroimaging. Definitions by clinical means alone can be imprecise and sometimes misleading. In general, stroke mortality rates have declined over recent decades. The overall case fatality (the proportion of deaths among all strokes) is roughly 20% within the first month, and subsequently increases around 5% per year. Large variations occur between countries both in stroke incidence, mortality, and case fatality. Mortality rates were 3.5-fold higher in low-income countries than in middle-income and high-income countries.

Stroke has a multifactorial origin and a plethora of putative and confirmed risk factors have been listed and tested in various types of studies. Well-known modifiable risk factors for stroke are virtually the same as those for cardiovascular disease in general: hypertension, smoking, dyslipidemia, diabetes, etc. Among non-modifiable risk factors old age, racial or ethnic factors, low birth weight, and genetic susceptibility play a role. In individuals with non-modifiable risk factors prevention focused on the modifiable ones is particularly important. Several prospective studies have shown that up to 70–80% of stroke events may be preventable, if people simultaneously adhere to several healthy lifestyle habits. Stroke risk assessment and prevention rely on risk profiles in a population. The Framingham Stroke Profile is widely used but hitherto has not been validated in many populations, but many other stroke risk scores have been developed in various populations.

A recent review indicated that about 10–20% of atherosclerotic ischemic strokes can probably be attributed to more recently established, probably causal risk factors for ischemic heart disease: raised ApoB/ApoA1 ratio, obesity, physical inactivity, psychosocial stress, and low fruit and vegetable intake. However, their causal role remains to be proven. While the importance of genes predisposing to stroke cannot be denied, the contribution of any single gene towards ischemic stroke is likely to be modest and apply in selected patients only and in combination with environmental factors or via other epistatic (gene–gene or gene–environmental) effects. The evidence is strong to state that the control of the established risk factors for stroke will result in prevention of a very large number of stroke events and premature deaths.

References

1. MONICA Manual, Part IV:Event Registration. Section 2: Stroke event registration data component. Office of Cardiovascular Diseases, World Health Organization; 1999 [cited 16 Oct 2008]. Available from: http://www.ktl.fi/publications/monica/manual/part4/iv-2.htm.

2. Feigin VL, Lawes CMM, Bennet DA, Parag V. Worldwide stroke incidence and early case fatality reported in 56 population-based studies: a systematic review. *Lancet Neurol* 2009; **8**:355–69.

3. Lopez AD, Mathers CD, Ezzati M, Jamison DT, Murray CJL. Global and regional burden of disease and risk factors, 2001: systematic analysis of population health data. *Lancet* 2006; **367**(9524):1747–57.

4. Strong K, Mathers C, Bonita R. Preventing stroke: saving lives around the world. *Lancet Neurol* 2007; **6**(2):182–7.

5. Beaglehole R, Ebrahim S, Reddy S, Voute J, Leeder S. Prevention of chronic diseases: a call to action. *Lancet* 2007; **370**(9605):2152–7.

6. Feigin VL, Lawes CM, Bennett DA, Anderson CS. Stroke epidemiology: a review of population-based studies of incidence, prevalence, and case-fatality in the late 20th century. *Lancet Neurol* 2003; **2**(1):43–53.

7. Johnston SC, Mendis S, Mathers CD. Global variation in stroke burden and mortality: estimates from monitoring, surveillance, and modeling. *Lancet Neurol* 2009; **8**:345–54.

8. Mathers C, Fat DM, Boerma JT. *The Global Burden of Disease: 2004 Update.* Geneva, Switzerland: World Health Organization; 2008.

9. Sacco RL, Kasner SE, Broderick JP, *et al.* An updated definition of stroke for the 21st century: a statement for healthcare professionals from the American Heart Association/American Stroke Association. *Stroke* 2013; **44**(7):2064–89.

10. Sarti C, Rastenyte D, Cepaitis Z, Tuomilehto J. International trends in mortality from stroke, 1968 to 1994. *Stroke* 2000; **31**(7):1588–601.

11. Mirzaei M, Truswell AS, Arnett K, *et al.* Cerebrovascular disease in 48 countries: secular trends in mortality 1950–2005. *J Neurol Neurosurg Psychiatry* 2012; **83**(2):138–45.

12. Sivenius J, Tuomilehto J, Immonen-Raiha P, *et al.* Continuous 15-year decrease in incidence and mortality of stroke in Finland: the FINSTROKE study. *Stroke* 2004; **35**(2):420–5.

13. Meretoja A, Kaste M, Roine RO, *et al.* Trends in treatment and outcome of stroke patients in Finland from 1999 to 2007. PERFECT Stroke, a nationwide register study. *Ann Med* 2011; **43**(Suppl 1):S22–30.

14. Liu L, Ikeda K, Yamori Y. Changes in stroke mortality rates for 1950 to 1997. A great slowdown of decline trend in Japan. *Stroke* 2001; **32**:1745–9.

15. Bonita R, Broad JB, Beaglehole R. Changes in stroke incidence and case-fatality in Auckland, New Zealand, 1981–91. *Lancet* 1993; **342**(8885):1470–3.

16. Derby CA, Lapane KL, Feldman HA, Carleton RA. Trends in validated cases of fatal and nonfatal stroke, stroke classification, and risk factors in southeastern New England, 1980 to 1991: data from the Pawtucket Heart Health Program. *Stroke* 2000; **31**(4):875–81.

17. Truelsen T, Prescott E, Gronbaek M, Schnohr P, Boysen G. Trends in stroke incidence. The Copenhagen City Heart Study. *Stroke* 1997; **28**(10):1903–7.

18. Thorvaldsen P, Asplund K, Kuulasmaa K, *et al.* Stroke incidence, case fatality, and mortality in the WHO MONICA Project. *Stroke* 1995; **26**:361–7.

19. Feigin VL, Wiebers DO, Whisnant JP, O'Fallon WM. Stroke incidence and 30-day case-fatality rates in Novosibirsk, Russia, 1982 through 1992. *Stroke* 1995; **26**(6):924–9.

20. Korv J, Roose M, Kaasik AE. Changed incidence and case-fatality rates of first-ever stroke between 1970 and 1993 in Tartu, Estonia. *Stroke* 1996; **27**(2):199–203.

21. Hong Y, Bots ML, Pan X, *et al.* Stroke incidence and mortality in rural and urban Shanghai from 1984 through 1991. Findings from a community-based registry. *Stroke* 1994; **25**(6):1165–9.

22. Sarti C, Stegmayr B, Tolonen H, *et al.* Are changes in mortality from stroke caused by changes in stroke event rates or case fatality? Results from the WHO MONICA Project. *Stroke* 2003; **34**(8):1833–40.

23. Asplund K, Hulter Åsberg K, Appelros P, *et al.* The Riks-Stroke story: building a sustainable national register for quality assessment of stroke care. *Int J Stroke* 2011; **6**(2):99–108.

24. Tu JV, Nardi L, Fang J, *et al.* National trends in rates of death and hospital admissions related to acute myocardial infarction, heart failure and stroke, 1994–2004. *CMAJ* 2009; **180**(13):E120–7.

25. Kelly PJ, Crispino G, Sheehan O, *et al.* Incidence, event rates, and early outcome of stroke in Dublin, Ireland: the North Dublin population stroke study. *Stroke* 2012; **43**:2042–7.

26. Rothwell PM, Coull AJ, Giles MF, *et al.* Change in stroke incidence, mortality, case-fatality, severity, and risk factors in Oxfordshire, UK from 1981 to 2004 (Oxford Vascular Study). *Lancet* 2004; **363**(9425):1925–33.

27. Heuschmann PU, Grieve A, Toschke AM, Rudd A, Wolfe CD. Ethnic group disparities in 10-year trends in stroke incidence and vascular risk factors: the South London Stroke Register (SLSR). *Stroke* 2008; **39**:2204–10.

28. Kulesh SD, Filina NA, Frantava NM, *et al.* Incidence and case-fatality of stroke on the East border of the European union. The Grodno Stroke Study. *Stroke* 2010; **41**:2726–30.

29. Goldstein LB, Adams R, Alberts MJ, *et al.*; American Heart Association; American Stroke Association Stroke Council. Primary prevention of ischemic stroke: a guideline from the American Heart Association/ American Stroke Association Stroke Council: cosponsored by the Atherosclerotic Peripheral Vascular Disease Interdisciplinary Working Group; Cardiovascular Nursing Council; Clinical Cardiology Council; Nutrition, Physical Activity, and Metabolism Council; and the Quality of Care and Outcomes Research Interdisciplinary Working Group. *Circulation* 2006; **113**(24):e873–923.

30. Brown RD, Whisnant JP, Sicks JD, O'Fallon WM, Wiebers DO. Stroke incidence, prevalence, and survival: secular trends in Rochester, Minnesota, through 1989. *Stroke* 1996; **27**(3):373–80.

31. Wolf PA, D'Agostino RB, O'Neal MA, *et al.* Secular trends in stroke incidence and mortality. The Framingham Study. *Stroke* 1992; **23**(11):1551–5.

32. Sacco RL, Boden-Albala B, Gan R, *et al.* Stroke incidence among white, black, and Hispanic residents of an urban community: the Northern Manhattan Stroke Study. *Am J Epidemiol* 1998; **147**(3):259–68.

33. Immonen-Raiha P, Sarti C, Tuomilehto J, *et al.* Eleven-year trends of stroke in Turku, Finland. *Neuroepidemiology* 2003; **22**(3):196–203.

34. Reeves MJ, Bushnell CD, Howard G, *et al.* Sex differences in stroke: epidemiology, clinical presentation, medical care, and outcomes. *Lancet Neurol* 2008; **7**(10):915–26.

35. Broderick J, Brott T, Kothari R, *et al.* The Greater Cincinnati/ Northern Kentucky Stroke Study: preliminary first-ever and total incidence rates of stroke among blacks. *Stroke* 1998; **29**(2):415–21.

36. Gorelick PB. Cerebrovascular disease in African Americans. *Stroke* 1998; **29**(12):2656–64.

37. Howard G, Anderson R, Sorlie P, *et al.* Ethnic differences in stroke mortality between non-Hispanic whites, Hispanic whites, and blacks. The National Longitudinal Mortality Study. *Stroke* 1994; **25**(11):2120–5.

38. Rosamond WD, Folsom AR, Chambless LE, *et al.* Stroke incidence and survival among middle-aged adults: 9-year follow-up of the Atherosclerosis Risk in Communities (ARIC) cohort. *Stroke* 1999; **30**(4):736–43.

39. Ingall T, Asplund K, Mahonen M, Bonita R. A multinational comparison of subarachnoid hemorrhage epidemiology in the WHO MONICA stroke study. *Stroke* 2000; **31**(5):1054–61.

40. Welin L, Svardsudd K, Wilhelmsen L, Larsson B, Tibblin G. Analysis of risk factors for stroke in a cohort of men born in 1913. *N Engl J Med* 1987; **317**(9):521–6.

41. Kiely DK, Wolf PA, Cupples LA, Beiser AS, Myers RH. Familial aggregation of stroke. The Framingham Study. *Stroke* 1993; **24**(9):1366–71.

42. Jousilahti P, Rastenyte D, Tuomilehto J, Sarti C, Vartiainen E. Parental history of cardiovascular disease and risk of stroke. A prospective follow-up of 14371 middle-aged men and women in Finland. *Stroke* 1997; **28**(7):1361–6.

43. Liao D, Myers R, Hunt S, *et al.* Familial history of stroke and stroke risk. The Family Heart Study. *Stroke* 1997; **28**(10):1908–12.

44. Barker DJ, Lackland DT. Prenatal influences on stroke mortality in England and Wales. *Stroke* 2003; **34**(7):1598–602.

45. Eriksson JG, Forsen T, Tuomilehto J, Osmond C, Barker DJ. Early growth, adult income, and risk of stroke. *Stroke* 2000; **31**(4):869–74.

46. Chiuve SE, Rexrode KM, Spiegelman D, *et al.* Primary prevention of stroke by healthy lifestyle. *Circulation* 2008; **118**(9):947–54.

47. Kurth T, Moore SC, Gaziano JM, *et al.* Healthy lifestyle and the risk of stroke in women. *Arch Intern Med* 2006; **166**(13):1403–9.

48. Weikert C, Berger K, Heidemann C, *et al.* Joint effects of risk factors for stroke and transient ischemic attack in a German population: the EPIC Potsdam Study. *J Neurol* 2007; **254**(3):315–21.

49. Stamler J, Stamler R, Neaton JD, *et al.* Low risk-factor profile and long-term cardiovascular and noncardiovascular mortality and life expectancy: findings for 5 large cohorts of young adult and middle-aged men and women. *JAMA* 1999; **282**(21):2012–18.

50. Zhang Y, Tuomilehto J, Jousilahti P, *et al.* Lifestyle factors on the risks of ischemic and hemorrhagic stroke. *Arch Intern Med* 2011; **171**:1811–18.

51. Tolonen H, Mahonen M, Asplund K, *et al.* Do trends in population levels of blood pressure and other cardiovascular risk factors explain trends in stroke event rates? Comparisons of 15 populations in 9 countries within the WHO MONICA Stroke Project. World Health Organization Monitoring of Trends and Determinants in Cardiovascular Disease. *Stroke* 2002; **33**(10):2367–75.

52. Rothwell PM, Warlow CP. Timing of TIAs preceding stroke: time window for prevention is very short. *Neurology* 2005; **64**(5):817–20.

53. Coull AJ, Rothwell PM. Underestimation of the early risk of recurrent stroke: evidence of the need for a standard definition. *Stroke* 2004; **35**(8):1925–9.

54. Rothwell PM. Incidence, risk factors and prognosis of stroke and TIA: the need for high-quality, large-scale epidemiological studies and meta-analyses. *Cerebrovasc Dis* 2003; **16**(Suppl 3):2–10.

55. Johnston SC, Gress DR, Browner WS, Sidney S. Short-term prognosis after emergency department diagnosis of TIA. *JAMA* 2000; **284**(22):2901–6.

56. Lovett JK, Dennis MS, Sandercock PA, *et al.* Very early risk of stroke after a first transient ischemic attack. *Stroke* 2003; **34**(8):e138–40.

57. Coull AJ, Lovett JK, Rothwell PM. Population based study of early risk of stroke after transient ischaemic attack or minor stroke: implications for public education and organisation of services. *BMJ* 2004; **328**(7435):326.

58. Hill MD, Yiannakoulias N, Jeerakathil T, *et al.* The high risk of stroke immediately after transient ischemic attack: a population-based study. *Neurology* 2004; **62**(11):2015–20.

59. Lisabeth LD, Ireland JK, Risser JM, *et al.* Stroke risk after transient ischemic attack in a population-based setting. *Stroke* 2004; **35**(8):1842–6.

60. Hankey GJ, Slattery JM, Warlow CP. Transient ischaemic attacks: which patients are at high (and low) risk of serious vascular events? *J Neurol Neurosurg Psychiatry* 1992; **55**(8):640–52.

61. Kernan WN, Viscoli CM, Brass LM, *et al.* The stroke prognosis instrument II (SPI-II): a clinical prediction instrument for patients with transient ischemia and nondisabling ischemic stroke. *Stroke* 2000; **31**(2):456–62.

62. Rothwell PM, Mehta Z, Howard SC, Gutnikov SA, Warlow CP. Treating individuals 3: from subgroups to individuals: general principles and the example of carotid endarterectomy. *Lancet* 2005; **365**(9455):256–65.

63. Rothwell PM, Giles MF, Flossmann E, *et al.* A simple score (ABCD) to identify individuals at high early risk of stroke after transient ischaemic attack. *Lancet* 2005; **366**(9479):29–36.

64. Grover SA, Lowensteyn I, Esrey KL, *et al.* Do doctors accurately

assess coronary risk in their patients? Preliminary results of the coronary health assessment study. *BMJ* 1995; **310**:975–8.

65. Montgomery AA, Fahey T, MacKintosh C, Sharp DJ, Peters TJ. Estimation of cardiovascular risk in hypertensive patients in primary care. *Br J Gen Pract* 2000; **50**:127–8.

66. Beswick AD, Brindle P, Fahey T, Ebrahim S. *A Systematic Review of Risk Scoring Methods and Clinical Decision Aids used in the Primary Prevention of Coronary Heart Disease*. London: Royal College of General Practitioners (UK) National Institute for Health and Clinical Excellence: Guidance; 2008.

67. Wolf PA, D'Agostino RB, Belanger AJ, Kannel WB. Probability of stroke: a risk profile from the Framingham Study. *Stroke* 1991; **22**(3):312–18.

68. D'Agostino RB, Wolf PA, Belanger AJ, Kannel WB. Stroke risk profile: adjustment for antihypertensive medication. The Framingham Study. *Stroke* 1994; **25**(1):40–3.

69. Wang TJ, Massaro JM, Levy D, *et al.* A risk score for predicting stroke or death in individuals with new-onset atrial fibrillation in the community: the Framingham Heart Study. *JAMA* 2003; **290**(8):1049–56.

70. Zhang XF, Attia J, D'Este C, Yu XH, Wu XG. A risk score predicted coronary heart disease and stroke in a Chinese cohort. *J Clin Epidemiol* 2005; **58**(9):951–8.

71. Lumley T, Kronmal RA, Cushman M, Manolio TA, Goldstein S. A stroke prediction score in the elderly: validation and Web-based application. *J Clin Epidemiol* 2002; **55**(2):129–36.

72. Gordon WJ, Polansky JM, Boscardin WJ, Fung KZ, Steinman MA. Coronary risk assessment by point-based vs. equation-based Framingham models: significant implications for clinical care. *J Gen Intern Med* 2010; **25**:1145–51.

73. Saaristo T, Peltonen M, Lindstrom J, *et al.* Cross-sectional evaluation of the Finnish Diabetes Risk Score: a tool to identify undetected type 2 diabetes, abnormal glucose tolerance and metabolic syndrome. *Diab Vasc Dis Res* 2005; **2**(2):67–72.

74. Kivipelto M, Ngandu T, Laatikainen T, *et al.* Risk score for the prediction of dementia risk in 20 years among middle aged people: a longitudinal, population-based study. *Lancet Neurol* 2006; **5**(9):735–41.

75. Silventoinen K, Pankow J, Lindstrom J, *et al.* The validity of the Finnish Diabetes Risk Score for the prediction of the incidence of coronary heart disease and stroke, and total mortality. *Eur J Cardiovasc Prev Rehabil* 2005; **12**(5):451–8.

76. Richards A, Eric M. Cheng EM. Stroke risk calculators in the era of electronic health records linked to administrative databases. *Stroke* 2013; **44**(2):564–9.

77. Fang MC, Go AS, Chang Y, *et al.* A new risk scheme to predict warfarin-associated hemorrhage: the ATRIA (Anticoagulation and Risk Factors in Atrial Fibrillation) study. *J Am Coll Cardiol* 2011; **58**:395–401.

78. Whisnant JP. Modeling of risk factors for ischemic stroke. The Willis Lecture. *Stroke* 1997; **28**(9):1840–4.

79. Hankey GJ. Potential new risk factors for ischemic stroke: what is their potential? *Stroke* 2006; **37**(8):2181–8.

80. Casas JP, Hingorani AD, Bautista LE, Sharma P. Meta-analysis of genetic studies in ischemic stroke: thirty-two genes involving approximately 18,000 cases and 58,000 controls. *Arch Neurol* 2004; **61**(11):1652–61.

81. Markus HS. Stroke genetics: prospects for personalized medicine. *BMC Med* 2012; **10**:113.

7

Common risk factors and prevention

Michael Brainin, Yvonne Teuschl, and Karl Matz

Introduction

The aim of primary prevention is to reduce the risk of first-ever stroke in asymptomatic people. Seven factors are regarded as potentially modifiable risk factors for vascular diseases: high blood pressure (BP), high cholesterol, smoking, excessive or heavy regular alcohol consumption, physical inactivity, overweight, and dietary factors. The strategy in primary prevention is to lower stroke risk attributed to these factors through education, lifestyle changes, and medication. Non-modifiable risk factors include old age and some genetic factors. The influence of other conditions such as arterial hypertension, atrial fibrillation, or diabetes mellitus can be lowered by controlling and treating the underlying disorder. Targets for stroke prevention can be directed either at the entire population or at high-risk individuals that are already suffering from disorders such as hypertension or diabetes mellitus. Usually, in general medicine, the latter approach is more prevalent. Therefore, issues relating to the high-risk approach of stroke prevention shall be the focus of this chapter.

The INTERSTROKE study is a large, recent case–control study including 3000 acute first-ever stroke cases recruited in 22 countries [1]. In this study five risk factors were identified that were associated with more than 80% of the population attributable risk of stroke: hypertension, current smoking, waist-to-hip ratio, diet risk score, and physical activity. Adding five additional risk factors (diabetes mellitus, alcohol intake, psychosocial factors, cardiac causes, and the ratio of ApoB to ApoA1) to the model explained up to 90% of the risk of stroke (see Figure 7.1).

Lifestyle factors

Stroke prevalence has been associated with individual lifestyle factors in several studies. Healthy lifestyle in general was considered in one large prospective cohort study of healthy women. In this study, healthy lifestyle, consisting of abstinence from smoking, low to normal body mass index (BMI), moderate alcohol consumption, regular exercise, and healthy diet, was found to be associated with a reduction in ischemic stroke (relative risk [RR] 0.3; 95% confidence interval [CI] 0.1–0.6) [2]. Using the data of two large cohort studies, the Nurses' Health Study (71 243 women) and the Health Professionals Follow-up Study (43 685 men), Chiuve et al. [3] defined a low-risk lifestyle score based on the five lifestyle components non-smoking, moderate activity ≥ 30 min/day, healthy diet, BMI < 25 kg/m^2, and modest alcohol consumption (men 5–30 g/day, women 5–15 g/day). The total number of low-risk factors was associated with a significantly reduced risk of total and ischemic stroke in men and women. Persons with low-risk lifestyle (all five low-risk lifestyle factors) had a decreased risk of stroke compared to persons fulfilling none of the low-risk lifestyle factors, RR 0.2 (95% CI 0.1–0.4) and RR 0.3 (95% CI 0.2–0.5) for women and men respectively. However, only 2% of women and 4% of men were at low risk for all five factors. Similarly, a large Finnish prospective cohort study (36 686 participants, 1478 stroke events) found that the number of healthy lifestyle indicators (smoking, BMI, physical activity, vegetable and alcohol consumption) is inversely associated with the risk of total, ischemic, and hemorrhagic stroke [4].

Lifestyle modifications have a high potential to prevent at low cost and low risk the development of

Textbook of Stroke Medicine, Second Edition, ed. Michael Brainin and Wolf-Dieter Heiss. Published by Cambridge University Press. © Michael Brainin and Wolf-Dieter Heiss 2014.

	Prevalence*			All stroke†		Ischemic stroke†		Intracerebral hemorrhagic stroke	
	Control (n=3000)	Ischemic stroke (n=2337)	Intracerebral hemorrhagic stroke (n=663)	Odds ratio (99% CI)	Population-attributable risk (99% CI)	Odds ratio (99% CI)	Population-attributable risk (99% CI)	Odds ratio (99% CI)	Population-attributable risk (99% CI)
Variable 1: hypertension									
A: self-reported history of hypertension	954/2996 (32%)	1277/2335 (55%)	399/662 (60%)	2.64 (2.26–3.08)	34.6% (30.4–39.1)	2.37 (2.00–2.79)	31.5% (26.7–36.7)	3.80 (2.96–4.78)	44.5% (37.2–52.0)
B: self-reported history of hypertension or blood pressure >160/90 mmHg	1109/3000 (37%)	1550/2337 (66%)	551/663 (83%)	3.89 (3.33–4.54)	51.8% (47.7–55.8)	3.14 (2.67–3.71)	45.2% (40.3–50.0)	9.18 (6.80–12.39)	73.6% (67.0–79.3)
Variable 2: smoking status									
Current smoker‡	732/2994 (24%)	868/2333 (37%)	207/662 (31%)	2.09 (1.75–2.51)	18.9% (15.3–23.1)	2.32 (1.91–2.81)	21.4% (17.5–25.8)	1.45 (1.07–1.96)	9.5% (4.2–20.0)
Variable 3: waist-to-hip ratio									
T2 vs. T1	989/2960 (33%)	768/2303 (33%)	266/655 (41%)	1.42 (1.18–1.71)	26.5% (18.8–36.0)$	1.34 (1.10–1.64)	26.0% (17.7–36.5)$	1.65 (1.22–2.23)	26.1% (14.1–43.3)$
T3 vs. T1	984/2960 (33%)	987/2303 (43%)	231/655 (35%)	1.65 (1.36–1.99)	–	1.69 (1.38–2.07)	–	1.41 (1.02–1.93)	–
Variable 4: diet risk score									
T2 vs. T1	1064/2982 (36%)	842/2303 (37%)	271/658 (41%)	1.35 (1.12–1.61)	18.8% (11.2–29.7)$	1.29 (1.06–1.57)	17.3% (9.4–29.6)$	1.53 (1.13–2.08)	24.1% (11.9–42.7)$
T3 vs. T1	904/2982 (30%)	807/2303 (35%)	221/658 (34%)	1.35 (1.11–1.64)	–	1.34 (1.09–1.65)	–	1.41 (1.01–1.97)	–
Variable 5: regular physical activity¶	362/2994 (12%)	193/2334 (8%)	45/662 (7%)	0.69 (0.53–0.90)	28.5% (14.5–48.5)	0.68 (0.51–0.91)	29.4% (14.5–50.5)	0.70 (0.44–1.13)	27.6% (6.8–66.6)
Variable 6: diabetes mellitus	350/2999 (12%)	495/2336 (21%)	68/662 (10%)	1.36 (1.10–1.68)	5.0% (2.6–9.5)	1.60 (1.29–1.99)	7.9% (5.1–12.3)	‖	‖
Variable 7: alcohol intake‡									
1–30 drinks per month	524/2989 (18%)	338/2326 (15%)	121/660 (18%)	0.90 (0.72–1.11)	3.8% (0.9–14.4)$	0.79 (0.63–1.00)	1.0% (0.0–83.8)$	1.52 (1.07–2.16)	14.6% (8.5–24.0)$
>30 drinks per month or binge drinker	324/2989 (11%)	383/2326 (16%)	108/660 (16%)	1.51 (1.18–1.92)	–	1.41 (1.09–1.82)	–	2.01 (1.35–2.99)	–
Variable 8: psychosocial factors									
A: psychosocial stress	440/2987 (15%)	465/2324 (20%)	124/654 (19%)	1.30 (1.06–1.60)	4.6% (2.1–9.6)	1.30 (1.04–1.62)	4.7% (2.0–10.2)	1.23 (0.89–1.69)	3.5% (0.7–16.3)
B: depression	424/2995 (14%)	489/2320 (21%)	100/645 (16%)	1.35 (1.10–1.66)	5.2% (2.7–9.8)	1.47 (1.19–1.83)	6.8% (3.9–11.4)	‖	‖
Variable 9: cardiac causes**	140/3000 (5%)	321/2337 (14%)	28/662 (4%)	2.38 (1.77–3.20)	6.7% (4.8–9.1)	2.74 (2.03–3.72)	8.5% (6.4–11.2)	‖	‖
Variable 10: ratio of ApoB to ApoA1††									
T2 vs. T1	695/2091 (33%)	501/1698 (30%)	136/468 (29%)	1.13 (0.90–1.42)	24.9% (15.7–37.1)$	1.30 (1.01–1.67)	35.2% (25.5–46.3)$	‖	‖
T3 vs. T1	696/2091 (33%)	825/1698 (49%)	165/468 (35%)	1.89 (1.49–2.40)	–	2.40 (1.86–3.11)	–	‖	‖

Table 2: Risk of stroke associated with risk factors in the overall population (multivariable analyses)

All models were adjusted for age, sex, and region. T=tertile. Apo=apolipoprotein. *Data were missing for some individuals: seven for smoking status, 82 for waist-to-hip ratio, 57 for diet risk score, ten for physical activity, three for diabetes mellitus, 25 for alcohol intake, 35 for psychosocial stress, 40 for depression, one for cardiac causes, and 1743 for apolipoprotein concentrations: these individuals were excluded from the denominator in percentage calculations. †Individual risk-factor estimates for variables 1–9 are derived from the multivariable model, including all variables (1A and 2–9). For intracerebral hemorrhagic stroke, the multivariable model included variables 1A, 2–5, 7, and 8A. ‡Comparator for current smoker and alcohol intake is never or former. $ For variables expressed in tertiles, population-attributable risk was calculated from T2 plus T3 versus T1. ¶For the protective factor of physical activity, population-attributable risks are provided for the group without this factor. ‖Odds ratio and population-attributable risk was not calculated because the variable was not significant in univariate analyses and so was excluded from multivariable analyses. **Includes atrial fibrillation or flutter, previous myocardial infarction, rheumatic valve disease, or prosthetic heart valve. ††Estimate derived from multivariable model, including all variables (1A and 2–10; n=4257).

Figure 7.1. Risk of stroke associated with individual risk factors in the overall population. Reproduced with permission from O'Donnell et al. [1].

stroke risk factors such as diabetes, dyslipidemia, obesity, and hypertension. Thus, they should be an important issue in stroke prevention.

Five low-risk lifestyle factors with a high potential to prevent stroke:

- non-smoking
- moderate activity ≥30 min/day
- healthy diet
- BMI <25 kg/m^2
- modest alcohol consumption.

Cigarette smoking

Smoking is a well-documented preventable risk factor of stroke. Large observational studies have shown cigarette smoking to be an independent risk factor for stroke in both men and women with current smokers having a 2- to 4-fold increased risk of stroke compared with non-smokers (Figure 7.2) [e.g. 1, 5–7]. A meta-analysis of 22 studies indicates an overall risk increase for stroke (RR 1.5; 95% CI 1.4–1.6) [8]. Smoking causes changes in BP and weight; adjusted for age, BP, and obesity stroke risk was RR 2.6 (95% CI 2.3–2.9). A dose–response relationship was identified ranging from RR 2.5 (1–14 cigarettes/day) to RR 3.8 (≥25 cigarettes/day) [8].

Stroke risk for smokers as compared to non-smokers differed between stroke types, being highest for subarachnoid hemorrhages (SAH) (odds ratio [OR] 2.9; 95% CI 2.5–3.5), nearly 2-fold for ischemic stroke (OR 1.9; 95% CI 1.7–2.2) and no clear relationship for intracerebral hemorrhages (ICHs) (OR 0.7; 95% CI 0.6–1.0) [8]. Smoking is a well-established risk factor for ischemic stroke [8]. A meta-analysis focusing only on SAH found a RR of 1.9 (95% CI 1.5–2.3) for two longitudinal studies and an odds ratio of 3.5 (95% CI 2.9–4.3) for seven case–control studies [9]. Association of smoking and ICHs is less well established. One meta-analysis studying the risk factors for ICH found an adjusted RR for current smokers of 1.3 (95% CI 1.1–1.6; 13 studies) and an adjusted RR of 1.1 (95% CI 0.9–1.3; 12 studies) for ever having smoked [10]. Two large prospective studies, the Physicians' Health Study [11] and the Women's Health Study [12], found a positive dose-dependent association of ICH risk and smoking in men and women. The age and risk factors adjusted RR were 2.1 (95% CI 1.1–4.1) and 2.9 (95% CI 1.1–7.5) for heavy smokers (≥20 cigarettes/day), 1.8 (95% CI 0.6–5.7) and 2.4 (95% CI 0.7–8.3) for light smokers (<20 cigarettes/day), and 0.8 (95% CI 0.5–1.2) and 1.3 (95% CI 0.6–2.6) for past smokers compared to never smokers,

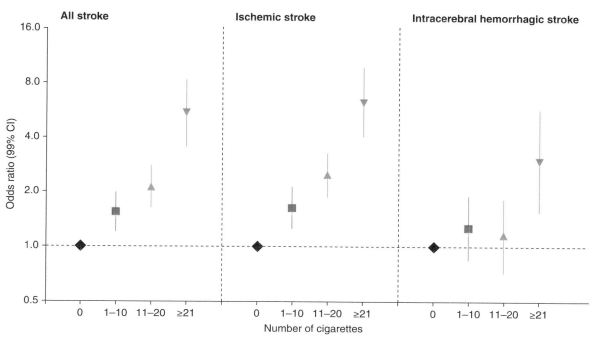

Figure 7.2. Risk of stroke associated with number of cigarettes smoked for all stroke, ischemic stroke, and intracerebral hemorrhagic stroke. Reproduced with permission from O'Donnell et al. [1].

for men and women respectively. On the other hand a pooled analysis of the the Atherosclerosis Risk in Communities (ARIC) study and the Cardiovascular Health Study (CHS) did not find an independent relationship between smoking and ICH [13].

Non-smokers exposed to tobacco smoke were estimated to absorb only the equivalent of 0.1–1 cigarette based on urine nicotine. Nevertheless passive smoking was associated with a greater progression in atherosclerosis [14]. Never smokers exposed to tobacco smoke had in the period of 3 years a mean increase of intimal-medial thickness (IMT) of the carotid artery of 31.6 μm (SD ± 2.0) compared to 25.9 μm (SD ± 2.1; p = 0.010) for non-smokers not exposed to smoke. The mean increase of IMT for current smokers was 43.0 μm (SD ± 1.9) [14]. Only a few studies investigated stroke risk due to environmental tobacco smoke exposure. A meta-analysis of 16 studies of variable design and quality suggests that spousal cigarette smoking is associated with an increased stroke risk (RR 1.3; 95% CI 1.2–1.4). The relative risk of stroke found for the highest level of exposure was 1.6 (95% CI 1.3–1.8) [15].

Smoking may have additive effects and many potentiate the effects of other risk factors. In the Oslo study, a large cohort study, BP of fatal stroke cases was higher than BP of other participants, but the absolute difference was larger for non-smokers than for smokers. This may suggest a lower tolerance for high BP in smokers [16]. Similar effects were found for BMI and blood glucose level. Differences in BMI and blood glucose level between fatal stroke cases and other men were only found for non-smokers [16]. An interaction between smoking and the use of oral contraceptives was noted for women. Compared to non-smoking women not using oral contraceptives, smoking women not using oral contraceptives had an increased risk of ischemic stroke (OR 1.2; 95% CI 0.7–2.1); non-smoking women using oral contraceptives had a 2.1 increased risk (95% CI 1.0–4.5), but smoking women using oral contraceptives had a 7.2 higher risk (95% CI 3.2–16.1) [17]. A similar but weaker synergistic effect was observed for hemorrhagic stroke [18].

Smoking cessation reduces stroke risk rapidly. In a meta-analysis total stroke risk was 1.2 (95% CI 1.1–1.3) in former smokers [8]. In the Framingham Study stroke risk had decreased 5 years after quitting smoking to the level of non-smokers [5]. In the Nurses' Health Study total and ischemic stroke excess risk nearly disappeared after 2 years and relative risk

for former smokers compared to never smokers was 1.4 (95% CI 1–1.7) while it was 2.6 (95% CI 2.1–3.2) in current smokers [6]. In a pooled analysis of three large Japanese cohort studies age-adjusted risk for stroke mortality had declined 5–9 years after smoking cessation by 23% in women and by 10% in men, and after 10–15 years it was decreased by 35% in men and 49% in women and no longer differed from people who had never smoked [7].

The benefits of quitting smoking are evident; however, due to its addictive effect the success in smoking cessation is only modest. Several behavioral and pharmacological therapies are available to assist smokers in quitting and their effects are the subject of a number of Cochrane reviews (e.g. [19–22]). All forms of nicotine replacement therapy (nicotine gum, transdermal patches, nasal spray, inhalers, tablets) are effective in increasing abstinence from smoking (RR 1.6; 95% CI 1.5–1.7) [19]. The antidepressants bupropion (RR 1.6; 95% CI 1.5–1.9) and nortriptyline (RR 2.0; 95% CI 1.5–2.8) are also successful for smoking cessation. Their effect seems, however, to be independent of their antidepressant effect and they are of similar efficacy to nicotine replacements [20]. The nicotine receptor partial agonist varenicline was also found to be more effective in 12 months abstinence when compared with a placebo or with bupropion [21]. Psychosocial interventions such as behavioral therapy, self-help, or telephone counseling are effective but have to be intensive [22].

> Stroke risk for smokers is 2.9-fold for subarachnoid hemorrhages and nearly 2-fold for ischemic stroke. Even passive smoking was associated with increased risk for stroke.

Alcohol consumption

Excessive alcohol drinking increases all-cause mortality, as well as the risk of coronary heart disease and stroke [23]. A meta-analysis including 35 observational studies found for a consumption of more than 60 g of ethanol/day (approximately six drinks) an increased risk of ischemic stroke (RR 1.7; 95% CI 1.3–2.2) and hemorrhagic stroke (RR 2.2; 95% CI 1.5–3.2) [24].

The relationship between alcohol and overall and ischemic stroke risk was described as J-shaped [23, 24]. This suggests that benefits overcome the harmful effect of alcohol at light to moderate alcohol consumption. Light alcohol consumption (<12 g/day) was associated with a reduction in all stroke (RR 0.83; 95% CI 0.75–0.91) and ischemic stroke (RR 0.80; 95% CI 0.67–0.96), and moderate consumption (12–24 g/day) with a reduction in ischemic stroke (RR 0.72; 95% CI 0.57–0.91) [24]. A positive linear relationship was found between alcohol consumption and hemorrhagic stroke [23, 24]. The relative risk reduction for total stroke for light alcohol drinking (<12 g/day) seems to be larger for women (RR 0.7; 95% CI 0.6–0.7) than for men (RR 0.9; 95% CI 0.8–1) [24].

The apparently positive effect of light to moderate alcohol consumption is still under discussion. Beneficial effects on lipids, hemostatic factors, insulin sensitivity, inflammatory markers, and flow-mediated vasodilation have been reported. Especially the flavonoids of red wine have been presumed to be involved in preventing the formation of atherosclerotic plaques [25]. Comparing the type of alcoholic beverage consumed, wine seems to be associated with the lowest risk of stroke (e.g. [26]). The pattern of drinking seems to influence the vascular risk; binge drinking, even when alcohol consumption was otherwise light, increases the risk of ischemic and total stroke [23, 27]. It has been suggested that alcohol is a trigger for ischemic stroke onset, and that stroke risk is elevated 2- to 3-fold after alcohol abuse within 24 hours (10–120 g) or within one week (150–400 g) preceding stroke [28].

Heavy alcohol intake and binge drinking increase heart rate, blood pressure, and the risk of hypertension and atrial fibrillation, thereby increasing stroke risk; this seems to be especially true for hemorrhagic stroke [29, 30]. In hypertensive subjects stroke risk was increased significantly by heavy drinking. In a 26-year Japanese prospective cohort study hemorrhagic stroke risk (RR 3.1; 95% CI 1.1–9.1) and to a lesser extent ischemic stroke risk (RR 2.0; 95% CI 1.1–3.6) were increased significantly in hypertensive heavy drinkers compared to non-drinking and light-drinking hypertensive subjects, whereas for non-hypertensive persons the increased risks of hemorrhagic stroke (RR 1.7; 95% CI 0.6–4.9) and ischemic stroke (RR 1.4; 95% CI 0.8–2.5) attributed to heavy drinking were not significant [30]. Reducing excessive alcohol intake was found to reduce systolic BP by 3.8 mmHg in four randomized controlled intervention studies [31].

Heavy long-term alcohol consumption (>36 g/day or more than three drinks/day) and episodic heavy drinking increase the risk of atrial fibrillation, a major risk factor of stroke [32].

Excessive alcohol drinking increases all-cause mortality, as well as the risk of coronary heart disease and stroke, but benefits overcome the harmful effect at light to moderate alcohol consumption levels. Anyhow, binge drinking is a trigger for ischemic stroke onset (stroke risk is elevated 2- to 3-fold after alcohol abuse within 24 hours).

Obesity

A high BMI ($\geq 25\,kg/m^2$) is associated with an increased risk of stroke in men [33, 34] and women [35, 36]. Ischemic stroke rate increases in a dose-dependent manner with BMI [33, 36–38]. The relationship between hemorrhagic stroke and BMI is less clear. Some studies found no influence of BMI on hemorrhagic stroke risk [34–36, 37], whereas others found an increased risk of hemorrhagic stroke for people with elevated BMI [33, 38].

Abdominal adiposity (measured by waist-to-hip ratio) has been suggested to be a better indicator for stroke risk than overall body mass (measured by BMI) [1, 36, 39]. However, after adjusting for other risk factors, risk prediction models using waist-to-hip ratio, waist circumference, or BMI to assess obesity did not differ in a clinically significant way [40, 41].

Obesity is associated with an increased risk of hypertension, diabetes, dyslipidemia, atrial fibrillation, and obstructive sleep apnea. Adjusting for these confounding risk factors often attenuates the effect of body mass [33–35, 38–40]. It is still under discussion whether obesity is an independent risk factor of stroke or mediated through BP, diabetes, and cholesterol levels [40].

Weight reduction was associated with improvement in BP, insulin sensitivity, blood glucose level, triglyceride and high-density lipoprotein (HDL) concentration, and markers for inflammation. In a meta-analysis systolic BP was reduced by 4.4 mmHg and diastolic BP by 3.6 mmHg for an average weight loss of 5.1 kg [42]. However, no randomized controlled trial has tested the effect of weight reduction in obese adults on stroke risk [43].

Combined interventions including dietary and exercise strategies with cognitive-behavioral therapy were the most successful for weight loss [44]. Increasing the intensity of psychological intervention resulted in greater weight reduction [44].

Obesity (high body mass index or high waist-to-hip ratio) is associated with an increased risk of stroke.

Physical inactivity

Several prospective longitudinal population studies have shown the protective effect of regular physical activity for stroke in women and men [45]. However, a recent meta-analysis suggests that higher level of physical activity may be required in women than in men to achieve a significant reduction in stroke risk [46]. In a meta-analysis of 18 cohort and 5 case–control studies, physically highly active individuals had a lower risk of stroke and lower stroke mortality than those with low activity (RR 0.7; 95% CI 0.7–0.8). Similarly, moderately active individuals had a lower risk of stroke, compared with those who were inactive (RR 0.8; 95% CI 0.7–0.9) [47].

A similar relationship was found in ischemic stroke for high versus low activity (RR 0.8; 95% CI 0.7–0.9) and for moderate versus low activity (RR 0.9; 95% CI 0.8–1.1) [47]. Only a few studies investigated the effect of activity on hemorrhagic stroke. However, in a meta-analysis high and moderate activity significantly decreased hemorrhagic stroke risk when compared with low activity (RR 0.7; 95% CI 0.5–0.9 and RR 0.9; 95% CI 0.6–1.1) [47].

Additionally, leisure-based physical activity (2–5 hours per week) has been independently associated with a reduced severity of ischemic stroke at admission and better short-term outcome [48].

Some studies found a dose–response relationship between stroke risk and different levels of activity [49–51]; others found a U-shaped relationship or no difference between moderate and high physical activity [52, 53]. This may be explained by different definitions of physical activity and levels of activity. Additionally, there may be different metabolic effects of different types of exercise. Overall only a few studies have evaluated the influence of occupational physical activity; the definitions of activity levels and activity types vary considerably and the amount of activity is generally self-assessed. Commuting physical activity (walking or cycling to work) may also reduce stroke risk [51]. Study results on the influence of the type of activity on stroke risk are inconsistent (a meta-analysis distinguishing between leisure and occupational physical activity found a protective effect of both activity types) [54]. People active at work had a decreased risk for ischemic (RR 0.6; 95% CI 0.4–0.8) and hemorrhagic stroke (RR 0.3; 95% CI 0.1–0.8), and those physically active during leisure time had a decreased risk for ischemic (RR 0.8; 95%

CI 0.7–0.9) and hemorrhagic stroke (RR 0.7; 95% CI 0.6–1.0). No randomized controlled trial has studied the effect of regular controlled exercises on stroke risk. There is not enough evidence for the type and intensity of fitness training protecting best against stroke.

The favorable effect of physical activity is at least partly mediated through beneficial effects on other risk factors. Physical activity decreases body weight and BP, and increases serum HDL cholesterol and glucose tolerance [55, 56]. Additionally, physically more active people were found to be more often non-smokers [53].

> Regular physical activity has a protective effect for stroke, probably mediated through beneficial effects on other risk factors.

Dietary factors

Poor dietary habits contribute to the development of other stroke risk factors such as obesity, diabetes, hypertension, and dyslipidemia. Changes in dietary habits therefore have high potential for reducing stroke risk. Different foods and nutrients have been suggested to influence stroke risk via several mechanisms, e.g. by influencing BP, insulin resistance, inflammation risk, platelet function, endothelial function, and oxidation [57].

Fruits, vegetables, whole grain

In large epidemiological studies, high fruit and vegetable intake was associated in a dose-dependent fashion with decreased risk of stroke. A meta-analysis including nine cohort studies found that persons eating more than five servings of fruit or vegetables per day had a decreased relative risk of stroke (RR 0.7; 95% CI 0.7–0.8) compared to people eating fewer than three servings. This effect was significant for both ischemic and hemorrhagic stroke [58]. In the Nurses' Health Study including 75 596 women and the Health Professionals Follow-up Study including 38 683 men ischemic and total stroke risk were reduced respectively by 7% and 3% in women and by 4% and 5% in men for each increment of one serving of fruits and vegetables per day [59]. Combining both studies the quintile with the highest intake of fruits and vegetables had a decreased relative risk of stroke (RR 0.69; 95% CI 0.52–0.92) compared to the lowest quintile. In a meta-analysis of seven cohort studies whole grain intake was associated with a reduction in cardiovascular disease but not stroke [60]. Generally, persons with higher fruit and vegetable intake were more likely to be non-smokers, engaged in more physical activity, and more highly educated [59].

Fish, omega 3 fatty acids

The consumption of oily fish or long chain omega 3 fatty acids has been suggested to decrease the risk of vascular disease by lowering serum lipids, decreasing BP, decreasing platelet aggregation, improving vascular reactivity, and decreasing inflammation. Ecological studies raised the concern that high fish consumption may increase the risk of hemorrhagic stroke. A recent meta-analysis of 21 prospective cohort studies (675 048 participants, 25 320 cerebrovascular events) found a moderate but significant reduced risk of stroke when comparing the lowest category of fish intake with the highest (RR 0.88; 95% CI: 0.84–0.93) [61]. The effects for ischemic and hemorrhagic strokes were similar. The effect of long chain omega 3 fatty acid on stroke risk was however not significant [61]. Possible explanations of the benefit of fish consumption compared to omega 3 fatty acids consumption may come from additional beneficial nutrients of fish (e.g. vitamins B and D), or a reduced intake of unhealthy food (red meat), or result from an association with higher socioeconomic status. Another concern was raised on the negative effect of methyl mercury contamination in fish. An evaluation of all risks and benefits of fish intake indicates that for modest fish consumption (1–2 servings/week) the benefits of fish intake exceed the potential risks; people with very high consumption should limit some fish species with high mercury levels [62].

Sodium, potassium, calcium, magnesium

Observational studies found an association between high sodium intake and stroke incidence [63]. On the other hand, a meta-analysis of randomized controlled trials showed no strong evidence for the effect of salt reduction on cardiovascular morbidity. This results probably from insufficient statistical power (6500 participants; 293 cardiovascular events) [64]. The observed positive effect of salt reduction is at least partly mediated by the well-studied positive relationship between salt intake and BP [65]. A reduction in salt intake in hypertensive persons (median urinary sodium reduction by 75 mmol/day or 4.4 g/day)

reduced systolic BP by 5.4 mmHg and diastolic BP by 2.8 mmHg. In normotensive individuals systolic and diastolic BP were reduced by 2.4 mmHg and 1.0 mmHg respectively [66]. The Dietary Approaches to Stop Hypertension (DASH) trial, a randomized controlled study including 412 participants, found strong evidence for the benefit of low sodium intake [67]. Participants were randomized to one of three sodium intake levels and either the DASH diet (rich in vegetables and fruits, and low in dairy fat products and total and saturated fat and cholesterol) or a control diet (a typical American diet). Sodium reduction as well as the DASH diet reduced BP significantly.

Epidemiological studies found an inverse relationship between intake of potassium and risk of stroke, especially in ischemic stroke. In a meta-analysis of 10 prospective studies a 1000 mg/day increase in potassium was associated with 11% decrease in stroke risk [68]. In particular, increased potassium intake reduces BP in people with hypertension without having an adverse effect on blood lipid concentration, catecholamine concentrations, or renal function [69]. Dietary calcium, especially from dairy sources has been found to be inversely associated with BP and with lower incidence of stroke in populations with low to moderate calcium intake and in Asian populations. The evidence is only moderate and may be confounded by other nutrients in dairy food [70]. Dietary magnesium has been found to be modestly inversely associated with the incidence of ischemic stroke in prospective cohort studies (RR for an increase in intake of 100 mg magnesium/day 0.91; 95% CI 0.87–0.96) [71].

Coffee, tea, chocolate

Coffee, tea, and chocolate consumption have been associated with lower rates of stroke. Favorable effects are probably not mediated by an effect on BP but by the antioxidant capacity of polyphenolic compounds. A meta-analysis of 11 prospective cohort studies (479 689 participants; 10 003 cases of strokes) suggests a weak inverse association of moderate coffee consumption (3–4 cups/day) with stroke [72]. Nevertheless there might be concerns on deleterious physiological effects in the hour after consumption that may trigger stroke onset. Consuming ≥3 cups of green or black tea per day reduced the risk of stroke by 21% as shown by a meta-analysis of 10 observational studies (194 965 participants, 4 378 strokes) [73]. A combined analysis of five observational studies (131 345 participants, 4 260 stroke cases) showed a 19% decreased relative risk of stroke in the highest compared to the lowest category of chocolate consumption [74]. However, no information of the type of chocolate consumed is available, and harmful effects resulting from the high sugar, saturated fat, and caloric content of commercially available chocolate should be considered.

Diet

Different nutrients and aliments cannot be seen independently of each other and thus the effect of different diets has been investigated. The DASH diet (see above) was associated with a significant decrease in BP [67]. Fung et al. used the individual information on food intake of the Nurses' Health Study to classify individuals' alimentation according to the DASH-style diet. Women with a dietary pattern more similar to the DASH diet had a lower stroke risk, and this effect increased linearly with an adjusted RR of 0.8 (95% CI 0.7–1.0) for the quintile with the highest intake of a DASH-style diet compared to the quintile with the lowest intake of a DASH-style diet [75]. A meta-analysis of three cohort studies (including [75]) found that adherence to a DASH-style diet significantly decreases stroke risk [76]. A Mediterranean-style diet rich in α-linolenic acid, olive oil, canola oil, fish, fruits, vegetables, and whole grains and low in saturated fat has been found to be successful for the prevention of cardiovascular diseases. In a meta-analysis of seven prospective cohort studies a 2-point increase of adherence to a Mediterranean diet was associated with a significantly reduced incidence of cardiovascular diseases (RR = 0.90; 95% CI: 0.87–0.93) [77]. Results of a recent randomized controlled primary prevention trial, the PREDIMED trial, showed that a Mediterranean diet supplemented with extra-virgin olive oil or mixed nuts can reduce stroke incidence when compared to a control group advised to reduce dietary fat. [78]. On the other hand, a randomized controlled trial including 48 835 women with dietary interventions consisting of total fat reduction to 20% of energy intake, and an increased intake of fruits, vegetables, and grain did not result in a reduced incidence of coronary events and stroke [79]. This may suggest that the amount of total fats consumed may be less important than the type of fats.

A diet low in sodium, high in potassium, and rich in fruits and vegetables, whole grains, cereal fiber, and fatty fish has the highest potential to reduce stroke risk.

Furthermore, coffee, tea, and chocolate consumption have been associated with lower rates of stroke.

Postmenopausal estrogen replacement therapy

Until menopause women generally suffer from a lower rate of vascular diseases, including ischemic stroke [80]. This has been attributed to a protective effect of estrogen and thus research has focused on the beneficial effect of postmenopausal hormone therapy for the prevention of cardiovascular diseases and stroke. However, the Women's Health Initiative (WHI), a large randomized trial of 16 608 generally healthy postmenopausal women, showed that oral conjugated equine estrogen plus progestin increased the risk of ischemic stroke by 44% [81]. More recent studies and meta-analyses confirmed that estrogen-alone or estrogen–progestin therapy had no effect for primary prevention of cardiovascular diseases and increased stroke incidence by more than 30% [82, 83]. Similarly, a meta-analysis of nine observational studies indicated an increased risk of stroke – especially of ischemic stroke – in women using hormone replacement therapy, with RR for overall and ischemic stroke respectively of 1.1 (95% CI 1.0–1.2) and 1.2 (95% CI 1.0–1.4) [84]. Recent but limited evidence suggests that the risk of stroke is not increased in healthy postmenopausal women under 60 at low risk of cardiovascular disease taking a low dose of transdermal estradiol (≤50 μg/day) for a short time. Thus, current research focuses on optimal dose, duration, route of administration, and timing of initiation of hormone replacement therapy [80, 83].

Selective estrogen receptor modulators (SERMs) are a new class of drugs used for hormone replacement therapy lacking the steroid structure of estrogens but able to bind directly to estrogen receptors. To date few studies have investigated the effect of SERMs on stroke risk. In a meta-analysis of nine trials raloxifene had no effect on stroke but doubled the risk of venous thromboembolism [85]. In the Raloxifene Use for The Heart (RUTH) trial including 10 101 postmenopausal women with coronary heart disease or multiple risk factors for coronary heart disease the risk of fatal stroke was increased [86]. A meta-analysis (nine trials) investigating the risk of ischemic stroke in tamoxifen treatment for breast cancer found an increase of overall (RR 1.4; 95% CI 1.1–1.7) and ischemic stroke risk (RR 1.8; 95% CI 1.4–2.4) [87].

One trial comparing bazedoxifene to raloxifene found also an increased risk of venous thromboembolism [88]. In the Postmenopausal Evaluation and Risk-reduction with Lasofoxifene (PEARL) trial, lasofoxifene reduced the risk of stroke, whereas the risk of deep vein thrombosis was increased [89].

> Hormone replacement therapy is associated with an increased risk of stroke, but whether dose, duration, route of administration and timing of initiation of hormone replacement therapy reduces the risk is still being investigated.

Diseases and pathological conditions

Hypertension

Elevated BP is the best-documented treatable risk factor for stroke. Worldwide, about 54% of strokes and 13.5% of deaths are attributed to high BP (systolic BP >115 mmHg; [90]). High BP (BP>115/75 mmHg) is strongly and directly related to vascular and overall mortality without evidence of any threshold (Figure 7.3) [91]. Starting at a BP of 115/75 mmHg, stroke mortality risk increases steeply in an approximately log-linear relationship with BP [91]. Age attenuates this relationship and stroke risk increases with every 10 mmHg of systolic BP by 40–50%, 30–40%, and 20–30% for the age groups <60, 60–69, and ≥70 respectively [92].

Lowering BP substantially reduces stroke and coronary risks. A meta-analysis of randomized controlled trials showed a 41% (33–48%) reduction in stroke for a BP reduction of 10 mmHg systolic or 5 mmHg diastolic (Figure 7.4) [93]. The benefit of BP reduction suggested by the results of clinical trials is therefore consistent with the relationship found in cohort studies.

As a consequence guidelines recommend lowering BP to 140/85 mmHg or below. The antihypertensive treatment should be more aggressive in persons at very high cardiovascular risk (especially diabetic

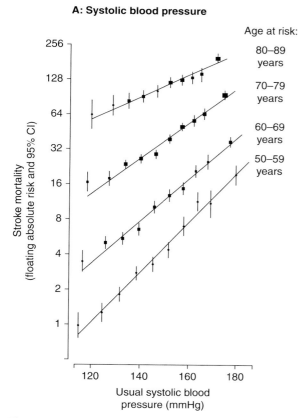

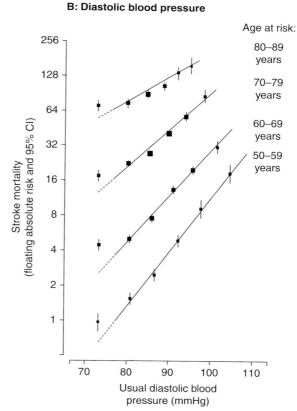

Figure 7.3. Age-specific stroke mortality associated with usual blood pressure, with data from prospective cohort study. Reproduced with permission from Lewington *et al.* [91].

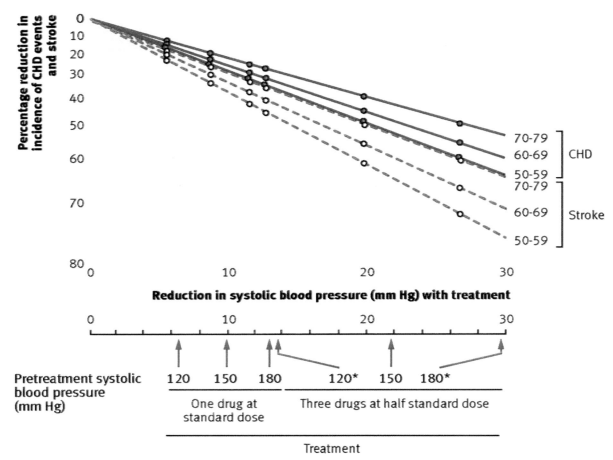

Figure 7.4. Reduction in incidence of coronary heart disease (CHD) events and stroke in relation to reduction in systolic blood pressure according to dose and combination of drugs, pretreatment systolic blood pressure, and age. Reproduced with permission from Law *et al.* [93].

patients) and cut-off limits set to 130–139 mmHg for systolic and 85–89 mmHg for diastolic BP [94]. In a meta-analysis more intensive regimes targeting BP levels of <135/85 mmHg were associated with a 24% lower risk of stroke [95], but available data for possible side-effects are limited. Lifestyle changes are recommended as part of the therapy. A combination of two or more antihypertensive agents is often necessary and preferable to achieve these targets [94].

Achieving BP reduction seems more important than the choice of the antihypertensive drug. To compare the effect of the different classes of BP-lowering drugs (angiotensin-converting enzyme [ACE] inhibitors, calcium antagonists, angiotensin-receptor blockers [ARBs], and thiazide diuretics and/or beta-adrenergic receptor blockers) the Blood Pressure Lowering Treatment Trialists' (BPLTT) Collaboration performed a large meta-analysis including 29 randomized trials and more than 160 000 participants [96, 97]. No antihypertensive drug class was found to be superior in reducing stroke risk [92, 96, 97]. Similarly, a Cochrane review showed that compared to placebo all first-line antihypertensive drug classes reduced the risk of stroke: thiazides (19 trials; RR 0.63; 95% CI 0.57–0.71), beta-blockers (5 trials; RR 0.83; 95% CI 0.72–0.97), ACE inhibitors (3 trials; RR 0.65; 95% CI 0.52–0.82), and calcium-channel blocker (1 trial; RR 0.58; 95% CI 0.41–0.84) [98].

As the strength in the association between BP and stroke risk attenuates with age, one might expect differences in the effect of BP-lowering drugs in older patients. Additionally the prevalence of systolic hypertension (systolic BP >140 mmHg and diastolic BP <90 mmHg) increases with age. In elderly subjects, controlling hypertension regardless of whether it is isolated systolic hypertension or not has been shown to be beneficial [99]. A meta-analysis including 31 trials with more than 190 000 participants found no evidence for the advantage of a specific antihypertensive drug class according to age (younger or older than 65 years) [100].

The Hypertension in the Very Elderly Trial (HYVET), a randomized controlled trial, showed that even hypertensive patients older than 80 years benefit from BP-lowering therapy by a reduction in non-fatal stroke rate (RR 0.7; 95% CI 0.5–1.0) and stroke mortality (RR 0.6; 95% CI 0.4–1.0) [101].

> Elevated blood pressure (BP) is the best-documented treatable risk factor for stroke. Lowering BP reduces stroke risk by 41% for every 10 mmHg systolic BP reduction.

Diabetes mellitus

Diabetes is a well-documented risk factor for stroke. In a meta-analysis of 102 prospective studies (530 083 participants) the hazard ratio for ischemic stroke was 2.3 (95% CI 2.0–2.7) and 1.6 (95% CI 1.2–2.1) for hemorrhagic stroke in people with versus those without diabetes [102].

There is insufficient evidence from randomized trials that improving glucose control reduces stroke. A meta-analysis of nine randomized controlled trials (59 197 participants, 2037 stroke events) found that intensive control of glucose compared to standard care had no effect on stroke incidence [103].

In addition to an increased stroke risk subjects with type 2 diabetes have an increased prevalence of other stroke risk factors such as obesity, hyperlipidemia, hypertension, and atrial fibrillation [104–106]. Intensive multiple risk factor therapy and especially lifestyle modification can decrease the risk of cardiovascular events (including stroke) in people with type 2 diabetes [107, 108].

Hypertension and diabetes are highly correlated [105]. In diabetic patients BP should be lowered to 130–139 mmHg for systolic and 85–89 mmHg for diastolic BP [94].

Dyslipidemia in type 2 diabetes is characterized by an increased blood triglyceride concentration and reduced HDL cholesterol concentration. However, total and low-density lipoprotein (LDL) cholesterol concentrations do not differ from the general population [106]. Treatment with statins reduces LDL

cholesterol and stroke risk similarly to results seen in non-diabetic persons. A meta-analysis of four randomized controlled trials (10 187 participants) testing statin therapy for primary prevention of major cardiovascular and cerebrovascular events in diabetic patients found a significant relative risk reduction in fatal and non-fatal stroke (RR 0.69; 95% CI 0.51–0.92) [109].

> There is insufficient evidence that improving glucose control reduces stroke.
> Blood pressure (BP) target in hypertensive diabetic patients should be 130–139 mmHg systolic and 85–89 mmHg diastolic BP.
> Treatment of diabetic patients with statins reduced the risk of stroke by 31%.

Dyslipidemia

Older epidemiological studies found no relationship between total serum cholesterol level and overall stroke incidence [110]. This might be due to different relationships for ischemic and intracerebral hemorrhages. In prospective cohort studies stroke risk was found to be positively associated with serum cholesterol level in ischemic stroke but negatively for intracerebral hemorrhages [111].

Age, sex, and vascular risk factors can modify the relationship between blood cholesterol and vascular mortality. A meta-analysis of 61 observational prospective studies analyzed the influence of blood cholesterol on vascular mortality by distinguishing different age classes, sex, and different levels of BP [111]. Overall the association between total blood cholesterol and stroke mortality was weak; a positive association was only found in the age group 45–59. For ischemic stroke this association was weakly positive in middle age (40–59) and may be accounted for by an association between total cholesterol and BP. For hemorrhagic stroke the association was negative and only found for older participants (70–79). The relationship between total blood cholesterol and stroke mortality is highly dependent on BP. For systolic BP levels below 145 mmHg this association was positive, for higher BP levels the relationship was negative. These relationships are similar for both stroke types but stronger in hemorrhagic stroke.

Insufficient data are available to identify a relationship between LDL cholesterol and stroke incidence [112]. HDL, in contrast, was found to be negatively associated with total and ischemic stroke incidence in several prospective cohort studies [111]. No such relationship was found for hemorrhagic stroke.

In contrast to the partly inconsistent findings from epidemiological studies, randomized controlled trials found a clear positive effect of cholesterol-lowering statin (3-hydroxy-3-methylglutaryl coenzyme A (HMG-CoA) reductase inhibitors) therapy on the incidence of ischemic stroke. This effect may not only derive from lower lipid levels but also from anti-inflammatory and antithrombotic properties of statins. In a Cochrane review of 18 randomized primary prevention trials (56 934 participants) statin treatment reduced the risk of fatal and non-fatal stroke by RR 0.78 (95% CI 0.68–0.89) when compared to placebo, with no evidence for serious harm [113]. The Cholesterol Treatment Trialists' (CTT) Collaboration reported in a meta-analysis including individual patient data of 27 randomized trials a reduction of stroke risk by 15% per 1.0 mmol/l LDL reduction (RR 0.85; 95% CI 0.80–0.89). In particular, this analysis showed that persons with a low level of cardiovascular risk (predicted 5-year risk <10%) profit similarly to persons with higher vascular risk [114]. Observational studies have raised concerns about a higher incidence of hemorrhagic strokes. A meta-analysis of 31 randomized trials found no difference in incidence of intracerebral hemorrhages (676 cases) in the active treatment group compared to controls (OR 1.08; 95% CI 0.88–1.32; p = 0.47) [115]. The risk of intracerebral hemorrhages was not related to the degree of LDL reduction. However, the risk of bleedings might be different in Asian populations where hemorrhagic strokes are more common. Because of the linear relationship between risk reduction in stroke and LDL cholesterol level, a more intensive statin therapy might be indicated. A meta-analysis of 10 mainly secondary prevention trials for coronary heart disease (41 778 participants) found a significant reduction of fatal and non-fatal stroke (RR 0.86; 95% CI 0.77–0.96) for more intensive statin therapy compared to less intensive therapy [116].

Among other lipid-lowering therapies used in primary stroke prevention were niacin, gemfibrozil, clofibrate, bezafibrate, and lifestyle modifications. A meta-analysis of 11 trials (9 959 subjects) found that niacin was associated with a significant reduction in cardiovascular events but not with stroke incidence (OR 0.88; 95% CI 0.5–1.54) [117]. Fibrates are effective in elevating HDL cholesterol, lowering triglyceride concentration, and reducing LDL cholesterol. However, a meta-analysis of ten randomized, partly secondary prevention trials (37 791 patients) comparing fibrate therapy with placebo found no effect on stroke incidence (RR 1.02; 95% CI 0.90–1.16) [118]. In a meta-analysis including 38 primary and secondary stroke prevention trials using different lipid-lowering therapies, the most effective in reducing stroke risk were statins [119]. For non-statin drugs no significant effect on stroke incidence was found [119]. The effect of diet (seven trials) was strongest, but highly variable and therefore insignificant (OR 0.6; 95% CI 0.3–1.1; p = 0.11). At the same time the cholesterol-lowering effect was highest for statins (21.8% in statins compared to 8.3% in non-statin drugs). Taking all lipid-lowering therapies together a strong correlation was found between stroke incidence and final cholesterol level ($r^2 = 0.48$) [119].

Recent studies suggest that myalgias may occur in a substantial number of patients treated with statins. In contrast, severe myopathy is a rare and generally self-limited side-effect of statin medications [120]. The notion that statins might be associated with an increased risk of intracranial hemorrhage was not substantiated in a recent, large meta-analysis [121].

> Randomized controlled trials found a clear positive effect of cholesterol-lowering statin therapy on the incidence of ischemic stroke. Niacin or fibrates showed no effect on stroke incident.

Atrial fibrillation

Atrial fibrillation (AF) is a strong independent risk factor for ischemic stroke [122]. The prevalence of AF increases with age, ranging from 0.1% among persons younger than 55 years to 9% among persons older than 80 years; it is almost 4% for persons older than 60 years [123]. AF is therefore primarily a risk factor in the older population.

Strokes associated with AF generally have a higher mortality and poorer functional outcome [124]. In the Framingham Study the risk of ischemic stroke was nearly 5-fold for subjects with AF [122]. However, stroke risk is highly variable in patients with AF and depends on sex, age, and the presence of other stroke risk factors; for those older than 75 years without prior stroke or transient ischemic attack (TIA) the stroke rate ranged from 3.2% to 5.2% per year [125].

Risk assessment is particularly important to balance potential benefits and risks of chronic anti-thrombotic therapy. Risk stratification should be used to determine whether patients should be given oral anticoagulation, aspirin, or nothing. Several schemes to stratify stroke risk in patients with AF have been proposed and tested [126]. A review comparing 12 stratification schemes found substantial differences between them [126]. Using 11 different schemes to classify individual stroke risk in a common test cohort resulted in 7–42% of the patients being categorized as at low risk, and 11–77% being at high risk [126]. These differences between risk stratification schemes probably contribute to confusion and the inconsistent use of anticoagulant treatment.

Therefore, the actual guidelines for the management of AF of the European Society of Cardiology recommend the use of the CHAD2DS2-VASc (Cardiac failure, Hypertension, Age ≥75 [doubled], Diabetes, Stroke [doubled]-Vascular disease, Age 65–74, and Sex category [female]) score for a risk factor-based assessment in patients with non-valvular AF [127]. Oral anticoagulation (e.g. adjusted-dose vitamin K antagonist) is recommended for patients with one "major" risk factor (prior stroke, TIA, thromboembolism, age ≥75 years) or ≥2 "clinically relevant non-major" risk factors (heart failure, hypertension, diabetes, age 65–75, female sex, vascular disease). For patients with one "clinically relevant non-major" risk factor anticoagulation or aspirin is recommended depending on other risk factors, complications, bleeding risk, and patients' preferences. Thus, antithrombotic therapy is recommended in all patients with AF and without contraindication unless they are younger than 65 and truly low risk (e.g. women <65 years with no other risk factor) [127].

Stroke risk for patients with paroxysmal or persistent AF is comparable to the risk in patients with permanent AF [127]. Patients with a prosthetic heart valve, with or without AF, should receive long-term anticoagulation with a target international normalized ratio (INR) based on the prosthesis type [127].

Stroke risk in patients with AF is markedly decreased by the use of oral anticoagulation. A meta-analysis of 29 randomized trials including more than 28 000 participants with at least 3 months' follow-up showed that antiplatelet agents compared to a placebo or no treatment reduced relative stroke risk by 22% (95% CI 6%–35%) in patients with non-valvular AF [128]. For primary prevention this corresponds to an absolute risk reduction of 0.8% per year. Compared to the control group, adjusted-dose

warfarin (target INR 2.0–3.0) reduced stroke risk relatively by 64% (95% CI 49%–74%); this corresponds to an absolute risk reduction of 2.7% in primary prevention. In direct comparison adjusted-dose warfarin proved to be more effective than antiplatelet therapy at reducing stroke (RR reduction 39%; 95% CI 18%–52%) [128]. Major extracranial bleeding events and intracranial hemorrhages were rare and therefore risk estimates are imprecise. However, the increase in absolute risk of major extracranial hemorrhage was less than the absolute reduction in stroke risk [128]. A Cochrane review including 9598 patients with non-valvular AF and no history of stroke or TIA found a risk reduction of ischemic stroke of OR 0.5 (95% CI 0.4–0.7) for oral anticoagulants compared to antiplatelet therapy and an increased risk of intracranial hemorrhages of OR 2.0 (95% CI 1.2–3.3) [129].

There have been concerns because participants of clinical trials are usually highly selected and especially very old persons, with the highest risk of AF, stroke, and hemorrhages, are generally not included. However, the results of these randomized trials have been found to translate well into clinical practice. Warfarin therapy compared to no treatment or aspirin was associated with a 51% reduced risk of thromboembolism (95% CI 39%–60%) in a cohort of persons with non-valvular AF [130]. Intracranial hemorrhages were rare but slightly higher for warfarin (adjusted hazard ratio 2.0; 95% CI 1.2–3.1; 0.46 vs. 0.23 per 100 person-years). The risk of non-intracranial major hemorrhages was not increased [130]. The risk of major hemorrhages increases with older age; however, this was independent of the use of warfarin [131]. The WASPO (Warfarin vs. Aspirin for Stroke Prevention in Octogenarians) [132] and BAFTA (Birmingham Atrial Fibrillation Treatment of the Aged) [133] trials showed that warfarin was safe and effective in older individuals.

New types of oral anticoagulants have recently been tested in phase III clinical trials. They can be classified into direct thrombin inhibitors (dabigatran) and into factor Xa inhibitors (e.g. rivaroxaban, apixaban). All trials showed noninferiority for the prevention of stroke and systemic embolism compared to warfarin. These agents offer the potential for enhanced efficacy, as well as an improved safety profile. Their indication is limited to AF (permanent or paroxysmal) and to patients with a creatinine clearance >30 ml/min [134]. So far no head to head trial has been done; however, an indirect comparison analysis of these three drugs showed differences in their efficacy and safety for primary prevention [135].

Atrial fibrillation is a strong independent risk factor for ischemic stroke, which is markedly decreased by oral anticoagulation. New oral anticoagulants are now available that are more effective and have an improved safety profile compared to vitamin K antagonists.

Obstructive sleep apnea

Obstructive sleep apnea (OSA) has been identified as an often undiagnosed risk factor for cardiovascular diseases and ischemic stroke. In a meta-analysis of five cohort studies (8435 participants) OSA was associated with a significant increased risk for stroke (OR 2.24; 95% CI 1.57–3.19) [136]. However, not all studies were adjusted for potential confounding risk factors. Thus it is still debated whether OSA is an independent risk factor for stroke or mediated through other major vascular risk factors such as obesity, hypertension, and diabetes. About 50% of OSA patients are hypertensive [137] and 15–30% suffer from type 2 diabetes [138].

Obesity is the most important risk factor for OSA and indeed lifestyle changes and weight loss can improve the symptoms of OSA [139]. However, the primary therapy for OSA is the application of

TABLE 3. Regression Coefficients Expressing Performance Decrements (in SD Units) for Each 10% Increment in 10-Year Risk of Stroke*			
Psychometric Test	β†	SE	P
Similarities (abstract reasoning ability)	−0.111	0.032	0.0005
Paired Associates Learning (new learning and memory)	−0.024	0.034	0.4879
Verbal Memory Composite‡	−0.041	0.029	0.1626
Visual-Spatial Memory and Organization Composite	−0.150	0.026	<0.0001
Visual Reproductions–Immediate Recall	−0.172	0.033	<0.0001
Visual Reproductions–Delayed Recall	−0.141	0.033	<0.0001
Visual Reproductions–Delayed Recognition	−0.139	0.034	<0.0001
Hooper Visual Organization Test	−0.138	0.033	<0.0001
Concentration, Visual Scanning and Tracking Composite	−0.138	0.029	<0.0001
Trail-Making Test A (log transformation)	−0.144	0.034	<0.0001
Trail-Making Test B (log transformation)	−0.129	0.032	<0.0001

Scores on the Wide Range Achievement Test–Reading were unrelated to FSRP.

*Persons with a history of dementia or stroke were excluded.

†Regression coefficients are adjusted for age, sex, and education level.

‡None of the tests of Logical Memory (Immediate Recall, Delayed Recall and Delayed Recognition) were associated with the FSRP (P>0.12).

Figure 7.5. In stroke- and dementia-free individuals, higher 10-year risk for stroke is associated with performance decrements in multiple cognitive domains. Regression coefficients expressing performance decrements (in SD Units) for each 10% increment in 10-year risk of stroke. FSRP = Framingham Stroke Risk Profile. Reproduced with permission from Elias et al. [141].

continuous positive airways pressure (CPAP) via a nasal mask. The major problem of CPAP is related to patients' acceptance of the facial mask [137]. CPAP has been shown to improve the symptoms of OSA and to reduce BP. A meta-analysis of 28 randomized trials (1948 patients) found a mean reduction in diurnal systolic BP of 2.58 mmHg (95% CI 1.59–3.57 mmHg) and in diastolic BP of 2.01 mmHg (95% CI 1.18–2.84 mmHg) for positive air pressure treatment compared to controls [140].

There are however only few data on the effect of CPAP on cardiovascular risk and no prospective randomized trial has tested the effect of OSA treatment on stroke risk.

> OSA was associated with a significant increased risk for stroke, but whether OSA is an independent risk factor for stroke or mediated through other major vascular risk factors is not clear.

Risk factors and cognition

Vascular risk factors have mostly been studied for the incidence risk of stroke but recently their contribution to the development of cognitive decline has also been noted. Interaction of vascular risks with neurodegenerative diseases such as Alzheimer dementia has been confirmed. While the vascular prevention issues involved in prevention of Alzheimer's and mixed dementia are of great importance, their role and separate risks will not be covered in this chapter. It is noteworthy though, that accumulating vascular risk factors already have measureable effects on cognitive performance. In the Framingham cohort, vascular high-risk persons showed a significantly higher impairment of cognitive performance (Figure 7.5) [141]. This was observed for tests indexing visual-spatial memory, attention, organization, scanning, and abstract reasoning. This has been confirmed in another cross-sectional study of middle-aged persons [142]. It is therefore important to recognize the needs for early preventive measures already in younger high-risk persons.

Chapter summary

Five low-risk **lifestyle factors** with a high potential to prevent stroke:
- Non-smoking – stroke risk for smokers increases 2.9-fold for subarachnoid hemorrhages and 2-fold for ischemic stroke, but there is no clear

relationship for intracerebral hemorrhages. The relative risk of passive smoking for stroke can be as high as 1.6.
- Modest alcohol consumption – excessive alcohol drinking increases all-cause mortality, as well as the risk of coronary heart disease and stroke. But benefits overcome the harmful effect of alcohol at light to moderate alcohol consumption.
- Body mass index (BMI) <25 kg/m^2 – a high BMI is associated with an increased risk of stroke. Abdominal adiposity (as measured by waist-to-hip ratio) has been suggested to be an even better indicator for stroke risk than overall body mass (as measured by BMI).
- Moderate activity ≥30 min/day – regular physical activity has a protective effect for stroke.
- Healthy diet – a diet low in sodium, high in potassium, and rich in fruits and vegetables, whole grains, cereal fiber, and fatty fish has the highest potential to reduce stroke risk.

These five lifestyle modifications contribute to the reduction of other stroke risk factors such as diabetes, hypertension, and dyslipidemia.

Diseases and pathological conditions
- Elevated blood pressure (BP) is the best-documented treatable risk factor for stroke. Lowering BP substantially reduces stroke with a risk reduction of 31% for every 10 mmHg reduction of systolic BP. Guidelines recommend lowering BP to 140/85 mmHg or below. No antihypertensive drug class was found to be superior in reducing stroke risk.
- There is insufficient evidence from randomized trials that improving glucose control reduces stroke. Cardiovascular mortality associated with different blood cholesterol levels was three times higher in diabetic compared to non-diabetic men. Treatment of diabetic patients with statins reduced the risk of stroke by 24–33%.
- In prospective cohort studies stroke risk was found to be weakly positively associated with serum cholesterol level in ischemic stroke but negatively for intracerebral hemorrhages. High-density lipoprotein (HDL) was found to be negatively associated with total and ischemic stroke incidence. Randomized controlled trials found a clear positive effect of cholesterol-lowering statin therapy on the incidence of ischemic stroke.
- Atrial fibrillation (AF, permanent, paroxysmal, or persistent) is a strong independent risk factor for ischemic stroke (risk = nearly 5-fold). Stroke risk

in patients with AF is markedly decreased by the use of oral anticoagulation (primary prevention: absolute risk reduction of 0.8% per year, warfarin being more effective than antiplatelet therapy).

- Obstructive sleep apnea is associated with a significant risk of stroke. It is not clear if it is an independent risk factor or if increased incidence is mediated through other vascular risk factors associated with obstructive sleep apnea.

Reduction of risk factors and treatment of pathological conditions associated with cerebrovascular disease are the most important interventions for stroke prevention.

References

1. O'Donnell MJ, Xavier D, Liu L, *et al.* Risk factors for ischemic and intracerebral *hemorrhagic* stroke in 22 countries (the INTERSTROKE study): a case-control study. *Lancet* 2010; **376**:112–23.

2. Kurth T, Moore S, Gaziano J, *et al.* Healthy lifestyle and the risk of stroke in women. *Arch Intern Med* 2006; **166**:1403–9.

3. Chiuve SE, Rexrode KM, Spiegelman D, *et al.* Primary prevention of stroke by healthy lifestyle. *Circulation* 2008; **118**:947–54.

4. Zhang Y, Tuomilehto J, Jousilahti P, *et al.* Lifestyle factors on the risks of ischemic and hemorrhagic stroke. *Arch Intern Med* 2011; **171**:1811–18.

5. Wolf PA, D'Agostino RB, Kannel WB, Bonita R, Belanger AJ. Cigarette smoking as a risk factor for stroke. The Framingham Study. *JAMA* 1988; **259**:1025–9.

6. Kawachi I, Colditz GA, Stampfer MJ, *et al.* Smoking cessation in relation to total mortality rates in women. A prospective cohort study. *Ann Intern Med* 1993; **119**:992–1000.

7. Honjo K, Iso H, Tsugane S, *et al.* The effects of smoking and smoking cessation on mortality from cardiovascular disease among Japanese: pooled analysis of three large-scale cohort studies in Japan. *Tob Control* 2010; **19**:50–7.

8. Shinton R, Beevers G. Meta-analysis of relation between cigarette smoking and stroke. *BMJ* 1989; **298**:789–94.

9. Teunissen LL, Rinkel GJ, Algra A, van Gijn J. Risk factors for subarachnoid hemorrhage: a systematic review. *Stroke* 1996; **27**:544–9.

10. Ariesen MJ, Claus SP, Rinkel GJ, Algra A. Risk factors for intracerebral hemorrhage in the general population: a systematic review. *Stroke* 2003; **34**:2060–5.

11. Kurth T, Kase CS, Berger K, *et al.* Smoking and the risk of hemorrhagic stroke in men. *Stroke* 2003; **34**:1151–5.

12. Kurth T, Kase CS, Berger K, *et al.* Smoking and risk of hemorrhagic stroke in women. *Stroke* 2003; **34**:2792–5.

13. Sturgeon JD, Folsom AR, Longstreth WT Jr, *et al.* Risk factors for intracerebral hemorrhage in a pooled prospective study. *Stroke* 2007; **38**:2718–25.

14. Howard G, Wagenknecht LE, Burke GL, *et al.* Cigarette smoking and progression of atherosclerosis: The Atherosclerosis Risk in Communities (ARIC) Study. *JAMA* 1998; **279**:119–24.

15. Lee PN, Forey BA. Environmental tobacco smoke exposure and risk of stroke in nonsmokers: a review with meta-analysis. *J Stroke Cerebrovasc Dis* 2006; **15**:190–201.

16. Håheim LL, Holme I, Hjermann I, Leren P. Smoking habits and risk of fatal stroke: 18 years follow up of the Oslo Study. *J Epidemiol Community Health* 1996; **50**:621–4.

17. WHO Collaborative Study of Cardiovascular Disease and Steroid Hormone Contraception. Ischemic stroke and combined oral contraceptives: results of an international, multicentre, case-control study. *Lancet* 1996; **348**:498–505.

18. WHO Collaborative Study of Cardiovascular Disease and Steroid Hormone Contraception. Hemorrhagic stroke, overall stroke risk, and combined oral contraceptives: results of an international, multicentre, case-control study. *Lancet* 1996; **348**:505–10.

19. Stead LF, Perera R, Bullen C, *et al.* Nicotine replacement therapy for smoking cessation. *Cochrane Database Syst Rev* 2012; **11**:CD000146.

20. Hughes JR, Stead LF, Lancaster T. Antidepressants for smoking cessation. *Cochrane Database Syst Rev* 2007; **1**:CD000031.

21. Cahill K, Stead LF, Lancaster T. Nicotine receptor partial agonists for smoking cessation. *Cochrane Database Sys Rev* 2012; **4**:CD006103.

22. Barth J, Critchley J, Bengel J. Psychosocial interventions for smoking cessation in patients with coronary heart disease. *Cochrane Database Syst Rev* 2008; **1**:CD006886.

23. Mazzaglia G, Britton AR, Altmann DR, Chenet L. Exploring the relationship between alcohol consumption and non-fatal or

fatal stroke: a systematic review. *Addiction* 2001; **96**:1743–56.

24. Reynolds K, Lewis B, Nolen JD, *et al.* Alcohol consumption and risk of stroke: a meta-analysis. *JAMA* 2003; **289**:579–88.

25. de Lange DW, Hijmering ML, Lorsheyd A, *et al.* Rapid intake of alcohol (binge drinking) inhibits platelet adhesion to fibrinogen under flow. *Alcohol Clin Exp Res* 2004; **28**:1562–8.

26. Truelsen T, Gronbaek M, Schnohr P, Boysen G. Intake of beer, wine, and spirits and risk of stroke: the Copenhagen city heart study. *Stroke* 1998; **29**:2467–72.

27. Hillbom M, Numminen H, Juvela S. Recent heavy drinking of alcohol and embolic stroke. *Stroke* 1999; **30**:2307–12.

28. Guiraud V, Amor MB, Mas JL, Touzé E. Triggers of ischemic stroke: a systematic review. *Stroke* 2010; **41**:2669–77.

29. Wannamethee SG, Shaper AG. Patterns of alcohol intake and risk of stroke in middle-aged British men. *Stroke* 1996; **27**: 1033–9.

30. Kiyohara Y, Kato I, Iwamoto H, Nakayama K, Fujishima M. The impact of alcohol and hypertension on stroke incidence in a general Japanese population. The Hisayama Study. *Stroke* 1995; **26**:368–72.

31. Dickinson HO, Mason JM, Nicolson DJ, *et al.* Lifestyle interventions to reduce raised blood pressure: a systematic review of randomized controlled trials. *J Hypertens* 2006; **24**:215–33.

32. Djoussé L, Levy D, Benjamin EJ, *et al.* Long-term alcohol consumption and the risk of atrial fibrillation in the Framingham Study. *Am J Cardiol* 2004; **93**:710–13.

33. Kurth T, Gaziano J, Berger K, *et al.* Body mass index and the risk of stroke in men. *Arch Intern Med* 2002; **162**:2557–62.

34. Jood K, Jern C, Wilhelmsen L, Rosengren A. Body mass index in mid-life is associated with a first stroke in men: a prospective population study over 28 years. *Stroke* 2004; **35**:2764–9.

35. Kurth T, Gaziano J, Rexrode K, *et al.* Prospective study of body mass index and risk of stroke in apparently healthy women. *Circulation* 2005; **111**:1992–8.

36. Hu G, Tuomilehto J, Silventoinen K, *et al.* Body mass index, waist circumference, and waist-hip ratio on the risk of total and type-specific stroke. *Arch Intern Med* 2007; **167**:1420–7.

37. Rexrode KM, Hennekens CH, Willett WC, *et al.* A prospective study of body mass index, weight change, and risk of stroke in women. *JAMA* 1997; **277**:1539–45.

38. Song YM, Sung J, Davey Smith G, Ebrahim S. Body mass index and ischemic and hemorrhagic stroke: a prospective study in Korean men. *Stroke* 2004; **35**:831–6.

39. Suk SH, Sacco RL, Boden-Albala B, *et al.*; Northern Manhattan Stroke Study. Abdominal obesity and risk of ischemic stroke: the Northern Manhattan Stroke Study. *Stroke* 2003; **34**:1586–92.

40. Emerging Risk Factors Collaboration, Wormser D, Kaptoge S, *et al.* Separate and combined associations of body-mass index and abdominal adiposity with cardiovascular disease: collaborative analysis of 58 prospective studies. *Lancet* 2011; **377**:1085–95.

41. Gelber RP, Gaziano JM, Orav EJ, *et al.* Measures of obesity and cardiovascular risk among men and women. *J Am Coll Cardiol* 2008; **52**:605–15.

42. Neter J, Stam B, Kok F, Grobbee D, Geleijnse J. Influence of weight reduction on blood pressure: a meta-analysis of randomized controlled trials. *Hypertension* 2003; **42**:878–84.

43. Curioni C, Andre C, Veras R. Weight reduction for primary prevention of stroke in adults with overweight or obesity. *Cochrane Database Syst Rev* 2006; 4:CD006062.

44. Shaw K, Gennat H, O'Rourke P, Del Mar C. Exercise for overweight or obesity. *Cochrane Database Syst Rev* 2006; 4:CD003817.

45. Li J, Siegrist J. Physical activity and risk of cardiovascular disease —a meta-analysis of prospective cohort studies. *Int J Environ Res Public Health* 2012; **9**:391–407.

46. Diep L, Kwagyan J, Kurantsin-Mills J, Weir R, Jayam-Trouth A. Association of physical activity level and stroke outcomes in men and women: a meta-analysis. *J Womens Health (Larchmt)* 2010; **19**:1815–22.

47. Lee C, Folsom A, Blair S. Physical activity and stroke risk: a meta-analysis. *Stroke* 2003; **34**:2475–81.

48. Deplanque D, Masse I, Lefebvre C, *et al.* Prior TIA, lipid-lowering drug use, and physical activity decrease ischemic stroke severity. *Neurology* 2006; **67**:1403–10.

49. Wannamethee G, Shaper AG. Physical activity and stroke in British middle aged men. *BMJ* 1992; **304**:597–601.

50. Hu FB, Stampfer MJ, Colditz GA, *et al.* Physical activity and risk of stroke in women. *JAMA* 2000; **283**:2961–7.

51. Hu G, Sarti C, Jousilahti P, *et al.* Leisure time, occupational, and commuting physical activity and the risk of stroke. *Stroke* 2005; **36**:1994–9.

52. Lee IM, Paffenbarger RS Jr. Physical activity and stroke incidence: the Harvard Alumni Health Study. *Stroke* 1998; **29**:2049–54.

53. Lee IM, Hennekens CH, Berger K, Buring JE, Manson JE. Exercise and risk of stroke in male physicians. *Stroke* 1999; **30**:1–6.

135

54. Wendel-Vos GC, Schuit AJ, Feskens EJ, et al. Physical activity and stroke: a meta-analysis of observational data. *Int J Epidemiol* 2004; **33**:787–98.

55. Cornelissen VA, Fagard RH. Effects of endurance training on blood pressure, blood pressure-regulating mechanisms, and cardiovascular risk factors. *Hypertension* 2005; **46**:667–75.

56. Shaw K, Gennat H, O'Rourke P, Del Mar C. Exercise for overweight or obesity. *Cochrane Database Syst Rev* 2006; 4:CD003817.

57. Ding EL, Mozaffarian D. Optimal dietary habits for the prevention of stroke. *Semin Neurol* 2006; **26**:11–23.

58. He FJ, Nowson CA, MacGregor GA. Fruit and vegetable consumption and stroke: meta-analysis of cohort studies. *Lancet* 2006; **367**:320–6.

59. Joshipura KJ, Ascherio A, Manson JE, et al. Fruit and vegetable intake in relation to risk of ischemic stroke. *JAMA* 1999; **282**:1233–9.

60. Mellen PB, Walsh TF, Herrington DM. Whole grain intake and cardiovascular disease: a meta-analysis. *Nutr Metab Cardiovasc Dis* 2008; **18**:283–90.

61. Chowdhury R, Stevens S, Gorman D, et al. Association between fish consumption, long chain omega 3 fatty acids, and risk of cerebrovascular disease: systematic review and meta-analysis. *BMJ* 2012; **345**:e6698.

62. Mozaffarian D, Rimm EB. Fish intake, contaminants, and human health: evaluating the risks and the benefits. *JAMA* 2006; **296**:1885–99.

63. Strazzullo P, D'Elia L, Kandala NB, Cappuccio FP. Salt intake, stroke, and cardiovascular disease: meta-analysis of prospective studies. *BMJ* 2009; **339**:b4567.

64. Taylor RS, Ashton KE, Moxham T, Hooper L, Ebrahim S. Reduced dietary salt for the prevention of cardiovascular disease. *Cochrane Database Syst Rev* 2011; 7:CD009217.

65. Stamler J. The INTERSALT Study: background, methods, findings, and implications. *Am J Clin Nutr* 1997; **65**:626S–42S.

66. He FJ, Li J, Macgregor GA. Effect of longer term modest salt reduction on blood pressure: Cochrane systematic review and meta-analysis of randomised trials. *BMJ* 2013; **346**:f1325.

67. Sacks FM, Svetkey LP, Vollmer WM, et al.; DASH-Sodium Collaborative Research Group. Effects on blood pressure of reduced dietary sodium and the Dietary Approaches to Stop Hypertension (DASH) diet. DASH-Sodium Collaborative Research Group. *N Engl J Med* 2001; **344**:3–10.

68. Larsson SC, Orsini N, Wolk A. Dietary potassium intake and risk of stroke: a dose-response meta-analysis of prospective studies. *Stroke* 2011; **42**:2746–50.

69. Aburto NJ, Hanson S, Gutierrez H, et al. Effect of increased potassium intake on cardiovascular risk factors and disease: systematic review and meta-analyses. *BMJ* 2013; **346**:f1378.

70. Larsson SC, Orsini N, Wolk A. Dietary calcium intake and risk of stroke: a dose-response meta-analysis. *Am J Clin Nutr* 2013; **97**:951–7.

71. Larsson SC, Orsini N, Wolk A. Dietary magnesium intake and risk of stroke: a meta-analysis of prospective studies. *Am J Clin Nutr* 2012; **95**:362–6.

72. Larsson SC, Orsini N. Coffee consumption and risk of stroke: a dose-response meta-analysis of prospective studies. *Am J Epidemiol* 2011; **174**:993–1001.

73. Arab L, Liu W, Elashoff D. Green and black tea consumption and risk of stroke: a meta-analysis. *Stroke* 2009; **40**:1786–92.

74. Larsson SC, Virtamo J, Wolk A. Chocolate consumption and risk of stroke: a prospective cohort of men and meta-analysis. *Neurology* 2012; **79**:1223–9.

75. Fung TT, Chiuve SE, McCullough ML, et al. Adherence to a DASH-style diet and risk of coronary heart disease and stroke in women. *Arch Intern Med* 2008; **168**:713–20.

76. Salehi-Abargouei A, Maghsoudi Z, Shirani F, Azadbakht L. Effects of Dietary Approaches to Stop Hypertension (DASH)-style diet on fatal or nonfatal cardiovascular diseases–Incidence: a systematic review and meta-analysis on observational prospective studies. *Nutrition* 2013; **29**:611–18.

77. Sofi F, Abbate R, Gensini GF, Casini A. Accruing evidence on benefits of adherence to the Mediterranean diet on health: an updated systematic review and meta-analysis. *Am J Clin Nutr* 2010; **92**:1189–96.

78. Estruch R, Ros E, Salas-Salvadó J, et al. Primary prevention of cardiovascular disease with a Mediterranean diet. *N Engl J Med* 2013; **368**:1279–90.

79. Howard B, Van Horn L, Hsia J, et al. Low-fat dietary pattern and risk of cardiovascular disease: The Women's Health Initiative Randomized Controlled Dietary Modification Trial. *JAMA* 2006; **295**:655–66.

80. Lisabeth L, Bushnell C. Stroke risk in women: the role of menopause and hormone therapy. *Lancet Neurol* 2012; **11**:82–91.

81. Wassertheil-Smoller S, Hendrix SL, Limacher M, et al. Effect of estrogen plus progestin on stroke in postmenopausal women: the Women's Health Initiative: a randomized trial. *JAMA* 2003; **289**:2673–84.

82. Sare GM, Gray LJ, Bath PM. Association between hormone replacement therapy and subsequent arterial and venous vascular events: a meta-analysis. *Eur Heart J* 2008; **29**:2031–41.

83. Marjoribanks J, Farquhar C, Roberts H, Lethaby A. Long term hormone therapy for perimenopausal and postmenopausal women. *Cochrane Database Syst Rev* 2012; 7:CD004143.

84. Nelson HD, Humphrey LL, Nygren P, Teutsch SM, Allan JD. Postmenopausal hormone replacement therapy: scientific review. *JAMA* 2002; **288**:872–81.

85. Villiers TJ. Clinical issues regarding cardiovascular disease and selective estrogen receptor modulators in postmenopausal women. *Climacteric* 2009; **12**:S108–11.

86. Barrett-Connor E, Mosca L, Collins P, *et al.*; Raloxifene Use for The Heart (RUTH) Trial Investigators. Effects of raloxifene on cardiovascular events and breast cancer in postmenopausal women. *N Engl J Med* 2006; **355**:125–37.

87. Bushnell CD, Goldstein LB. Risk of ischemic stroke with tamoxifen treatment for breast cancer: a meta-analysis. *Neurology* 2004; **63**:1230–3.

88. Silverman SL, Christiansen C, Genant HK, *et al.* Efficacy of bazedoxifene in reducing new vertebral fracture risk in postmenopausal women with osteoporosis: results from a 3 year randomized, placebo and active controlled clinical trial. *J Bone Miner Res* 2008; **23**:1923–34.

89. Cummings SR, Ensrud K, Delmas PD, *et al.* Lasofoxifene in postmenopausal women with osteoporosis. *N Engl J Med* 2010; **362**:686–96.

90. Lawes CM, Vander Hoorn S, Rodgers A; International Society of Hypertension. Global burden of blood-pressure-related disease, 2001. *Lancet* 2008; **371**:1513–18.

91. Lewington S, Clarke R, Qizilbash N, Peto R, Collins R. Age-specific relevance of usual blood pressure to vascular mortality: a meta-analysis of individual data for one million adults in 61 prospective studies. *Lancet* 2002; **360**:1903–13.

92. Lawes CM, Bennett DA, Feigin VL, Rodgers A. Blood pressure and stroke: an overview of published reviews. *Stroke* 2004; **35**:1024.

93. Law MR, Morris JK, Wald NJ. Use of blood pressure lowering drugs in the prevention of cardiovascular disease: meta-analysis of 147 trials in the context of expectations from prospective epidemiological studies. *BMJ* 2009; **338**:b1665.

94. Mancia G, Laurent S, Agabiti-Rosei E, *et al.* Reappraisal of European guidelines on hypertension management: a European Society of Hypertension Task Force document. *J Hypertens* 2009; **27**:2121–58.

95. Lv J, Neal B, Ehteshami P, *et al.* Effects of intensive blood pressure lowering on cardiovascular and renal outcomes: a systematic review and meta-analysis. *PLoS Med* 2012; **9**:e1001293.

96. Neal B, MacMahon S, Chapman N; Blood Pressure Lowering Treatment Trialists' Collaboration Effects of ACE inhibitors, calcium antagonists, and other blood-pressure-lowering drugs: results of prospectively designed overviews of randomised trials. Blood Pressure Lowering Treatment Trialists' Collaboration. *Lancet* 2000; **356**:1955–64.

97. Turnbull F; Blood Pressure Lowering Treatment Trialists' Collaboration. Effects of different blood-pressure-lowering regimens on major cardiovascular events: results of prospectively-designed overviews of randomised trials. *Lancet* 2003; **362**:1527–35.

98. Wright JM, Musini VM. First-line drugs for hypertension. *Cochrane Database Syst Rev* 2009; 3:CD001841.

99. Staessen J, Fagard R, Thijs L, *et al.* Randomised double-blind comparison of placebo and active treatment for older patients with isolated systolic hypertension. The systolic hypertension in Europe (syst-eur) trial investigators. *Lancet* 1997; **350**:757–64.

100. Blood Pressure Lowering Treatment Trialists' Collaboration, Turnbull F, Neal B, *et al.* Effects of different regimens to lower blood pressure on major cardiovascular events in older and younger adults: meta-analysis of randomized trials. *BMJ* 2008; **336**:1121–3.

101. Beckett NS, Peters R, Fletcher AE, *et al.*; HYVET Study Group. Treatment of hypertension in patients 80 years of age or older. *N Engl J Med* 2008; **358**:1887–98.

102. Emerging Risk Factors Collaboration, Sarwar N, Gao P, *et al.* Diabetes mellitus, fasting blood glucose concentration, and risk of vascular disease: a collaborative meta-analysis of 102 prospective studies. *Lancet* 2010; **375**:2215–22.

103. Zhang C, Zhou YH, Xu CL, Chi FL, Ju HN. Efficacy of intensive control of glucose in stroke prevention: a meta-analysis of data from 59,197 participants in 9 randomized controlled trials. *PLoS One* 2013; **8**:e54465.

104. Huxley RR, Filion KB, Konety S, Alonso A. Meta-analysis of cohort and case-control studies of type 2 diabetes mellitus and risk of atrial fibrillation. *Am J Cardiol* 2011; **108**:56–62.

105. Kannel WB, Wilson PW, Zhang TJ. The epidemiology of impaired glucose tolerance and hypertension. *Am Heart J* 1991; **121**:1268–73.

106. UK Prospective Diabetes Study 27. Plasma lipids and lipoproteins

at diagnosis of NIDDM by age and sex. *Diabetes Care* 1997; **20**:1683–7.

107. Gaede P, Lund-Andersen H, Parving HH, Pedersen O. Effect of a multifactorial intervention on mortality in type 2 diabetes. *N Engl J Med* 2008; **358**:580–91.

108. Sone H, Tanaka S, Iimuro S, *et al.* Long-term lifestyle intervention lowers the incidence of stroke in Japanese patients with type 2 diabetes: a nationwide multicentre randomized controlled trial (the Japan Diabetes Complications Study). *Diabetologia* 2010; **53**:419–28.

109. de Vries FM, Denig P, Pouwels KB, Postma MJ, Hak E. Primary prevention of major cardiovascular and cerebrovascular events with statins in diabetic patients: a meta-analysis. *Drugs* 2012; **72**:2365–73.

110. Prospective studies collaboration. Cholesterol, diastolic blood pressure, and stroke: 13,000 strokes in 450,000 people in 45 prospective cohorts. *Lancet* 1995; **346**:1647–53.

111. Lewington S, Whitlock G, Clarke R, *et al.*; Prospective Studies Collaboration. Blood cholesterol and vascular mortality by age, sex, and blood pressure: a meta-analysis of individual data from 61 prospective studies with 55,000 vascular deaths. *Lancet* 2007; **370**:1829–39.

112. Shahar E, Chambless LE, Rosamond WD, *et al.*; Atherosclerosis Risk in Communities Study. Plasma lipid profile and incident ischemic stroke: the Atherosclerosis Risk in Communities (ARIC) study. *Stroke* 2003; **34**:623–31.

113. Taylor F, Huffman MD, Macedo AF, *et al.* Statins for the primary prevention of cardiovascular disease. *Cochrane Database Syst Rev* 2013; **1**:CD004816.

114. Cholesterol Treatment Trialists' (CTT) Collaborators, Mihaylova B, Emberson J, *et al.* The effects of lowering LDL cholesterol with statin therapy in people at low risk of vascular disease: meta-analysis of individual data from 27 randomized trials. *Lancet* 2012; **380**:581–90.

115. McKinney JS, Kostis WJ. Statin therapy and the risk of intracerebral hemorrhage: a meta-analysis of 31 randomized controlled trials. *Stroke* 2012; **43**:2149–56.

116. Mills EJ, O'Regan C, Eyawo O, *et al.* Intensive statin therapy compared with moderate dosing for prevention of cardiovascular events: a meta-analysis of >40 000 patients. *Eur Heart J* 2011; **32**:1409–15.

117. Lavigne PM, Karas RH. The current state of niacin in cardiovascular disease prevention: a systematic review and meta-regression. *J Am Coll Cardiol* 2013; **61**:440–6.

118. Zhou YH, Ye XF, Yu FF, *et al.* Lipid management in the prevention of stroke: a meta-analysis of fibrates for stroke prevention. *BMC Neurol* 2013; **13**:1.

119. Corvol JC, Bouzamondo A, Sirol M, *et al.* Differential effects of lipid-lowering therapies on stroke prevention: a meta-analysis of randomized trials. *Arch Intern Med* 2003; **163**:669–76.

120. Mammen AL, Amato AA. Statin myopathy: a review of recent progress. *Curr Opin Rheumatol* 2010; **22**:644–50.

121. McKinney JS, Kostis WJ. Statin therapy and the risk of intracerebral hemorrhage: a meta-analysis of 31 randomized controlled trials. *Stroke* 2012; **43**:2149–56.

122. Wolf PA, Abbott RD, Kannel WB. Atrial fibrillation as an independent risk factor for stroke: the Framingham Study. *Stroke* 1991; **22**:983–8.

123. Go AS, Hylek EM, Phillips KA, *et al.* Prevalence of diagnosed atrial fibrillation in adults: national implications for rhythm management and stroke prevention: the AnTicoagulation and Risk Factors in Atrial Fibrillation (ATRIA) Study. *JAMA* 2001; **285**:2370–5.

124. Lamassa M, Di Carlo A, Pracucci G, *et al.* Characteristics, outcome, and care of stroke associated with atrial fibrillation in Europe: data from a multicenter multinational hospital-based registry (The European Community Stroke Project). *Stroke* 2001; **32**:392–8.

125. Stroke Risk in Atrial Fibrillation Working Group. Independent predictors of stroke in patients with atrial fibrillation: a systematic review. *Neurology* 2007; **69**:546–54.

126. Stroke Risk in Atrial Fibrillation Working Group. Comparison of 12 risk stratification schemes to predict stroke in patients with nonvalvular atrial fibrillation. *Stroke* 2008; **39**:1901–10.

127. European Heart Rhythm Association; European Association for Cardio-Thoracic Surgery, Camm AJ, *et al.* Guidelines for the management of atrial fibrillation: the Task Force for the Management of Atrial Fibrillation of the European Society of Cardiology (ESC). *Eur Heart J* 2010; **31**:2369–429.

128. Hart RG, Pearce LA, Aguilar MI. Meta-analysis: antithrombotic therapy to prevent stroke in patients who have nonvalvular atrial fibrillation. *Ann Intern Med* 2007; **146**:857–67.

129. Aguilar MI, Hart R, Pearce LA. Oral anticoagulants versus antiplatelet therapy for preventing stroke in patients with non-valvular atrial fibrillation and no history of stroke or transient ischemic attacks. *Cochrane Database Syst Rev* 2007; **3**:CD006186.

130. Go AS, Hylek EM, Chang Y, *et al.* Anticoagulation therapy for stroke prevention in atrial fibrillation: how well do randomized trials translate into clinical practice? *JAMA* 2003; **290**:2685–92.

131. Fang MC, Go AS, Hylek EM, *et al.* Age and the risk of warfarin-associated hemorrhage: the anticoagulation and risk factors in atrial fibrillation study. *J Am Geriatr Soc* 2006; **54**:1231–6.

132. Rash A, Downes T, Portner R, *et al.* A randomised controlled trial of warfarin versus aspirin for stroke prevention in octogenarians with atrial fibrillation (WASPO). *Age Ageing* 2007; **36**:151–6.

133. Mant J, Hobbs FD, Fletcher K, *et al.* Warfarin versus aspirin for stroke prevention in an elderly community population with atrial fibrillation (the Birmingham Atrial Fibrillation Treatment of the Aged Study, BAFTA): a randomised controlled trial. *Lancet* 2007; **370**:493–503.

134. Wisler JW: Clinical trials update : recent and ongoing studies in anticoagulation for atrial fibrillation. *Open Access J Clin Trials* 26 2013; **5**:101–10.

135. Rasmussen LH, Larsen TB, Graungaard T, Skjøth F, Lip GY. Primary and secondary prevention with new oral anticoagulant drugs for stroke prevention in atrial fibrillation: indirect comparison analysis. *BMJ* 2012; **345**:e7097.

136. Loke YK, Brown JW, Kwok CS, Niruban A, Myint PK. Association of obstructive sleep apnea with risk of serious cardiovascular events: a systematic review and meta-analysis. *Circ Cardiovasc Qual Outcomes* 2012; **5**:720–8.

137. Somers VK, White DP, Amin R, *et al.* Sleep apnea and cardiovascular disease: an American Heart Association/ American College of Cardiology Foundation Scientific Statement from the American Heart Association Council for High Blood Pressure Research Professional Education Committee, Council on Clinical Cardiology, Stroke Council, and Council on Cardiovascular Nursing. In collaboration with the National Heart, Lung, and Blood Institute National Center on Sleep Disorders Research (National Institutes of Health). *Circulation* 2008; **118**:1080–111.

138. Pamidi S, Tasali E. Obstructive sleep apnea and type 2 diabetes: is there a link? *Front Neurol* 2012; **3**:126.

139. Thomasouli MA, Brady EM, Davies MJ, *et al.* The impact of diet and lifestyle management strategies for obstructive sleep apnoea in adults: a systematic review and meta-analysis of randomised controlled trials. *Sleep Breath* 2013; **17**:925–35.

140. Montesi SB, Edwards BA, Malhotra A, Bakker JP. The effect of continuous positive airway pressure treatment on blood pressure: a systematic review and meta-analysis of randomized controlled trials. *J Clin Sleep Med* 2012; **8**:587–96.

141. Elias MF, Sullivan LM, D'Agostino RB, *et al.* Framingham stroke risk profile and lowered cognitive performance. *Stroke* 2004; **35**:404–9.

142. Joosten H, van Eersel MEA, Gansevoort RT, *et al.* Cardiovascular risk profile and cognitive function in young, middle-aged, and elderly subjects. *Stroke* 2013; **44**:1543–9.

Cardiac diseases relevant to stroke

Claudia Stöllberger and Josef Finsterer

Introduction

Cardiac diseases can be relevant to stroke in different respects:

- In embolic stroke, cardiac diseases may be the cause of embolism, such as atrial fibrillation (AF), endocarditis, left ventricular aneurysm, or cardiomyopathies such as left ventricular hypertrabeculation/non-compaction (LVHT).
- Brady- and tachyarrhythmias may compromise cerebral blood flow.
- Cardiac diseases may coexist, and influence the clinical course and rehabilitation, such as coronary heart disease or dilated cardiomyopathy (dCMP).
- In some instances, cardiac diseases may be the consequence of the stroke, such as stroke-induced transient left ventricular dysfunction, also referred to as Takotsubo cardiomyopathy (TTC).
- Congenital abnormalities such as patent foramen ovale (PFO) or atrial septal aneurysm (ASA) may implicate paradoxical embolism.

Several diseases may coexist in a single patient, such as coronary heart disease and AF. Thus, from a pragmatic point of view, this chapter aims to focus on the most frequent and controversially discussed cardiac abnormalities in stroke patients.

Rhythm disturbances

Atrial fibrillation

AF is a cardiac arrhythmia, defined by the absence of P waves and varying RR distances in the electrocardiogram. AF is a common arrhythmia and its prevalence increases with age up to 9% at age 80–89 years

(Figure 8.1). Approximately 85% of the individuals with AF are between 65 and 85 years of age [1]. Apart from hemodynamic consequences due to the loss of atrial contraction and symptoms, such as palpitations, AF may lead to embolic stroke or peripheral or mesenteric embolism. Compared to patients with sinus rhythm, patients with AF due to rheumatic heart disease, particularly mitral stenosis, have a 17-fold increased risk of stroke, whereas patients with non-rheumatic AF have a 5-fold increased risk of stroke [2]. Among all ischemic strokes, up to 31% are due to embolic complications of AF [3]. Effective methods of detecting AF in stroke patients are warranted since patients with AF after ischemic stroke are at high risk of suffering recurrent strokes, irrespective of whether AF is permanent or paroxysmal.

Diagnosing paroxysmal atrial fibrillation

Whereas diagnosis of permanent AF is easily feasible from the 12-lead electrocardiogram, identifying paroxysmal AF in stroke patients is still a challenge. A review comprising five studies analyzed the diagnostic yield of monitoring devices for detecting paroxysmal AF in 736 stroke patients: Holter monitoring over 24–72 hours detected AF in 4.6%, whereas 4-day or 7-day event loop recorders detected AF in an additional 6–8% after negative Holter monitoring [4]. A further study applied 7-day event recording at 0, 3, and 6 months and detected AF in 14% of patients with an initial negative Holter [5]. Interestingly, frequent supraventricular ectopic beats (>70 during a 24-hour Holter) were predictors of AF [5]. Another study found that the combined use of Holter and serial electrocardiograms within the first 3 days gave a better rate of AF detection (14%) than serial electrocardiograms alone (11%) [6].

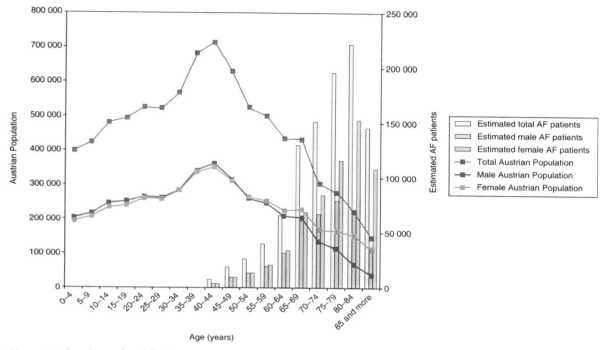

Figure 8.1. Prevalence of atrial fibrillation according to age ranges in the Austrian population according to an estimation for the US population [1].

Future developments for detection of paroxysmal atrial fibrillation

Detection of paroxysmal AF is impeded by the available monitoring devices. The electrodes may cause skin irritation, making it difficult to wear them for long periods. Event loop recorders miss asymptomatic AF because they rely on the patient's recognition of symptoms. Improved methods for detecting AF are currently being evaluated in pilot trials, such as a 30-day cardiac event monitoring belt in the EMBRACE study or the Reveal XT [7]. The Reveal XT (Medtronic Inc.) is an implantable event-triggered recorder which detects and monitors atrial and ventricular tachycardias. Using a special algorithm, the device is able to detect AF episodes, and determining their time of onset and duration (Figure 8.2). Ongoing studies are evaluating the use of this implantable loop recorder for the diagnosis of paroxysmal AF in patients with stroke. In a cohort study of 51 patients with ischemic stroke for which no cause had been found following appropriate vascular and cardiac imaging and at least 24 hours of cardiac rhythm monitoring, the implantable loop recorder was applied and detected AF in 26% [8].

Left atrial appendage occlusion for stroke prevention in atrial fibrillation

Surgical or percutaneous closure of the left atrial appendage (LAA) is considered an alternative to oral anticoagulation (OAC) to prevent strokes in AF. The Watchman left atrial appendage occluder has been compared with warfarin in the PROTECT-AF trial and has been shown to be noninferior to warfarin [9, 10]. However, there are several concerns about the rationale and safety of LAA occlusion.

There is no evidence that embolism in AF exclusively derives from LAA thrombi. When prospectively investigating clinically stable outpatients with AF and with no recent embolism by transesophageal echocardiography, the prevalence of LAA thrombi was only 2.5%, and during a follow-up of 58 months LAA thrombus did not predict stroke/embolism [11].

The LAA has properties which may impede the completion of the occlusion. The LAA myocardium has a higher distensibility than the left atrial myocardium. Progressive dilatation of the LAA occurs in AF, possibly leading to leakage of a primarily completely closed LAA. Incomplete LAA closure creates a pouch

141

with stagnant blood flow, which enhances thrombus formation (Figure 8.3).

Even if technical improvements lead to a more effective LAA occlusion, potential further side-effects have to be considered. The LAA plays an important role in hemodynamic and body fluid regulation. LAA elimination may impede physiological regulation of heart failure and thirst-perception [12]. The LAA is a

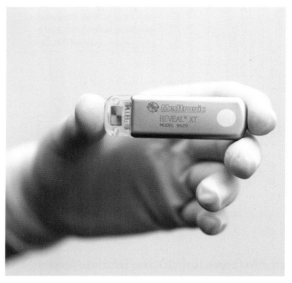

Figure 8.2. The Reveal XT (Medtronic Inc.) is an implantable device that records the cardiac rhythm for up to 3 years. Ongoing studies are evaluating these implantable loop recorders for the diagnosis of paroxysmal atrial fibrillation in patients with stroke.

place of secretion of atrial natriuretic peptide (ANP). ANP contributes to physiological control of lipid mobilization in humans so LAA elimination might promote development of obesity [13]. In view of global warming and the obesity epidemic, LAA elimination is a highly questionable procedure for stroke prevention.

Ablation of atrial fibrillation for stroke prevention

Radiofrequency catheter ablation (RFA) of AF is a recently proposed interventional method to cure AF. There are concerns, however, whether RFA is a safe and effective therapy to prevent strokes.

The targets of RFA are myocardial sleeves near the junction of the pulmonary veins with the left atrium and autonomic ganglia in the left atrial posterior wall, all located epicardially. The RFA catheter, however, is introduced into the left atrium and thus radiofrequency energy is delivered from the endocardial surface with the aim of creating transmural lesions. Thus, RFA can only be performed successfully when affecting the epicardial side of the left atrial wall. Therefore the rate of procedural complications, including pericardial tamponade and life-threatening atrio-esophageal fistula, is considerably high [14, 15].

Since AF is not only an electrical problem, the targets of RFA are not well defined. AF results from long-standing arterial hypertension, and ischemic and valvular heart disease leading to structural abnormalities such as atrial myocardial fibrosis. Since RFA does not abolish myocardial fibrosis it can be

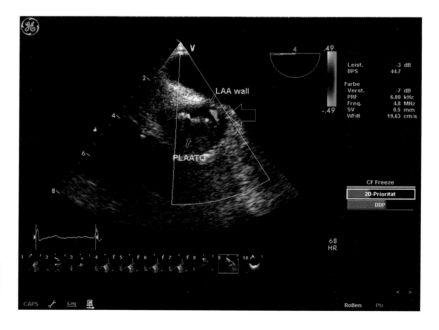

Figure 8.3. Transesophageal echocardiographic picture of the left atrium and left atrial appendage with a percutaneously implanted left atrial appendage occluder (PLAATO device) showing a small jet by color Doppler sonography (arrow) between the PLAATO device and the left atrial appendage (LAA) wall. This jet was not visible at PLAATO implantation but was only detected after 24 months.

expected that ectopic activity may arise from other non-ablated regions and that AF may recur. These considerations are supported by the low long-term efficacy of RFA, especially in permanent AF and structural heart disease [14].

The mean age of patients in whom RFA has been performed so far is 50–63 years [14]. The success rate of RFA is low when the patient is over 65 years [15]. The prevalence of AF, however, increases with advancing age (Figure 8.1) [1]. Thus, the proportion of AF patients who might profit from RFA is much lower than the proportion of those who might not.

Possible candidates for RFA tend to have a low risk of embolic stroke since they are below 65 years and mostly have AF without cardiovascular diseases. RFA, however, increases the risk of stroke periprocedurally due to endocardial lesions. OAC for at least 3 months is usually recommended to prevent thrombus formation on the ablation lines [14, 15]. It has also been emphasized that recurrent AF is more frequently clinically silent after than before RFA [16]. As a consequence it is uncertain whether OAC can be stopped at all after RFA. Furthermore, the transseptal puncture during RFA creates interatrial shunts, and it is at present unknown whether these shunts are clinically relevant in terms of paradoxical embolism. Thus, RFA may create new potential sources of arterial embolism.

We doubt that RFA prevents stroke in AF for the following reasons:

- The majority of AF patients are too old for RFA.
- Candidates for RFA belong to a subgroup with a low risk of embolism.
- The RFA procedure itself may increase the embolic risk.
- At present it is uncertain how long this embolic risk persists after the procedure.

Atrial fibrillation (AF) may lead to embolic stroke. Patients with AF have a 5-fold (non-rheumatic AF) to 17-fold increased risk of stroke (embolism due to rheumatic heart disease).

Bradycardia and tachycardia

If brady- or tachycardia is observed in a stroke patient, the initial diagnostic steps are very similar and aim to assess the clinical severity and to differentiate between cardiac and non-cardiac causes. A suggested practical approach to stroke patients with brady- or tachycardia is given in Table 8.1.

Brady- or tachycardias cause symptoms such as dizziness, light-headedness, or fainting spells. These

Table 8.1. Practical approach to stroke patients with brady- or tachycardia

Assessment of vital signs

Measurement of blood pressure

Registration of a 12-lead electrocardiogram

Measurement of the QT interval according to Bazett's formula: $QTc = QT/\sqrt{RR}$

Registration of the body temperature

Blood tests (electrolytes, blood cell count, D-dimer, C-reactive protein, thyroid function tests)

Assessment of current and previous medication

symptoms may erroneously be interpreted as epileptic seizures. Thus, Holter monitoring to detect recurrent episodes of brady- or tachycardia may be useful in patients with suggestive symptoms. The electroencephalogram is usually normal in these patients.

Bradycardia

Bradycardia is defined as a heart rate <50 beats per minute, and becomes symptomatic only when the rate drops significantly. Bradycardia may be due to cardiac and non-cardiac causes. Non-cardiac causes comprise side-effects of drugs, and disorders such as hypothyroidism, hypothermia, electrolyte disturbances, and increased parasympathetic tone. Furthermore, the brain may be involved in cardiovascular regulation, and the insular cortex is assumed to play a role in rhythm control [17]. Cardiac causes of bradycardia include acute or chronic coronary heart disease, valvular heart disease, and degenerative primary electrical disease. Performing a standard electrocardiogram enables one to diagnose more precisely the type of bradycardia as sinus bradycardia, atrioventricular block, sinus arrest, or AF, and to look for signs of acute myocardial ischemia and to assess whether QT prolongation is present, which is a potentially life-threatening situation [18].

Tachycardia

Tachycardia is defined as a heart rate >100 beats per minute. Like bradycardia, tachycardia may be caused by non-cardiac and cardiac causes. Non-cardiac causes of tachycardia in stroke patients comprise fever, hypovolemia, anemia, hyperthyroidism, pulmonary embolism, pain, alcohol withdrawal, bronchospasm, side-effects of drugs, and rebound in patients previously treated with beta-blocking agents. Cardiac causes of tachycardia are the same as for bradycardia, and the clinical consequences range from palpitations to sudden cardiac death.

> Brady- or tachycardia causes symptoms such as dizziness, light-headedness, or fainting spells. These symptoms may erroneously be interpreted as epileptic seizures.

QT prolongation

Prolongation of ventricular repolarization manifests as a prolongation of the QT interval on the electrocardiogram. QT prolongation may be associated with torsades de pointes tachycardia. Torsades de pointes are often self-limiting and are associated with palpitations, dizziness, or syncope. Degeneration into ventricular fibrillation and sudden cardiac death can occur. In addition to the congenital long QT syndrome many drugs, such as antiarrhythmic drugs class IA and III, antibiotics, antihistamines, neuroleptics, and antidepressants, are known to prolong the QT interval. Information about QT-prolonging drugs can be obtained from the internet (www.torsades.org). Most of these drugs block a specific potassium channel substantially involved in ventricular repolarization. Cardiovascular diseases induce a higher susceptibility to drug-induced prolongation of the QT interval. Correctable factors include hypokalemia, concomitant administration of different QT-prolonging drugs, and bradycardia. In 30–40% of the patients with stroke the QT interval is prolonged [19, 20]. QT prolongation in stroke may be due to cardiovascular comorbidity, concomitant drug intake, and metabolic disturbances, but may also originate from an ischemic cerebral region, especially the insular region [17, 19].

If QT prolongation is observed in a stroke patient, triggering factors should be screened and, if possible, eliminated. Special care should be taken with patients with QT prolongation associated with bradycardia because it entails the risk of torsades de pointes [18]. In these patients the heart rate should be raised to >80 beats per minute and implantation of a pacemaker is recommended.

> Stroke is associated with QT prolongation in 30–40% of patients.

Coronary heart disease
Coexistence of coronary heart disease and stroke

There is a frequent coexistence of coronary heart disease and stroke, most probably due to common atherosclerotic risk factors such as arterial hypertension, diabetes mellitus, smoking, and hypercholesterolemia. A history of symptomatic coronary heart disease, either myocardial infarction or angina pectoris, is found in up to 33% of patients with ischemic stroke [21]. An autopsy study of patients with fatal stroke found coronary plaques in 72%, coronary stenosis in 38%, and myocardial infarction in 41% [22]. Two-thirds of the myocardial infarctions in that study were clinically silent [22]. Coronary heart disease, however, is not only a frequent finding at autopsy but also influences the prognosis of patients surviving a stroke. Five-year follow-up studies have shown that survivors of ischemic stroke are more likely to die of cardiac causes than of recurrent stroke [21, 23]. These results stress the importance for the neurologist to be aware of cardiac symptoms in stroke patients and for the cardiologist to apply cardioprotective measures for stroke patients.

> There is a frequent coexistence of coronary heart disease and stroke, most probably due to common atherosclerotic risk factors.

Diagnosis of coronary heart disease in stroke patients

When caring for stroke patients in the acute or rehabilitation phase, it is necessary to be aware of clinical symptoms of myocardial ischemia such as chest pain or exertional dyspnea, or electrocardiographic abnormalities such as ST-depression, T-wave abnormalities, or newly developing Q-waves [20]. The detection of myocardial injury can be improved by measuring serum levels of troponin T or troponin I biomarkers which are found to be highly specific for myocardial necrosis [24]. Elevated troponin levels in stroke patients with signs or symptoms of myocardial ischemia should entail rhythm monitoring and cardiological consultation regarding further therapeutic and diagnostic measures, including coronary angiography and percutaneous coronary intervention. Stroke patients with normal troponin levels but signs and symptoms suggestive of myocardial ischemia should also be referred to the cardiologist, because stress testing might be indicated. In acute stroke patients without a history or signs of coronary heart disease, however, elevated troponin levels are not indicators of silent coronary heart disease, but rather of a bad prognosis due to heart and renal failure [25]. Troponin positivity may also indicate myocardial involvement in a neuromuscular disease [26].

Myocardial infarction as a cause of embolism

Cardiogenic embolism from a left ventricular thrombus may occur as a complication of acute or subacute myocardial infarction or due to a ventricular aneurysm in the chronic phase of a large, mainly anterior wall infarction [27]. The incidence of left ventricular thrombi early after myocardial infarction has declined in recent years, most probably due to changes in the acute therapy of myocardial infarction, which now comprises intensive anticoagulant therapy and percutaneous coronary interventions [28]. However, left ventricular thrombi may still be detected in patients after myocardial infarction, especially if revascularization in the acute phase has not been performed or was unsuccessful or if the myocardial infarction affected large parts of the left ventricle. Thus, imaging studies to look for left ventricular thrombi, preferentially transthoracic echocardiography, should be performed in all stroke patients with a history or electrocardiographic signs of previous myocardial infarction.

> Acute or subacute myocardial infarction and ventricular aneurysms can be a cause of embolic stroke.

Valvular heart disease

Infective endocarditis and stroke

Ischemic and hemorrhagic strokes occur in 10–23% of patients with endocarditis and cluster during the period of untreated infection [29–31]. Among patients with endocarditis and stroke, the mitral valve seems to be more frequently affected than the aortic valve [30, 31]. Native valves as well as prosthetic valves may be affected by endocarditis, leading to stroke. Stroke patients with prosthetic valves have a worse prognosis than patients with native valves [32, 33].

Diagnosis of infective endocarditis

Despite the availability of echocardiography, laboratory, and microbiological investigations, considerable delay occurs until infective endocarditis is diagnosed. Between onset of the symptoms and diagnosis a mean interval of 31 days has been reported [34]. This is due to the unspecific symptoms of endocarditis such as prolonged flu-like disease, generalized weakness, and fatigue. Embolic events such as stroke are frequently the cause of hospital admission in these patients [29]. Thus, endocarditis has to be considered as a

differential diagnosis in all stroke patients, and symptoms suggestive of endocarditis should be asked for at admission. The suspicion of endocarditis should increase if elevated blood sedimentation rate, leukocytosis, or elevated C-reactive protein is found or if the patient has fever. Blood cultures should be taken in these patients before initiation of antibiotic therapy. In most of the cases with stroke and suspected endocarditis transesophageal echocardiography is necessary because of its better visualization of the valves, valve prosthesis, and vegetation to confirm or exclude the diagnosis (Figure 8.4).

Therapy of infective endocarditis

Antibiotic therapy is the main therapy for infective endocarditis. The risk of stroke in infective endocarditis has been shown to decrease rapidly within 1 week after the initiation of antibiotic therapy [29]. However, if there are large vegetations or destruction of the valves leading to heart failure cardiac surgery may be necessary. In the past, cardiac surgeons have frequently been reluctant to operate on infective endocarditis patients with acute stroke because of concerns about cerebral bleeding complications because of anticoagulation during the cardiopulmonary bypass. However, delay in surgical intervention can lead to the death of patients who might have benefited from surgery. Although no prospective data are available, a retrospective study of patients with infective endocarditis and stroke undergoing cardiac surgery has shown that mortality was 18%, complete neurological recovery was achieved in 70% of the survivors, and secondary cerebral hemorrhage due to cardiac surgery occurred less frequently than was previously thought [35]. A further study showed that there is no apparent survival benefit in delaying surgery when indicated in infective endocarditis patients after ischemic stroke [36]. Based on these findings we recommend that in the event of infective endocarditis in a stroke patient the neurologist, cardiologist, microbiologist, and cardiac surgeon should discuss together the optimal therapeutic management. The therapy should be planned with consideration of the clinical course, the echocardiographic findings, the microorganism involved, the response to antibiotic therapy, and the neurological condition.

> Strokes occur in 10–23% of patients with endocarditis, especially of the mitral valve. Endocarditis must be considered as a differential diagnosis in all stroke patients if laboratory signs of inflammation are present.

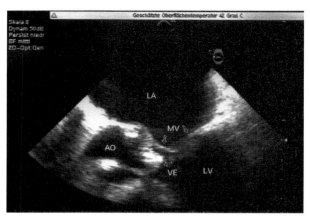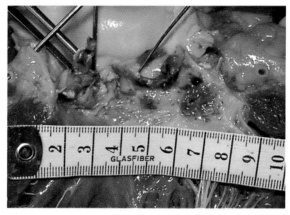

Figure 8.4. Transesophageal echocardiographic picture (left) and autopsy specimen (right) of a patient with embolic stroke and aortic valve endocarditis. LA = left atrium, MV = mitral valve, LV = left ventricle, VE = vegetation, AO = aortic valve.

Stroke after heart valve surgery

After heart valve surgery patients are at increased risk of thromboembolism, due to either thrombus formation on the artificial valve, infective endocarditis, or AF. The embolic risk varies according to the type of surgery (repair versus replacement), the type of replaced valve (bioprosthesis versus mechanical prosthesis), and the affected valve (mitral versus aortic valve). Approximately 20% of patients with aortic or mitral valve prosthesis have an embolic stroke within 15 years after valve replacement [37].

Valve repair

Valve repair is nowadays the preferred surgical correction of mitral regurgitation. Long-term follow-up studies have shown that after mitral repair, the risk of ischemic stroke is similar to that in the general population [38]. However, mitral repair is not always technically feasible, and AF may develop postoperatively, especially when the left atrium is already enlarged before surgery.

Bioprosthesis

Generally, the embolic risk is lower in patients with bioprostheses than with mechanical prostheses. Prostheses in the aortic position have a lower embolic risk than in the mitral position [37]. A disadvantage of bioprostheses is their propensity to degenerate, necessitating reoperation [39]. Furthermore, as in patients after valve repair, AF may

develop, especially after mitral valve surgery, and further increase embolic risk.

Mechanical valve prosthesis

Patients with mechanical prostheses have a higher embolic risk with mitral than with aortic valve replacement [37]. Preoperative left ventricular dysfunction has been identified as an additional risk factor for stroke in patients with mitral prostheses. Patients with a mechanical valve prosthesis and poorly controlled OAC are at increased risk of ischemic stroke as well as bleeding, including cerebral bleeding [39, 40].

> After heart valve surgery patients are at increased risk of thromboembolism.

Patent foramen ovale

In utero, the foramen ovale serves as a physiological conduit for right-to-left shunting. Once the pulmonary circulation is established after birth, left atrial pressure increases and allows functional closure of the foramen ovale. This is followed by anatomical closure of the septum primum and septum secundum. In about 25% of humans, the closure is incomplete, and PFO remains as a flap-like opening, permitting right-to-left shunting when the right atrial pressure exceeds the left atrial pressure. Transesophageal echocardiography (TEE) is considered the method of choice for diagnosing PFO, although there is considerable interobserver ($\kappa = 0.77$) and intraobserver ($\kappa = 0.82$) variability in the diagnosis [41].

Paradoxical embolism

Several retrospective and case–control studies in patients with cryptogenic stroke found that the prevalence of PFO is 30–46% and thus higher than in the general population [42–44]. Paradoxical embolism has been assumed to be the underlying pathomechanism. However, only few of the reported cases of cryptogenic stroke in patients with PFO meet the criteria for the diagnosis of paradoxical embolism, which are: systemic embolism without a cardiac source, presence of venous thrombosis or pulmonary embolism, and an intracardiac defect which will permit right-to-left shunting. Screening especially for venous thromboembolism has been performed only rarely. The results of these studies highlight the importance of searching for venous thromboembolism early after stroke (Table 8.2). Delays in venous diagnostic evaluation may account for negative or confusing results.

Stroke risk and PFO

It is uncertain whether the recurrence rate of stroke in patients with cryptogenic stroke is dependent on the presence of a PFO. In a prospective randomized study, the recurrence rate of stroke was the same in those with or without PFO in those treated with either warfarin or aspirin [44]. Whether subjects from the general population with PFO have an increased risk of ischemic stroke has been studied by two prospective cohort studies, which unanimously found that PFO was not a risk factor for future cerebrovascular events [45, 46]. Overall, it has not been demonstrated that patients with PFO are at increased risk of recurrent stroke. Furthermore, it is uncertain how many strokes in PFO patients are due to paradoxical embolism and how to treat paradoxical embolism. Surgical or interventional closure of PFO is increasingly performed as a measure to prevent recurrent stroke in patients with suspected paradoxical embolism. However, three recently published randomized trials examining the efficacy of a PFO device have shown that PFO closure offers no benefit for patients with cryptogenic stroke compared to medical therapy [47–49].

Interventional PFO closure might even create new cardiac sources for embolism. Thrombus formation may occur on the left side of the occlusion device and lead to arterial embolism, especially in patients with coagulopathies [50, 51].

> In patients with cryptogenic stroke the prevalence of patent foramen ovale (PFO) is 30–46%, but patients with PFO are not at increased risk of recurrent stroke and PFO closure offers no benefit compared to medical therapy.

Table 8.2. Studies investigating the venous system in suspected paradoxical embolism

Author (year)	Patients	Technique	Days between event and investigation	Prevalence of thrombosis,%	Location of thrombosis, n
[77] (1991)	23	V	2–210	26	Femoral, 3
					Iliac, 3
[78] (1993)	42	V	0–90	60	Calf, 13
					Popliteal, 2
					Femoral, 8
					Iliac, 1
[79] (1993)	13	V	0–28	0	0
[80] (1994)	17	R	ND	35	ND
[81] (1994)	16	V or D	ND	31	ND
[82] (1994)	27	V or D	ND	11	ND
[83] (1994)	18	V	1–300	11	ND
[84] (1997)	53	V	1–15	9	ND
[85] (2004)	46	MRV	2 ± 0.67	20	Pelvic, 9

Notes: V = venography; R = radioisotope venography; ND = data not given; D = duplex sonography; MRV = magnetic resonance venography.

Atrial septal aneurysm

An ASA is diagnosed echocardiographically if the atrial septum appears abnormally redundant and mobile. Unfortunately, there are no uniform echocardiographic criteria for this abnormality. The etiology of ASA is unknown. ASA is frequently associated with PFO. It is uncertain whether strokes in ASA are due to paradoxical embolism or other mechanisms. The prevalence of ASA, as assessed by echocardiography in the general population, is 1–2% and depends on the echocardiographic criteria. Furthermore, interobserver ($\kappa = 0.45$) and intraobserver ($\kappa = 0.74$) variability in diagnosing ASA is high [41]. Similarly to PFO, ASA has been found to be closely associated with cryptogenic stroke in retrospective and case–control studies, but failed to be identified as a risk factor for future stroke in prospective randomized or population-based studies [44, 48, 49]. Due to the rarity of ASA it will be difficult to perform adequately powered studies. Development of uniformly accepted diagnostic criteria would facilitate research into ASA.

> Atrial septal aneurysm has been found to be closely associated with cryptogenic stroke but is not a risk factor for future stroke.

Dilated cardiomyopathy

dCMP is a cardiac condition characterized by dilatation of the cardiac cavities (LVEDD >57 mm), reduced systolic function (FS <25%), and normal coronary angiography [52]. dCMP is frequently associated with cardiac rhythm abnormalities and intraventricular thrombus formation. Whether dCMP without AF is associated with an increased risk of stroke or embolism is under debate. At least in patients with dCMP and documented intracardiac thrombus formation the risk of stroke or embolism is regarded as being increased. The prevalence of intra-atrial thrombi in patients with dCMP is estimated to be 20–25% and the prevalence of intraventricular thrombi 50% [53]. During an observational period of 31 months 5% of the patients with dCMP developed a stroke [54]. Among 846 patients with ischemic stroke dCMP was found in 19%, who all had benefits from OAC [55]. Single cases with dCMP who developed ischemic stroke have also been reported, such as two patients with dCMP from cardiac involvement in Duchenne muscular dystrophy [56]. OAC is recommended for secondary stroke prevention in patients with dCMP and intracardiac thrombus formation [53, 57]. OAC is recommended for primary prevention in patients with AF and dCMP. For patients with sinus rhythm, the recently published WARCEF study showed no significant overall difference in the primary outcome endpoint (ischemic stroke, intracerebral hemorrhage, or death from any cause) between treatment with warfarin and treatment with aspirin. A reduced risk of ischemic stroke with warfarin was offset by an increased risk of major hemorrhage. Thus, the choice between warfarin and aspirin in these patients should be individualized [58].

Restrictive cardiomyopathy

Restrictive cardiomyopathy (rCMP) is diagnosed echocardiographically if there is enlargement of both atria, normal systolic function and wall thickness, and a restrictive filling pattern (deceleration time <150 ms) [59]. The cause of rCMP may be idiopathic or rCMP may be a cardiac manifestation of systemic diseases such as amyloidosis, sclerodermia, sarcoidosis, hemochromatosis, Churg–Strauss syndrome, hypereosinophilic syndrome, hyperoxaluria, cystinosis, Gaucher's disease, Fabry's disease, Noonan's syndrome, Werner's syndrome, reactive arthritis, pseudoxanthoma elasticum, various neuromuscular disorders, carcinoid, or lymphoma [59, 60]. Compared to patients with dCMP, patients with rCMP are assumed to have a worse prognosis regarding morbidity and mortality [60]. Whether rCMP is associated with an increased risk of ischemic stroke is unknown, but single cases with rCMP have been described who developed an ischemic stroke [61]. In a study of 15 patients with amyloidosis 60% developed an arterial thromboembolic event, three of whom had an ischemic stroke and two of whom transient ischemic attacks [62]. Most probably these embolic events have their source in the enlarged left atrium and are aggravated by AF, which develops frequently in rCMP patients [59].

Takotsubo cardiomyopathy

TTC, also known as apical ballooning, is a reversible neuromyocardial failure which resembles acute myocardial infarction clinically and electrophysiologically in patients with normal coronary arteries [63]. TTC is clinically characterized by sudden onset of anginal chest pain, dyspnea, or syncope. Initially, the ECG shows ST elevation, which turns into negative

T-waves a few hours or days later, which may persist for months [64, 65]. Reversible akinesia or hypokinesia affects most frequently the left ventricular apex but rarely also the midventricular segments: the non-affected ventricular segments show hypercontrac-tility. Cardiac enzymes, such as creatine phosphoki-nase, and troponin might be slightly elevated. Coronary angiography shows no stenoses of the cor-onary arteries. The cause and pathogenesis of TTC are unknown, but it may be triggered by physical or emo-tional stress, most probably due to catecholamine tox-icity [66]. TTC has been described in association with many diseases including pheochromocytoma, lymph-oma, alcohol withdrawal, plasmapheresis, intestinal perforation, severe knee joint pain, overexertion, amyotrophic lateral sclerosis, subarachnoidal hemor-rhage, anesthesia, ventricular tachycardia, pneumo-thorax, pulmonary embolism, maline myopathy, tracheostomy, metabolic myopathy, epileptic seizures, and ischemic stroke [67, 68]. Stroke, however, may be also a consequence of TTC. TTC results in signifi-cantly reduced systolic function and wall motion abnormalities, which may give rise to thrombus for-mation and lastly cardioembolic events. Thromboem-bolism or transient ischemic attacks have been reported associated with TTC [69].

Left ventricular hypertrabeculation/ non-compaction

LVHT is characterized by a meshwork of interwoven myocardial strings, lined with endocardium, which constitutes a spongy myocardial layer clearly distinct from the normal compacted myocardium (Figure 8.5) [70]. The non-compacted to compacted layer ratio required to fulfill the diagnostic criteria is >2, although there is no consensus about the echocardio-graphic criteria to define LVHT [70]. Consensus, however, exists that LVHT is most easily diagnosed on echocardiography. LVHT is most frequently located in the apex of the left ventricle and over the lateral wall, but usually spares the middle and basal parts of the septum. LVHT is frequently associated with heart failure and systolic dysfunction, which have been also identified as prognostic factors in LVHT [71]. Because of the heterogeneous genetic background of LVHT it does not seem to represent a distinct cardiomyopathy but is rather the result of an attempt to compensate for an insufficiently con-tracting myocardium or possibly the result of myo-carditis. LVHT is associated with neuromuscular disorders (NMDs) in up to 82% of the cases, if sys-tematically searched for [72]. Among all NMDs, Barth syndrome is the one most frequently associated with LVHT [73].

No consensus has been reached so far as to whether LVHT is associated with an increased risk of stroke/embolism or not. In a study on 62 patients with LVHT no increased risk of these patients developing stroke/embolism as compared with age, sex, and left ventricular fractional shortening matched controls was found [70]. In a retrospective study of 144 patients with LVHT stroke was found on imaging studies in 15% of them [74]. Though stroke/embolism has been reported in single patients with LVHT, we regard it as not justified to generally propose OAC for

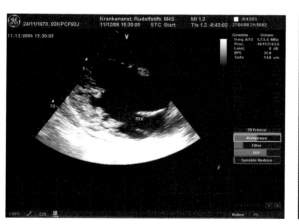
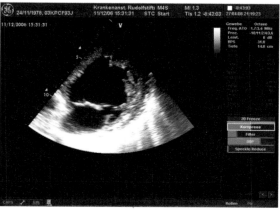

Figure 8.5. Transthoracic echocardiographic parasternal long axis view (left) and apical four-chamber view (right) showing left ventricular hypertrabeculation/non-compaction involving the posterobasal and lateral wall (left).

149

LVHT patients, unless there is concomitant AF, severely reduced left ventricular systolic function, or any other established indication of OAC. So far there is no evidence for a general clotting defect in LVHT patients requiring OAC [70].

Endomyocardial fibrosis

Endomyocardial fibrosis is a rare disease in European countries and is more prevalent in sub-Saharan Africa [75]. The etiology of endomyocardial fibrosis is unknown. Immunological, infectious, and toxicological etiologies are assumed [75]. Clinically, endomyocardial fibrosis is characterized by severe congestive heart failure with only moderately increased heart size. Systolic performance is normal or only slightly depressed despite severe restriction of filling, atrioventricular valve regurgitation, or both. Echocardiography may reveal partial obliteration of the right or left ventricle [75]. Endocardial resection with atrioventricular valve replacement is the treatment of choice, with appreciable postoperative improvement and a 10-year survival of approximately 70% [75]. Whether there is a generally increased risk of stroke in patients with endomyocardial fibrosis is unknown, but single patients have been reported who developed an ischemic stroke. Among these is one who developed multiple ischemic strokes in association with endomyocardial fibrosis from schistosomiasis and one with multiple cerebellar and cerebral infarctions from endomyocardial fibrosis associated with hypereosinophilic syndrome [76].

Chapter summary

Rhythm disturbances

Atrial fibrillation (AF) may lead to embolic stroke or peripheral or mesenteric embolism. Patients with AF have a 5-fold (non-rheumatic AF) to 17-fold increased risk of stroke (embolism due to rheumatic heart disease). Diagnosis of permanent AF is feasible from the 12-lead electrocardiogram, and paroxysmal AF can be diagnosed with 24–72-hour Holter monitoring or 7-day event loop recorders. Implantable loop recorders may facilitate the detection of AF.

Brady- or tachycardia causes symptoms such as dizziness, light-headedness, fainting spells. These symptoms may erroneously be interpreted as epileptic seizures.

QT prolongation: stroke is associated with QT prolongation in 30–40% of patients. QT prolongation in stroke may be due to cardiovascular comorbidity, concomitant drug intake, and metabolic disturbances, but may also be due to the affected brain region, especially the insular region. QT prolongation may be associated with torsades de pointes tachycardia, which manifests as palpitations, dizziness, or syncope. Degeneration into ventricular fibrillation and sudden cardiac death can occur.

Coronary heart disease

There is a frequent coexistence of coronary heart disease and stroke, most probably due to common atherosclerotic risk factors. Suspected coronary heart disease should lead to cardiological consultation for further therapeutic and diagnostic measures, including coronary angiography and percutaneous coronary intervention. Acute or subacute myocardial infarction and ventricular aneurysms can also be a cause of embolic stroke.

Valvular heart disease

Ischemic and hemorrhagic strokes occur in 10–23% of patients with endocarditis, especially of the mitral valve. Diagnosis of infective endocarditis is difficult. Thus, endocarditis has to be considered as a differential diagnosis in all stroke patients if laboratory signs of inflammation are present.

After heart valve surgery patients are at increased risk of thromboembolism. The embolic risk varies according to the type of surgery (repair versus replacement), the type of replaced valve (bioprosthesis versus mechanical prosthesis), and the affected valve (mitral versus aortic valve).

Patent foramen ovale (PFO)

In about 25% of humans the foramen ovale remains open, permitting right-to-left shunting when the right atrial pressure exceeds the left atrial pressure. In patients with cryptogenic stroke the prevalence of PFO is 30–46% (paradoxical embolism from venous thrombosis), but it has not been demonstrated that patients with PFO are at increased risk of recurrent stroke. Randomized trials have shown that percutaneous PFO closure offers no benefit after ischemic stroke compared with medical therapy.

Atrial septal aneurysms (ASM)

An ASM is diagnosed echocardiographically if the atrial septum appears abnormally redundant and mobile. Similarly to PFO, ASM has been found to be closely associated with cryptogenic stroke in retrospective and case–control studies, but failed to be identified as a risk factor for future stroke in prospective randomized or population-based studies.

It is unknown whether conditions such as dilated cardiomyopathy, restrictive cardiomyopathy, Takotsubo cardiomyopathy (a reversible neuromyocardial failure, which resembles acute myocardial infarction clinically and electrophysiologically in patients with normal coronary arteries), left ventricular hypertrabeculation /non-compaction, or endomyocardial fibrosis raise the risk of stroke independently of the presence of atrial fibrillation.

References

1. Feinberg WM, Blackshear JL, Laupacis A, et al. Prevalence, age distribution, and gender of patients with atrial fibrillation. *Arch Intern Med* 1995; **155**:469–73.

2. Wolf PA, Dawber TR, Thomas HE Jr, Kannel WB. Epidemiologic assessment of chronic atrial fibrillation and risk of stroke: The Framingham Study. *Neurology* 1978; **28**:973–7.

3. Steger C, Pratter A, Martinek-Bregel M, et al. Stroke patients with atrial fibrillation have a worse prognosis than patients without: data from the Austrian Stroke registry. *Eur Heart J* 2004; **25**:1734–40.

4. Liao J, Khalid Z, Scallan C, et al. Non-invasive cardiac monitoring for detecting paroxysmal atrial fibrillation or flutter after acute ischemic stroke. A systematic review. *Stroke* 2007; **38**:2935–40.

5. Wallmann D, Tüller D, Wustmann K, et al. Frequent atrial premature beats predict paroxysmal atrial fibrillation in stroke patients. An opportunity for a new diagnostic strategy. *Stroke* 2007; **38**:2292–4.

6. Douen AG, Pageau N, Medic S. Serial electrocardiographic assessments significantly improve detection of atrial fibrillation 2.6-fold in patients with acute stroke. *Stroke* 2008; **39**:480–2.

7. Spring M, Dorian P, Fry B, et al. A 30-day cardiac event monitor belt for recording paroxysmal atrial fibrillation after a cerebral ischemic event. The EMBRACE Pilot Study. *Stroke* 2008; **39**:571–2.

8. Cotter PE, Martin PJ, Ring L, et al. Incidence of atrial fibrillation detected by implantable loop recorders in unexplained stroke. *Neurology* 2013; **80**:1546–50.

9. Holmes DR, Reddy VY, Turi ZG, et al. Percutaneous closure of the left atrial appendage versus warfarin therapy for prevention of stroke in patients with atrial fibrillation: a randomised non-inferiority trial. *Lancet* 2009; **374**:534–42.

10. Reddy VY, Doshi SK, Sievert H, et al. Percutaneous left atrial appendage closure for stroke prophylaxis in patients with atrial fibrillation: 2.3-Year Follow-up of the PROTECT AF (Watchman Left Atrial Appendage System for Embolic Protection in Patients with Atrial Fibrillation) Trial. *Circulation* 2013; **127**:720–9.

11. Stöllberger C, Chnupa P, Kronik G, et al. Transesophageal echocardiography to assess embolic risk in patients with atrial fibrillation. *Ann Intern Med* 1998; **128**:630–8.

12. Stöllberger C, Schneider B, Finsterer J. Elimination of the left atrial appendage to prevent stroke or embolism? Anatomic, physiologic, and pathophysiologic considerations. *Chest* 2003; **124**:2356–62.

13. Moro C, Crampes F, Sengenes C, et al. Atrial natriuretic peptide contributes to physiological control of lipid mobilization in humans. *FASEB J* 2004; **18**:908–10.

14. Weerasooriya R, Khairy P, Litalien J, et al. Catheter ablation for atrial fibrillation: are results maintained at 5 years of follow-up? *J Am Coll Cardiol* 2011; **57**:160–6.

15. Lee SH, Tai CT, Hsieh MH, et al. Predictors of early and late recurrence of atrial fibrillation after catheter ablation of paroxysmal atrial fibrillation. *J Interv Card Electrophysiol* 2004; **10**:221–6.

16. Hindricks G, Piorkowski C, Tanner H, et al. Perception of atrial fibrillation before and after radiofrequency catheter ablation: relevance of asymptomatic arrhythmia recurrence. *Circulation* 2005; **112**:307–13.

17. Oppenheimer S. Cerebrogenic cardiac arrhythmias: cortical lateralization and clinical significance. *Clin Auton Res* 2006; **16**:6–11.

18. Topilski I, Rogowski O, Rosso R, et al. The morphology of the QT interval predicts torsade de pointes during acquired bradyarrhythmias. *J Am Coll Cardiol* 2007; **49**:320–8.

19. Tatschl C, Stöllberger C, Matz K, et al. Insular involvement is associated with QT prolongation: ECG abnormalities in patients with acute stroke. *Cerebrovasc Dis* 2006; **21**:47–53.

20. Fure B, Bruun Wyller T, Thommessen B. Electrocardiographic and troponin T changes in acute ischemic stroke. *J Intern Med* 2006; **259**:592–7.

21. Dhamoon MS, Tai W, Boden-Albala B, *et al*. Risk of myocardial infarction or vascular death after first ischemic stroke. The Northern Manhattan Study. *Stroke* 2007; **38**:1752–8.

22. Gongora-Rivera F, Labreuche J, Jaramillo A, *et al*. Autopsy prevalence of coronary atherosclerosis in patients with fatal stroke. *Stroke* 2007; **38**:1203–10.

23. Hankey GJ, Majrozik K, Broadhurst RJ, *et al*. Five-year survival after first-ever stroke and related prognostic factors in the Perth Community Stroke Study. *Stroke* 2000; **31**:2080–6.

24. Barber M, Morton JJ, Macfarlane PW, *et al*. Elevated troponin levels are associated with sympathoadrenal activation in acute ischemic stroke. *Cerebrovasc Dis* 2007; **23**:260–6.

25. Jensen JK, Kristensen SR, Bak S, *et al*. Frequency and significance of troponin T elevation in acute ischemic stroke. *Am J Cardiol* 2007; **99**:108–12.

26. Finsterer J, Stöllberger C, Krugluger W. Cardiac and noncardiac, particularly neuromuscular, disease with troponin-T positivity. *Neth J Med* 2007; **65**:289–95.

27. Vaitkus PT, Barnathan EX. Embolic potential, prevention and management of mural thrombus complicating anterior myocardial infarction: a meta-analysis. *J Am Coll Cardiol* 1993; **22**:1004–9.

28. Zielinska M, Kaczmarek K, Tylkowski M. Predictors of left ventricular thrombus formation in acute myocardial infarction treated with successful primary angioplasty with stenting. *Am J Med Sci* 2008; **335**:171–6.

29. Dickerman SA, Abrutyn E, Barsic B, *et al*. The relationship between the initiation of antimicrobial therapy and the incidence of stroke in infective endocarditis: an analysis from the ICE prospective cohort study (ICE-PCS). *Am Heart J* 2007; **154**:1086–94.

30. Cabell CH, Pond KK, Peterson GE, *et al*. The risk of stroke and death in patients with aortic and mitral valve endocarditis. *Am Heart J* 2001; **142**:75–80.

31. Anderson DJ, Goldstein LB, Wilkinson WE, *et al*. Stroke location, characterization, severity, and outcome in mitral vs aortic valve endocarditis. *Neurology* 2003; **61**:1341–6.

32. Thuny F, Avierinos JF, Tribouilloy C, *et al*. Impact of cerebrovascular complications on mortality and neurologic outcome during infective endocarditis: a prospective multicentre study. *Eur Heart J* 2007; **28**:1155–61.

33. Wang A, Athan E, Pappas PA, *et al*. Contemporary clinical profile and outcome of prosthetic valve endocarditis. *JAMA* 2007; **297**:1354–61.

34. Schulz R, Werner GS, Fuchs JB, *et al*. Clinical outcome and echocardiographic findings of native and prosthetic valve endocarditis in the 1990s. *Eur Heart J* 1996; **17**:281–8.

35. Ruttmann E, Willeit J, Ulmer H, *et al*. Neurological outcome of septic cardioembolic stroke after infective endocarditis. *Stroke* 2006; **37**:2094–9.

36. Barsic B, Dickerman S, Krajinovic V, *et al*. Influence of the timing of cardiac surgery on the outcome of patients with infective endocarditis and stroke. *Clin Infect Dis* 2013; **56**:209–17.

37. Ruel M, Masters RG, Rubens FD, *et al*. Late incidence and determinants of stroke after aortic and mitral valve replacement. *Ann Thorac Surg* 2004; **78**:77–84.

38. Russo A, Grigioni F, Avierinos JF, *et al*. Thromboembolic complications after surgical correction of mitral regurgitation. *J Am Coll Cardiol* 2008; **51**:1203–11.

39. Kulik A, Bédard P, Lam BK, *et al*. Mechanical versus bioprosthetic valve replacement in middle-aged patients. *Eur J Cardiothorac Surg* 2006; **30**:485–91.

40. Will MB, Bernacca GM, Bell EF, *et al*. Our inability to predict thromboembolic events after prosthetic valve surgery. *J Heart Valve Dis* 2006; **15**:570–80.

41. Cabanes L, Coste J, Derumeaux G, *et al*. Interobserver and intraobserver variability in detection of patent foramen ovale and atrial septal aneurysm with transesophageal echocardiography. *J Am Soc Echocardiogr* 2002; **15**:441–6.

42. Lechat P, Mas JL, Lascault G, *et al*. Prevalence of patent foramen ovale in patients with stroke. *N Engl J Med* 1988; **318**:1148–52.

43. Lamy C, Giannesini C, Zuber M, *et al*. Clinical and imaging findings in cryptogenic stroke patients with and without patent foramen ovale. The PFO-ASA Study. *Stroke* 2002; **33**:706–11.

44. Homma S, Sacco RL, Di Tullio MR, *et al*.; PFO in Cryptogenic Stroke Study (PICSS) Investigators. Effect of medical treatment in stroke patients with patent foramen ovale. Patent Foramen Ovale in Cryptogenic Stroke Study. *Circulation* 2002; **105**:2625–31.

45. Di Tullio MR, Sacco RL, Sciacca RR, *et al*. Patent foramen ovale and the risk of ischemic stroke in a multiethnic population. *J Am Coll Cardiol* 2007; **49**:797–802.

46. Meissner I, Khandheria BK, Heit JA, *et al*. Patent foramen ovale: innocent or guilty? Evidence from a prospective population-based study. *J Am Coll Cardiol* 2006; **47**:440–5.

47. Furlan AJ, Reisman M, Massaro J, *et al*. Closure or medical therapy for cryptogenic stroke with patent

foramen ovale. *N Engl J Med* 2012; **366**:991–9.

48. Carroll JD, Saver JL, Thaler DE, *et al.* Closure of patent foramen ovale versus medical therapy after cryptogenic stroke. *N Engl J Med* 2013; **368**:1092–100.

49. Meier B, Kalesan B, Mattle HP, *et al.* Percutaneous closure of patent foramen ovale in cryptogenic embolism. *N Engl J Med* 2013; **368**:1083–91.

50. Abaci A, Unlu S, Alsancak Y, *et al.* Short and long term complications of device closure of atrial septal defect and patent foramen ovale: meta-analysis of 28,142 patients from 203 studies. *Catheter Cardiovasc Interv* 2013; **82**:1123–38. doi: 10.1002/ccd.24875.

51. Stöllberger C, Finsterer J, Krexner E, *et al.* Stroke and peripheral embolism from an Amplatzer septal occluder 5 years after implantation. *J Neurol* 2008; **255**:1270–1.

52. Burkett EL, Hershberger RE. Clinical and genetic issues in familial dilated cardiomyopathy. *J Am Coll Cardiol* 2005; **45**:969–81.

53. Gibelin P. Anticoagulant treatment and dilated cardiomyopathy. *Arch Mal Coeur Vaiss* 1995; **88**(Suppl 4):617–21.

54. Crawford TC, Smith WT 4th, Velazquez EJ, *et al.* Prognostic usefulness of left ventricular thrombus by echocardiography in dilated cardiomyopathy in predicting stroke, transient ischemic attack, and death. *Am J Cardiol* 2004; **93**:500–3.

55. Abreu TT, Mateus S, Correia J. Therapy implications of transthoracic echocardiography in acute ischemic stroke patients. *Stroke* 2005; **36**:1565–6.

56. Ikeniwa C, Sakai M, Kimura S, *et al.* Two cases of Duchenne muscular dystrophy complicated with dilated cardiomyopathy and

cerebral infarction. *No To Shinkei* 2006; **58**:250–5.

57. McCabe DJ, Rakhit RD. Antithrombotic and interventional treatment options in cardioembolic transient ischemic attack and ischemic stroke. *J Neurol Neurosurg Psychiatry* 2007; **78**:14–24.

58. Homma S, Thompson JL, Pullicino PM, *et al.* Warfarin and aspirin in patients with heart failure and sinus rhythm. *N Engl J Med* 2012; **366**:1859–69.

59. Stöllberger C, Finsterer J. Extracardiac medical and neuromuscular implications in restrictive cardiomyopathy. *Clin Cardiol* 2007; **30**:375–80.

60. Artz G, Wynne J. Restrictive cardiomyopathy. *Curr Treat Options Cardiovasc Med* 2000; **2**:431–8.

61. Salih MA, Al-Jarallah AS, Abdel-Gader AG, *et al.* Cardiac diseases as a risk factor for stroke in Saudi children. *Saudi Med J* 2006; **27** (Suppl 1):S61–8.

62. Hausfater P, Costedoat-Chalumeau N, Amoura Z, *et al.* AL cardiac amyloidosis and arterial thromboembolic events. *Scand J Rheumatol* 2005; **34**:315–19.

63. Stöllberger C, Finsterer J, Schneider B. Tako-tsubo-like left ventricular dysfunction: clinical presentation, instrumental findings, additional cardiac and non-cardiac diseases and potential pathomechanisms. *Minerva Cardioangiol* 2005; **53**:139–45.

64. Abe Y, Kondo M, Matsuoka R, *et al.* Assessment of clinical features in transient left ventricular apical ballooning. *J Am Coll Cardiol* 2003; **41**:737–42.

65. Gianni M, Dentali F, Grandi AM, *et al.* Apical ballooning syndrome or takotsubo cardiomyopathy: a systematic review. *Eur Heart J* 2006; **27**:1523–9.

66. Ueyama T, Senba E, Kasamatsu K, *et al.* Molecular mechanism of emotional stress-induced and catecholamine-induced heart attack. *J Cardiovasc Pharmacol* 2003; **41**(Suppl 1):S115–18.

67. Finsterer J, Stöllberger C, Sehnal E, *et al.* Apical ballooning (Takotsubo syndrome) in mitochondrial disorder during mechanical ventilation. *J Cardiovasc Med (Hagerstown)* 2007; **8**:859–63.

68. Porto I, Della Bona R, Leo A, *et al.* Stress cardiomyopathy (tako-tsubo) triggered by nervous system diseases: A systematic review of the reported cases. *Int J Cardiol* 2013; **167**:2441–8.

69. Mitsuma W, Kodama M, Ito M, *et al.* Thromboembolism in Takotsubo cardiomyopathy. *Int J Cardiol* 2010; **139**:98–100.

70. Stöllberger C, Finsterer J. Left ventricular hypertrabeculation/noncompaction. *J Am Soc Echocardiogr* 2004; **17**:91–100.

71. Stöllberger C, Winkler-Dworak M, Blazek G, *et al.* Prognosis of left ventricular hypertrabeculation/noncompaction is dependent on cardiac and neuromuscular comorbidity. *Int J Cardiol* 2007; **121**:189–93.

72. Stöllberger C, Finsterer J, Blazek G. Left ventricular hypertrabeculation/noncompaction and association with additional cardiac abnormalities and neuromuscular disorders. *Am J Cardiol* 2002; **90**:899–902.

73. Finsterer J, Stöllberger C, Blazek G. Prevalence of Barth syndrome in adult left ventricular hypertrabeculation/noncompaction. *Scand Cardiovasc J* 2008; **42**:157–60.

74. Stöllberger C, Blazek G, Dobias C, *et al.* Frequency of stroke and embolism in left ventricular hypertrabeculation/

153

noncompaction. *Am J Cardiol* 2011; **108**:1021–3.

75. Bukhman G, Ziegler J, Parry E. Endomyocardial fibrosis: still a mystery after 60 years. *PLoS Negl Trop Dis* 2008; **2**:e97.

76. Sarazin M, Caumes E, Cohen A, *et al.* Multiple microembolic borderzone brain infarctions and endomyocardial fibrosis in idiopathic hypereosinophilic syndrome and in *Schistosoma mansoni* infestation. *J Neurol Neurosurg Psychiatry* 2004; **75**:305–7.

77. Gautier JC, Dürr A, Koussa S, *et al.* Paradoxical cerebral embolism with a patent foramen ovale. A report of 29 patients. *Cerebrovasc Dis* 1991; **1**:193–202.

78. Stöllberger C, Slany J, Schuster I, *et al.* The prevalence of deep venous thrombosis in patients with suspected paradoxical embolism. *Ann Intern Med* 1993; **119**:461–5.

79. Ranoux D, Cohen A, Cabanes L, *et al.* Patent foramen ovale: is stroke due to paradoxical embolism? *Stroke* 1993; **24**:31–4.

80. Itoh T, Matsumoto M, Handa N, *et al.* Paradoxical embolism as a cause of ischemic stroke of uncertain etiology. A transcranial Doppler sonographic study. *Stroke* 1994; **25**:771–5.

81. Hanna JP, Sun JP, Furlan AJ, *et al.* Patent foramen ovale and brain infarct. Echocardiographic predictors, recurrence, and prevention. *Stroke* 1994; **25**:782–6.

82. Klötzsch C, Janßen G, Berlit P. Transesophageal echocardiography and contrast-TCD in the detection of a patent foramen ovale: experiences with 111 patients. *Neurology* 1994; **44**:1603–6.

83. Rohr-Le Floch J. Foramen ovale perméable et embolie paradoxale: une hypothèse controversée. *Rev Neurol (Paris)* 1994; **150**:282–5.

84. Lethen H, Flachskampf FA, Schneider R, *et al.* Frequency of deep vein thrombosis in patients with patent foramen ovale and ischemic stroke or transient ischemic attack. *Am J Cardiol* 1997; **80**:1066–9.

85. Cramer SC, Rordorf G, Maki JH, *et al.* Increased pelvic vein thrombi in cryptogenic stroke. Results of the Paradoxical Emboli from Large Veins in Ischemic Stroke (PELVIS) Study. *Stroke* 2004; **35**:46–50.

Common stroke syndromes

Céline Odier and Patrik Michel

Introduction

The approach to neurovascular disease has considerably changed over the last decade. With advances in neuroimaging, localization of the lesion has become easier. However, clinical recognition of stroke syndromes is still very important for several reasons.

First, in the acute phase, it enables diagnosis, exclusion of stroke imitators (migraine, epilepsy, posterior reversible encephalopathy syndrome (PRES), anxiety, psychogenic, etc.), and recognition of rare manifestations of stroke, such as cognitive-behavioral presentations which are easily misdiagnosed.

Second, it contributes to the planning of acute interventions by localizing the stroke (anterior versus posterior circulation or cortical versus subcortical involvement) and by interpretation of imaging abnormalities. Each subtype of stroke may benefit from intravenous thrombolysis for example, but only some subtypes, such as proximal intracranial occlusion, may be appropriate candidates for acute endovascular recanalization.

Third, during hospitalization, localization helps to direct the subsequent workup. If a cardioembolic etiology is suspected, for instance, it would lead to more intensive cardiac investigations, such as transesophageal echography or repeated 24-hour cardiac rhythm recording. In contrast, if a lacunar etiology is presumed, the cardiac investigation may remain limited.

Fourth, it also allows the clinician to anticipate, recognize, and treat complications related to a specific stroke type, such as large fluctuations in the lacunar "capsular warning syndrome" or brainstem compression from cerebellar edema.

Finally, making the correct diagnosis means choosing the appropriate secondary prevention. In the presence of a significant carotid stenosis, endarterectomy may be very effective if the recent stroke occurred in the territory distal to the stenosis, but of limited effectiveness if another territory is involved.

Several classifications for stroke territory, mechanism, and etiology exist. The TOAST classification [1] is most frequently used for stroke mechanism, but is partially outdated (Table 9.1). A modification of it (SS-TOAST) adds a variety of clinical and radiological criteria and seems more accurate [2]. The greater difficulty in using it has been improved by a recently published computer algorithm. The Oxfordshire method defines four subtypes of strokes according to clinical presentation attributed to a vascular territory: lacunar infarcts (LACI), total anterior circulation infarcts (TACI), partial anterior circulation infarcts (PACI), and posterior circulation infarcts (POCI).

In this chapter, we will discuss classic presentations of anterior circulation, posterior circulation, lacunar, watershed, and hemorrhagic strokes and try to identify clinical clues which can improve the diagnosis.

Anterior circulation syndromes

The anterior circulation refers to the part of the brain perfused by the carotid arteries. There are five main intracranial branches, which are from proximal to distal: ophthalmic, posterior communicating (PCoA), anterior choroidal (AChA), anterior cerebral (ACA) and middle cerebral (MCA) arteries. In some individuals, 2–10% according to different authors [3, 4], the posterior cerebral artery (PCA) comes from the carotid artery, via a large PCoA, while the proximal PCA originating from the basilar artery is hypo- or aplastic. In these cases, the anterior circulation irrigates the PCA territory. This variant of the circle of Willis is also known as a fetal origin of the PCA.

Textbook of Stroke Medicine, Second Edition, ed. Michael Brainin and Wolf-Dieter Heiss. Published by Cambridge University Press. © Michael Brainin and Wolf-Dieter Heiss 2014.

Table 9.1. Stroke categories according to the TOAST classification.

1. Large-vessel disease

2. Small-vessel disease

3. Cardioembolism

4. Other etiology

5. Undetermined or multiple possible etiologies

The anterior circulation can be subdivided into two systems, the leptomeningeal artery system vascularizing the cortex, the adjacent white matter and the AChA, and the deep perforating artery system, perfusing the basal ganglia, the centrum semiovale and the parts of internal capsule.

Middle cerebral artery (MCA)

The middle cerebral artery (MCA) is also designated the Sylvian artery, from Jacques Dubois, known as Jacobus Sylvius (1489–1555), a linguist and anatomist in Paris. The artery is subdivided into the M1 segment, from which start the deep perforating lenticulostriate arteries, the M2 segment, corresponding to the segment after the bifurcation into superior and inferior divisions, and the M3 segment, including the insular part. The M4 segments, the leptomeningeal arteries, arise from the M3 segments and are named orbitofrontal, prefrontal, precentral, central sulcus, anterior parietal, posterior parietal, angular and temporal arteries, with important variations in their territories.

The MCA territory is the one most frequently affected by acute strokes. MCA territory infarcts can be subtle or a devastating clinical syndrome, depending on the site of the occlusion, the extent of ischemia, the etiology, and the collateral arterial network. As collateral networks are highly variable, an occlusion of the same artery at the same place may lead to quite variable severity of the stroke and of prognosis. Large infarcts are defined as involvement of two of the three MCA territories (deep, superior and inferior divisions) and "malignant MCA stroke" as complete or near complete MCA territory infarction with ensuing mass effect from brain edema.

Clinically, a patient with an *acute complete MCA* infarction presents contralateral hemiparesis, hemihypesthesia, hemianopsia, and ipsilateral conjugated eye and head deviation (the patient looks at his/her lesion). The patient is usually awake or presents mild drowsiness or agitation, particularly with a right infarct. Cognitive signs are always present: in the case of a left lesion, aphasia, and most of the time global, ideomotor apraxia. In the case of a right lesion, contralateral multimodal hemineglect (visual, motor, sensitive, visual, spatial, auditive), anosognosia (denial of illness), anosodiaphoria (indifference to illness), asomatognosia (lack of awareness of a part of one's own body) and confusional state are seen. This picture suggests an M1 occlusion with or without carotid occlusion and is associated with a rather unfavorable prognosis. Particularly in younger people, malignant stroke with brain edema may develop, leading to high intracranial pressure and subsequent subfacial, uncal and transtentorial herniation. The clinical deterioration occurs typically within 48–72 hours, when vigilance decreases and initial signs worsen. New cortical symptoms may occur because of infarction of ACA or PCA arteries, which become compressed against inter-hemispheric falx and cerebellar tentorium, respectively. When the herniation of the medial temporal lobe continues, the uncus compresses the third cranial nerve, leading to an ipsilateral fixed mydriasis and the contralateral cerebral peduncle is compressed against the cerebellar tentorium, leading to ipsilateral corticospinal signs, such as Babinski's sign and paresis (Kernohan notch). A bilateral ptosis has also been described as an imminent sign of temporal herniation, mostly in a right malignant MCA infarct [5]. Early recognition of patients at risk enables the medical team to propose a hemicraniectomy for selected patients, a treatment which has proved highly effective if performed within 48 hours and before those signs occur [6].

A *complete superficial MCA* infarct, sparing the lenticulostriated arteries, suggests a thrombus in a distal part of the MCA trunk, at the bifurcation of the artery (proximal M2 segment). Motor and sensitive functions of the lower limbs are less involved than the face and arms. If leg involvement is important and persistent, concomitant ischemia in the internal capsule (AChA) or in the ACA territory should be suspected. The visual field deficit may be a contralateral homonymous hemianopia or a quadrantanopsia. The deviation of the head and the eyes is more transitory and the sensitive deficit is less severe. Cognitive deficits are similar to an M1 occlusion but often less pronounced or rapidly improving.

An infarct of the *superior* (sometimes called *anterior*) M2 division of the MCA manifests itself clinically with contralateral isolated brachiofacial paresis, partial brachiofacial sensitive loss (mainly tactile and discriminative modalities), transient conjugate ipsilateral eye and head deviation and aphasia (aphemia or Broca aphasia) frequently associated with buccolingual apraxia in the case of left infarcts and various degrees of multimodal hemineglect, anosognosia, anosodiaphoria, confusion and monotone language in right lesions. Visual fields are usually spared.

In the presence of an infarct of the *inferior* (sometimes called *posterior*) M2 division of the MCA, less frequent than superior division infarction, the presentation includes contralateral homonymous hemianopsia or upper quadrantanopsia, mild or transient brachiofacial paresis and cognitive disturbances, which are the dominant part of the picture. With a left lesion, Wernicke's aphasia or conduction aphasia are observed and with a right lesion, hemineglect, constructional and clothing dyspraxia, spatial disorientation, behavioral changes, confusional state, hallucination, delusions and amusia may be present.

Involvement of one of the *leptomeningeal branches* (M3 or M4) can produce highly circumscribed infarcts accompanied by specific neurological deficits and is most of the time related to embolism. For example, an isolated Wernicke's aphasia occurs with occlusion of the left posterior temporal branch and suggests strongly a cardioembolic mechanism, particularly in the elderly.

The *lenticulostriate arteries* vascularize the basal ganglia and parts of the internal capsule. Ischemia in their territory can therefore produce severe deficits with a very small-volume lesion. Cortical signs are absent or minor, except in the case of deafferentation of the cortex by interruption of subcortical cortical pathways. Clinical signs include proportional hemiparesis, hemihypesthesia, dysarthria, hypophonia, and occasionally abnormal movements in the case of involvement of basal ganglia.

The *centrum ovale* receives its blood supply from medullary perforating arteries coming principally from leptomeningeal arteries. Small infarcts (less than 1.5 cm) usually present as lacunar syndromes but deficits are often less proportional than in pontine or internal capsule lacunes.

Etiology in the deep perforator territories of the MCA is mostly lipohyalinosis and local arteriolosclerosis, in contrast with larger and multiple infarcts, which are embolic from an arterial or cardiac source. Both small and larger lesions may occur in the border zone area between the deep (leptomeningeal) and superficial (meningeal) arteries from hemodynamic mechanisms (see below).

> The MCA territory is the one most frequently affected by acute strokes. Symptoms of an *acute complete MCA infarction*: contralateral hemiparesis, hemihypesthesia, hemianopsia, ipsilateral conjugated eye and head deviation (the patient looks at his/her lesion); plus, in the case of a left lesion, aphasia, and in the case of a right lesion, contralateral multimodal hemineglect. Malignant stroke with brain edema may develop, leading to high intracranial pressure and subsequent herniation.

Infarctions of the lower arterial segments show similar symptoms, but not the complete picture.

Anterior cerebral artery (ACA)

The ACA is subdivided into the A1 segment (before the anterior communicating artery (ACoA)), followed by the A2 segment (after the ACoA), then A3 segments. The A1 segment has deep perforating arteries, named the medial lenticulostriate arteries, and gives rise to the recurrent artery of Heubner (raH), which supplies the caudate head, the genu and anterior arm of the internal capsule and the supero-anterior putamen. Both the lenticulostriate arteries and the raH are particularly vulnerable during aneurysm surgery of the ACoA.

The clinical presentation of ACA infarcts includes weakness predominantly of the distal lower limb and to a lesser degree of the upper limb, motor hemineglect, transcortical motor aphasia and behavioral disturbances (with involvement of the supplementary motor area). Sensory hemisyndromes affecting mainly the contralateral leg are also described. Sphincter dysfunction, mutism, anterograde amnesia, grasping, and behavioral disturbances are particularly frequent in ischemia of the deep perforating arteries and the raH. Involvement of the corpus callosum can produce the callosal disconnection syndrome, secondary to interruption of the connection of physical information from the right hemisphere to cognitive center in the left hemisphere. Therefore, it is restricted to the left hand, which presents ideomotor apraxia, agraphia, tactile anomia (inability to name objects placed into the left palm) and the alien-hand syndrome.

> *ACA infarcts* cause weakness predominantly of the distal lower limb and to a lesser degree of the upper limb, motor hemineglect and transcortical motor aphasia.

157

Anterior choroidal artery (AChA)

The boundaries of the territory supplied by the AChA are still controversial [7], probably reflecting interpersonal variants. The artery vascularizes to a variable degree the inferior posterior and retrolenticular part of the internal capsule, the tail of the caudate nucleus, part of the lenticular nucleus, the posterior corona radiata, the lateral geniculate body, and the beginning of the optic radiations. Clinically less important are variable contributions to the vascular supply of the uncus, amygdala, hippocampus, optic tract, parts of midbrain (substantia nigra, cerebral peduncle), subthalamic region, and choroid plexus.

In the majority of patients, the presentation is a lacunar syndrome: pure motor or sensorimotor hemiparesis and less frequently a pure sensory deficit or an ataxic hemiparesis syndrome.

A rarer but typical presentation of AChA infarcts is the triad of contralateral severe hemiparesis, hemihypesthesia and upper quadrantanopsia or contralateral versus ipsilateral hemianopsia (in the case of lateral geniculate body or optic tract, respectively) without cognitive disturbances, in contrast with MCA infarction. A rare but specific visual field defect is a homonymous defect in the upper and lower quadrants with sparing of a horizontal sector [8].

Rarely, cognitive signs occur in AChA infarcts secondarily to involvement of thalamocortical pathways, including hemineglect and constructional apraxia with right lesion and thalamic aphasia (fluent language with relatively preserved comprehension and repetition but anomia, jargon speech and semantic paraphasic errors) with left infarct. AchA infarct may therefore imitate incomplete MCA strokes.

> Lacunar syndrome within AChA territory causes most frequently pure motor or sensorimotor hemiparesis.
> A rarer but typical presentation of AChA infarcts is the triad of contralateral severe hemiparesis, hemihypesthesia, and upper quadrantanopsia.

Internal carotid artery (ICA)

The manifestations of acute internal carotid occlusion are quite variable, depending on the collateral status and pre-existing carotid stenosis. *Embolic occlusion of the ICA*, either proximally or distally, usually leads to severe stroke, showing concomitant signs of all anterior circulation arteries. Consciousness is usually more decreased and leg weakness more severe and persistent than in isolated proximal MCA occlusion.

In contrast, a progressive atherosclerotic occlusion is usually less severe, with a classic subacute two-phase presentation. It may even be asymptomatic. Retinal ischemia from carotid emboli may be transient (amaurosis fugax) or persistent (central retinal artery occlusion or branch retinal artery occlusion). It often occurs in isolation and requires urgent workup including detailed ophthalmological examination, carotid imaging, and a search for Horton's arteritis. In the case of a chronic ICA stenosis or occlusion, hemodynamic stress such as hypotension can lead to a watershed stroke.

In rare situations, an individual can present a *limb-shaking TIA*, which manifests as a choreic or a coarse tremor-like abnormal movement of variable frequency and several minutes' duration, mostly of the upper extremity. It typically occurs when an orthostatic stress leads to a hypoperfusion of the brain [9] secondary to carotid severe stenosis.

> *Embolic occlusion of the ICA*, either proximally or distally, usually leads to severe stroke, showing concomitant signs of all anterior circulation arteries. A *progressive atherosclerotic occlusion* is usually less severe, with a classic subacute two-phase presentation or even asymptomatic. Retinal ischemia from carotid emboli may be transient (amaurosis fugax) or persistent.

Posterior circulation syndromes

The posterior circulation is also called the vertebrobasilar circulation. The two vertebral arteries leave the subclavian arteries, pass through transverse foramina in the apophysis of the sixth to the second cervical vertebra, enter the cranium through the foramen magnum, and join together to form the basilar artery (BA). The BA gives several paramedian and circumferential branches as well as four cerebellar arteries, and then splits into two PCAs at the level of the cerebellar tentorium. There exist numerous individual variations, the clinically most important being the fetal origin of the PCAs from the carotid arteries (via the PCoA).

Clinical clues to differentiate posterior from anterior circulation strokes

Important clinical symptoms and signs point to a posterior circulation stroke and should be recognized. Preceding TIAs and strokes in the days and hours before are more frequent in the posterior circulation. Similarly, headache is more frequent in the posterior circulation, is typically ipsilateral to the infarct, and may have features of primary headaches such as migraine [10].

Past diplopia, tilt of the vision, true rotatory or linear vertigo, drunken-type gait, hiccup, bilateral or crossed motor or sensory symptoms, initial decreased level of consciousness and amnesia should be actively searched for in the history of stroke patients.

On exam, a disconjugate gaze strongly suggests a brainstem lesion. It may occur as a fixed misalignment of the ocular axis, such as in vertical skew deviation of the eyes as part of the ocular tilt reaction. Alternatively, it is due to a paresis of one or several orbital muscles as a result of an infarct of a single nucleus or its intra-axial fascicle (cranial nerves III, IV or VI), or from connections in between these nuclei (such as in internuclear ophthalmoplegia).

Gaze paresis may also be conjugate in brainstem lesions. If the eyes are deviated toward the hemiparesis, i.e. there is "wrong-way eye deviation" if compared to a hemispheric lesion in the MCA territory, the eyes cannot be directed to the other side because the command centers allowing this action are damaged in the pons (for saccades: parapontine reticular formation, PPRF; and for pursuit: parts of the nucleus of the VI) or the midbrain (parts of the nucleus of the VI). Contrarily to most supratentorial infarcts, this eye deviation cannot be overcome with oculovestibular reflexes ("doll's eyes maneuver"). A lateral medullary lesion (Wallenberg syndrome) leads to an ipsilateral deviation of the eyes, however, and is usually accompanied by a marked horizontal or horizonto-rotatory nystagmus.

A vertical gaze paresis (upwards, downwards, or both) points to a dorsal mesencephalic lesion and may be associated with a caudal paramedian thalamic infarct, especially if downgaze palsy is also present.

A nystagmus of central origin may be recognized by its direction (vertical, multidirectional gaze-evoked or pendular), the absence of nausea despite clear-cut nystagmus with primary gaze, and its lack of improvement with fixation. However, it should be underlined that a medullary or a cerebellar stroke can mimic a peripheral nystagmus and that vestibular ischemia from an anterior inferior cerebella artery (AICA) may result in a peripheral vestibular lesion.

An ocular tilt reaction is characterized by the triad of skew deviation (downward displacement of the axis of the globe ipsilateral to the lesion), conjugate ocular torsion towards the side of the lesion and head tilt to the side of the lesion. Visual tilt of the environment towards the side of the lesion is frequently associated and may result in "upside-down vision". The ocular tilt reaction may be caused by peripheral lesion of the vestibular apparatus or the central vestibular connections including vestibular nuclei, vestibulocerebellum, and the medial longitudinal fascicle (MLF) up to the interstitial nucleus of Cajal.

Another visual sign is Horner's syndrome, consisting of myosis, mild ptosis of the upper and lower eyelid, and hemifacial anhidrosis. It occurs with an ipsilateral dorsolateral brainstem, upper cervical, or thalamic lesion, but may also occur due to a carotid dissection, the peripheral sympathetic fibers surrounding the carotid artery.

Motor, cerebellar, and sensitive signs are less specific in brainstem lesions, but the presence of bilateral or crossed signs is suggestive. The former is due to the bilateral supply of the brainstem by one midline artery (the BA). The latter is caused by ischemia of cranial nerves and fascicles that produce ipsilateral signs and simultaneous damage to the long sensory and motor tracts that cross in the caudal parts of the brainstem. Truncular ataxia is quite characteristic of brainstem lesions, and acute unilateral deafness (with or without vertigo) suggests ischemia in the AICA territory.

Despite these clinical clues, lacunar brainstem infarcts may be indistinguishable from supratentorial ones, and proximal PCA occlusion may mimic MCA infarction. In the latter situation, hemiparesis results from ischemia to the cerebral peduncles, cognitive signs and eye deviation from thalamic involvement, and hemianopia from thalamic or hemispheric PCA ischemia. If somnolence, early anisocoria or vertical gaze palsy are present, posterior circulation stroke is more probable than carotid territory stroke.

Clinical symptoms and signs that point to a posterior circulation stroke: preceding TIAs and strokes in the days and hours before the infarct, headache, typically ipsilateral to the infarct, a disconjugate gaze or a conjugate gaze paresis with the eyes deviated toward the hemiparesis (brainstem lesion), a vertical gaze paresis (dorsal mesencephalic lesion), nystagmus, ocular tilt reaction (triad of skew deviation, conjugate ocular torsion towards the side of the lesion, and head tilt to the side of the lesion), Horner's syndrome (myosis, mild ptosis of the upper and lower eyelid, and hemifacial anhidrosis), bilateral or crossed motor, cerebellar, and sensitive signs, truncular ataxia, acute unilateral deafness, somnolence and early anisocoria.

159

The vertebral artery (VA) and the posterior inferior cerebellar artery (PICA)

The vertebral arteries give origin to two arteries before joining to form the basilar artery: the anterior spinal artery, which supplies the medial medulla oblongata and the upper cervical cord, and the PICA, which supplies the inferior cerebellum and the dorsolateral medulla. The latter structure may also receive direct (long circumferential) branches from the vertebral artery. Three classic clinical syndromes are recognized in their territory: the medial medullary stroke (or Déjerine syndrome); the dorsolateral medullary stroke (or Wallenberg syndrome); and the hemimedullary stroke (or Babinski-Nageotte syndrome).

The medial medullary stroke is a rare stroke syndrome and classically includes contralateral hemiparesis sparing the face (corticospinal tract), contralateral lemniscal sensory loss (medial lemniscus) and ipsilateral tongue paresis (nucleus of hypoglossal nerve and tract). The dorsolateral medullary stroke is the most common of those three syndromes and is named the Wallenberg syndrome, after Adolf Wallenberg (1862–1946), a German neurologist. Wallenberg syndrome and an infarct in the inferior cerebellum stroke can be seen in isolation or together, the latter being usually the case if the vertebral artery is occluded. Wallenberg's syndrome includes ipsilateral thermoalgesic facial deficit (spinal trigeminal nucleus and tract), contralateral thermoalgesic deficit (spinothalamic tract), dysphagia, dysphonia due to palatal and vocal cord weakness (ambiguous nucleus), ipsilateral ataxia (inferior cerebellar peduncle), severe nausea, vomiting, nystagmus, ocular and truncular ipsipulsion (vestibular nuclei) and ipsilateral Horner's sign (descending sympathetic tract). Hiccup is common, and may be refractory to treatment. If a Wallenberg's syndrome is present, the presence or absence of an inferior cerebellar lesion cannot be determined clinically.

Inferior cerebellar lesions in the PICA territory without involvement of the dorsolateral medulla present with vertigo, nausea, vomiting, nystagmus, ipsilateral limb ataxia, severe gait ataxia, and ocular/truncular ipsipulsion. A deceptive appearance of PICA stroke is the isolated vertigo presentation, which can mimic a vestibular neuronitis. One clue which can help to make the correct diagnosis is the presence of an unusual nystagmus, which will be purely horizontal or direction-changing, and

preservation of the vestibulo-ocular reflex with the head thrust (Halmagyi) maneuver. This maneuver should not be applied in patients with suspected vertebral artery dissection.

Isolated inferior cerebellar infarcts usually have a good outcome. However, in the case of large PICA infarcts, a post-infarct edema can provoke brainstem compression, obstruction of the fourth ventricle with subsequent hydrocephalus and tonsillar (downward) or transtentorial (upward) herniation. In the first case, the patient develops paresthesia in the shoulder, neck stiffness up to opisthotonos, no motor responses, small and unreactive pupils, ataxic then superficial respiratory pattern, Cushing's triad (hypertension, bradycardia, apnea) and finally cardio-respiratory arrest. With transtentorial herniation, lethargy and coma are accompanied by central hyperventilation, upward gaze paralysis, unreactive, mid-position pupils and decerebration.

The hemimedullary syndrome is very rare and includes Wallenberg's presentation with Déjerine's syndrome, leading to contralateral motor and all-modalities sensory deficits, ipsilateral tongue, pharynx and vocal cord weakness and facial thermoalgesic deficit, ipsilateral ataxia and Horner's syndrome.

> Dorsolateral medullary stroke (or Wallenberg syndrome) is the most common brainstem syndrome of vertebral artery involvement.

The anterior inferior cerebellar artery (AICA)

The AICA vascularizes the dorsolateral inferior pons, the antero-inferior cerebellum, the cochlea, the labyrinth, and the VIIIth cranial nerve. Major variations of the extent of cerebellar supply by the three cerebellar arteries may make localization to the AICA difficult unless certain cranial nerve deficits are present.

The classic AICA syndrome includes vertigo with vomiting and nystagmus (vestibular nuclei, vestibular nerve or labyrinthine artery), ipsilateral deafness with tinnitus (cochlear nerve or cochlear artery), ipsilateral peripheral-type facial palsy (facial nucleus or fascicle of VII), ipsilateral facial hypesthesia (trigeminal nuclei or fascicle), ipsilateral Horner's syndrome (descending sympathetic tract), ipsilateral ataxia, dysarthria (middle cerebellar peduncle and cerebellum) and contralateral thermoalgesic sensory deficit (spinothalamic tract). It is frequently misdiagnosed as Wallenberg syndrome, but the main clinical distinctions are the hearing loss and the peripheral-type facial palsy. Occasionally, horizontal ipsilateral gaze palsy or dysphagia are also present. More rarely, AICA territory stroke can present as an isolated vertigo or isolated cerebellar syndrome.

The superior cerebellar artery (SCA)

An isolated SCA syndrome is rare, but the territory is regularly involved in distal basilar artery occlusion. The SCA syndrome includes ipsilateral limb and gait ataxia and important dysarthria. Nystagmus (middle and/or superior cerebellar peduncle, superior cerebellum and vermis), ipsilateral Horner's syndrome (descending sympathetic tract), contralateral fourth palsy (IV nucleus), and contralateral thermoalgesic sensory deficit (spinothalamic tract) may be present. Other signs have been described, such as ipsilateral choreiform abnormal movements or palatal myoclonus (superior cerebellar peduncle interrupting the dentatorubral pathway), sleep abnormalities, and partial contralateral deafness (lateral lemniscus). Given its close relationship to the distal basilar artery, SCA strokes are very frequently embolic (from an arterial or cardiac source).

The basilar artery (BA)

The BA lies on the ventral surface of the brainstem and vascularizes the pons, the mesencephalon and the middle and upper cerebellum through the AICA and SCA. Its territory can be subdivided into three parts on a ventro-dorsal level [11]. The anteromedial territory receives its blood supply from the paramedian arteries, the anterolateral territory from the short circumferential arteries (or anterolateral arteries) and the dorsolateral territory from the long circumferential arteries (or posterolateral arteries) as well as from the cerebellar arteries. In ventral paramedian lesions, hemiparesis is the most severe. In anterolateral lesions, the motor deficit is mild and can predominate in the leg (crural dominant hemiparesis), reflecting the topographical orientation of the fibers (leg – lateral, arm – medial) [12]. Dorsolateral lesions often involve the spinothalamic tract and lateral part of the medial lemniscus, while paramedian infarcts involve the medial part of the medial lemniscus. Involvement of the tegmentum implies more sensory, cranial nerves and oculomotor deficits.

Stroke severity in the BA territory is highly variable: it can present with isolated neurological deficits in the case of penetrator occlusions of lacunar origin or can be devastating when the artery itself is acutely occluded. Different eponym syndromes have been described in the literature, corresponding to circumscribed lesions and precise deficits (see Table 9.2)

Occlusion of the basilar artery mostly results in a devastating stroke with severe disability or death. About half of individuals present premonitory signs and symptoms, especially if atherosclerosis of the vertebral or basilar artery is the cause. Some symptoms are nonspecific, such as paresthesias, dysarthria, ("herald") hemiparesis or dizziness. More specific prodromes are mentioned above, and also include pathological laughter ("fou rire prodromique")[13] as well as pseudoseizures with tonic spasm of the side which will become paretic [14]. Rapid identification of basilar artery ischemia can help to provide aggressive therapy by i.v. or i.a. thrombolysis before a catastrophic picture of a locked-in syndrome or coma. Indeed, it has been shown that vessel recanalization and low NIHSS on admission were independent predictors of favorable outcome [15].

Less severe pontine stroke syndromes are listed in Table 9.2. Severe pontine strokes are characterized by a locked-in syndrome that involves quadriplegia, bilateral face palsy, and horizontal gaze palsy. Consciousness and vertical gaze are usually spared unless the midbrain is involved. Therefore, careful examination of voluntary up- and downgaze in a seemingly comatose patient may establish preserved consciousness and communication.

Distal basilar territory stroke usually leads to midbrain ischemia and is therefore characterized by ocular manifestations, such as disorders of reflex and voluntary vertical gaze, skew deviation, disorder of convergence with pseudosixth palsy in the presence of hyperconvergence, Collier sign (upper eyelid retraction), and small pupils with diminished reaction to light because of interruption of the afferent limb of the pupillary reflex. Small midbrain lesions may result in nuclear or fascicular third nerve palsies. Nuclear palsy is recognizable by bilateral upgaze paresis and bilateral ptosis as the medial subnucleus of the III innervates the contralateral superior rectus muscle and the central nucleus innervates both levator palpebrae superioris. Other classic midbrain syndromes can be found in Table 9.2. Hypersomnolence or coma usually requires extension of the ischemia into the thalamic territory as part of the "top of the basilar syndrome" [16].

Atherosclerosis and embolism are the two major mechanisms of basilar artery stroke and occlusion.

161

Table 9.2. Selected brainstem syndromes with their eponyms.

Eponym	Site	Cranial nerves	Tracts	Signs
Weber	Base of midbrain	III	Corticospinal	Oculomotor palsy with crossed hemiplegia
Claude	Midbrain tegmentum	III	Red nucleus and brachium conjunctivum	Oculomotor palsy with contralateral cerebellar ataxia and tremor
Benedikt	Midbrain tegmentum	III	Red nucleus	Oculomotor palsy, contralateral abnormal movements
Nothnagel	Midbrain tectum	Unilateral or bilateral III	Superior cerebellar peduncles	Oculomotor palsy, ipsilateral cerebellar ataxia
Parinaud	Dorsal midbrain			Paralysis of upward gaze, light-near dissociation, retraction nystagmus, eyelid retraction, lid lag
Raymond	Ventral caudal pons	VI	Corticospinal tract	Abduction palsy and crossed hemiplegia
Millard-Gubler	Caudal ventral medial pons	VII, VI (fascicles)	Corticospinal tract	Abduction and peripheral facial palsy, contralateral hemiplegia
Foville	Caudal tegmental medial pons	VI nucleus, VII, PPRF	Corticospinal tract, medial lemniscus, MLF	Gaze and peripheral facial palsy, contralateral hemiparesis (and hypesthesia, INO)
Raymond-Cestan	Rostral dorsal pons	(PPRF and VI nucleus)	Spinothalamic tract and edial lemniscus (corticospinal tract)	Ataxia with "rubral" tremor, contralateral all sensory modalities deficit (contralateral hemiparesis, ipsilateral gaze palsy)
Marie-Foix	Lateral caudal pons (AICA)		Middle cerebellar peduncle, corticospinal, spinothalamic tracts	Ipsilateral ataxia, contralateral hemiparesis and spinothalamic sensory loss
Wallenberg	Medulla, lateral tegmentum	Spinal V, IX, X, XI	Lateral spinothalamic tract, descending sympathetic fibers, spino- and olivocerebellar tracts	Ipsi V, IX, X, XI palsy, Horner's, cerebellar ataxia. Contralateral pain and temperature deficit
Déjerine	Medial medullary syndrome	XII	Corticospinal, lemniscus median	Ipsilateral tongue palsy, contralateral hemiplegia and lemniscal sensory loss
Opalski	Submedullary syndrome	V, IX, X, XI	Corticospinal tract below the pyramid	Ipsilateral hemiplegia with Wallenberg syndrome
Babinski-Nageotte	Hemimedullary syndrome			Combination of Wallenberg's, Déjerine's and Opalski's syndromes

Common sites of atherothrombotic stenosis are the origin of vertebral arteries (which can lead to artery-to-artery embolism), the intracranial part of the VA, where thrombus frequently extends into the caudal part of the BA, between the union of VA and AICA, and the midpart of the BA [17]. Embolic clots may arise from vertebral or basilar atherosclerosis or from aortic or cardiac sources. They are a regular cause of distal vertebral and proximal BA occlusions, and the predominant cause of distal BA occlusions.

Another less common cause of BA strokes is the dolichoectasic basilar or vertebral arteries. They have been documented in up to 10% and are related to the presence of vascular risk factors and an increased risk for lacunar stroke [18].

> Rapid identification of basilar artery ischemia can help to provide timely aggressive therapy by i.v. or i.a. thrombolysis before a catastrophic picture develops.

The posterior cerebral artery (PCA)

The PCA is subdivided into four segments with associated clinical presentation. An occlusion of the proximal segment (P1 or precommunal) usually causes a total PCA infarction, including upper midbrain, variable parts of the thalamus and posterior hemispheric territory. Occlusions of the P2 (or postcommunal) segment before the branching of the thalamogeniculate arteries provoke ischemic lesions in the lateral thalamus and the hemispheric PCA territory. Lastly, cortical PCA branch occlusion causes diverse cortical lesions in the superficial PCA territory, including the occipital, postero-inferior temporal and variable part of the posterior parietal lobes.

Sensory symptoms are quite common in PCA infarcts and are usually related to laterothalamic involvement. Motor symptoms are infrequent and minor [19] and are mostly related to laterothalamic edema affecting the posterior internal capsule or to ischemia of the cerebral peduncles. In the latter situation, a patient may present severe contralateral hemiplegia, hypesthesia and hemianopsia, mimicking an MCA stroke as mentioned above.

Bilateral PCA infarcts are typical of the "top of the basilar syndrome", which may also include dyschromatopsia, visual agnosia or alexia-without agraphia with a left lesion, spatial disorientation (topographagnosia), palinopsia, amusia, Balint syndrome (asimultanognosia or incapacity to see a scene as a whole, ocular apraxia or poor hand–eye coordination and optic ataxia or apraxia of gaze), metamorphosia, and prosopagnosia [16]. The syndrome of bilateral PCA strokes must be distinguished from PRES (posterior reversible encephalopathy syndrome) and venous thrombosis, all of which can cause headaches, central visual loss, and decreased level of consciousness.

The source of PCA strokes is embolic in the majority of cases, i.e. from cardiac sources, and proximal vertebrobasilar and aortic atherothrombotic disease. Rarer causes include dissections, fetal origin of PCA, and migrainous stroke.

> Sensory symptoms (visual loss, hemianopsia) are quite common in PCA infarcts, while motor symptoms are infrequent and minor. The "top of the basilar syndrome" causes headaches, central visual loss, and decreased level of consciousness.

The thalamus

The thalamus is a centrally situated structure with extensive reciprocal connections with the cortex, basal ganglia, and brainstem nuclei. Therefore it can mimic cortical and subcortical strokes in the anterior or posterior circulation and is also called "the great imitator". Its vascularization is subdivided into four territories correlated with the organization of the thalamic nuclei [20] (Figure 9.1):

- the tuberothalamic (or polar) artery
- the thalamogeniculate (or inferolateral) artery
- the paramedian arteries
- the posterior choroidal artery (PChA).

The thalamus is essentially fed by the posterior circulation via branches from the PCA (P1 and P2 segments),

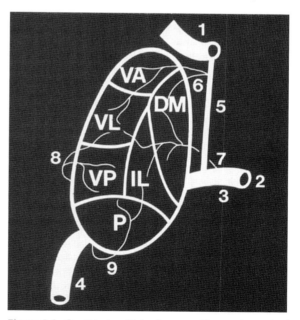

Figure 9.1. Carotid artery (1); basilar artery (2); posterior cerebral segment P1 (3); segment P2 (4); posterior communicating artery (5); tuberothalamic artery (6); paramedian arteries (7); thalamogeniculate artery (8); posterior choroidal artery (9). Source: Barth *et al.* in: Bogousslavsky J, Caplan L, eds. *Stroke Syndromes*. Cambridge: Cambridge University Press; 2001: 461.

the PCoA and the PChA. Only blood going to the lateral geniculate body (via the AChA) and the anterior thalamus (via the PCoA) may stem from the carotid system.

There are inter-individual variations in thalamic supply, leading to variable clinical presentations and prognosis. For example, Percheron reported that the paramedian arteries may arise from a unique P1 segment or from a vascular arcade connecting both P1 segments [21].

The tuberothalamic (or polar) artery arises from the PCoA and irrigates the anterior nuclei, the ventral anterior nucleus, amygdalofugal pathway, mamillothalamic tract, rostral part of the ventrolateral nucleus, ventral pole of the medial dorsal nucleus and ventral part of the internal medullary lamina. It is absent in about a third of the population, in which case the paramedian arteries vascularize its territory. Infarction results in anterograde amnesia (mostly reversible if unilateral), automatic-voluntary dissociation with facial paresis for emotional movement, personality changes, mild contralateral hemiparesis or clumsiness. Cognitive and behavioral disturbances include temporospatial disorientation, euphoria, misjudgment, lack of spontaneity, apathy, emotional unconcern, and a unique behavioral pattern, named palipsychism [21]. Individuals present a disorganized speech with grammatically correct phrases, but with intrusions of unrelated themes, which have usually been discussed previously. With a left lesion, buccofacial or limb apraxia and thalamic aphasia can occur with reduced fluency, anomia, phonological and semantic paraphasia, perseveration, impaired comprehension, acalculia with preservation of reading and repetition. Visual-spatial disturbances are present with a right lesion.

The thalamogeniculate (or inferolateral) arteries are a group of 5–10 arteries arising from the P2 segment of the PCA. The principal branches supply the ventrolateral nucleus and the ventroposterior nuclei, while the medial branches supply the medial geniculate body and the inferior branches the rostral and lateral pulvinar, as well as the laterodorsal nucleus. The clinical presentation can include contralateral hemihypesthesia, involving one or several sensory modalities. It may be associated with choreoathetoid movements, hemiataxia, slight transient hemiparesis, and thalamic astasia. Thalamic astasia is characterized by disequilibrium backwards or toward the side contralateral to the lesion in the absence of

significant motor deficit and is thought to result from interruption of the dentatorubrothalamic pathway. Sensory deficits are heterogeneous. Individuals describe paresthesias without objective deficit, particularly in the cheiro-oral region, or a "mid-line split", defined by a subjective sensation of an abrupt stopping of the deficit on the midline of the trunk. Pseudoradicular sensory deficit is also suggestive of a thalamic involvement. Subsequent to, or rarely in the acute phase of, an inferolateral infarct, some individuals develop paroxysmal stimulus-sensitive, severe and refractory pain in the affected hemibody side with vasomotor disturbances and choreoathetoid movements, named the thalamic pain syndrome of Déjerine-Roussy. The "thalamic hand", described by Foix and Hillemand, is flexed, pronated and the thumb is buried beneath the other fingers [20]. Behavioral disturbances are infrequent in inferolateral stroke and include soft executive dysfunction and affective changes, resembling those found after cerebellar stroke [21].

The paramedian arteries arise from the P1 segment of the PCA. The inferior and middle rami irrigate parts of the midbrain and the pons, while the superior ramus irrigates a variable extent of thalamus but mostly the dorsomedial nucleus, the intra-laminar nuclei and internal medullary lamina. Infarctions also tend to involve the medial midbrain. The classic features consist of a triad with an initial decreased level of consciousness with or without fluctuations, vertical gaze abnormalities and cognitive impairment, which become more obvious after the resolution of the somnolence. Bilateral involvement is evidently more severe. Cognitive disturbances consist mostly of personality changes with disinhibited behavior, impulsivity, apathy and even loss of psychic self-activation associated with amnesia similar to Korsakoff syndrome. This picture of amnesia and behavioral disturbances is recognized as a "thalamic dementia". However, severe persistent amnestic syndrome is observed only with concomitant lesion of the anterior nucleus. With unilateral infarction, a left–right asymmetry is obvious in language versus visual-spatial impairment. The aphasia, named adynamic aphasia [20], is characterized by a reduced verbal fluency, with perseveration and paraphasic errors but with a relatively preserved syntax, comprehension, and repetition. Hypophonia and dysarthria can be associated.

The fourth territory is irrigated by the PChA, arising from the P2 segment of the PCA, and is subdivided into medial and lateral branches. They supply the pulvinar, part of the lateral and medial geniculate body, the posterior parts of the intralaminar nuclei, and lateral dorsal and lateral posterior nuclei. They also irrigate posterior portions of medial temporal structures, parts of midbrain and probably the subthalamic nucleus. The clinical syndrome is characterized by visual field defects, decreased optokinetic nystagmus contralaterally to the lesion, contralateral hemisensory loss with mild hemiparesis, and transcortical aphasia. Visual field deficits include homonymous quadrantanopsia, superior or inferior, and a homonymous horizontal wedge-shaped sectoranopsia, which is highly suggestive of a lateral geniculate body lesion irrigated by the PChA. On the other hand, a homonymous visual defect in the upper and lower quadrants sparing a horizontal sector is highly characteristic of vascular lesions in the lateral geniculate body irrigated by the AChA [22]. Some individuals, in the event of pulvinar involvement, develop delayed contralateral hyperkinetic movements, including ataxia, rubral tremor, dystonia, myoclonus and chorea, a syndrome named the "jerky dystonic unsteady hand". No specific behavioral disturbance is described, but some spatial neglect was associated with right pulvinar lesions.

Ischemia in the thalamus can mimic cortical and subcortical strokes in the anterior or posterior circulation. Depending on the location there can be additional symptoms (e.g. amnesia, cognitive impairment, decreased level of consciousness, personality changes, hemiataxia, pain).

Lacunar stroke syndromes

Lacunes are defined as small subcortical infarcts less than 1.5 cm in diameter occurring in perforator territories. Together with leukoaraiosis, microbleeds, and "hypertensive" (deep) intracerebral hemorrhages, they are part of the spectrum of small-vessel disease. This disease is tightly related to chronic hypertension, but diabetes, male gender, increasing age, smoking, previous lacunar TIA or stroke, and coronary artery disease are also risk factors. About 20% of all strokes are considered to be of lacunar origin, and it is estimated that only one of five lacunes is symptomatic. Lacunes result most frequently from occlusion of a single penetrating artery from lipohyalinosis within the artery. Other mechanisms include

microatheromas, occlusion of the penetrator orifice from a large plaque in the mother artery, microembolism, vasculitis, hypercoagulable states or genetic disease (CADASIL) and are present in up to a third of patients [23].

Five main classical lacunar syndromes are recognized:

- pure motor hemiparesis
- pure sensory stroke
- sensorimotor stroke
- dysarthria–clumsy hand syndrome
- ataxic hemiparesis.

Pure motor hemiparesis and ataxic hemiparesis are most frequently due to an infarct in the internal capsule, corona radiata, or basis pontis. The deficit is usually proportional, involving face, arm and leg to the same extent. Pure sensory stroke is usually related to a lesion in the ventroposterior nucleus of the thalamus, and less frequently the corona radiata. Sensorimotor stroke may result from a lesion of the internal capsule, and rarely from the paramedian pons. Dysarthria–clumsy hand syndrome is due most of the time to a lacunar infarct in the basis pontis, less frequently to a lesion in the internal capsule or cerebral peduncle. Therefore, a lacunar stroke in a specific location may lead to different lacunar stroke syndromes. Similarly, it has to be repeated that non-lacunar strokes and small intracerebral hemorrhages may present as lacunar syndromes, underlining the need for appropriate neuroimaging of all patients suspected of stroke.

Many other lacunar syndromes have been described. They include isolated dysarthria, facial paresis, pure motor hemiparesis with internuclear ophthalmoplegia, isolated third nerve palsy, pure motor hemiparesis with transient subcortical aphasia, isolated ataxia and hemichorea-hemiballismus [24], and many of the syndromes in Table 9.2. Hemichorea-hemiballismus is a classic presentation of a lacunar infarct in the subthalamic nucleus, but lesions in the basal ganglia may also cause it.

Ischemic lacunar strokes have some characteristic clinical features. They often progress during the first 24–48 hours after onset or can fluctuate considerably. If a severe hemiplegia alternates repeatedly with normal function, the phenomenon is called "capsular warning syndrome", resulting usually from a lacune in the internal capsule. About half of these fluctuating patients will end with a lacunar stroke within 24–48 hours. The pathogenesis is not clear but seems to be rather electro-physiological, given its stereotyped fluctuations, and the absence of response to antithrombotic medication and to elevation of perfusion pressure. In the acute setting, individuals with presumed lacunar strokes should be treated with intravenous thrombolysis whenever possible, as overall they respond as well as do patients with other stroke subtypes.

Although lacunar infarcts have better recovery and lower mortality rate during the first year, small-vessel disease carries a high risk of vascular death, recurrent stroke, and development of cognitive disturbances [25].

> Lacunes are small subcortical infarcts less than 1.5 cm in diameter occurring in perforator territories. Five main classic lacunar syndromes are recognized:
> - pure motor hemiparesis
> - pure sensory stroke
> - sensorimotor stroke
> - dysarthria–clumsy hand syndrome
> - ataxic hemiparesis.

Watershed infarcts (WS)

Watershed (or borderzone) infarcts represent about 5% of all strokes. They involve the junction of distal regions of two arterial systems. Pathophysiologically, systemic hemodynamic failure, tight stenosis (or occlusion) of a cervical or intracranial artery [26], or embolic occlusion of an intracerebral artery are implicated. Recently, a combination of these mechanisms has been proposed [27]: hypoperfusion due to severe arterial stenosis or occlusion would impair the reserve of brain areas becoming more susceptible to the effect of microemboli, and low flow with stagnation of blood would increase clot formation and decrease wash-out of emboli.

WS infarcts have been studied best in the anterior circulation in relationship to severe stenosis or occlusion of the ICA. Two typical patterns are observed: cortical WS (CWS) and the internal WS (IWS) strokes. The CWS area is located superficially in the cortex between the MCA, ACA and PCA territories. Strokes appear radiologically as wedges extending from the prefrontal or parieto-occipital cortex down to the frontal and occipital horns of the lateral ventricle respectively. The IWS area is situated in an anterior–posterior orientation in the centrum semiovale and along the lateral ventricle [28]. Incomplete

IWS strokes may appear as a small single lesion or as a chain-like (or rosary-like) pattern in this deep territory. There is better evidence that IWS stroke, particularly rosary-like infarction in the centrum semiovale, has an association with hemodynamic failure rather than with embolic mechanisms.

Clinical presentation of WS infarction is heterogeneous and depends on the location of ischemic changes. Signs and symptoms may be bilateral in the case of systemic hypotension or unilateral in the case of unilateral carotid severe stenosis or occlusion. The classic picture of a bilateral deep anterior IWS stroke, the "man-in-the-barrel" with proximal weakness of upper and lower limbs, is rare. Posterior infarction is classically associated with Balint's syndrome (asimultagnosia, optic ataxia, and ocular apraxia). If an arterial pathology is present, onset can be less abrupt than in embolic strokes and can fluctuate with changes of blood pressure and body position. Infratentorially, WS strokes are not well investigated.

The watershed area in the upper spinal cord is thought to be on the thoracic level T4 to T6 because of paucity of blood supply [29] and in the lumbosacral segments due to the high concentration of neurons and higher metabolic demands [30].

> Watershed (or borderzone) infarcts involve the junction of distal regions of two arterial systems. The clinical presentation is heterogeneous and depends on the location of ischemic changes.

Chapter summary

Anterior circulation syndromes
The anterior circulation refers to the part of the brain perfused by the carotid arteries.

Middle cerebral artery (MCA)
The MCA territory is the one most frequently affected by acute strokes. MCA territory infarcts can be subtle or a devastating clinical syndrome, depending on the site of the occlusion, the extent of ischemia, the etiology, and the collateral arterial network.

Symptoms of an *acute complete MCA* infarction: contralateral hemiparesis, hemihypesthesia, hemianopsia, ipsilateral conjugated eye and head deviation (the patient looks at his/her lesion); plus, in the case of a left lesion, aphasia, and in the case of a right lesion, contralateral multimodal hemineglect. Malignant stroke with brain edema may develop, leading to high intracranial pressure and subsequent herniation.

Infarctions of the lower arterial segments show similar symptoms, but not the complete picture (e.g. isolated brachiofacial paresis with or without visual field symptoms).

Internal carotid artery (ICA)

Embolic occlusion of the ICA, either proximally or distally, usually leads to severe stroke, showing concomitant signs of all anterior circulation arteries. A *progressive atherosclerotic occlusion* is usually less severe, with a classic subacute two-phase presentation, or even asymptomatic. Retinal ischemia from carotid emboli may be transient (amaurosis fugax) or persistent (central retinal artery occlusion or branch retinal artery occlusion).

Posterior circulation syndromes

The two vertebral arteries leave the subclavian arteries and join together to form the basilar artery.

Clinical symptoms and signs that point to a posterior circulation stroke: preceding TIAs and strokes in the days and hours before the infarct, headache, typically ipsilateral to the infarct, a disconjugate gaze or a conjugate gaze paresis with the eyes deviated toward the hemiparesis (brainstem lesion), a vertical gaze paresis (dorsal mesencephalic lesion), nystagmus, ocular tilt reaction (triad of skew deviation, conjugate ocular torsion towards the side of the lesion, and head tilt to the side of the lesion), Horner's syndrome (myosis, mild ptosis of the upper and lower eyelid, and hemifacial anhydrosis), bilateral or crossed motor, cerebellar and sensitive signs, truncular ataxia, acute unilateral deafness, somnolence and early anisocoria.

Lacunar stroke syndromes

Lacunes = small subcortical infarcts less than 1.5 cm in diameter occurring in perforator territories. Five main classic lacunar syndromes are recognized:

- pure motor hemiparesis
- pure sensory stroke
- sensorimotor stroke
- dysarthria–clumsy hand syndrome
- ataxic hemiparesis.

Ischemic lacunar strokes have some characteristic clinical features. They often progress during the first 24–48 hours after onset or can fluctuate considerably.

Watershed infarcts

Watershed (or borderzone) infarcts involve the junction of distal regions of two arterial systems. The clinical presentation is heterogeneous and depends on the location of ischemic changes. The classic picture of a bilateral deep anterior IWS stroke, the "man-in-the-barrel" with proximal weakness of upper and lower limbs, is rare.

References

1. Rovira A, Grive E, Rovira A, Alvarez-Sabin J. Distribution territories and causative mechanisms of ischemic stroke. *Eur Radiol* 2005; **15**(3):416–26.

2. Ay H, Furie KL, Singhal A, *et al.* An evidence-based causative classification system for acute ischemic stroke. *Ann Neurol* 2005; **58**(5):688–97.

3. van der Lugt A, Buter TC, Govaere F, *et al.* Accuracy of CT angiography in the assessment of a fetal origin of the posterior cerebral artery. *Eur Radiol* 2004; **14**(9):1627–33.

4. Brandt T, Steinke W, Thie A, Pessin MS, Caplan LR. Posterior cerebral artery territory infarcts: clinical features, infarct topography, causes and outcome. Multicenter results and a review of the literature. *Cerebrovasc Dis* 2000; **10**(3):170–82.

5. Averbuch-Heller L, Leigh RJ, Mermelstein V, Zagalsky L, Streifler JY. Ptosis in patients with hemispheric strokes. *Neurology* 2002; **58**(4):620–4.

6. Vahedi K, Hofmeijer J, Juettler E, *et al.* Early decompressive surgery in malignant infarction of the middle cerebral artery: a pooled analysis of three randomised controlled trials. *Lancet Neurol* 2007; **6**(3): 215–22.

7. Hamoir XL, Grandin CB, Peeters A, *et al.* MRI of hyperacute stroke in the AChA territory. *Eur Radiol* 2004; **14**(3):417–24.

8. Helgason CM. A new view of anterior choroidal artery territory infarction. *J Neurol* 1988; **235**(7):387–91.

9. Baumgartner RW, Baumgartner I. Vasomotor reactivity is exhausted in transient ischemic attacks with limb shaking. *J Neurol Neurosurg Psychiatry* 1998; **65**(4): 561–4.

10. Brandt T, Steinke W, Thie A, Pessin MS, Caplan LR. Posterior cerebral artery territory infarcts: clinical features, infarct topography, causes and outcome. Multicenter results and a review of the literature. *Cerebrovasc Dis* 2000; **10**(3): 170–82.

11. Tatu L, Moulin T, Bogousslavsky J, Duvernoy H. Arterial territories of human brain: brainstem and cerebellum. *Neurology* 1996; 47(5):1125–35.

12. Kataoka S, Miaki M, Saiki M, *et al.* Rostral lateral pontine infarction: neurological/topographical correlations. *Neurology* 2003; 61(1):114–17.

13. Wali GM. "Fou rire prodromique" heralding a brainstem stroke. *J Neurol Neurosurg Psychiatry* 1993; 56(2):209–10.

14. Bassetti C, Bogousslavsky J, Barth A, Regli F. Isolated infarcts of the pons. *Neurology* 1996; 46(1):165–75.

15. Arnold M, Nedeltchev K, Schroth G, *et al.* Clinical and radiological predictors of recanalization and outcome of 40 patients with acute basilar artery occlusion treated with intra-arterial thrombolysis. *J Neurol Neurosurg Psychiatry* 2004; 75(6):857–62.

16. Caplan LR. "Top of the basilar" syndrome. *Neurology* 1980; 30(1):72–9.

17. Idicula TT, Joseph LN. Neurological complications and aspects of basilar artery occlusive disease. *Neurologist* 2007; 13(6):363–8.

18. Pico F, Biron Y, Bousser MG, Amarenco P. Concurrent dolichoectasia of basilar and coronary arteries. *Neurology* 2005; 65(9):1503–4.

19. Brandt T, Steinke W, Thie A, Pessin MS, Caplan LR. Posterior cerebral artery territory infarcts: clinical features, infarct topography, causes and outcome. Multicenter results and a review of the literature. *Cerebrovasc Dis* 2000; 10(3):170–82.

20. Schmahmann JD. Vascular syndromes of the thalamus. *Stroke* 2003; 34(9):2264–78.

21. Carrera E, Bogousslavsky J. The thalamus and behavior: effects of anatomically distinct strokes. *Neurology* 2006; 66(12):1817–23.

22. Brazis PW, Masdeu JC, Biller J. *Localization in Clinical Neurology.* Lippincott Williams & Wilkins; 2006: 155.

23. Baumgartner RW, Sidler C, Mosso M, Georgiadis D. Ischemic lacunar stroke in patients with and without potential mechanism other than small-artery disease. *Stroke* 2003; 34(3):653–9.

24. Arboix A, Lopez-Grau M, Casasnovas C, *et al.* Clinical study of 39 patients with atypical lacunar syndrome. *J Neurol Neurosurg Psychiatry* 2006; 77(3):381–4.

25. Norrving B. Lacunar infarcts: no black holes in the brain are benign. *Pract Neurol* 2008; 8(4):222–8.

26. Bogousslavsky J, Regli F. Unilateral watershed cerebral infarcts. *Neurology* 1986; 36(3):373–7.

27. Caplan LR, Hennerici M. Impaired clearance of emboli (washout) is an important link between hypoperfusion, embolism, and ischemic stroke. *Arch Neurol* 1998; 55(11):1475–82.

28. Momjian-Mayor I, Baron JC. The pathophysiology of watershed infarction in internal carotid artery disease: review of cerebral perfusion studies. *Stroke* 2005; 36(3):567–77.

29. Novy J, Carruzzo A, Maeder P, Bogousslavsky J. Spinal cord ischemia: clinical and imaging patterns, pathogenesis, and outcomes in 27 patients. *Arch Neurol* 2006; 63(8):1113–20.

30. Duggal N, Lach B. Selective vulnerability of the lumbosacral spinal cord after cardiac arrest and hypotension. *Stroke* 2002; 33(1):116–21.

Less common stroke syndromes

Wilfried Lang

Introduction

This chapter deals with focal brain ischemia, either TIA or ischemic stroke. Causes, mechanisms, and clinical syndromes of brain hemorrhage are described elsewhere. This chapter is divided into three parts. The first part focuses on an uncommon mechanism of focal brain ischemia, which is low flow. Most TIA and ischemic strokes are caused by embolism or *in situ* artery occlusion. Hemodynamic causes of focal brain ischemia are less common. Second, uncommon clinical presentations of focal brain ischemia are described. In the third part, uncommon causes of TIA and ischemic stroke are presented together with associated clinical syndromes.

Uncommon mechanism of stroke: low flow

Ischemic strokes and transient ischemic attacks caused by low cerebral flow – anterior circulation

Most ischemic strokes and transient ischemic attacks are caused by embolic and acute, *in situ* (usually thrombotic) occlusion of an artery in the brain. However, in some patients severe stenosis or occlusion of carotid or vertebral arteries may cause a critical reduction of blood flow, particularly when collateral circulation is compromised because the circle of Willis is incomplete or diseased. Mechanisms to compensate for the reduction of blood flow are vasodilatation by autoregulation and an increase of the oxygen extraction fraction. If the vascular bed is maximally dilated the supplied brain is particularly vulnerable to any fall in perfusion pressure. Under these circumstances a small drop in systemic blood pressure may cause transient or permanent focal ischemia.

Boundary-zone infarcts

The evidence that at least some boundary-zone infarcts are caused by low flow rather than acute arterial occlusion is that a sudden, profound and relatively prolonged hypotension (e.g. as a result of cardiac arrest or cardiac surgery) sometimes causes infarction bilaterally in the posterior boundary zones between the supply territories of the middle cerebral artery (MCA) and the posterior cerebral artery in the parieto-occipital regions. The clinical features include visual disorientation and agnosia, and amnesia.

Hemianopia is the most common symptom in unilateral posterior boundary-zone infarction, usually with macular sparing and predominating in the lower quadrant. Brachiofacial hypoesthesia is frequent, while motor weakness is rare and remains mild. In the dominant hemisphere, lesions manifest as either isolated word-finding difficulty or transcortical sensory aphasia (impaired comprehension but preserved word repetition and speech output). In the non-dominant hemisphere contralateral hemispatial neglect and anosognosia are usually found.

Anterior boundary-zone infarction is recognized in severe carotid stenosis or occlusion. The boundary zone is located in the frontoparasagittal region, between the supply territories of the MCA and the anterior cerebral artery in the frontoparasagittal region. The clinical features are contralateral weakness of the leg, more than the arm and sparing the face, some impaired sensation of the same distribution and transcortical motor aphasia (intact comprehension and repetition with impaired speech output), which may be preceded by mutism if in the dominant hemisphere.

There is an internal or subcortical boundary zone in the corona radiate and centrum semiovale, lateral and/or above the lateral ventricle. This lies between the supply areas of the lenticulostriate perforating branches from the MCA trunk and the medullary perforating arteries which arise from the cortical branches of the MCA and the anterior and, perhaps, posterior cerebral arteries. Infarction can occur within this internal boundary zone, usually causing lacunar or partial anterior circulation syndrome, in association with severe carotid disease and sometimes an obvious hemodynamic precipitating cause.

A sudden and profound hypotension sometimes causes **boundary-zone infarction**.

A fall in cerebral perfusion pressure as a cause of focal brain ischemia should be suspected if the symptoms start under certain circumstances [1]:

- on standing up very quickly, even if postural hypotension cannot be demonstrated in the clinic
- immediately after a heavy meal
- in very hot weather
- with exercise, coughing, or hyperventilation
- during Valsalva maneuver (but embolism is another possibility)
- during a clinically obvious episode of cardiac dysrhythmia (chest pain, palpitations, etc.) but embolism from heart is also possible
- during operative hypotension
- if the patient has recently been started on or increased the dose of any drug likely to cause hypotension.

Limb-shaking TIA

A transient ischemic attack which is typically associated with severe large artery disease with exhausted hemodynamic reserve is "limb-shaking TIA". It is characterized by 30–60 sec episodes of repetitive jerking movements of contralateral arm and/or leg and has been described with carotid occlusion but also with stenosis of intracranial vessels, e.g. middle cerebral artery or anterior cerebral artery. "Limb-shaking TIA" is elicited in situations which dispose to low flow, e.g. orthostatic dysregulation, hyperventilation in Moyamoya disease, or by carotid compression. The symptoms usually point towards a seizure-like activity and are often misdiagnosed as focal seizures. In contrast to seizure activity, limb shaking shows no somatotopic spread of movement

activity (no Jacksonian march) and usually has a low frequency (about 3 Hz). It is reported that limb shaking disappears with revascularization, e.g. carotid endarterectomy or extracranial–intracranial bypass (Figure 10.1).

A transient ischemic attack which is typically associated with severe large artery disease with exhausted hemodynamic reserve is "**limb-shaking TIA**".

Ischemic ophthalmopathy

Another symptom of low flow is monocular transient retinal ischemia occurring when looking into bright light. Objects appear bleached and a brief visual loss may follow. This symptom has been related to retinal claudication: an increase in the metabolic demand during exposure to bright light cannot be met because of an already marginal perfusion. Ischemic ophthalmopathy is a specific, concomitant disorder of uncompensated, critically reduced perfusion pressure due to internal carotid artery occlusive disease. Quite characteristic is the history of a gradual, progressive loss of visual acuity, occasionally with bouts of obscuration, leading to a slowly progressive, irreversible damage of the retinal neuronal layer. Further typical findings are neovascularization of the retina and iris (rubeosis iris) [2].

Ischemic strokes and transient ischemic attacks caused by low cerebral flow – posterior circulation
Rotational vertebral artery occlusion (RVAO) and stroke

Rotational vertebral artery occlusion (RVAO) is caused by mechanical compression of vertebral arteries during head rotation. The vertebral artery is usually compressed at the atlantoaxial C1–C2 level. Tendinous insertions, osteophytes or degenerative changes resulting from cervical spondylosis may be the cause of compression. Most RVAO patients exhibit an ipsilateral stenosis or vessel malformation (e.g. hypoplasia) and a contralateral dominant vertebral artery. With ispilateral head rotation, the (contralateral) dominant vertebral artery is compressed. The leading symptom is vertigo, followed by tinnitus. Video-oculography showed that RVAO is associated with a mixed downbeat torsional and horizontal beating nystagmus which may spontaneously reverse direction [3]. The labyrinth is predominantly supplied

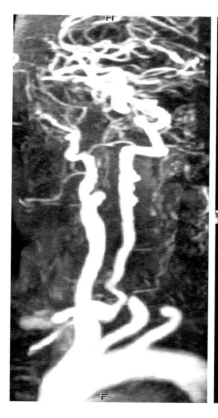

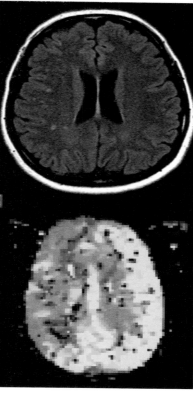

Figure 10.1. Limb-shaking TIA. A 55-year-old woman with risk factors (metabolic syndrome, smoking) presented with a limb shaking of the left leg when standing. The right internal carotid artery (ICA) was occluded. Occlusion was presumably acute. Territory of the ICA was supplied from the left ICA via the anterior communicating artery. There was no collateral blood flow from the posterior communicating artery. Initially, the symptom was considered to be focal epileptic. Perfusion MR showed reduction of blood flow in the anterior territory of the right middle cerebral artery and the right anterior cerebral artery.

by the internal auditory artery, which is usually a branch of the anterior inferior cerebellar artery (AICA). As AICA usually takes off the basilar artery at its lower portion, reduced blood flow from the vertebral artery would result in ischemia. Approximately 50% of RVAO patients treated conservatively suffered from infarction or residual neurological deficits [4]. Brief episodes of rotational vertigo can also be caused by compression of the vestibular nerve as caused by close contact with intracranial vessels, particularly the posterior inferior cerebellar artery (PICA).

> **Rotational vertebral artery occlusion** (RVAO) is caused by mechanical compression of vertebral arteries during head rotation. The leading symptom is vertigo, followed by tinnitus.

Drop attack and vertebrobasilar ischemia

"Drop attacks" are episodes of sudden loss of postural tone which cause the subject to fall to the ground without apparent loss of consciousness, vertigo or other sensation. The attack occurs without warning and is not induced by a change of posture or movement of the head. The patient may be unable to rise

immediately after the fall despite being uninjured. Not a single patient in the New England Medical Center Posterior Circulation Registry had a drop attack as the only symptom of posterior circulation ischemia [5]. With vertebrobasilar ischemia, sudden falls are usually preceded by and associated with symptoms such as vertigo, diplopia or blurred vision (Figure 10.2). A "drop attack" has been described in a patient with parasagittal motor cortex/subcortex ischemia in the territory of both anterior cerebral arteries [6].

> In "drop attacks" a sudden loss of postural tone causes a fall to the ground without loss of consciousness.

Subclavian steal syndrome and hemodynamic effects of proximal vertebral artery disease

Most patients with subclavian artery stenosis or occlusion are asymptomatic. In a large series, only 15 out of 324 patients (4.6%) had objective signs of brachial ischemia such as aching after exercise or coolness of the arm. Among 116 patients with unilateral steal as shown by ultrasonography none had

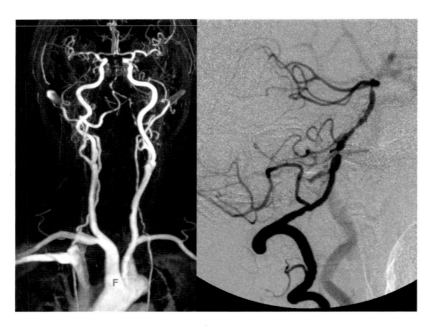

Figure 10.2. Drop attack. An 82-year-old woman with insulin-dependent diabetes mellitus suffered from recurrent short episodes with nausea, vertigo (sensation of being turned around), sweating, blurred vision, weakness and sudden falling without losing consciousness. Episodes were particularly frequent after reduction of elevated blood pressure. Stenosis of the basilar artery proximal to the AICA (anterior inferior cerebellar artery) was assumed to be the cause of these drop attacks. Symptoms disappeared after stent-PTA of the stenosis.

symptoms of brain ischemia [7]. Among more than 400 patients with posterior circulation TIAs or ischemic stroke only two had symptoms (TIAs) attributable to significant subclavian or innominate artery disease [8]. Symptoms which have been associated with decreased anterograde flow or retrograde flow in the vertebral artery are episodes with dizziness, diplopia, decreased vision or oszillopsia. The attacks are brief and may be elicited by exercise of the arm. A difference in the wrist or the antecubital pulses and a difference of blood pressure between the two arms are reliable signs which indicate subclavian steal syndrome. Causes of stenosis or occlusion of the vertebral artery are: arteriosclerosis, Takayashu disease and temporal arteritis or mechanical trauma, as have been reported by bowlers or baseball pitchers.

> Most patients with subclavian artery stenosis or occlusion are asymptomatic. Associated symptoms may include episodes with dizziness, diplopia, decreased vision or oszillopsia.

Severe stenosis or occlusion of the proximal vertebral artery is more likely to be a cause of embolism than to have hemodynamic effects: among 407 patients in the New England Medical Center Posterior Circulation Registry 80 of 407 patients had severe stenosis or occlusion of the proximal vertebral artery. In 45 of the 80 (56%) embolization was the most likely cause of cerebral ischemia. Only in 13 of 80 were hemodynamic effects considered to be the cause of cerebral

ischemia. Twelve of these 13 patients had severe bilateral occlusive disease of the vertebral artery [8].

Hyperviscosity and low flow

Blood flow in the brain is determined by the size of blood vessels, blood pressure and hemorrheological factors of the blood. Abnormal changes of blood plasma with hematological disease (e.g. Waldenstrom's macroglobulinemia or paraproteinemia), increase in cell counts (e.g. in diseases such as polycythemia vera, erythrocytosis or hyperleukotic leukemias), and decreased red cell deformability (sickle-cell anemia, spherocytosis, hemoglobinopathies) lead to a hyperviscous state [9].

Cerebral blood flow is diminished with high hematocrit as found in polycythemia vera. Symptoms are often unspecific, such as headache, dizziness or vertigo, paresthesias, blurred vision or tinnitus. Low flow and/or increased coagulability may be the cause of focal brain ischemia. Different ischemic patterns have been described, such as lacunar infarction, boundary infarction, Binswanger's disease or large artery (territorial) infarction. In sickle-cell anemia, deformability of red cells is decreased. This may cause damage in the microcirculation, particularly in the boundary zones between major arterial territories. But large-artery occlusive disease, occasionally with the development of moyamoya, was also found.

Plasma hyperviscosity syndrome is a clinical entity with mucous membrane bleeding, blurred vision, visual loss, lethargy, headache, dizziness, vertigo, tinnitus, paresthesias, and occasionally seizures.

> Abnormal changes of blood plasma lead to a **hyperviscous state** and cerebral blood flow can be diminished. Symptoms are often unspecific, such as headache, dizziness or vertigo, paresthesias, blurred vision or tinnitus.

Uncommon clinical presentations of stroke

The capsular warning syndrome

A small infarct in the internal capsule is considered to be caused by the occlusion of a single lenticulostriate artery which arises from the mainstem of the middle cerebral artery (MCA). This infarct typically presents with "pure motor hemiparesis". The term "capsular warning syndrome" describes the phenomenon in which the infarct may be preceded by repetitive, stereotypic transient ischemic attacks with "pure motor hemiparesis" ("lacunar TIAs"). This burst of hemiplegic TIAs is limited in time and lasts about 24–48 hours. The risk of developing a lacunar infarct is about 40% within the next few days. *In situ* small-vessel disease (microatheroma or lipohyalinosis) is considered to be the most likely mechanism. Alternatively, it has been suggested that an atheroma in the MCA may cause a high-grade obstruction at the origin of the single lenticulostriate artery [10] (Figure 10.3).

Bilateral blindness: "top of the basilar artery"

Sudden cortical blindness is a rare symptom of TIA or stroke and has been explained by an occlusion of the "top of the basilar artery" at the origin of the posterior

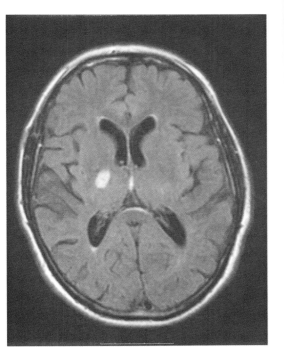

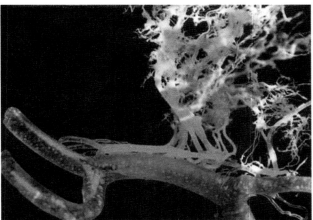

perforating lenticulostriate arteries

main branches

MCA

● occlusion of a perforator

Figure 10.3. Capsular warning sign. A 65-year-old with hypercholesterolemia was referred to the hospital because of a sudden weakness of left face, arm and leg. He was unable to walk. He was dysarthric. Symptoms disappeared after about 10 minutes but over the next 5 hours he had four further identical episodes lasting for several minutes. The next day he suffered a lacunar stroke in the internal capsule with persisting pure motor hemiparesis. It is assumed that the occlusion of a single perforating artery (lenticulostriate artery) was the cause of the lacunar infarct.

cerebral arteries [11]. The visual field defects may be quite asymmetric and variable. Symptoms may be transient (TIA) or persisting. Even when severe cortical blindness is present, patients may retain some ability to avoid bumping into objects and may blink to visual threat. This so-called blind sight is probably explained by some sparing of the visual cortex and by preservation of the so-called second visual system, which is composed of the superior colliculi and their projections to peristriate cortex (Figure 10.4). Embolism from the heart or the proximal vertebrobasilar artery is the cause of this sign [12]. Other symptoms of bilateral ischemia in the territory of the PCA may be: memory loss, usually involving both anterograde and retrograde amnesia, and agitated delirium. In cases of persistent amnesia, bilateral infarction of the mesial temporal lobe was described [8].

> Bilateral blindness can be due to occlusion of the basilar artery at the bifurcation to the posterior cerebral arteries.

Amnesia

Personal (autobiographical) memories depend on the ability to encode, store and retrieve information which we consciously experience ("autobiographic episodes"). The cognitive system representing this ability is termed episodic memory. It can be tested by questions about recent personal history or more

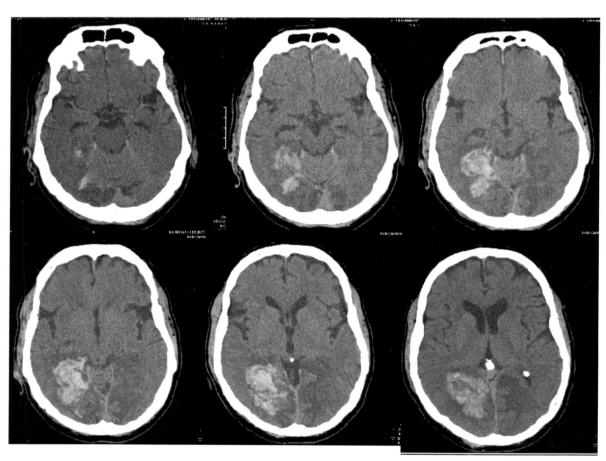

Figure 10.4. "Blind sight". A 65-year-old patient with known Parkinson's disease and vascular risk factors (diabetes mellitus, hypertension, obesity and smoking) suddenly lost muscle tone and consciousness. On admission he was awake, responded to verbal commands and was partially oriented. Pupils were mid-dilated, response to light was reduced. He reported not seeing anything with either eye. There was no weakness of the limbs. Although without conscious visual perception he was able to unconsciously prevent himself from bumping into objects when walking. When showing him different numbers of fingers he mentioned not seeing the fingers but his performance of rating the number of presented fingers was much above chance. CCT showed a bilateral infarction in the territory of the posterior cerebral artery with hemorrhage on the right side. The primary visual cortex of each side was damaged.

systematically by presenting a list of words and by testing free recall of them after a few minutes. The anatomical structures underlying episodic memory are the Papez circle (hippocampus, parahippocampus, ento- and perirhinal cortex, cingulate gyrus, fornix, nucleus anterior thalami, mamillothalamic tracts and mammillary bodies), the basolateral limbic circuit (dorso-medial thalamic nucleus and amygdala) and the basal forebrain. Input from this system is necessary to ensure that the multimodal information from the environment which is processed and integrated in the neocortical association areas becomes memorable and retrievable. A disorder of the system underlying episodic memory causes anterograde amnesia. The arterial blood supply of the anatomical structures subserving episodic memory has many sources, particularly the anterior cerebral artery and the anterior communicating artery (basal forebrain and fornix), posterior communicating artery (parts of the thalamus), posterior cerebral artery (hippocampus and parahippocampal gyrus), anterior choroidal artery (anterior hippocampus and adjacent cortex) and posterior choroidal artery (parts of the fornix).

There are three uncommon but relevant stroke syndromes which cause amnesia:

- bilateral infarcts of the medio-basal temporal lobe
- bilateral thalamic infarcts and
- subarachnoid hemorrhage from aneurysm of the anterior communicating artery.

Memory defects can follow unilateral or bilateral infarcts of the medio-basal temporal lobe but are more common with left-sided and bilateral lesions. Recall of memories is mainly based on two processes, judgements that something is familiar and the conscious recollection of an episode with all attributes. Depending on the site of the lesion, recognition of familiarity or conscious recollection may be more disturbed. Furthermore, left-sided infarcts are known to cause predominantly verbal amnesia whereas right-sided lesions may disturb visuo-spatial memories. Embolism from the heart or proximal vertebrobasilar artery is typically found to be the cause of bilateral infarcts.

Infarcts in the anterior and dorsomedial thalamus can produce severe memory deficits which are almost always accompanied by other neurological and neuropsychological symptoms such as attentional deficits, language disturbance, neglect or executive dysfunctions. If amnesia is the leading clinical symptom TIA or stroke has to be distinguished from transient global amnesia (TGA). TIA and stroke are either accompanied by other neuropsychological symptoms or can be demonstrated with brain imaging.

Amnesia can be caused by temporal lobe or thalamic infarcts.

Reduced vigilance or coma as the leading symptom

Bilateral paramedian thalamic infarction can result from an occlusion of a single thalamic-subthalamic artery which branches from the posterior cerebral artery (PCA). Patients can be hypersomnolent or comatose as if being in an anoxic or metabolic coma without localizable neurological signs. After regaining consciousness, disturbance of vertical gaze function (upgaze palsy, combined up- and downgaze palsy or skew deviation) and neuropsychological deficits may become apparent.

Coma is more frequently found in patients with acute occlusion of the basilar artery in whom ischemia involves the bilateral pontine tegmentum. But here, additional neurological signs such as ophthalmoplegia and bilateral extensor plantar reflexes indicate brainstem ischemia.

Coma is frequently found in basilar artery occlusion.

Agitation and delirium as the presenting symptom

According to the American Psychiatric Association (1987) delirium is defined as a clinical symptom with the following symptoms and signs:

- reduced ability to maintain attention to external stimuli and to appropriately shift attention to new stimuli
- disorganized thinking as indicated by irrelevant or incoherent speech
- symptoms such as reduced level of consciousness, perceptual disturbances (misinterpretations, illusions or hallucinations), disturbances of sleep–wake cycle, increased or decreased psychomotor activity, disorientation to time, place, or person, memory impairment
- clinical features developing over a short time and tending to fluctuate over the course of a day.

Agitation and/or delirium may be the leading or the only symptom of acute stroke. It is uncommon and may not be considered a clinical manifestation of stroke. In a retrospective analysis, 19 of 661 stroke patients (3%) presented with delirium [13]. Right hemisphere infarcts that include the hippocampus, amygdala, entorhinal and perirhinal cortex and their underlying white matter have been found to be most frequently associated with agitation and delirium.

Isolated cranial nerves

Stroke in the brainstem is typically indicated by (a) ipsilateral cranial nerve (III–XII) palsy (single or multiple) together with contralateral motor or sensory deficit, (b) bilateral motor and/or sensory deficits or (c) disorders of conjugate eye movements. Rarely, cranial nerve palsy without any sensory or motor deficits may indicate a focal brainstem ischemia. Two out of 22 patients with focal ischemic lesions in the mesencephalon had an isolated palsy of the oculomotor nerve [14]. Thömke *et al.* [15] studied 29 patients with diabetes mellitus and oculomotor

nerve palsy. In five patients a focal ischemic lesion in the mesencephalon was causal for the deficit. Isolated palsy of the trochlear nerve has been described with focal hemorrhage or ischemia in the mesencephalon. Isolated palsy of the abducens, trigeminal, facial nerve and even of the vestibular part of the vestibulocochlear nerve is caused by focal hemorrhage or ischemia in the pons [16]. Ischemia may be caused by low flow in boundary zones.

Focal brainstem ischemia may cause isolated cranial nerve palsy.

Akinesia or involuntary movements

Acute hypokinetic or hyperkinetic movement disorders are an uncommon but sometimes the leading symptom of stroke.

Acute akinesia or hypokinesia of the contralateral part of the body is found after ischemic lesions of the medial part of the frontal lobe [17] (Figure 10.5). The supplementary motor area (SMA) is the medial part of

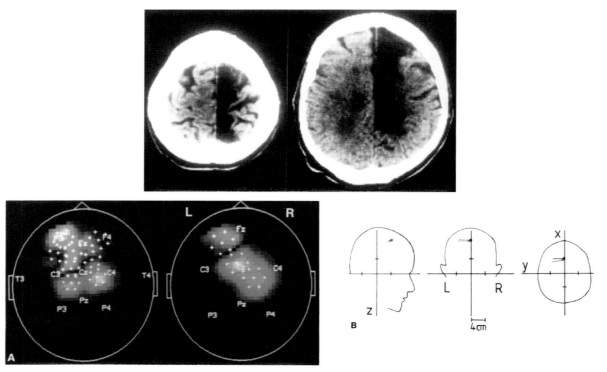

Figure 10.5. Contralateral akinesia/hypokinesia. A patient suffered from a large infarction in the territory of the right anterior cerebral artery (ACA). His left arm was spontaneously not used but showed forced grasping reflexes to visual and tactile stimuli. The patient participated in an experiment with measurements of magnetic fields of the brain preceding spontaneous movements of the right index finger. With movements of the right finger an activation in the intact left supplementary motor area (SMA) preceding the onset of movement by more than 1 second was shown [17].

the premotor cortex and is supplied by the anterior cerebral artery. It is part of a neuronal loop which involves frontal cortex, basal ganglia and thalamus. The SMA receives excitatory input from the ventro-lateral thalamus. Lesions of the SMA in the left hemi-sphere cause a lack of spontaneous speech (transcortical motor aphasia) with preserved comprehension and repetition and a hypokinesia/akinesia of contralateral body. Usually, these symptoms are transient. Lesions of the right SMA are associated with hypokinesia/akinesia of the left part of the body. Bilateral lesions of the mesial frontal cortex are known to cause severe akinetic states. Typically there is a marked contrast between the paucity or absence of spontaneous movements and the pre-served or even exaggerated ability to respond to external visual or tactile clues ("forced grasping"). Response to external stimuli helps to distinguish motor hypokinesia/akinesia from motor neglect. Motor (hemi-) neglect may be an isolated symptom but is mainly part of a neglect syndrome which is characterized by a reduction of focal attention.

Hemichorea-hemiballism is the most frequently reported acute involuntary movement disorder in acute stroke. It has classically been described after an acute small deep infarct in the subthalamic nucleus [18].

> Akinesia can be caused by lesions in the medial frontal lobe.

Focal paresis

Weakness of one side of the body is the most frequent symptom of TIA or stroke. Typically either one part or several parts of the body are involved (face, arm, leg, face + arm, face + arm + leg). It is more uncommon in focal brain ischemia for isolated movements such as extension of fingers and hand or movements of the tongue to be the only symptom (Figure 10.6).

Uncommon causes of stroke and associated clinical syndromes

Stroke manifestations of systemic disease

Infective and non-infective endocarditis: multi-territorial pattern of ischemic stroke

Endocarditis of the heart and its valves in particular can be classified into infective and non-infective types. The vast majority of endocarditis is secondary to infections caused by bacterial (*Staphylococcus*

aureus, coagulase-negative *Staphylococcus* or *Entero-coccus*) or, rarely, fungal (*Candida*, *Aspergillus*) organisms [19]. Cerebral embolism from infected valves is the central mechanism of neurological injury in patients with infective endocarditis. Embolic debris from infected valves typically lodges in the distal branches of the middle cerebral artery [20]. Over 50% of patients had infarcts involving more than one arterial territory [21]. Besides brain and retinal ischemia, other cerebrovascular complications include intracranial hemorrhage and subarachnoid hemorrhage [22]. Mycotic aneurysms are often assumed to be the cause of cerebral hemorrhage. They are thought to develop after septic microembolism to the vaso vasorum of cerebral vessels. But mycotic aneurysms are found in less than 3% of hemorrhages. More common mechanisms of hemorrhage include hemorrhagic transformation of the ischemic infarc-tion, septic endarteritis and non-aneurysmal arterial erosion at the site of the previous embolic occlusion, and concurrent antithrombotic medication use [23].

Non-infective endocarditis is termed non-bacterial thrombotic endocarditis (NBTE). It is characterized by the accumulation of sterile platelet and fibrin aggre-gates on the heart valves to form small vegetations. About 50% of NBTE cases occur in association with cancer, especially mucin-producing adenocarcinomas (particularly pancreatic carcinoma and non-small-cell lung cancer) and hematological malignancies (lymph-oma and leukemia [24]). Although only less than 2% of patients with cancer have NBTE, up to 50% of these patients with NBTE suffer from stroke [25]. A significant proportion of patients with NBTE have other disorders, including rheumatic heart disease, rheumatological diseases such as lupus (where it is referred to as Lipman-Sacks endocarditis), AIDS, gas-trointestinal diseases such as cirrhosis, and severe sys-temic illness, such as burns or sepsis [26]. Small and large multi-territorial infarction is a radiographic sign in NBTE [27]. Thus, encephalopathy rather than focal deficits may be the initial clinical presentation.

> Endocarditis of various origins typically causes multi-territorial infarctions.

Inflammatory vasculopathies and connective tissue disease: a chronic and multisystemic disease

Inflammatory vasculopathies and connective tissue disease are Takayashu's arteritis, systemic lupus erythematosus (SLE), antiphospholipid antibody

177

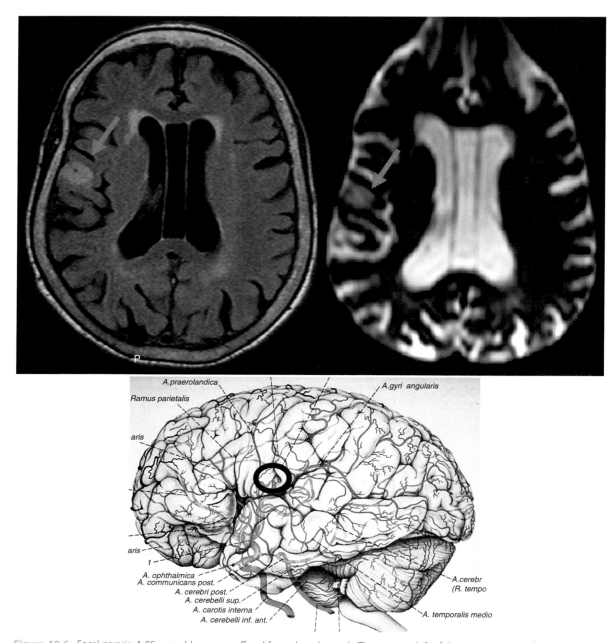

Figure 10.6. Focal paresis. A 95-year-old woman suffered from slurred speech. There was a shift of the tongue to the left side. Diffusion-weighted imaging showed a small cortical lesion in the frontal operculum which was most likely caused by a cardiac embolism because of atrial fibrillation.

syndrome, Sneddon syndrome, primary systemic vasculitis (classic polyarteritis nodosa, microscopic polyangiitis, Churg-Strauss syndrome, Wegener's granulomatosis), Sjögren syndrome, Behçet disease, primary angiitis of the central nervous system, and paraneoplastic vasculitis. Warlow *et al.* [1] have summarized clinical clues which may in general indicate inflammatory vasculopathies and connective tissue disease. Patients may present with TIA and stroke but also with encephalopathy:

- preceding or accompanying systemic features such as weight loss, headache, malaise, skin rash, livedo reticularis, arthropathy, renal failure and fever
- lack of any other obvious or more common cause of stroke
- younger patient in most cases (an exception being giant cell arteritis)
- a raised ESR and C-reactive protein
- anemia and leukocytosis in the routine blood screening tests
- when there is diagnostic suspicion, specified immunological tests such as raised serum antiphospholipid, double-stranded DNA and antineutrophil cytoplasmic antibodies (ANCAs).

Among those diseases, giant cell arteritis and systemic lupus erythematosus are uncommon but not rare and will be presented in more detail.

Giant cell arteritis is also known as temporal arteritis, cranial arteritis, or Horton's disease. The annual incidence increases with age from 2.6/100 000 for those aged between 50 and 59 years to 44.6/100 000 for those older than 80 years. Headache, especially in the night, located in the temporal region, fever, weight loss, fatigue and malaise or arthralgia and jaw claudication are the predominating symptoms. Most patients with giant cell arteritis have symptoms of polymyalgia rheumatica, which may precede the headache. A raised ESR (over 50 or even 100 mm in the first hour) is also indicative.

Ischemic symptoms of the retina and the brain usually develop late in the course of disease. But stroke may even be the first indication of disease. Giant cell arteritis involves the ophthalmic, posterior ciliary and central retinal arteries, which causes infarction of the optic nerve. It may also involve intracranial vessels, particularly the extradural vertebral arteries, which may cause stroke. Diplopia and ophthalmoplegia may develop but are mainly caused by necrosis of the extraocular muscles and not by brainstem ischemia.

Systemic lupus erythematosus is a chronic autoimmune disease affecting mainly young women. It much more often causes a generalized subacute or chronic encephalopathy than focal ischemic or hemorrhagic cerebral episodes. Intimal proliferation involving small vessels may represent florid or healed vasculitic lesions. Large artery occlusions can be explained in some patients by cardiac sources (NBTE: non-bacterial thrombotic embolism). Most patients have circulating antinuclear antibodies. A raised antinuclear factor is highly sensitive but not specific. Double-stranded DNA and anti-Sm antibodies are much more specific but are found in less than half of cases. A high proportion of patients also have antiphospholipid antibodies, which seem to be particularly associated with cardiac valvular vegetations and arterial thrombosis. The antiphospholipid syndrome cannot be diagnosed on the basis of a raised single titer of antibody in the serum. The titer must be substantially raised on several occasions and must be associated not only with ischemic stroke but also with other manifestations of disease such as deep venous thrombosis, recurrent miscarriage, livedo reticularis, cardiac valvular vegetations, migraine-like headache, thrombocytopenia, or hemolytic anemia.

> Inflammatory vasculopathies require special diagnostic tests.

Intracranial vasculopathies caused by virus and bacterial infection
Varicella zoster virus vasculopathy

Varicella zoster virus (VZV) vasculopathy may often be clinically silent but may present with stroke and can be diagnosed because of the following symptoms, signs and findings (for review: Nagel *et al.* [28]). (1) About two-thirds of patients have a history of zoster rash, particularly ophthalmic-distribution zoster or a history of chicken pox. There is a delay between the onset of zoster/chicken pox and the onset of stroke averaging 4.1 months (range between same day and 2.5 years). But about one-third of patients with a pathologically and virologically verified disease have no history of zoster rash or chicken pox. (2) Angiographic evidence of narrowing in cerebral arteries may be found in MR angiography. In vascular studies 70% had vasculopathies. Different patterns of vascular lesions have been found. There was pure large artery disease in 13%, pure small artery disease in 37% and a mixed vascular pathology in most patients (50%). (3) Varicella zoster virus as the cause of stroke can be proven by examinations of the cerebrospinal fluid: 67% of patients have a pleocytosis (>5 white blood cells/mm^3). Thus, some patients may even have no pleocytosis. Specific antibodies (anti-VZV-IgG) with proven intrathecal synthesis were found in 93% of patients, and VZV-DNA in 30%. A negative result

179

for both VZV DNA and anti-VZV-IgG antibody in CSF can reliably exclude the diagnosis of VZV vasculopathy.

Chronic bacterial, meningeal infections

Ischemic stroke complicates chronic meningeal infections which cause inflammation and thrombosis of arteries and veins on the surface of the brain. With tuberculous meningitis, infection is predominantly located at the base of the brain and vasculitis causes thrombosis in the large intracranial arteries and territorial infarction. Different vascular territories may be involved depending on the spatial extent of the meningeal infection. Tuberculous meningitis has to be considered as a clinical syndrome when one of the following criteria accompanies ischemic stroke [29]:

- medical history with manifestation of tuberculosis in the lungs or in a different organ (this manifestation may have been many decades ago)
- one or more symptoms indicating chronic meningeal infection such as headache or subfebrile temperature preceding stroke
- other signs indicating a process in the basal meninges such as lesion of cranial nerves or development of hydrocephalus as a consequence of an obstruction of the basal cisterns.

In addition there may be more unspecific signs as well, such as loss of appetite, drowsiness or myalgia. Contrast-enhanced magnetic resonance imaging may show up the basal meningitis. The cerebrospinal fluid shows mild to moderate pleocytosis with white blood cells up to $300/mm^3$, the glucose is reduced with subacute infections and protein is elevated as a sign of the disturbed circulation of the cerebrospinal fluid. Infection with tuberculosis can be proven by cytology (Ziehl–Neelsen), culture, detection of DNA (PCR) or antigen.

Syphilitic meningovasculitis

Syphilitic meningovasculitis may be the first clinical presentation of an infection with *Treponema pallidum*. The primary infection with a syphilitic lesion in the mucosa may have been months to years ago. Syphilitic meningovasculitis presents with an obliteration of small or middle-sized large vessels; rarely are large arteries involved. The territory of the middle cerebral artery is mainly involved. Infected vessels and their vasa vasorum together with lymphocytic infiltration cause a slow progression of stenosis leading to

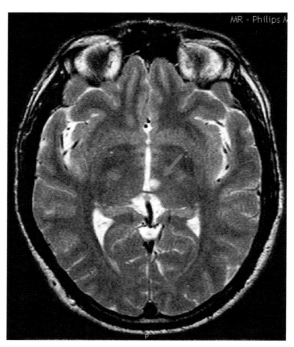

Figure 10.7. Meningovascular syphilis. The patient presented with the following signs: awake but apathic, decreased episodic memory, complete upgaze palsy, incomplete downgaze palsy, disturbed converge of eyes, contraversive ocular tilt reaction (tendency to fall to the right side and skew deviation). Pupils were reactive to light. There was a minimal hemiparesis shown up by a tendency to pronate with the right arm. MR shows a vascular lesion in the territory of the left thalamic-subthalamic artery. This lesion was caused by meningovascular syphilis proved by intrathecal production of specific antibodies (FTA-Abs) and mild pleocytosis.

occlusion. Patients may present with signs of meningeal (meningo-encephalitic) inflammation such as headache, dizziness, feeling sick, sleep disorder, change of personality, apathy, and deficits of episodic memory. Ischemic stroke can be preceded by TIA. Usually, the size of ischemic infarcts is small. There may be lesions of the cranial nerves because of the associated meningitis (Figure 10.7). Documentation of the intrathecal production of specific antibodies is required for a definite diagnosis of syphilitic meningovasculitis. Pleocytosis in the CSF together with specific antibodies in the serum can be taken as evidence of a likely syphilitic meningovasculitis. Other mechanisms of stroke associated with syphilis are mesaaortitis luetica with aortic dissection and endocarditis.

Viral and bacterial infections can cause specific vasculopathies.

Hereditary causes of stroke (single gene disorders) and their clinical presentation

CADASIL (cerebral autosomal dominant arteriopathy with subcortical infarcts and leukoencephalopathy), Fabry disease and MELAS (mitochondrial encephalopathy lactic acidosis and stroke) are genetic disorders associated with their own clinical and radiological presentation.

CADASIL

Genetic and pathological research suggests that the accumulation of the ectodomain of the NOTCH 3 protein is associated with severe ultrastructural alterations of the arteriolar wall [30]. The earliest clinical manifestation of CADASIL is migraine with aura at a mean age of 28 years. The aura may be visual or sensory but the frequency of attacks with basilar, hemiplegic and prolonged aura is high. At a mean age of 41 years, stroke becomes manifest in the course of disease. Two-thirds of patients present with lacunar syndromes such as pure motor, ataxic hemiparesis, pure sensory or sensory motor stroke. With increasing load of subcortical white matter lesion, vascular dementia with deficits of executive functions, and attentional and memory deficits develops (mean age of 50 years). Twenty percent of patients have severe mood disorders, and focal or generalized seizures have been observed in about 8% of patients.

Microangiopathy or small-vessel disease (SVD) is the morphological presentation of the disease with multiple lacunar lesions and extensive white matter hyperintensities (WMHs), which may be accompanied by evidence of microbleeds (MBs). A first hint for CADASIL is the presence of extensive morphological abnormalities with SVD in the absence of vascular risk factors, especially in younger patients. Not infrequently, such a constellation may lead to a false suspicion of multiple sclerosis. Further evidence comes from the distribution of WMHs. In CADASIL, WMHs are characteristically located in the white matter of the anterior temporal lobe and the external capsule as early as in the third decade [31]. Location of WMHs and age of onset are unusual for other SVDs (Figure 10.8).

> CADASIL is a rare genetic disorder causing small-vessel disease and multiple white matter lesions in young adults.

Fabry disease

Fabry disease, also Anderson–Fabry disease or angiokeratomy corporis diffusum, is an X-linked lysosomal storage disorder. Alpha-galactosidase deficiency leads to accumulation of glycolipids, mainly in endothelial and smooth muscle cells. A more recent study of 721 sufferers from acute cryptogenic stroke aged 18 to 55 years showed a rare but not negligible frequency of Fabry disease, which was 4.9% in male and 2.4% in female stroke patients [32]. The patients are mainly young and present with a variety of symptoms and signs which are caused by deposition of glycolipids in the tissue: skin manifestation with angiokeratomas (mainly in the bathing-trunk area) and hypohydrosis,

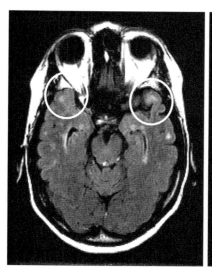 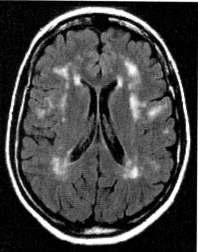

Figure 10.8. CADASIL. Extensive morphological abnormalities are found in CADASIL despite the absence of vascular risk factors, particularly in younger patients. White matter hyperintensities (WMHs) are characteristically located in the white matter of the anterior temporal lobe and the external capsule, which is unusual for other small-vessel diseases. (Courtesy of Professor Franz Fazekas, University of Graz.)

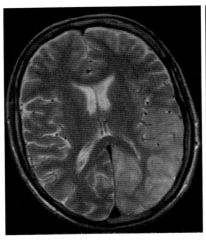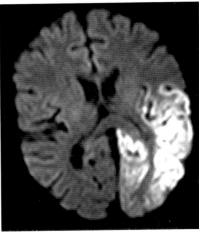

Figure 10.9. MELAS. MELAS-related brain lesions appear bright on diffusion-weighted imaging (right-hand picture). A hint towards the correct diagnosis is that MELAS lesions usually tend to cross the known borders of the vascular territories of the brain. In this patient, the two vascular territories, posterior cerebral artery and middle cerebral artery, of the left hemisphere are involved. (Courtesy of Professor Franz Fazekas, University of Graz.)

small fiber neuropathy with burning pain and paresthesias in hands and feet, renal dysfunction or failure, vessel ectasia (particular basilar artery), corneal dystrophy, cardiomyopathy, and stroke.

The early presence of incidental WMHs has been observed and there appears to be a predisposition for infarction to occur in the vertebrobasilar system. Vascular ectasia up to the megadolichobasilar artery has also been reported. The most specific abnormality, however, appears to be a hyperintense signal of the pulvinar thalami on T1-weighted images [33]. Up to one-quarter of patients with Fabry disease may show this abnormality, which could be a consequence of microvascular calcification. Clinically silent or manifest strokes, both cortical and subcortical, are caused by occlusion of small vessels or by extasia of larger vessels, embolism from the heart, and rarely by intracranial hemorrhage.

> Fabry disease presents with a variety of symptoms, including stroke.

MELAS (mitochondrial encephalopathy lactic acidosis and stroke)

MELAS is a mitochondrial disorder that causes stroke-like syndromes in young patients, occurring as early as the teenage years, with transient or permanent hemianopia, aphasia or hemiparesis. Sudden episodes of headache and seizure or vomiting occur. Blood lactate levels are elevated, indicating dysfunction of the respiratory chain. Most commonly, MELAS is associated with a mitochondrial DNA point mutation at position 3243 within the tRNA encoding gene. Many different phenotypes, alone or

in combinations, have been reported with this mutation (hearing impairment, cognitive decline, progressive external ophthalmoplegia, or epilepsy).

MELAS-related brain lesions appear bright on diffusion-weighted imaging with reduced diffusity on corresponding ADC maps and are thus frequently mistaken for acute infarction [34]. A hint towards the correct diagnosis comes from the fact that MELAS lesions usually tend to cross the known borders of the vascular territories of the brain and have a variable ADC. Posterior parietal and occipital locations appear to be most frequent (Figure 10.9). The lesions may also subside without remaining signal changes, which would be quite unusual for infarction, and have a tendency to slowly progress or to reoccur at other sites, sometimes within relatively short intervals of days to weeks [35]. Besides increased levels of lactate in the CSF during the attack, MR spectroscopy may also serve to demonstrate increased lactate in the brain parenchyma and cerebral lesions as well as in the CSF [36]. The most likely origin of stroke-like episodes is a sudden metabolic failure with loss of function and transient or persistent cellular damage.

> MELAS is a mitochondrial disorder causing stroke-like syndromes, red-ragged fibers, myopathy and lactacidosis.

Arterial dissection: uncommon clinical presentations

Bogousslavsky *et al.* [37] found an incidence of arterial dissection of 2.5% in 1200 consecutive first stroke patients. Under the age of 45 the incidence of cervical artery dissection (CAD) is much higher at 10–25% and CAD is the second leading cause of stroke in younger adults [38]. Most patients with dissections are between 30 and 50 years of age, and the mean age is approximately 40 years. The annual incidence of cervical internal carotid artery dissection was found to be 3.5 per 100 000 in those older than 20 years, and the annual incidence of vertebral artery dissection 1.5 per 100 000 [39]. Extracranial ICA dissection typically occurs about 2 cm distal to the bifurcation, near the C2/C3 vertebral level, and extends superiorly for a variable distance. The vertebral artery is most mobile and susceptible to mechanical injury at the C1/C2 level.

Predisposing factors for CAD are trauma (mild or trivial, major, iatrogenic), arteriopathies (e.g. fibromuscular dysplasia, Ehlers Danlos syndrome, Marfan syndrome), migraine, recent infection or drugs (cocaine). Estimates of dissection risk after chiropractic manipulation vary widely with the study methodology but range from 1 in 5.85 million manipulations to as many as 1 in 20 000 manipulations. One study found connective tissue disorders in one-fourth of patients with cervical artery dissections after chiropractic manipulations [40].

Arterial dissections usually arise from an intimal tear that allows the development of an intramural hematoma (false lumen). In some patients, no communication between the true and the false lumen can be demonstrated, suggesting that some dissections are the result of a primary intramedial hematoma. Subintimal dissections are more likely to cause luminal stenosis. Subadventitial dissections may cause arterial dilatation (aneurysms). Mechanisms of ischemic stroke are either hemodynamic compromise secondary to luminal narrowing or occlusion or embolism from thrombus within the true lumen. The absence of an external elastic lamina and a thin adventitia makes intracranial arteries prone to subadventitial dissection and subsequent subarachnoid hemorrhage. SAH is reported in about one-fifth of intracranial ICA dissections and in more than half of intracranial vertebral artery dissections [41].

Saver and Easton [42] summarized symptoms and signs of ICA dissection:

- ischemic stroke (46%)
- TIA (30%)
- unusual and sharp pain in the face or in the neck on the side ipsilateral to ICA dissection (21%)
- pulsatile tinnitus alone when carotid dissection spreads distally to the base of the skull (2%)
- partial Horner's syndrome as a result of damage to the sympathetic nerve fibers around the dissected ICA (32%) and
- ipsilateral palsies of one or more cranial nerves (IX, X, XI, XII), particularly the hypoglossus (XII), as a result of nerve compression (3%) at the base of the skull (Figure 10.10).

Baumgartner et al. [43] have reported that dissections causing ischemic events are more often associated with occlusion and stenosis greater than 80% and that

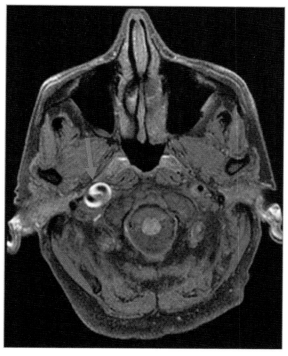

Figure 10.10. Collet Sicard syndrome in dissection of the internal carotid artery. A 60-year-old man noticed right-sided neck pain, ipsilateral headache, problems with swallowing and tongue movements and dysarthria (hoarseness). Some weeks later he was admitted to a neurological department and presented with right-sided glossopharyngeal and spinal accessory nerve lesions (moderate paresis of the upper portion of the trapezius and the sternocleidomastoid muscles), hypoglossus and recurrent nerve palsies. MRI showed a dissection of the right internal carotid artery in its very distal extracranial section with a prominent subadventitial wall hematoma and expansion of the vessel diameter but without relevant narrowing of the lumen. There was a prominent coiling of the internal carotid artery in the area of dissection. The combination of lower cranial nerve palsies (IX to XII) is commonly referred to as Collet Sicard syndrome. (Courtesy of Dr Michael Spiegel, University of Innsbruck.)

dissections that do not cause ischemic events are more often associated with Horner's syndrome and lower cranial nerve palsies.

> Cervical artery dissection is the second leading cause of stroke in young adults.

Symptoms and signs of extracranial vertebral dissection are [42]:

- ischemic stroke (75%)
- TIA (25%)
- head or neck pain (75%)
- rarely: cervical nerve root lesions (C5 and C6) as caused by ischemia or pressure from the bulging arterial wall.

Aortic arch dissection can cause generalized brain hypoxemia and low-flow infarction as a result of systemic hypotension caused by cardiac tamponade, acute aortic regurgitation or myocardial infarction. Dissection may spread out into the major neck arteries and may cause occlusion with low flow or TIA and ischemic stroke by embolism. Clues for the diagnosis of aortic dissection are [1]:

- sudden and severe anterior chest pain and/or interscapular pain which may move as the dissection extends
- syncope
- hypotension
- diminished, unequal or absent arterial pulses and blood pressure in the arms and sometimes legs
- acute aortic regurgitation and cardiac failure
- simultaneous or sequential ischemia in carotid, subclavian, vertebral, spinal, coronary and other aortic branches if the dissection extends over several centimeters.

Moyamoya

The first report of a patient was published in 1957 by Takeuchi and Shimizu [44] with the diagnosis "bilateral hypoplasia of the internal carotid arteries". This was a 29-year-old man who had been suffering from visual disturbance and hemiconvulsive seizures since the age of 10 years.

Moyamoya is defined by a pattern of severe stenosis or occlusion of one or more often of both internal carotid arteries with additional involvement of the circle of Willis. It may progress after diagnosis. Small collaterals develop from the lenticulostriate, thalamoperforating and pial arteries at the base of the brain, from leptomeningeal collaterals of the posterior cerebral artery or from branches of the external cerebral artery (orbital, ethmoidal or transdural). The pattern of collaterals looks like a puff of smoke (moyamoya in Japanese) in the basal ganglia region on the cerebral angiogram. Moyamoya is mostly, but not entirely, found in Japanese and other East Asian subjects. The annual incidence in Japan has been calculated to be 0.35/100 000 persons. It is mainly familial or congenital but can be caused by various disorders (meningeal or nasopharyngeal infection, vasculitis, irradiation, trauma, a generalized fibromuscular dysplasia, sickle-cell disease or neurofibromatosis, drugs such as cocaine).

The mechanism of brain ischemia is low flow. The vascular reserve capacity is exhausted and ischemia can be provoked by conditions which induce vasodilatation, such as hyperventilation, and are often precipitated by infection in the upper respiratory airway. Children present with recurrent focal cerebral ischemia and infarction, cognitive impairment, headache, seizure and, occasionally, involuntary movements. Adults can present with either focal brain ischemia (TIA, stroke; 63.4%), hemorrhage (21.6%), epileptic seizures (7.6%) or others (e.g. cognitive impairment, headache; 7.5%) [45].

> Moyamoya is characterized by stenosis/occlusion of both internal carotid arteries and a network of collaterals ("haze"). It is mostly, but not exclusively, found in Japan.

Migraine and stroke

The prevalence of migraine with aura is about 4%. An aura is defined as a neurological symptom which is localizable in the brain, develops gradually over 5–20 minutes and lasts less than 1 hour. Aura can be classified into:

- typical aura with visual, hemiparesthetic, aphasic or hemiparetic (hemiplegic) symptoms and signs
- prolonged aura (lasting longer than 1 hour but less than 7 days with normal brain imaging)
- basilar aura
- migraine aura without headache
- migraine with acute aura onset.

With migrainous infarction the symptoms associated with the typical aura are not fully reversible after 7 days and/or there is an infarct on brain imaging. The following criteria have to be fulfilled:

- patient has previously fulfilled criteria for migraine with neurological aura
- the present attack is typical of previous attacks, but neurological deficits are not completely reversible within 7 days or/and neuroimaging demonstrates ischemic infarction in the relevant area
- other causes of infarction have been ruled out by appropriate investigations (particularly other causes which are associated with migraine, such as CADASIL, MELAS or antiphospholipid syndrome, or which may mimic migraine such as arterial dissection).

A migrainous stroke often results in a homonymous hemianopia and rarely causes persisting and severe disability. Arterial occlusion has rarely been demonstrated and it is not clear why it occurs. "Vasospasm" is often postulated and is said to have been observed in the retinal circulation during transient monocular blindness in a few patients. A migrainous stroke should never be a diagnosis of desperation when no other cause of ischemic stroke can be found, but a positive statement to describe a characteristic clinical syndrome in the absence of no more likely causes of stroke [1].

> A migrainous stroke only rarely causes persisting deficits.

Chapter summary

- An uncommon mechanism of brain ischemia: low flow. In some patients severe stenosis or occlusion of carotid or vertebral arteries may cause a critical reduction of blood flow; a drop in systemic blood pressure may cause transient or permanent focal ischemia. A sudden and profound hypotension sometimes causes **boundary-zone infarction**. A fall in cerebral perfusion pressure as a cause of focal brain ischemia should be suspected if the symptoms start under certain circumstances, such as after cardiac arrest or cardiac surgery, on standing up very quickly, or with exercise, coughing or hyperventilation. Syndromes of low flow may include **"limb-shaking TIA"**, **monocular transient retinal ischemia**, **rotational vertebral artery occlusion** and **"drop attacks"**. Abnormal changes of blood plasma with hematological disease (e.g. paraproteinemia), increase of cell counts (e.g. polycythemia vera) and decreased

red cell deformability (e.g. sickle-cell anemia) lead to a **hyperviscous state** and cerebral blood flow can be diminished, causing unspecific symptoms such as headache, dizziness or vertigo, paresthesias, blurred vision or tinnitus.
- Uncommon clinical presentations of stroke
  - Include sudden cortical blindness, akinesia, agitation and delirium, as well as isolated cranial nerve palsy.
- Uncommon causes of stroke
  - Infective or non-infective **endocarditis** can lead to cerebral embolism from the valves of the heart, resulting in a multi-territorial pattern of stroke.
  - **Inflammatory vasculopathies** (e.g. giant cell arteritis, systemic lupus erythematosus, polyarteritis nodosa, paraneoplastic vasculitis). In giant cell arteritis infarction of the optic nerve can develop. Systemic lupus erythematosus more often causes a generalized subacute or chronic encephalopathy than focal ischemic or hemorrhagic cerebral episodes. A raised antinuclear factor, double-stranded DNA, anti-Sm antibodies or antiphospholipid antibodies can frequently be found.
  - **Varicella zoster virus (VZV) vasculopathy** may present with stroke. Diagnosis: history of zoster rash, particularly ophthalmic-distribution zoster or a history of chicken pox, MR angiographic evidence of narrowing in cerebral arteries, pleocytosis and anti-VZV-IgG and VZV DNA in the cerebrospinal fluid.
  - **Tuberculous meningitis** (inflammation and thrombosis of arteries and veins on the surface of the brain can lead to ischemic stroke). Diagnosis: medical history of tuberculosis, symptoms indicating chronic meningeal infection, lesion of cranial nerves or development of hydrocephalus, cytology (Ziehl–Neelsen), culture, detection of DNA (PCR) or antigen.
  - **Syphilitic meningovasculitis** presents with an obliteration of small or middle-sized large vessels; rarely are large arteries involved. Usually, the size of ischemic infarcts is small. Diagnosis: intrathecal production of specific antibodies or pleocytosis in the CSF with specific antibodies in the serum.
  - **CADASIL** (cerebral autosomal dominant arteriopathy with subcortical infarcts and leukoencephalopathy) manifests with migraine with aura at a mean age of 28 years.

At a mean age of 41 years, stroke (small-vessel disease with multiple lacunar lesions) becomes manifest.

- Patients with **Fabry disease** (an X-linked alpha-galactosidase deficiency leads to an accumulation of glycolipids) are young and present with a variety of symptoms: angiokeratomas, small fiber neuropathy, renal failure, cardiomyopathy, and stroke.
- **MELAS** (mitochondrial encephalomyopathy lactic acidosis and stroke) is a mitochondrial disorder that causes stroke-like syndromes in young patients, occurring as early as the teenage years, with transient or permanent hemianopia, aphasia or hemiparesis. The most likely origin of stroke-like episodes is a sudden metabolic failure with loss of function and transient or persistent cellular damage.
- **Cervical artery dissection** (CAD) is the second leading cause of stroke in younger adults. Ischemic stroke can also be a symptom of **extracranial vertebral dissection. Aortic arc dissection** can cause low-flow infarction or ischemic stroke by embolism.
- **Moyamoya** is mostly found in East Asians and shows a pattern of severe stenosis or occlusion of one or both internal carotid arteries; the mechanism of brain ischemia is low flow.
- A **migrainous** stroke often results in a homonymous hemianopia and rarely causes persisting and severe disability.

References

1. Warlow C, van Gijn J, Dennis M, *et al. Stroke*, 3rd edn. Oxford: Blackwell; 2008.

2. Ringelstein ER, Stögbauer F. Border zone infarcts. In: Bogousslavsky J, Caplan L, eds. *Stroke Syndromes*, 2nd edn. Cambridge: Cambridge University Press; 2001: 564–83.

3. Choi KD, Shin HY, Kim JS, *et al.* Rotational vertebral artery syndrome: oculographic analysis of nystagmus. *Neurology* 2005; **65**:1287–90.

4. Kuether TA, Nesbit GM, Clark GM, Barnell SL. Rotational vertebral artery occlusion: a mechanism of vertebrobasilar insufficiency. *Neurosurgery* 1997; **41**:427–32.

5. Caplan LR, Wityk RJ, Glass TA, *et al.* New England Medical Center Posterior Circulation registry. *Ann Neurol* 2004; **56**:389–98.

6. Gerstner E, Liberato B, Wright CB. Bi-hemispheric anterior cerebral artery with drop attack and limb shaking TIAs. *Neurology* 2005; **65**:174.

7. Hennerici M, Klemm C, Rautenberg W. The subclavian steal phenomenon: a common vascular disorder with rare neurological deficits. *Neurology* 1988; **38**:669–73.

8. Caplan LR. *Posterior Circulation Disease. Clinical Findings, Diagnosis, and Management.* Boston: Blackwell; 1996.

9. Dashe JF. Hyperviscosity and stroke. In: Bogousslavsky J, Caplan L, eds. *Uncommon Causes of Stroke* Cambridge: Cambridge University Press; 2001: 100–10.

10. Donnan GA, O'Malley HM, Quang L, Hurley S, Bladin PF. In: Donnan GA, Norrving B, Bamford J, Bogousslavsky J, eds. *Subcortical Stroke*, 2nd edn. Oxford: Oxford University Press; 2002: 175–84.

11. Caplan LR. "Top of the basilar" syndrome. *Neurology* 1980; **30**:72–9.

12. Fisher CM. The posterior cerebral artery syndrome. *Can J Neurol Sci* 1986; **13**:232–9.

13. Dunne JW, Leedman PJ, Edis RH. Inobvious stroke: a cause of delirium and dementia. *Austr N Z J Med* 1986; **16**:771–8.

14. Bogousslavsky J, Maeder P, Regli F, Meuli R. Pure midbrain infarction: clinical syndromes, MRI, and etiological patterns. *Neurology* 1994; **44**:2032–40.

15. Thömke F, Tettenborn B, Hopf HC. Third nerve palsy as the sole manifestation of midbrain ischemia. *Neuro-ophthalmology* 1995; **15**:327–35.

16. Thömke F. Brainstem diseases causing isolated ocular nerve palsies. *Neuro-ophthalmology* 2002; **28**:53–67.

17. Lang W, Cheyne D, Kristeva R, *et al.* Three-dimensional localization of SMA activity preceding voluntary movement – A study of electric and magnetic fields in a patient with infarction of the right supplementary motor area. *Ex Brain Res* 1991; **87**:688–95.

18. Gheka J, Bogousslavsky J. Abnormal movements. In: Bogousslavsky J, Caplan L, eds. *Stroke Syndromes*, 2nd edn. Cambridge: Cambridge University Press; 2001: 162–82.

19. Prabhakaran S. Neurologic complications of endocarditis. *Continuum* 2008; **14**:53–74.

20. Jones HR, Siekert RG. Neurological manifestations of infective endocarditis. Review of clinical and therapeutic challenges. *Brain* 1989; **112**:1295–315.

21. Anderson DJ, Goldstein LB, Wilkinson WE, *et al.* Stroke location, characterization, severity, and outcome in mitral vs. aortic valve endocarditis. *Neurology* 2003; **61**:1341–6.

22. Hart RG, Foster JW, Luther MF, Kanter MC. Stroke in infective endocarditis. *Stroke* 1990; **21**:695–700.

23. Hart RG, Kagan-Hallett K, Joerns SE. Mechanisms of intracranial hemorrhage in infective endocarditis. *Stroke* 1987; **18**:1048–56.

24. Biller J, Challa VR, Toole JF, Howard VJ. Nonbacterial thrombotic endocarditis. A neurological perspective of clinicopathological correlations of 99 patients. *Arch Neurol* 1982; **39**:95–8.

25. Rogers LR, Cho ES, Kempin S, Posner JB. Cerebral infarction from non-bacterial thrombotic endocarditis. Clinical and pathological study including the effects of anticoagulation. *Am J Med* 1987; **83**:746–56.

26. Lopez JA, Ros RS, Fishbein MC, Siegel RJ. Nonbacterial thrombotic endocarditis: a review. *Am Heart J* 1987; **113**:773–84.

27. Singhal AB, Topcuoglu MA, Buonanno FS. Acute ischemic stroke patterns in infective and nonbacterial thrombotic endocarditis: a diffusion-weighted magnetic resonance imaging study. *Stroke* 2002; **33**:1267–73.

28. Nagel MA, Cohrs RJ, Mahalingam R, *et al.* The varizella zoster virus vasculopathies – clinical, CSF, imaging, and virologic features. *Neurology* 2008; **70**:853–60.

29. Schmutzhard E. *Entzündliche Erkrankungen des Nervensystems.* Stuttgart: Thieme; 2000.

30. Joutel A, Corpechot C, Ducros A, *et al.* Notch3 mutations in CADASIL, a hereditary adult-onset condition causing stroke and dementia. *Nature* 1996; **383**:707–10.

31. van den Boom, Lesnik Oberstein S, Ferrari M, Haan M. Cerebral autosomal dominant arteriopathy with subcortical infarcts and leukoencephalopathy: MR imaging findings at different ages – 3rd–6th decades. *Radiology* 2003; **229**:683–90.

32. Rolfs A, Böttcher T, Zschiesche M, *et al.* Prevalence of Fabry disease in patients with cryptogenic stroke: a prospective study. *Lancet* 2005; **366**:1794–6.

33. Takanashi J, Barkovich A, Dillon W, *et al.* T1 hyperintensity in the pulvinar: a key imaging feature for diagnosis of Fabry disease. *Am J Neuroradiol* 2003; **24**:916–21.

34. Mizrachi I, Gomez-Hassan D, Blaivas M, Trobe J. Pitfalls in the diagnosis of mitochondrial encephalopathy with lactic acidosis and stroke-like episodes. *J Neuro-ophthalmol* 2006; **26**:38–43.

35. Iizuka T, Sakai F, Kan S, Suzuki N. Slowly progressive spread of the stroke-like lesions in MELAS. *Neurology* 2003; **61**:1238–44.

36. Möller H, Kurlemann G, Pützler M, *et al.* Magnetic resonance spectroscopy in patients with MELAS. *J Neurol Sci* 2005; **229**–230:131–9.

37. Bogousslavsky J, Despland PA, Regli F. Spontaneous carotid dissection with acute stroke. *Arch Neurol* 1987; **44**:137–40.

38. Bogousslavsky J, Pierre P. Ischemic stroke in patients under age 45. *Neurol Clin* 1992; **10**:113.

39. Schievink WI. Spontaneous dissection of the carotid and vertebral arteries. *N Engl J Med* 2001; **344**:898.

40. Zweifler RM, Silverboard GS. Arterial dissections. In: Mohr JP, Choi DW, Grotta JC, *et al.*, eds. *Stroke: Pathophysiology, Diagnosis, and Management,* 4th edn. New York: Churchill Livingstone; 2004: 549–73.

41. Friedman AH, Drake CG. Subarachnoid hemorrhage from intracranial dissecting aneurysm. *J Neurosurg* 1984; **60**:325.

42. Saver JL, Easton JD. Dissections and trauma of cervicocerebral arteries. In: Barnett HJM, Mohr JP, Stein BM, *et al.*, eds. *Stroke: Pathophysiology, Diagnosis and Management,* 3rd edn. New York: Churchill Livingstone; 1998: 769.

43. Baumgartner RW, Arnold M, Baumgartner I, *et al.* Carotid dissection with and without events: local symptoms and cerebral artery findings. *Neurology* 2001; **57**:827.

44. Takeuchi K, Shimizu K. Hypoplasia of the bilateral internal carotid arteries. *No To Shinkei* 1957; **9**:37.

45. Adams HP. Moya-moya. In: Bogousslavsky J, Caplan J, eds. *Uncommon Causes of Stroke.* Cambridge: Cambridge University Press; 2001: 241.

Intracerebral hemorrhage

Corina Epple, Michael Brainin, and Thorsten Steiner

Introduction

Intracerebral hemorrhages (ICHs) account for 10–17% of all strokes [1]. Hemorrhages into the brain occur unexpectedly and are often lethal events. Typical warning signs are not known; rarely a feeling of unsteadiness, dizziness, or a tingling sensation can precede an ICH, but such symptoms do not have localizing value such as in ischemia, where stroke-like warning signs (transient attacks) can occur days or weeks before the onset of a stroke. Often enough only a history of elevated blood pressure is known. Thus, for most patients, it comes "out of the blue." Today, patients with ICH represent a growing workload on any stroke emergency ward or stroke unit. Stroke physicians and stroke nurses should be trained to manage not only ischemic strokes but also ICHs because of their differing risks, varying prognosis, and high proportion of complications. Therefore, ICH patients often require a different intensity of observation and separate management.

Etiology

Epidemiology

ICH, like ischemic stroke, has a clear age-dependent incidence rate, occurring slightly earlier in life than ischemic attacks. Most population-based registries report an incidence of 10–15 per 100 000 per year, and variations exist towards higher rates in some populations. A decrease of rates has been reported over time from several regions of the world. The incidence of ICH is influenced by racial factors and was found to be higher in Black, Hispanic, and Asian populations compared with White populations. While the exact reasons for this decline are not known, it is reasonable to assume that a decline in rates as well as

severity of arterial hypertension has significantly contributed to the declining rate of ICH [2–4].

Classification

The classification of ICH is confusing and difficult, due to the mostly unknown pathophysiology. ICHs can be distinguished by etiology and localization. Concerning localization we differentiate between lobar bleeding and ICHs in deep brain structures, as basal ganglia and thalamic bleedings. This determination is almost entirely due to etiological factors, because deep ICHs are often associated with hypertension, although hypertension is not the reason for ICHs but induces the causative arteriosclerotic microangiopathy. For this reason, deep ICHs in combination with hypertension are also termed "typical" ICHs. More than 50% of ICHs are associated with hypertension. Other typical hypertensive bleedings are located in the cerebellum and the brainstem. The term "spontaneous ICH" emphasizes that apart from hypertension no reason for the bleeding has been found.

Lobar bleedings are often associated with structural lesions, such as cerebral amyloid angiopathy (CAA), neoplasmas, arteriovenous malformations (AVMs) and are often seen in elderly patients. Lobar bleedings are often termed "atypical" ICH [5, 6]. About 30–40% of all ICHs occur in the basal ganglia, 20–30% in the thalamus, 35–45% are lobar and about 10% occur in the cerebellum and pons (Table 11.1). The striatum (caudate nucleus and putamen) is the most common site of "spontaneous" ICH [7, 8].

The commonly used classification into primary (due to hypertension and/or CAA) and secondary ICH is obsolete and should be avoided, because it mixes etiology and risk factors of ICH. Secondary ICH may be caused by arterial disease (such as CAA,

Table 11.1. Distribution by site of 1539 cases of ICH from the Austrian Stroke Registry (seen at stroke units between 2003 and 2007) and 464 cases of ICH from an Italian population-based registry by Sacco et al. (between 1994 to 1998) [1].

	Austrian Stroke Registry		Sacco et al. 2009	
	N (1539)	(%)	N (464)	(%)
Putaminal/thalamic	704	(45.7)	205	(44.2)
Lobar	528	(34.3)	210	(45.3)
Cerebellar	72	(4.7)	28	(6.0)
Pontine	58	(3.8)	16	(3.5)
Miscellaneous	177	(11.5)	5	(1.1)

Table 11.2. Classification of underlying ICH etiology

Arterial disease	Small-vessel disease	Acquired small-vessel disease Amyloid angiopathy Genetic small-vessel disease Intracranial aneurysm Moyamoya Vasculitis Reversible cerebral vasoconstrictive syndrome Secondary hemorrhagic transformation of brain infarct
	Large-vessel disease	
Venous disease	Acute intracranial venous and/or sinus thrombosis	
Vascular malformation	Arteriovenous malformation Dural arteriovenous fistula Cerebral cavernous malformation	
Hemostatic disorder	Hematological disease	Congenital factor VII deficiency, hemophilia, thrombocytopenia, etc.
	Iatrogenic disorders	VKA, FX-Inhib., F-II-Inhib., antiplatelet agents, etc.
ICH in the context of other disease and condition	Substance abuse Infective endocarditis Neoplasms	
Cryptogenic	Cause suspected but not detectable with currently available diagnostic tests	

small-vessel disease, intracranial aneurysms, vasculitis, or moyamoya), venous disease (such as sinus venous thrombosis), vascular malformations, hemostatic disorders (such as hematological disease or iatrogenic disorders, for example with a vitamin K antagonists [VKA]), or ICH in the context of other disease (such as trauma, neoplasms, substance abuse). Table 11.2 indicates an overview of classification of underlying ICH etiology (Figure 11.1).

Intracerebral hemorrhage, which accounts for 10–17% of all strokes, can have multiple etiologies and various, modifiable risk factors, hypertension and cerebral amyloid angiopathy being the most frequent ones.

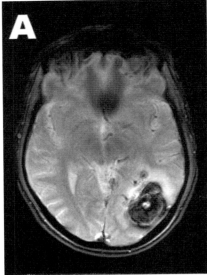

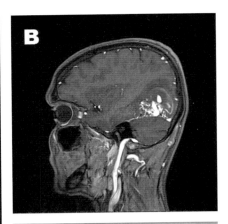

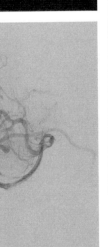

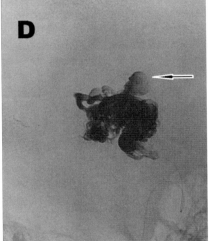

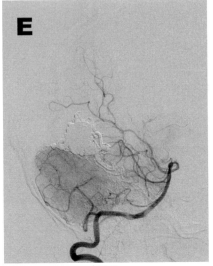

Figure 11.1. AVM: (A) MRI with blood-sensitive gradient echo sequence (GRE) showing a left temporo-occipital ICH. (B) T1 after gadolinium reveals a false aneurysm extending into ICH. (C) DSA lateral view with 4 cm nidus fed by multiple temporal feeders coming from P3 segment and superficial/deep venous drainage (Spetzler-Martin grade 4). (D) During transarterial embolization of false aneurysm and parts of the nidus (arrow marks the rupture point) (E) Lateral view with Onyx cast after complete embolization. (Courtesy of Dr.med. Markus Möhlenbruch, Neuroradiology, Klinikum Frankfurt Höchst/Heidelberg University Hospital).

OAC-ICH

The use of oral anticoagulants (OACs) such as warfarin or phenprocoumon, also a contributing rather than a causative factor, does not only lead to a higher incidence of ICH, but also to hematoma expansion in 27–54% of the cases, and well beyond the 24-hour time window where most of hematoma expansion occurs in spontaneous ICH [9]. This might at least partially explain a substantial increase in mortality of up to 70%. Underlying causes of spontaneous ICH and OAC-ICH might be the same, with anticoagulant therapy being only a precipitating factor [10–12].

Another issue arising from clinical practice comes from the increasing incidence of anticoagulation-associated ICH in elderly people with atrial fibrillation and other cardiac diseases. While in many cases it is often not evident whether anticoagulation (especially when within the therapeutic range) is the cause of ICH and thus can be rated as a "complication" of therapy, ICH might equally often be considered a failure of anticoagulation therapy resulting from insufficient protection of the brain. Then, an ischemic infarct turning into a secondary hemorrhage is visible upon first imaging. Due to the primary ischemic lesions rapidly turning hemorrhagic, the true incidence of secondary hemorrhagic infarcts is probably higher than was previously thought. Genetic tests or markers of primary hemorrhage would in the future be helpful in making important distinctions between primary and secondary hemorrhages into the brain but are not yet applicable for routine use [13].

Mortality and prognostic factors

Although mortality due to ICH has been reduced over the last 10 years it is still about 20–30% (approaching 50%) within 3 months with severe disability in the majority of survivors [1]. Half of the deaths occur within the acute phase, especially in the first 2 days. Early mortality, which is mostly reported as 30-day mortality, is higher than in ischemic stroke and largely depends on bleeding volume. In the cerebral hemispheres, a volume of over 60 ml carries an unfavorable prognosis and is seen for deep hemorrhage (93%), and slightly less often for lobar bleeding (71%). Smaller bleedings show better prognosis and less early mortality [14–16].

One multivariate analysis showed that independent prognostic factors of 30-day mortality are ICH volume, Glasgow Coma Score on admission, age over 80 years, infratentorial origin of ICH, and presence of intraventricular blood [17]. The parenchymal volume of the hemorrhage is the most decisive prognostic component. Total volumes of more than 60 ml cannot be compensated by intracranial compartmental reserve capacity. Decompensation will lead to herniation of the medial temporal lobe and downward shift with compression of the brainstem. It is also well known that hemorrhages into the thalamic region tend to rupture into the ventricles after some hours or days, and this is manifested as a dramatic clinical event with sudden deterioration [18].

It is worth noting that in one study a decreased mortality rate was seen when ICH patients are cared for in a setting of a neurological/neurosurgical intensive care unit (ICU) compared to treatment in a general ICU [19]. Also a treatment in a stroke unit compared with treatment on a general medical ward showed a reduced 30-day mortality (39% vs. 63%) [20]. It is generally believed that ICH survivors have better neurological and functional prognoses than the survivors of ischemic stroke [21].

Also hematoma growth was shown to be a crucial and independent predictor of early neurological deterioration and is associated with increased mortality and poor functional outcome [22]. A pooled individual patient meta-analysis showed that for each 10% increase in ICH growth, there was a 5% increased hazard of death, a 16% greater likelihood of worsening by 1 point on the mRS (modified Rankin Scale), or 18% greater likelihood of moving from independence to assisted independence or from assisted independence to poor outcome on the Barthel Index [23]. These findings indicate that early extension of the initial hematoma boundaries has substantial clinical implications.

> The incidence of ICH is 10 per 100 000 per year; early mortality is up to 50% within the first month. Factors determining prognosis are ICH volume, hematoma expansion, presence of intraventricular blood, infratentorial origin of ICH, Glasgow Coma Score on admission, and age over 80 years.

Risk factors

Genetics of spontaneous ICH

Monogenic disorders associated with spontaneously occurring ICH are not known. No genetic markers exist to date. But some disorders convey an increased risk of ICH, and have more frequent microscopic bleeding, such as hereditary CAA, CADASIL (cerebral autosomal dominant arteriopathy with silent infarcts and leukoaraiosis), and collagen type IV A1-associated vasculopathy. Morbus Fabry and ApoE ε2 and ε4 genotype are associated specifically with lobar ICH [24]. Genetic screening and counseling might be reasonable for pedigrees of patients with some very rare and selected cases. Defining the more complex genetics of spontaneous ICH, however, will probably require defining multiple common genetic variants with weaker effects. While investigations of genetic risk factors for spontaneous ICH have thus far been limited to candidate gene polymorphisms, whole-genome association studies are being undertaken in spontaneous ICH. They are likely to generate novel insights into cerebral bleeding risks and strategies for prevention [25].

Hypertension, smoking, alcohol, cholesterol, and other risk factors

Hypertension is the most common risk factor for spontaneous ICH and the frequency has been estimated to be between 70% and 80%. The pathophysiological role of hypertension is supported by the high frequency of left ventricular hypertrophy in autopsy of patients with ICH. The role of hypertension and the beneficial effect of antihypertensive treatment with regard to risk of ICH were verified in several large clinical trials. In the PROGRESS trial the relative risk of ICH was reduced by 76% in comparison with the placebo-treated group after 4 years of follow-up [26].

Other risk factors for ICH in addition to old age, hypertension, and ethnicity include cigarette smoking and excessive alcohol consumption. Both the Physicians' Health Study and the Women's Health Study confirmed the role of smoking as a risk factor for ICH. For men smoking 20 cigarettes or more the relative risk of ICH was 2.06 (95% confidence interval [CI] 1.08–3.96) and for women smoking 15 cigarettes or more the relative risk was 2.67 (95% CI 1.04–6.90) [27, 28].

Several studies document an increased risk of ICH in relation to regular alcohol consumption and that spontaneous ICH can also be triggered by binge drinking [29]. A recently published trial showed that alcohol abuse is associated with the occurrence of ICH in young age. In the study heavy drinkers (defined as alcohol consumption of more than 300 g ethanol/week) had their ICH at a median age of 60 years, 14 years before the non-heavy drinkers.

An empiric relation between heavy alcohol intake and arterial hypertension has been discussed. However, the underlying vasculopathy remains unexplored in these patients, although a small-vessel disease was suggested [30].

Anticoagulation increases the risk of ICH 8 to 11 times compared to that in patients of similar age who are not on anticoagulation [12, 31]. Previous medications, such as thrombolytics, also increase the risk of ICH.

While elevated cholesterol levels play a less significant role in ICH than in ischemia, statin use and/or very low levels of cholesterol have been questionable factors in increasing the risk of ICH. For example the SPARCL (Stroke Prevention by Aggressive Reduction in Cholesterol Levels) study showed a small increase in risk of ICH in ischemic stroke patients treated with atorvastatin [32]. Inferences made from observational data show that statin use prior to ICH does not influence mortality or functional outcome and statin use following ICH is not associated with an increased risk of ICH recurrence [33]. Westover at al. used a mathematical decision analysis and revealed a small amplification of the risk of recurrent ICH in survivors of prior hemorrhagic stroke by the use of statins. Therefore, the authors recommend avoiding statins after an ICH, particularly in survivors of lobar ICH, who are at highest risk of ICH recurrence. In the case of deep ICH the analysis showed a closer balance between statin's risks and benefits, so that statin therapy may be considered after deep ICH. Still, it remains unclear by which mechanism statins might amplify the risk of hemorrhagic stroke. So far antithrombotic and fibrinolytic effects have been discussed [34].

A variety of illicit drugs, such as amphetamine and cocaine, are known to cause ICH and this possibility should be kept in mind in young patients in whom other causes such as AVM or trauma have been excluded [35].

> Hypertension is the most common risk factor for spontaneous ICH. Further risk factors include old age, cigarette smoking, excessive alcohol consumption, anticoagulation, and illicit drugs such as amphetamine and cocaine.

Pathophysiology of ICH

Small-vessel disease

The "miliary aneurysms" described by Charcot and Bouchard in the small penetrating vessels of patients with intracerebral bleeding have been shown to be "false" aneurysms. The aneurysmal feature was based on the impression of irregularity of the penetrating vessels due to their intramural blood accumulation denoting penetration, leakage, and intima destruction. It was C.M. Fisher who concluded from the detailed study of two brains that hypertensive ICH most likely results from rupture of lipohyalinoic arteries followed by secondary arterial ruptures at the periphery of the enlarging hematoma in a cascade or avalanche fashion [31]. This observation of mechanical disruption and tearing of smaller vessels might account for the gradual development of ICH and can probably be considered the most relevant neuropathological correlate for the "growing" properties of hemorrhages (like a rolling snowball). The main histological findings in vessels of ICH patients include lipohyalinosis and media hypertrophy, as well as elongation of the deep penetrating arterioles of the brain. The lenticulostriate, thalamo-perforating, and basilar artery rami ad pontem are affected most often. In the cerebellum the arterioles supplying the area of the dentate nucleus are often involved, also the rami of the superior and posterior inferior cerebellar arteries. This demonstrates that the underlying cause of a hypertensive ICH is the arteriosclerotic microangiopathy and the hypertension only being a risk factor and not the bleeding cause, which can be ascertained by microbleeds in the basal ganglia in magnetic resonance imaging (MRI).

> Hypertensive ICH most likely results from rupture of lipohyalinoic arteries followed by secondary arterial ruptures at the periphery of the enlarging hematoma.

Cerebral amyloid angiopathy (CAA)

CAA refers to the deposition of amyloid proteins into the cerebral vessel walls with degenerative changes. Hereditary forms of CAA are known but CAA is most commonly sporadic and related to amyloid β (Aβ) peptide deposition. This deposition is seen in the walls of small arteries and arterioles of the leptomeninges, cerebral and cerebellar cortices, and less often in capillaries and veins. Overlaps with Alzheimer's disease (AD) are known and therefore old age and positive ApoE ϵ4 allele are major risk factors for both conditions. Although the metabolism and pathological triggers for CAA production and deposition are not well understood, CAA is now recognized as a major cause of non-hypertensive lobar cerebral

hemorrhage in the elderly. The overlaps of CAA and dementia are recognized though also less well understood.

CAA is a frequent finding particularly over the age of 70 years, differing only in amount and distribution. In elderly persons over the age of 90 years it is present in 50% of individuals and in AD patients it is present in over 80% of all neuropathological cases.

The biological and neuropathological interaction between Aβ deposition in primary degenerative diseases of the brain as well as in elderly patients with a high risk of parenchymal bleeding is a major focus of research. In one rare hereditary form with excessive CAA deposits, cognitive decline was independent of other Alzheimer-related pathological criteria, such as neurofibrillary tangles. Mounting evidence shows that drugs able to inhibit amyloid deposition seem to be an avenue for clinical therapy options for amyloid-associated progressive cognitive decline [36, 37].

CAA-associated hemorrhages account for the second largest group of hemorrhages after hypertension-associated bleedings and their rate depends on the case mix of elderly people at one stroke unit. Gradient echo (GRE) MRI can be useful for detecting silent hemorrhages in typical (cortical) areas and thus help to determine the diagnosis of CAA. Amyloid positron emission tomography (PET) imaging is currently being tested as a tool for direct diagnosis but so far no peripheral blood markers for CAA or CAA-related risk of ICH have been found; only some hereditary forms can be diagnosed from blood or other tissue samples.

> Cerebral amyloid angiopathy (CAA) refers to the deposition of amyloid proteins into the cerebral vessel walls with degenerative changes. CAA-associated ICH predominantly occur lobar.

Microbleeds

MRI visualizes acute and chronic hematomas, but also old, clinically non-apparent cerebral microbleeds that are not detected on computed tomography (CT). Microbleeds have a hypointense appearance on MRI and are usually smaller than 5–10 mm. Pathological studies have shown that microbleeds seen with GRE MRI usually correspond to hemosiderin-laden macrophages adjacent to small vessels and are indicative of previous extravasation of blood [38]. Microbleeds were seen in 83% (95% CI 71–90) of ICH cases with recurrent ICH [39].

193

(a) (b)

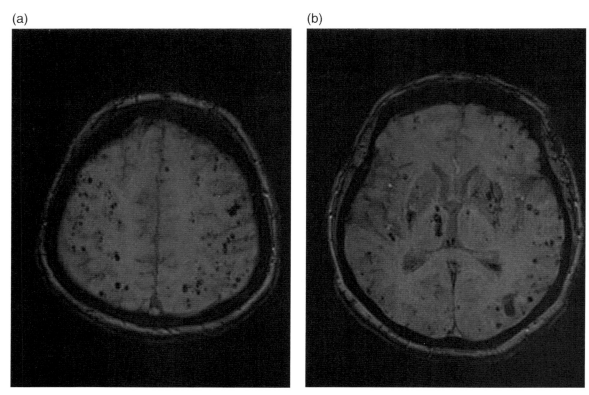

Figure 11.2. Microbleeds. MRI with blood-sensitive gradient echo (GRE) sequences. Lobar microbleeds are typical for CAA, whereas the microbleeds seen in deep regions refer to hypertension.

Hypertension, CAA, getting older, and, less commonly, CADASIL have been identified as important risk factors for microbleeds [40–42]. Microbleeds have been suggested as markers of a bleeding-prone angiopathy [43, 44]. The results of several case reports and small series suggest that patients with microbleeds might be at increased risk of hemorrhage when on antithrombotic or thrombolytic therapy. By contrast, the results of two large studies did not show an increased risk of hemorrhage in patients with microbleeds who were treated with intravenous tissue plasminogen activator [45, 46].

Although there are still many studies ongoing, microbleeds are considered to bear prognostic significance for any future bleeding event and have been confirmed as a common finding in patients with CAA, where they are most commonly found in lobar brain regions [36]. By contrast, in patients with ICH due to hypertensive disease, microbleeds are most commonly found in deep and infratentorial regions, although hypertension can also contribute to lobar microbleeds. A particularly noteworthy finding is that the total number of microbleeds predicts the risk of future symptomatic ICH in patients with lobar hemorrhage and probable CAA (Figure 11.2) [47].

> Old, clinically non-apparent cerebral microbleeds can be visualized on MRI, and have been suggested as markers of a bleeding-prone angiopathy.

Imaging

General recommendations

At many centers non-contrast CT is the imaging modality of choice for the assessment of ICH, owing to its widespread availability and rapid acquisition time. MRI has not been favored due to its higher costs and due to the fact that conventional T1-weighted and T2-weighted MRI pulse sequences are not sensitive to blood in the hyperacute stage. However, recent studies have impressively shown that blood-sensitive GRE sequences are as accurate as CT for the detection of parenchymal hemorrhage and far superior to CT for the detection of chronic hemorrhage [48, 49]. Table 11.3 outlines the MRI signals in T1-, T2- and

Table 11.3. MRI signal relative to brain in different ICH stages

	Hyperacute ICH (4–6 hours)	Acute stage (7–72 hours)	Early subacute stage (4–7 days)	Late subacute stage (1–4 weeks)	Early chronic stage (months)	Late chronic stage (months to years)
T1						
T2						
GRE						

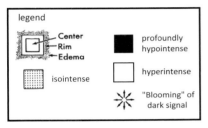

legend

Center / Rim / Edema

isointense

profoundly hypointense

hyperintense

"Blooming" of dark signal

Source: adapted from "Diagnostic Imaging: Brain" by Anne G. Osborn, Karen L. Salzman and A. James Barkovich; Lippincott Williams & Wilkins; 2nd annotated edition (2010)

GRE-weighted sequences relative to the different stages of the ICH. New MRI techniques, including magnetic resonance spectroscopy and diffusion tensor imaging, might have importance in the understanding of hemorrhagic injury and provide insights into the time course and pathophysiology of ICH [50].

In case of lobar bleedings with an underlying AVM, characteristic flow voids can be seen in the brain parenchyma on MRI. CT angiography or MR angiography might reveal the underlying vascular lesion; however, in some cases, catheter angiography is required and might need to be repeated if the results are initially negative owing to the mass effect of the hematoma. Findings from imaging such as pathological calcifications, presence of subarachnoid blood, vessel abnormalities, or an unusual location of hemorrhage can be considered to support an indication for direct catheter angiography. Cavernous malformation can usually be reliably diagnosed by means of GRE MRI, where one or more hypointense rings show due to hemosiderin from a previous bleeding.

Silent hemorrhages seen on blood-sensitive GRE sequences have also been found quite frequently and their clinical significance as risk factors has not been fully determined. They might be relevant markers of vascular risk factors or in patients already having suffered an ICH, and might signal an increased risk of further hemorrhage. This risk might also be increased in anticoagulation patients, but this has not yet been confirmed in controlled studies.

> Native CCT is sufficient to confirm the diagnosis of acute ICH. In case of deterioration follow-up imaging is required. In case of "atypical" ICH an underlying AVM or other reasons should be investigated by further diagnostics (MRI or CT angiography). A catheter angiography is necessary if no reason for bleeding was found in MRI.

Spot sign

Contrast extravasation on admission CT angiography (the so-called "spot sign") and a contrast extravasation in a post-contrast CT scan as a predictor of hematoma expansion were found in retrospective and prospective studies, recently extended to a proposed "spot sign score," which is used to grade the number of spot signs and their maximum dimension and attenuation. This is a reliable independent predictor of mortality and poor outcome among survivors in spontaneous ICH, but not

195

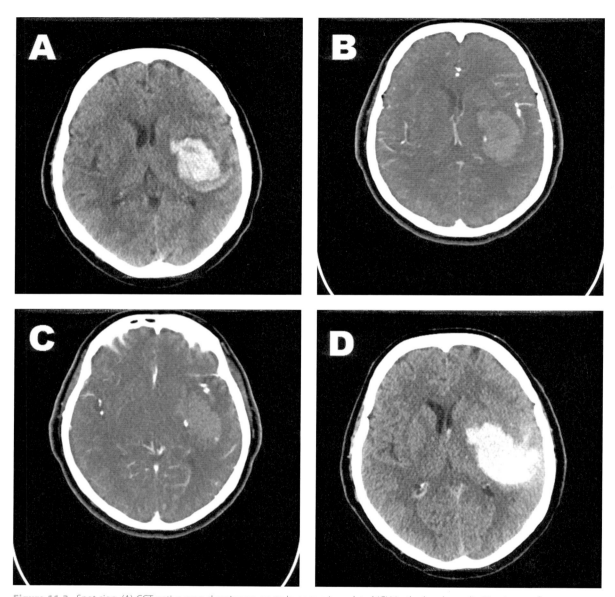

Figure 11.3. Spot sign. (A) CCT native scan showing an acute hypertension-related ICH in the basal ganglia 90 minutes after symptom onset (ICH volume 56 ml). (B and C) CT angiography (source images) showing two spot signs indicating extravasation of contrast media. (D) CCT 12 hours later showing a hematoma expansion (ICH volume 90 ml).

a predictor for hematoma expansion, whereas a contrast extravasation after CT angiography indicates active bleeding and is regarded as a potential sign for predicting hematoma expansion [51–53]. The PREDICT trial, a prospective multicenter observational study (including 228 patients for primary analysis), showed that the CTA spot sign is highly predictive of hematoma expansion for intraparenchymal and intraventricular hemorrhage (IVH) growth;

it is associated with larger hemorrhage and a poor prognosis. The usefulness of the CTA spot sign should be tested in proof-of-concept trials of hemostatic drugs in patients with ICH [54]. Further systematical and comparative validation of predictors of hematoma expansion is warranted as this might prevent delay of appropriate therapy but also influence estimates on prognosis or decisions to withdraw therapy (Figure 11.3).

Clinical syndromes

Clinical presentation of spontaneous ICH depends on site and size. Therefore, clinical investigation as well as neuroimaging is important for a reliable diagnosis. All attempts to make a probabilistic diagnosis on clinical grounds alone to differentiate between ischemic and hemorrhagic stroke have not been considered satisfactory [55].

Putaminal hemorrhages are the most frequent ones. If the hemorrhage spreads from the putamen into the thalamic region, they are called putaminothalamic. Then they show a large volume extending over the area of the basal ganglia and deep white matter of one hemisphere. Such an ICH can rupture into the lateral or third ventricles, giving rise to sudden posturing and coma. More often, progression is not abrupt but gradual and can be seen occurring over several hours, showing an increase of sensorimotor hemiparesis and a gradual decrease of alertness. Usually transition into drowsiness and stupor occurs in parallel with a decrease in motor function. If a progressive deterioration of consciousness is seen in a hemiparetic patient with a sensorimotor hemiparesis, this can give rise to suspicion of a growing hematoma. If no deterioration or progression occurs in the first hours or days, hemorrhages such as small or medium-sized putaminal bleedings also tend to remain stable after the first few days and cannot be distinguished from ischemic infarcts in the basal ganglia and capsular region on clinical grounds alone. They both present with sudden onset of sensorimotor hemiparesis of varying degree and can both be associated with additional hemispheric symptoms such as aphasia or neglect. This contradicts the prevailing opinion at some centers that "typical" hemiparetic strokes that remain stable can be reliably considered to be caused by ischemia and therefore do not need confirmation with neuroimaging. In general, there is also no medical rationale to restrict imaging to young patients or to patients with some other demographic or clinical feature.

ICH can also occur extremely abruptly and loss of consciousness can occur within minutes after onset. This is the case in large putaminal or thalamic hematomas that rupture into the ventricles, or in pontine hemorrhages extending over the midline.

Contralateral limb weakness and hemisensory symptoms are typical of middle-sized putaminal hemorrhages, whereas bleeding into the thalamus causes a distinct and total hemisensory loss and dense hemiplegia.

Conjugate eye deviation to the side of the bleeding signals extension into the frontal lobe. This is a sign either of frontal lobar hemorrhage or of a putaminal hemorrhage extending into the deep frontal white matter. In contrast, thalamic hemorrhage can be accompanied by a conjugate spasm of both eyes, appearing as a convergent downward gaze (the patient looks at his/her nose tip). The pupil which is smaller denotes the hemispheric side of the bleeding, and, when present, this invariably denotes involvement of subthalamic structures. Such cases have to be monitored closely because of the likelihood of rupture into the ventricles. This is the case when sudden, bilateral localizing signs appear and loss of consciousness is the rule.

Vomiting is a frequent sign of ICH but can also indicate ischemic stroke. It can be a prominent sign in posterior fossa hemorrhage, and, although patients with cerebellar hemorrhages almost always vomit early in the clinical course, it is not a reliable sign with either localizing or etiological value. Many patients with posterior fossa hemorrhage show severe impairment of sitting balance and ataxia that can be pronounced ipsilaterally. Close observation of vital parameters is crucial, as deterioration can be sudden or progressive over the first few days after onset. Evacuation of the hematoma can also become necessary after some days.

Contrasting with lay beliefs, headache is also not a cardinal symptom of ICH. Headache can occur in large hematomas and has no localizing value unless it is very severe and then indicates rupturing in cerebrospinal fluid space. In patients with loss of consciousness meningeal irritation must not be apparent.

> Clinical presentation of spontaneous ICH depends on localization and size. The most frequent putaminal hemorrhages show a sudden onset. Progressive deterioration of consciousness points to a growing hematoma, and sudden posturing and coma to a rupture of the bleeding into the lateral or third ventricle. Vomiting and headache are frequent, but not reliable, signs.

Complications

Hematoma expansion

An increase in the bleeding volume is an early complication of ICH. For a long time it was erroneously believed that the volume of a cerebral hematoma

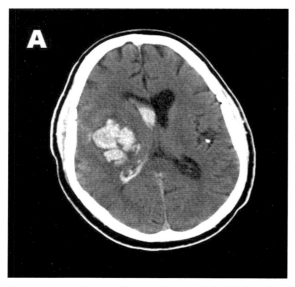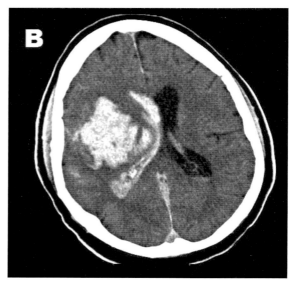

Figure 11.4. A 64-year-old man with acute right-sided hemiparesis and dysarthria; NIHSS score 9; prior acetylsalicylic acid use, hypertension not treated. (A) CCT shows a spontaneous ICH with IVH (hematoma volume 44 ml) one hour after onset. (B) 2 hours later the patient developed a clinical deterioration (NIHSS score 18) with systolic blood pressure >180 mmHg despite treatment with i.v. drugs. CCT shows a hematoma expansion (hematoma volume 95 ml).

was usually maximal at onset. Frequently observed deterioration during the first day was attributed to developing cerebral edema and mass effect surrounding the hemorrhage. However, serial CT scans showed that clinical deterioration is often attributed to hematoma expansion and this is also a reason for high mortality [56].

The pathophysiology behind early hematoma expansion is not well understood, and the frequency of increased bleeding is high. It is not clear whether it reflects leakage or rebleeding, or both. Several mechanisms of brain injury after ICH have been investigated, but most of these evolve too late to account for early hematoma expansion [57]. A role for disturbed autoregulation and uncontrolled perfusion pressure in hypertension as a driving force for further bleeding is conceivable but data on this are controversial. Brott *et al.* showed that "growth," defined as a 33% increase of hematoma volume on CT, occurred in 26% of 103 patients within 4 hours after the first symptoms. Another 12% had growth within the following 20 hours. Hemorrhage growth was significantly associated with clinical deterioration [58]. Enlargement of ICH is also seen when observation periods are extended up to 48 hours, though the frequency diminishes with time from onset of symptoms. Predictors of hemorrhage expansion include initial hematoma volume, early presentation, irregular shape, liver

disease, hypertension, hyperglycemia, alcohol use, and hypofibrinogenemia (Figure 11.4) [16].

Intraventricular hemorrhage (IVH)

Between 36% and 50% of patients with spontaneous ICH suffer additional IVH and the 30-day mortality rate was reported as 43% for patients with ICH and IVH compared with 9% in patients with isolated IVH [59]. Tuhrim *et al.* found that location of parenchymal origin of ICH, distribution of ventricular blood, and total volumes are predictors of outcome in patients with spontaneous ICH and intraventricular extension [59]. Furthermore, hydrocephalus was found to be an independent predictor of mortality.

Edema

Edema after ICH is observed in the acute and subacute phase and may increase up to 14 days [60]. Shrinking of the hematoma due to clot retraction leads to an accumulation of serum in the early phase [57]. Thrombin and several serum proteins were found to be involved in the inflammatory reaction of the perihematomal zone [61, 62]. Factors released from activated platelets at the site of bleeding, such as vascular endothelial growth factor, may interact with thrombin to increase vascular permeability and contribute to the development of edema [63].

Several studies in spontaneous ICH suggest that the role of perihematomal ischemia is small and has no great clinical importance [64].

> Frequent complications of ICH are an increase of the bleeding volume, intraventricular hemorrhage, hydrocephalus, and edema.

Therapeutic options

Therapeutic options can be divided into surgical and non-surgical approaches, whereas both might complement each other. Current treatment strategies might also be double-edged swords: surgical intervention can reduce bleeding size but can also lead to decompression of tissue and thereby enhance bleeding. Non-surgical intervention such as hemostasis might stop bleeding but might also compromise normal circulation. Therefore, the right balance and possibly the combination of current treatment regimes, as well as the evaluation of alternative future strategies, seem urgent.

Surgical approach

Insufficient evidence exists with regard to the efficacy of surgical treatment for spontaneous ICH, and whether or not surgical approaches are beneficial remains controversial. Surgical procedures with varying amounts of supportive evidence include conventional craniotomy, minimally invasive surgery, and decompressive craniectomy. The diverse methods of minimally invasive surgery include stereotactic guidance with aspiration and thrombolysis with alteplase or urokinase and image-guided stereotactic endoscopic aspiration.

The Surgical Trial in IntraCerebral Hemorrhage (STICH), currently the largest prospective trial on surgery in spontaneous ICH, failed to show an outcome benefit over conservative treatment [65]. A subgroup analysis showed that patients with superficial hematomas and without IVH presented a more encouraging picture of surgery. Thus we are still unable to specify potential candidates for the optimum surgical technique in current guidelines. The STICH II trial investigated the suggestion that patients with superficial lobar hematomas and no IVH might benefit from early hematoma evacuation (<12 hours after randomization) [66]. Unfortunately, STICH II also failed to demonstrate a benefit from hematoma evacuation. A previously published meta-analysis of 2186 cases concluded that in particular early surgery (<8 hours of ictus) is beneficial [67].

It has been shown that patients with smaller bleeds have a better clinical outcome and a lower mortality, which led to the hypothesis that methods of removing ICH in stable patients could result in lowered risk of mortality and improved outcome [68].

The combination of stereotactic minimally invasive aspiration and clot lysis with recombinant tissue plasminogen activator (rtPA) has been proposed, especially with regard to deep hematomas. Whether this approach can indeed lead to a better outcome is currently being investigated in the ongoing MISTIE trial combining stereotactic clot aspiration (starting 6 hours after clot stabilization) with different doses of rtPA (alteplase) within the first 72 hours from onset (NCT00224770) [69]. The specific objective of MISTIE is to test the efficacy and safety of this intervention and assess its ability to remove blood clots from brain tissue. The preliminary analysis suggests that minimally invasive surgery plus alteplase shows greater clots resolution than does conventional medical treatment. The treatment of spontaneous supratentorial ICH will remain controversial until a definitive prospective randomized controlled trial shows evidence in favor of a particular treatment. At present the recommendations for or against surgery are based on conflicting evidence. Also for intraventricular bleedings recommendations are difficult due to lack of evidence.

> The treatment of spontaneous supratentorial ICH remains controversial. Surgical procedures with varying amounts of supportive evidence include conventional craniotomy, minimally invasive surgery (including stereotactic guidance with aspiration and thrombolysis with alteplase or urokinase and image-guided stereotactic endoscopic aspiration), and decompressive craniectomy.

Non-surgical approach
Management of blood pressure

Many studies have shown an association between increased blood pressure (>140/90 mmHg) in the acute phase of ICH and hematoma expansion, perihematomal edema, and rebleeding [70, 71]. The mechanism for the acute increase of blood pressure after spontaneous ICH is unknown. However, it is proposed to be a multifactorial process that includes activation of the neuroendocrine systems (sympathetic nervous system, glucocorticoid system, or the rennin–angiotensin axis), increased cardiac output, and stress response to conditions such as increased intracranial pressure, headache, and urinary retention [72–74]. The poor outcome associated with increased blood pressure after ICH could be minimized with blood pressure monitoring and treatment aimed at optimizing cerebral perfusion while minimizing ongoing bleeding. Appreciating a slight effect of antihypertensives on hematoma expansion reduction in an overall weak or equivocal context of evidence and considering that autoregulation is often preserved in the acute phase (as opposed to the post-acute phase) of ICH and furthermore aggressive lowering of blood pressure theoretically carries the risk of cerebral ischemia in hypertensive patients, it seems reasonable to presently follow current guidelines and lower blood pressure cautiously [50, 75, 76]. The INTERACT-2 trial (second Intensive Blood Pressure Reduction in Acute Cerebral Hemorrhage Trial) looked at a clinical primary endpoint of death or major disability (MRS of 3–6) at 90 days. Though statistical significance was just missed for the primary endpoint, most other measurements do speak in favor of intensive blood pressure lowering: the predefined ordinal analysis of the MRS revealed a significant clinical benefit for patients with intensive blood pressure treatment, the analyses of prespecified subgroups (age, ethnicity, time to randomization, baseline blood pressure, history of hypertension, baseline NIHSS, hematoma volume and location), and safety outcome did not differ in the two groups [77]. The results of ATACH 2 (NCT 01176565) are awaited, and might further answer the question of whether there are other benefits of early systolic blood pressure reduction in patients with ICH, and provide clearer evidence for the target blood pressure and the choice of drugs, because the trial will look at the clinical effect of a stronger blood pressure treatment (treatment trigger threshold <180 mmHg within a shorter time frame (3 hours) compared to INTERACT-2. Pending these results, the American Heart Association/American Stroke Association (AHA/ASA) guidelines recommend blood pressure lowering if systolic blood pressure is >200 mmHg or MAP is >150 mmHg, and that acute lowering of systolic blood pressure is probably safe [72].

Effects of antagonization of anticoagulation and restoring of hemostasis

Underlying hemostatic abnormalities can contribute to ICH. Patients at risk include those on anticoagulant therapy, those with acquired or congenital coagulation factor deficiencies, and those with qualitative or quantitative platelet abnormalities. For patients with a coagulation factor deficiency or thrombocytopenia, replacement of the appropriate factor or platelets is indicated.

Vitamin K antagonist-associated ICH (VKA-ICH)

Experts agree that anticoagulation has to be reversed rapidly, but the chosen ways to achieve this differ greatly [78]. There is an ongoing controversy with regard to treatment and different guidelines are inconsistent on an international level. None of the treatment regimens have been proven to be more effective than another. It is customary to discontinue oral VKAs and substitute vitamin K, but this alone is insufficient for rapid normalization of coagulation, even when given intravenously, because it requires several hours to correct the international normalized ratio (INR). Therefore vitamin K cannot be considered as an antidote. Current questions arise on feasibility, safety, and efficacy of prothrombin-dependent coagulation factors in a concentrated form (PCC: prothrombin complex concentrate) versus unconcentrated "fresh-frozen plasma (FFP)" versus single factors such as recombinant coagulation factor VIIa (rFVIIa). Time to INR reversal seems to be the most important determinant, and minimizing delays in drug administration should have highest priority. The overall positive performance of PCCs compared with FFP and VKA might be because of faster INR reversal in the acute bleeding phase. This attribute of PCCs might be explained by a higher concentration of coagulation factors in PCCs compared with FFP, which contains all coagulation factors in a non-concentrated form [79]. The INCH (International normalized ratio (INR) Normalization in Coumadin-associated intracerebral Haemorrhage) trial, an ongoing multi center randomized controlled trial to compare FFP with PCC, has been initiated 2009 to answer the question of INR early reversal [80].

DOAC-associated ICH

New direct oral anticoagulants (DOAC) have been developed that directly inhibit the key coagulation factors thrombin or factor Xa. It is conceivable that the number of patients treated with DOAC will increase, due to the easy handling and the favorable risk–benefit profile compared with VKA. In an emergency setting of ICH under DOAC treatment physicians face the problem that routine coagulation tests such as partial thrombin time (PTT) and prothrombin time (PT, expressed as INR) may be within normal limits. Thus, oral anticoagulation in comatose or aphasic patients might go undetected unless laboratory methods such as ecarin clotting time (ECT), thrombin time (TT), or hemoclot assays are applied [81].

Although the data are limited, PCCs have been proposed as a plausible – but unproven – therapy for the rapid reversal of DOAC's anticoagulant effects. Some of the PCC preparations contain inactivated clotting factors, whereas others (activated PCC) contain activated clotting factors. The latter preparations may be more potent but also have higher thrombogenic potential [82]. Diuresis with intravenous fluids may enhance the renal excretion of dabigatran. Acute hemodialysis might also be useful if these measures do not stop the bleeding, because only about one-third of dabigatran is bound to plasma proteins and can therefore not be dialyzed, although this can take hours to begin and complete. Dialysis is not suitable for apixaban and rivaroxaban because of a plasma protein binding of 85–95%. Therefore, plasmapheresis seems more plausible in these cases. However, in the emergency setting, hemodialysis and plasmapheresis may be difficult [83, 84].

> On the one hand a high blood pressure as a driving force and on the other hand the persistence of leakage, especially in a compromised coagulation, are the two major pathophysiological considerations with regard to hematoma expansion that are deemed as potential treatment targets. Thus, lowering blood pressure, antagonizing anticoagulant therapy, and applying hemostatics as conservative principles have been tested in clinical trials of reasonable quality. For prevention of hematoma expansion after DOAC (direct oral anticoagulants)-associated intracerebral hemorrhage, it is plausible to discontinue DOAC and administer procoagulant coagulation factors (e.g. prothrombin complex concentrate), according to limited data.

Chapter summary

> Intracerebral hemorrhage (ICH) comes "out of the blue"; typical warning signs are not known. The volume of the hemorrhage into the brain is the most decisive prognostic component. ICHs associated with arterial hypertension are charactersistically localized in basal ganglia, thalamus, cerebellum, or brainstem. Lobar ICH are often associated with structural lesions.

Incidence: 10 per 100 000 persons per year. Early mortality: up to 50% within the first month (prognostic factors: ICH volume, Glasgow Coma Score on admission, age over 80 years, infratentorial origin of ICH, and presence of intraventricular blood).

Risk factors: hypertension is the most common risk factor. Further risk factors: old age, cigarette smoking, excessive alcohol consumption, anticoagulation, and illicit drugs such as amphetamine and cocaine.

Etiology: concerning localization we differentiate between lobar bleeding and ICH in deep brain structures, as basal ganglia and thalamic bleedings. Hypertensive ICH most likely results from rupture of lipohyalinoic arteries followed by secondary arterial ruptures at the periphery of the enlarging hematoma. Thirty percent are found in association with cerebral amyloid angiopathy (CAA). CAA refers to the deposition of amyloid proteins into the cerebral vessel walls with degenerative changes. CAA-associated ICH predominantly occurs in a lobar location. The common used classification into primary (due to hypertension and/or CAA) and secondary ICH is obsolete and should be avoided, because it mixes etiology and risk factors of ICH.

Imaging: Native CCT is sufficient for primary diagnostic. In the case of deterioration, follow-up imaging is required. In the case of atypical ICH an underlying arteriovenous malformation or other reasons should be investigated in further diagnostics (MRI or CT angiography). A catheter angiography is necessary if no reason for bleeding was found in MRI.

Clinical presentation of spontaneous ICH depends on site and size. Imaging (non-contrast CT) is necessary to differentiate ischemic infarcts from hemorrhage. Putaminal hemorrhages show a sudden onset of sensorimotor hemiparesis of varying degree and can be associated with additional hemispheric symptoms such as aphasia or neglect. Progressive deterioration of consciousness points to a growing hematoma, and sudden posturing and coma to a rupture of the bleeding into ventricles. Conjugate eye deviation to the side of the bleeding signals extension into the frontal lobe; a conjugate spasm of both eyes appearing as a convergent downward gaze signals thalamic hemorrhage. Vomiting and headache are frequent, but not reliable, signs with neither localizing nor etiological value.

Complications are due to increase of the bleeding, intraventricular hemorrhage, hydrocephalus, and edema.

Therapeutic options: Surgical approach: insufficient evidence exists with regard to the efficacy of surgical treatment for spontaneous ICH, and whether or not surgical approaches are beneficial remains controversial. Surgical procedures with varying amounts of supportive evidence include conventional craniotomy, minimally invasive surgery (including stereotactic guidance with aspiration and thrombolysis with alteplase or urokinase and image-guided stereotactic endoscopic aspiration), and decompressive craniectomy. **Non-surgical approach**: relates to general treatment (temperature, glucose, seizures). Hemostatic therapy may be considered in patient with OAC-ICH or within clinical trials of spontaneous ICH.

References

1. Sacco S, Marini C, Toni D, Olivieri L, Carolei A. Incidence and 10 year survival of intracerebral hemorrhage in a population-based registry. *Stroke* 2009; **40**:394–9.

2. Fang J, Alderman MH, Keenan NL, Croft JB. Declining US stroke hospitalization since 1997: National Hospital Discharge Survey, 1988–2004. *Neuroepidemiology* 2007; **29** (3–4):243–9.

3. Islam MS, Anderson CS, Hankey GJ, *et al*. Trends in incidence and outcome of stroke in Perth, Western Australia during 1989 to 2001: the Perth Community Stroke Study. *Stroke* 2008; **39** (3):776–82.

4. Sacco RL, Boden-Albala B, Gan R, *et al*. Stroke incidence among white, black, and Hispanic residents of an urban community: the Northern Manhattan Stroke Study. *Am J Epidemiol* 1998; **147**:259–68.

5. Knudsen KA, Rosand J, Karluk D, Greenberg SM. Clinical diagnosis of cerebral amyloid angiopathy: validation of the Boston criteria. *Neurology* 2001; **56**:537–9.

6. Lang EW, Ren Ya Z, Preul C, *et al*. Stroke pattern interpretation: the variability of hypertensive versus amyloid angiopathy hemorrhage. *Cerebrovasc Dis* 2001; **12**:121–30.

7. Chiquete E, Broderick J, Hennerici M. Hematoma growth is a determinant of mortality and poor outcome after intracerebral hemorrhage. *Neurology* 2006; **66**:1175–81.

8. Ruiz-Sandoval JL, Romero-Vargas S, Chiquete E. Hypertensive intracerebral hemorrhage in young people: previously unnoticed age-related clinical differences. *Stroke* 2006; **37**:2946–50.

9. Flaherty ML, Kissela B, Woo D, *et al*. The increasing incidence of anticoagulant-associated intracerebral hemorrhage. *Neurology* 2007; **68**:116–21.

10. Flibotte JJ, Hagan N, O'Donnell J, Greenberg SM, Rosand J. Warfarin, hematoma expansion and outcome of intracerebral hemorrhage. *Neurology* 2004; **63**:1059–64.

11. Hart RG, Boop BS, Anderson DC. Oral anticoagulants and intracranial hemorrhage. Facts and hypotheses. *Stroke* 1995; **26**:1471–7.

12. Rosand J, Hylek EM, O'Donnell HC, Greenberg SM. Warfarin-associated hemorrhage and cerebral amyloid angiopathy: a genetic and pathological study. *Neurology* 2000; **55**:947–51.

13. Rosell A, Cuadrado E, Ortega-Aznar A, *et al*. MMP-9-positive neutrophil infiltration is associated to blood-brain barrier breakdown and basal lamina type IV collagen degradation during hemorrhagic transformation after human ischemic stroke. *Stroke* 2008; **39**:1121–6.

14. Broderick J, Brott T, Duldner JE, Tomsick T, Huster G. Volume of intracerebral hemorrhage: a powerful and easy-to-use predictor of 30-day mortality. *Stroke* 1993; **24**:987–93.

15. Counsell C, Boonyakarnkul S, Dennis M, *et al*. Primary intracerebral haemorrhage in the Oxfordshire community stroke project, 2: prognosis. *Cerebrovasc Dis* 1995; **5**:26–34.

16. Fujii Y, Takeuchi S, Sasaki O, Minakawa T, Tanaka R. Multivariate analysis of predictors of hematoma enlargement in spontaneous intracerebral hemorrhage. *Stroke* 1998; **29**:1160–6.

17. Hemphill JC, Bonovich DC, Besmertis L, Manley GT, Johnston SC. The ICH score: a simple, reliable grading scale for intracerebral hemorrhage. *Stroke* 2001; **32**:891–7.

18. Steiner T, Schneider D, Mayer S, *et al.* Dynamics of intraventricular hemorrhage in patients with spontaneous intracerebral hemorrhage: risk factors, clinical impact, and effect of hemostatic therapy with recombinant activated factor VII. *Neurosurgery* 2006; **59**:767–74.

19. Diringer MN, Edwards DF. Admission to a neurological/neurosurgical intensive care unit is associated with reduced mortality rate after intracerebral hemorrhage. *Crit Care Med* 2001; **29**:635–40.

20. Rønning OM, Guldvog B, Stavem K. The benefit of an acute stroke unit in patients with intracranial haemorrhage: a controlled trial. *J Neurol Neurosurg Psychiatry* 2001; **70**:631–4.

21. Paolucci S, Antonucci G, Grasso MG, *et al.* Functional outcome of ischemic and hemorrhagic stroke patients after inpatient rehabilitation: a matched comparison. *Stroke* 2003; **34**:2861–5.

22. Leira R, Davalos A, Silva Y, *et al.* Early neurological deterioration in intracerebral hemorrhage: predictors and associated factors. *Neurology* 2004; **63**:461–7.

23. Davis SM, Broderick J, Hennerici M, *et al.* Hematoma growth is a determinant of mortality and poor outcome after intracerebral hemorrhage. *Neurology* 2006; **66**:1175–81.

24. Martini SR, Flaherty ML, Brown AM, *et al.* Risk factors for intracerebral hemorrhage differ according to hemorrhage location. *N Engl J Med* 2012; **79**:2275–82.

25. Rost NS, Greenberg SM, Rosand J. The genetic architecture of intracerebral hemorrhage. *Stroke* 2008; **39**(7):2166–73.

26. PROGRESS Collaborative Group. Randomised trial of a perindopril-based blood-pressure-lowering regimen among 6,105 individuals with previous stroke or transient ischemic attack. *Lancet* 2001; **358**:1033–41.

27. Kurth T, Kase CS, Berger K, *et al.* Smoking and risk of hemorrhagic stroke in women. *Stroke* 2003; **34**:2792–5.

28. Kurth T, Kase CS, Berger K, *et al.* Smoking and the risk of hemorrhagic stroke in men. *Stroke* 2003; **34**:1151–5.

29. Juvela S, Hillbom M, Palomaki H. Risk factors for spontaneous intracerebral hemorrhage. *Stroke* 1995; **26**:1558–64.

30. Casolla B, Dequatre-Ponchelle N, Rossi C. Heavy alcohol intake and intracerebral hemorrhage: characteristics and effect on outcome. *Neulogy* 2012; **79**:1109–15.

31. Kase CS, Mohr JP, Caplan LR. Intracerebral hemorrhage. In: Mohr JP, Choi DW, Grotta JC, Weir B, Wolf PA, eds. *Stroke: Pathophysiology, Diagnosis, and Management.* 4th edn: Philadelphia: Churchill Livingstone; 2004:327–76.

32. Stroke Prevention by Aggressive Reduction in Cholesterol Levels (SPARCL) Investigators. High-dose atorvastatin after stroke or transient ischemic attack. *N Engl J Med* 2006; **355**:549–59.

33. Fitzmaurice E, Wendell L, Snider R, *et al.* Effect of statins on intracerebral hemorrhage outcome and recurrence. *Stroke* 2008; **39**(7):2151–4.

34. Westover MB, Bianchi MT, Eckman MH, Greenberg SM. Statin use following intracerebral hemorrhage: a decision analysis. *Arch Neurol* 2011; **68**:573–9.

35. He J, Whelton PK, Vu B, Klag MJ. Aspirin and risk of hemorrhagic stroke: a meta-analysis of randomized controlled trials. *JAMA* 1998; **280**:1930–5.

36. Greenberg SM, Briggs ME, Hyman BT, *et al.* Apolipoprotein E epsilon 4 is associated with the presence and earlier onset of hemorrhage in cerebral amyloid angiopathy. *Stroke* 1996; **27**:1333–7.

37. McCarron MO, Nicoll JA. Apolipoprotein E genotype and cerebral amyloid angiopathy-related hemorrhage. *Ann N Y Acad Sci* 2000; **903**:176–9.

38. Fazekas F, Kleinert R, Roob G, *et al.* Histopathologic analysis of foci of signal loss on gradient-echo T2*-weighted MR images in patients with spontaneous intracerebral hemorrhage: evidence of microangiopathy-related microbleeds. *Am J Neuroradiol* 1999; **20**(4):637–42.

39. Cordonnier C, Al-Shahi Salman R, Wardlaw J. Spontaneous brain microbleeds: systematic review, subgroup analyses and standards for study design and reporting. *Brain* 2007; **130**:1988–2003.

40. Kinoshita T, Okudera T, Tamura H, Ogawa T, Hatazawa J. Assessment of lacunar hemorrhage associated with hypertensive stroke by echo-planar gradient-echo T2*-weighted MRI. *Stroke* 2000; **31**:1646–50.

41. Tsushima Y, Aoki J, Endo K. Brain microhemorrhages detected on T2*-weighted gradient-echo MR images. *Am J Neuroradiol* 2003; **24**:88–96.

42. Tsushima Y, Tamura T, Unno Y, Kusano S, Endo K. Multifocal low-signal brain lesions on T2*-weighted gradient-echo imaging. *Neuroradiology* 2000; **42**:499–504.

43. Kidwell CS, Saver JL, Villablanca JP. Magnetic resonance imaging detection of microbleeds before thrombolysis: an emerging application. *Stroke* 2002; **33**:95–8.

44. Wong KS, Chan YL, Liu JY, Gao S, Lam WW. Asymptomatic

microbleeds as a risk factor for aspirin-associated intracerebral hemorrhages. *Neurology* 2003; **60**:511–13.

45. Fiehler J, Albers GW, Boulanger JM. Bleeding risk analysis in stroke imaging before thrombolysis (BRASIL): pooled analysis of T2*-weighted magnetic resonance imaging data from 570 patients. *Stroke* 2007; **38**:2738–44.

46. Kakuda W, Thijs VN, Lansberg MG. Clinical importance of microbleeds in patients receiving IV thrombolysis. *Neurology* 2005; **65**:1175–8.

47. Greenberg SM, Eng JA, Ning M, Smith EE, Rosand J. Hemorrhage burden predicts recurrent intracerebral hemorrhage after lobar hemorrhage. *Stroke* 2004; **35**:1415–20.

48. Becker K, Tirschwell D. Intraparenchymal hemorrhage, bleeding, hemostasis, and the utility of CT angiography. *Int J Stroke* 2008; **3**:11–13.

49. Kidwell CS, Wintermark M. Imaging of intracranial haemorrhage. *Lancet Neurol* 2008; **7**:256–67.

50. Steiner T, Kaste M, Forsting M, *et al.* Recommendations for the management of intracranial haemorrhage – part 1: Spontaneous intracerebral haemorrhage. The European Stroke Initiative Writing Committee and the Writing Committee for the EUSI Executive Committee. *Cerebrovasc Dis* 2006; **22**:294–316.

51. Delgado Almandoz JE, Yoo AJ, Stone MJ, *et al.* Systematic characterization of the computed tomography angiography spot sign in primary intracerebral hemorrhage identifies patients at highest risk for hematoma expansion: the spot sign score. *Stroke* 2009; **40**:2994–3000.

52. Goldstein JN, Fazen LE, Snider R, *et al.* Contrast extravasation on CT angiography predicts hematoma expansion in intracerebral hemorrhage. *Neurology* 2007; **68**:889–94.

53. Li N, Wang Y, Wang W, *et al.* Contrast extravasation on computed tomography angiography predicts clinical outcome in primary intracerebral hemorrhage, a prospective study of 139 cases. *Stroke* 2011; **42**:3441–6.

54. Demchuk AM, Dowlatshahi D, Rodriguez-Luna D, *et al.* Prediction of haematoma growth and outcome in patients with intracerebral haemorrhage using the CT-angiography spot sign (PREDICT): a prospective observational study. *Lancet Neurol* 2012; **11**:307–14.

55. Weir CJ, Murray GD, Adams FG, *et al.* Poor accuracy of stroke scoring systems for differential clinical diagnosis of intracranial haemorrhage and infarction. *Lancet* 1994; **344**:999–1002.

56. Herbstein DJ, Schaumberg HH. Hypertensive intracerebral hematoma. An investigation of the initial hemorrhage and rebleeding using chronium CR 51-labeled erythrocytes. *Arch Neurol* 1974; **30**:412–14.

57. Xi G. Intracerebral hemorrhage: pathophysiology and therapy. *Neurocrit Care* 2004; **1**:5–18.

58. Brott T, Broderick J, Kothari R, *et al.* Early hemorrhage growth in patients with intracerebral hemorrhage. *Stroke* 1997; **28**:1–5.

59. Tuhrim S, Horowitz DR, Sacher M, Godbold JH. Volume of ventricular blood is an important determinant of outcome in supratentorial intracerebral hemorrhage. *Crit Care Med* 1999; **27**:617–21.

60. Gebel JM Jr, Jauch EC, Brott TG, *et al.* Relative edema volume is a predictor of outcome in patients with hyperacute spontaneous intracerebral hemorrhage. *Stroke* 2002; **33**:2636–41.

61. Castillo J, Davalos A, Alvarez-Sabin J, *et al.* Molecular signatures of brain injury after intracerebral hemorrhage. *Neurology* 2002; **58**:624–9.

62. Lee KR, Colon GP, Betz AL, *et al.* Edema from intracerebral hemorrhage: the role of thrombin. *J Neurosurg* 1996; **84**:91–6.

63. Sansing LH, Kaznatcheeva EA, Perkins CJ, *et al.* Edema after intracerebral hemorrhage: correlations with coagulation parameters and treatment. *J Neurosurg* 2003; **98**:985–92.

64. Schellinger PD, Fiebach JB, Hoffmann K, *et al.* Stroke MRI in intracerebral hemorrhage: is there a perihemorrhagic penumbra? *Stroke* 2003; **34**:1674–9.

65. Mendelow AD, Gregson B, Fernandes HM, *et al.* Early surgery versus initial conservative treatment in patients with spontaneous supratentorial intracerebral haematomas in the International Surgical Trial in Intracerebral Haemorrhage (STICH): a randomised trial. *Lancet* 2005; **365**:387–97.

66. Mendelow AD, Gregson BA, Rowan EN, *et al.* Early surgery versus initial conservative treatment in patients with spontaneous supratentorial lobar intracerebral haemotomas (STICH II): a randomized trial. *Lancet* 2013; **382**:397–408.

67. Gregson BA, Broderick JP, Auer LM, *et al.* Individual patient data subgroup meta-analysis of surgery for spontaneous supratentorial intracerebral hemorrhage. *Stroke* 2012; **43**:1496–504.

68. Lampl Y, Ronit G, Eshel T. Neurological and functional outcome in patients with supratentorial hemorrhages.

A prospective study. *Stroke* 1995; **26**:2249–53.

69. Morgan T, Zuccarello M, Narayan R, *et al.* Preliminary findings of the minimally-invasive surgery plus rtPA for intracerebral hemorrhage evacuation (MISTIE) clinical trial. *Acta Neurochir Suppl* 2008; **105**:147–51.

70. Anderson CS, Huang Y, Wang JG, *et al.* Intensive blood pressure reduction in acute cerebral haemorrhage trial (interact): a randomised pilot trial. *Lancet Neurol* 2008; **7**:391–9.

71. Qureshi AI, Tariq N, Divani AA, *et al.*, and the ATACH investigators. Antihypertensive treatment of acute cerebral hemorrhage (ATACH). *Crit Care Med* 2010; **38**:637–48.

72. Morgenstern LB, Hemphill JC 3rd, Anderson C, *et al.*, American Heart Association Stroke Council and Council on Cardiovascular Nursing. Guidelines for the management of spontaneous intracerebral hemorrhage: a guideline for healthcare professionals from the American Heart Association/ American Stroke Association. *Stroke* 2010; **41**:2108–29.

73. Ohwaki K, Yano E, Nagashima H, *et al.* Blood pressure management in acute intracerebral hemorrhage: relationship between elevated blood pressure and hematoma enlargement. *Stroke* 2004; **35**:1364–7.

74. Qureshi AI. Acute hypertensive response in patients with stroke: pathophysiology and management. *Circulation* 2008; **118**:176–87.

75. Broderick JP, Connolly ES, Feldman E, *et al.*; American Heart Association/American Stroke Association Stroke Council; American Heart Association/ American Stroke Association High Blood Pressure Research Council; Quality of Care and Outcomes in Research Interdisciplinary Working Group. Guidelines for the management of spontaneous intracerebral hemorrhage in adults. 2007 update: a guideline from the American Heart Association, American Stroke Association Stroke Council, High Blood Pressure Research Council, and the Quality of Care and Outcomes in Research Interdisciplinary Working Group. *Stroke* 2007; **38**: e391–413.

76. Diedler J, Sykora M, Rupp A, *et al.* Impaired cerebral vasomotor activity in spontaneous intracerebral hemorrhage. *Stroke* 2009; **40**:815–19.

77. Anderson CS, Heeley E, Huang Y, *et al.*; for the INTERACT-2 Investigaters. Rapid blood-pressure lowering in patients with acute intracerebral hemorrhage. *N Engl J Med* 2013; **368**:2355–65.

78. Aguilar MI, Hart RG, Kase CS, *et al.* Treatment of warfarin-associated intracerebral hemorrhage: literature review and expert opinion. *Mayo Clin Proc* 2007; **82**: 82–92.

79. Huttner HB, Schellinger PD, Hartmann M, *et al.* Hematoma growth and outcome in treated neurocritical care patients with intracerebral hemorrhage related to oral anticoagulant therapy. Comparison of acute treatment strategies using vitamin K, fresh frozen plasma, and prothrombin complex concentrates. *Stroke* 2006; **37**:1465–70.

80. Steiner T, Freiberger A, Griebe M, *et al.* International normalised ratio normalisation in patients with coumarin-related intracranial haemorrhages–the INCH trial: a randomised controlled multicentre trial to compare safety and preliminary efficacy of fresh frozen plasma and prothrombin complex – study design and protocol. *Int J Stroke* 2011; **6**(3):271–7.

81. Eerenberg ES, Kamphuisen PW, Sijpkens MK, *et al.* Reversal of rivaroxaban and dabigatran by prothrombin complex concentrate: a randomized, placebo-controlled, crossover study in healthy subjects. *Circulation* 2011; **124**:1573–9.

82. Leissinger CA, Blatt PM, Hoots WK, Ewenstein B. Role of prothrombin complex concentrates in reversing warfarin anticoagulation: a review of the literature. *Am J Hematol* 2008; **83**:137–43.

83. van Ryn J, Stangier J, Haertter S, *et al.* Dabigatran etexilate–a novel, reversible, oral direct thrombin inhibitor: interpretation of coagulation assays and reversal of anticoagulant activity. *Thromb Haemost* 2010; **103**:1116–27.

84. Wagner F, Peters H, Formella S, *et al.* Effective elimination of dabigatran with haemodialysis: a phase I single-centre study in patients with end stage renal disease. *American Heart Association Scientific Sessions* 13–15 November 2011 (Orlando, Florida). 2011.

Subarachnoid hemorrhage

Philipp Lichti and Thorsten Steiner

Definition

Subarachnoid hemorrhage (SAH) is an acute, arterial bleeding under the arachnoid mater, the spider-web-like membrane covering the brain and spinal cord. Interposed between the more superficial and much thicker dura mater and the deeper pia mater, the subarachnoid space is filled with cerebrospinal fluid (CSF), which allows the hematoma to expand quickly and cause the typical, acute meningeal symptoms. Besides the expansion of the blood within the subarachnoid space, an infiltration of the subdural space as well as the parenchyma is possible. The leading cause for a non-traumatic SAH is the rupture of an intracranial aneurysm, which accounts for about 80% of cases [1–2]. Treatments are based on randomized controlled trials and prospective cohort studies [3–4]. SAH still has a poor prognosis, which is influenced by vasospasm, hydrocephalus, and the delayed ischemic deficit.

Epidemiology

SAH is a severe and significant clinical picture. It accounts for 1–7% of all strokes [5], the incidence varies from 7 to 15 per 100 000 persons, with an overall incidence of 9.1 per 100 000 persons in most countries [6]. This accounts for approximately 25 000–30 000 cases of SAH in the United States and 36 000 in Europe per year. [1, 7]. Regionally higher incidences are reported from Finland and Norway [8, 9].

Also, SAH has a high social and economic importance, as the median age lies, in contrast to thromboembolic strokes, at 50–60 years [10]. The risk for women is 1.6 times that for men, depending on the hormone status [11]. Before the age of 40, SAH is more common in men, but after the age of 50 it is more common in woman [12]. The risk for Black populations is 2.1 times that of White populations [13].

There is an estimated number of unreported cases, about 1 out of 5, that die of SAH before arriving at a hospital. The following 3-months mortality is about 20%. Due to new developments, especially in the intensive care and neurosurgical treatment, the clinical outcome of SAH has improved, but morbidity is still as high as 30% and there is severe disability within 6 months. The morbidity and mortality depend on multiple factors. Causes of death in the hospital are: the primary impairment due to the hemorrhage (20%), secondary bleeding (20%), vasospasms (20%), hydrocephalus (20%), and surgery complications (20%).

> Subarachnoid hemorrhage (SAH) accounts for 1–7% of all strokes. The median age lies, in contrast to thromboembolic strokes, at 50–60 years. About 1 out of 5 cases die of SAH before arriving at a hospital. The following 3-months mortality is about 20%.

Risk factors

Risk factors can be divided into risk factors for aneurysm formation, aneurysm growth, and aneurysm rupture (SAH). These factors may be modifiable and not modifiable.

It is not yet clear whether the source of intracranial aneurysms is congenital or acquired. It seems that it is a multifactorial source of genetic and behavioral factors combined. Reports show that intracranial aneurysms run in families, so first-grade relatives have a 3–5 times higher risk [14] to a prevalence of 9.5%.

There is also an association with arteriovenous malformations and degenerating connective tissue disorders. Intracranial aneurysms occur in patients with autosomal dominant polycystic kidney disease

(ADPKD), who are more at risk of suffering an SAH [15]. Further connective tissue disorders associated with increased risk for SAH include Ehlers–Danlos syndrome (type IV), Marfan syndrome, pseudoxanthoma elasticum, and fibromuscular dysplasia [10].

Regarding modifiable risk factors, one is arterial hypertension and general atherosclerosis [16]. Hypertension is a risk factor for developing an aneurysm as well as aneurysm rupture. Toxic factors include alcohol consumption and cigarette smoking [17]. Cigarette smoking is the most important modifiable risk factor for aneurysm formation, growth, and rupture and should therefore be discouraged [18]. Other toxic risk factors are drug abuse, especially cocaine [19, 20], sympathomimetic agents, and amphetamines [21]. Anticoagulant therapy, as well as problems with blood clotting and pituitary apoplexy, can also cause an SAH [9].

> In summary, the most important modifiable risk factors for SAH are current cigarette smoking, hypertension, and excessive alcohol intake. The non-modifiable risk factors include sex, age, size of aneurysm, and family history. Risk factors for de novo formation of aneurysms are female sex, current cigarette smoking, arterial hypertension, age at diagnosis, family history, and connective tissue disorders. The main risk factor for aneurysm growth is current cigarette smoking.

Pathogenesis

In about 80% of all patients, an intracranial aneurysm is the cause of an SAH [22]. An aneurysm is a localized dilatation or ballooning of a blood vessel, due to a weakness of the elastic fibers. The most common form of intracranial aneurysm is of the saccular out-pouching with a spherical shape. The sizes vary from small aneurysms with a diameter of 15 mm over large (15–25 mm) to giant (25–50 mm) and super giant (over 50 mm). Approximately 70% of bleeding aneurysms are small (less than 12 mm), 25% are between 10 and 25 mm and only 2–4% are bigger than 25 mm. The saccular aneurysms show no tunica media or elastica in pathological processing, indicating that the weakness of the vessel wall is important in the genesis of aneurysms. Therefore, the risk factors (see above) are correlated with connective tissue disorders.

> In summary, ruptured and unruptured aneurysms combined, intracranial aneurysms occur in the ACA (anterior communicating artery) in 18%, the MCA (middle cerebral artery) in 15%, the ICA (internal carotid artery) in 50%, the PCoA (posterior communicating artery) in 14%, and the VBA (vertebral artery) in 17% [23]. Multiple aneurysms occurrence varies in incidence, with about 13% in angiographic studies and 22.7% at autopsy [24]. For hemodynamic reasons, the aneurysms develop at the junction spots of the main arteries. About 85% of the aneurysms are located at the anterior and about 15% at the posterior part of the circle of Willis.

Prognosis

Prognostic factors for mortality include age, the degree of the initial disturbance of consciousness, the amount of subarachnoid blood, and the localization of the aneurysm. Other determinants are sex (with a higher mortality rate in women [25, 26]), hypertension [27], and alcohol consumption [28]. Aneurysm of the posterior vascular territory and a great amount of blood in the cisterns and the ventricles have an inferior prognosis. Due to modern intensive care medicine and aneurysm treatment, the all in all mortality has improved, but stays high [5, 29]. Cumulative case fatality rates over time after SAH are as follows: day 1: 25–30%; week 1: 40–45%; first month: 50–60%; sixth month: 55–60%; year 1: 65%; and year 5: 65–70% [18, 30].

Of the surviving two-thirds of patients about 50% feature permanent disabilities. These include neuro-cognitive deficits, anxiety, and depression [31, 32]. Upon arrival in the hospital, patients with a poor initial grade (Hunt and Hess or World Federation of Neurosurgeons Scale [WFNS] grade IV and V) have the worst long-term functional outcomes and the highest mortality rate [33, 34].

An early and aggressive treatment of the SAH improves the long-term outcome [35, 36]. In general, hospitals with a high number of SAH cases (more than 18) show an improvement of long-term outcome [37].

Mortality is about one-third. The surviving two-thirds of patients feature about 50% permanent disabilities.

Clinical presentation

Ruptured intracranial aneurysm (RIA) (see Figure 12.1) needs to be differentiated from an *unruptured intracranial aneurysm* (UIA). A UIA is either asymptomatic and is detected by chance (e.g. in association with a RIA), or it becomes symptomatic by clinical signs other than bleeding, e.g. by cerebral nerve palsy, see below.

A

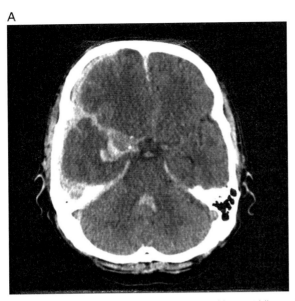

B

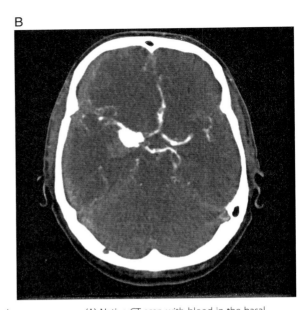

Figure 12.1. Subarachnoid hemorrhage caused by a middle cerebral artery aneurysm. (A) Native CT scan with blood in the basal subarachnoid spaces, the Sylvian fissure, and the fourth ventricle. The temporal horns are compressed. A large aneurysm of the middle cerebral artery, near the carotid-T can be found. (B) The same aneurysm in the CT angiography.

The symptoms of SAH range from subtle to the classic symptoms, including thunderclap headache. The thunderclap headache is a sudden onset pain, often described as the "worst possible headache." It is in most cases pulsating to the occipital region, similar to an abrupt hit on the head [2, 38]. Headache is reported in 95% of all patients with an SAH and about one-third have no other symptoms apart from the headache [22]. About half the patients suffer from initial unconsciousness and one-third of the patients suffer from focal signs beginning with the headache or soon afterwards [39, 40]. The impaired consciousness is most likely due to increasing intracranial pressure (ICP), which can be as high as the diastolic blood pressure. The increased ICP reduces the cerebral blood flow (CBF), which causes the unconsciousness. The reactive hyperemia, which follows, can end the unconsciousness. However, in severe cases of SAH unconsciousness may still persist [41].

Up to 60% of patients with SAH report a minor but unusual headache, occurring 6–20 days before the SAH, often referred to as "warning bleeding" [42]. It is proposed that the cause is a "warning leak," a drain or trickle bleeding of an aneurysm [43]. However, patients suffering from a prior headache before SAH do not differ regarding the clinical outcome from patients without prior headache. In contrast, a documented bleeding before the actual SAH does decrease the clinical outcome and it is therefore important to be distinguished from a "warning bleeding" [42].

Further warning signs for an imminent SAH can be caused by compression syndromes due to aneurysms, depending on the location [14]. These resemble symptomatic UIAs:

- Paresis or palsy of the oculomotor nerve, including mydriasis, in aneurysms of the posterior communicating artery (PCoA)
- Paresis of the abducens nerve, in aneurysms of the ICA (supraclinoid portion) or of the basilar artery
- Anopsia due to a compression of the optic chiasm or the optic nerve, in aneurysms of the supraclinoid portion of the ICA and
- Superior orbital fissure syndrome in aneurysms of the infraclinoid portion of the ICA.

The acute onset of the bleeding is often accompanied by nausea and vomiting. Meningeal signs develop mainly within the first hours as a result of the blood spreading in the spinal canal, so neck stiffness evolves usually within 6 hours after the initial onset of the SAH [44]. Epileptic grand mal seizures appear mostly in the first hour after initial onset and occur in about 20% of all patients [45]. A typical focal neurological sign such as sensor-motoric hemiparesis highly suggests an accompanying intracerebral hemorrhage. Cardiac dysfunctions accompany SAH in about 33% of cases, including arrhythmias and pulmonary edema [46].

Diagnosis

SAH is an acute medical emergency which requires an immediate transport to a hospital for further diagnosis and treatment. About 12% of all SAHs are overlooked and misdiagnosed. The most common causes for missing the diagnosis are: not undertaking of brain scans (mainly CT scan) and not performing lumbar puncture, if the scan is without pathological findings, leading to increased morbidity and mortality based on higher rebleeding rates [47].

The clinical prognosis can be assessed by the Glasgow Coma Scale (GCS) [48], the Hunt and Hess scale [49] and the WFNS [50]. Based on the GCS, the Prognosis on Admission of Aneurysmal Subarachnoid Haemorrhage (PAASH) scale shows good internal and external validity [18] and is slightly preferable over the WFNS [51]. Though extensively used in clinical practice, the Hunt and Hess scale should be abandoned and switched to the PAASH (Table 12.1).

The native CT scan is the most important diagnostic measurement if a SAH is suspected, because of its availability. The sensitivity is about 95% in the first 24 hours, but drops down in time to 50% after 7 days [52]. The initial CT can assess the severity, localization, and the focus of the bleeding. Possible regions of the aneurysm can be predicted:

- Blood focus in the frontal part of the hemispheric fissure is commonly associated with an aneurysm of the ACA, as is intraventricular hemorrhage.
- Blood focus in the Sylvian fissure is commonly associated with an aneurysm of the MCA, often combined with intracerebral hemorrhage.
- Massive blood in the subarachnoid space is a high risk for developing vasospasm or hydrocephalus.
- Blood in the fourth ventricle is commonly associated with aneurysm of the posterior inferior cerebellar artery (PICA) and likely to cause hydrocephalus.
- Small amounts of blood in the perimesencephalic cistern is often not associated with intracerebral aneurysm.

Further, to evaluate the likelihood of delayed cerebral ischemia (DCI) the radiological Fisher scale is used based on the amount and distribution of blood in the CT scan. The modified Fisher scale is used as a more accurate predictor of symptomatic vasospasm, with particular attention to thick cisternal and ventricular blood [53–55].

MRI scans, preferably with proton density-weighted, fluid-attenuated inversion recovery, diffusion-weighted imaging and gradient echo sequences, reveal similar results in detecting blood to CT scans in acute SAH and have a small advantage in detecting SAH after several days [56].

In the recent past, CT angiography (CTA) and magnetic resonance angiography (MRA) have

Table 12.1. The two SAH grading scales with criteria per grade and relation to outcome

Scale	Grade	Criteria	Proportion of patients with poor outcome	OR for poor outcome
WFNS	I	GCS 15	14.8%	Reference
	II	GCS 13–14, no focal deficit	29.4%	2.3
	III	GCS 13–14, focal deficit present	52.6%	6.1
	IV	GCS 7–12	58.3%	7.7
	V	GCS 3–6	92.7%	69
PAASH	I	GCS 15	14.8%	Reference
	II	GCS 11–14	41.3%	3.9
	III	GCS 8–10	74.4%	16
	IV	GCS 4–7	84.7%	30
	V	GCS 3	93.9	84

Poor outcome defined as GCS 1–3 or modified Rankin score 4–6 OR = odds ratio.
Data adapted from van Heuven *et al.* [51] and Steiner *et al.* [18].

improved both in availability and imaging technique and are used in support of catheter angiography. The sensitivity of a 3D time-of-flight (TOF) MRA in aneurysms ≥5 mm ranges from 85% to 100%, and for all aneurysms from 55% to 93%. The MRA is therefore useful for evaluate bigger, partly thrombotic aneurysms [57–60]. The sensitivity of a CTA ranges from 77% to 100% for all aneurysms and can give additional information such as wall calcification and intraluminal thrombosis [61–63]. A CTA is generally performed immediately after the initial native CT scan.

If the neuroimaging is negative in a patient with reasonable suspicion for an SAH, a lumbar puncture must be conducted. The CSF shows a consistent elevated erythrocyte count in all tubes (at least three should be attained). To differentiate a traumatic tap from SAH, xanthochromia (yellow-tinged appearance of the CSF) can be demonstrated after centrifugation; however, it may take up to 12 hours for xanthochromia to appear in the CSF. Another method to evaluate the CSF in SAH is spectrophotometry, with a sensitivity of 100% but a specificity of only 29–92% [64, 65]. The elevated number of erythrocytes causes a pleocytosis and elevated protein in the CSF.

Proving an SAH is the indication for a selective catheter cerebral angiography, including bilateral carotid and at least one vertebral artery injection. It is used to determine the aneurysm localization and

configuration and to look for multiple aneurysms, which occur at a rate of about 20%. Also, the collateral blood flow and the existence and magnitude of vasospasms can be evaluated [66]. If an initial angiography does not reveal an aneurysm, this might be because of vasospasm, local thrombosis, or inadequate technique. A second angiography should be performed after 1–2 weeks, with a 1–2% chance of detecting initially obscured aneurysms [67]. An example of an aneurysm can be seen in Figure 12.2.

Further lab diagnostics include blood count, inflammatory parameters, electrolytes, and coagulation parameters. Performing an initial ECG is important, as arrhythmias and ECG changes (including QU prolongation, Q waves, ST elevation) are reported in 40–70% of cases in the first hour after SAH onset [68].

Treatment

General treatment

The treatment of the SAH depends on the clinical and neuroradiological presentation. Patients suffering from a severe SAH should be monitored and treated in specialized intensive care units, or in an intermediate care facility of a stroke or neurovascular unit with the availability of vascular neurosurgeons and interventional neuroradiologists [69–71].

A
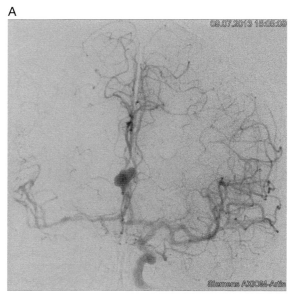

B
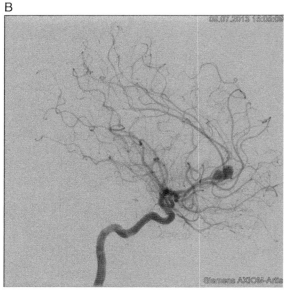

Figure 12.2. Digital subtraction angiography (DSA) showing a distal anterior cerebral artery aneurysm on the right side. The aneurysm has a size of 1.3 × 6 mm in maximum diameter. The right internal carotid artery was occluded prior to the SAH.

The first priority in the treatment of an SAH is the stabilization of the patient. This includes systemic oxygenation and hemodynamics to optimize cerebral perfusion and oxygen supply, control of the ICP, the blood pressure, and possible seizures, as well as prevention of aneurysm rebleeding [10]. Sedation and pain relief belong to the first measures (Table 12.2).

Table 12.2. Recommendations for monitoring and general management of patients with aneurysmal SAH

Monitoring

- Intensive continuous observation at least until occlusion of the aneurysm
- Continuous ECG monitoring
- Start with GCS, focal deficits, blood pressure and temperature at least every hour

Blood pressure

- Stop antihypertensive medication that the patient was using
- Do not treat hypertension unless it is extreme; limits for extreme blood pressures should be set on an individual basis, taking into account age of the patient, pre-SAH blood pressures, and cardiac history; systolic blood pressure should be kept below 180 mmHg, only until coiling or clipping of ruptured aneurysm, to reduce risk for rebleeding

Fluids and electrolytes

- Intravenous line mandatory
- Insert an indwelling urinary catheter
- Start with 3 liter/day (isotonic saline, 0.9%), and adjust infusion for oral intake
- Aim for normovolemia also in case of hyponatremia and compensate for fever
- Monitor electrolytes, glucose, and white blood cell count at least every other day

Pain

- Start with paracetamol (acetaminophen) 500 mg every 3–4 hours; avoid aspirin before aneurysm occlusion
- For severe pain, use codeine, tramadol (suppository or i.v.), or, as a last resort, piritramide (i.m. or i.v.)

Prevention of deep venous thrombosis and pulmonary embolism

- Compression stockings and intermittent compression by pneumatic devices in high-risk patients

Adapted from Steiner *et al.* [18].

To reduce the risk of a sudden increase of ICP, the patient should be kept in bed, defecation should be eased (laxatives), and pain treated early on (analgesics) until the aneurysm is occluded [18]. Antiemetic drugs should be given to awake people.

The level of conscious and the neurological status should be evaluated regularly at least for 7 days, depending on the severity of the SAH and the general clinical condition of the patient. The further monitoring includes a continuous blood pressure recording via an arterial line, and control of fluid balance via a bladder catheter.

Blood glucose should be regularly checked, as hyperglycemia develops in one-third of SAH patients and is independently associated with poor outcome [27, 72–74]. Hyperglycemia over 10 mmol/l should be treated.

About half of all patients with SAH develop fever, with about 20% percent showing no signs of infection. Fever in the absence of infection can be attributed to a systemic inflammatory reaction or to loss of central temperature control [75]. As fever is associated with poor outcome, increased temperature should be treated medically and physically [73].

High values of initial blood pressure, which frequently occur in patients with SAH, may increase the risk of early rebleeding. However, lowering the blood pressure aggressively increases the risk of secondary ischemia [76]. It is recommended to tolerate a systolic blood pressure up to 180 mmHg until coiling or clipping. It seems reasonable to decrease in moderate values, about as low as 25% of the initial pressure [18]. Systolic values of 140–160 mmHg are hence recommended. However the mean arterial pressure (MAP) should be higher than 90 mmHg to maintain CBF. MAP of 110 mmHg can be tolerated [10, 66, 77]. Applying analgesics and nimodipine often reduces the blood pressure without need of further antihypertensive treatment. If needed, urapidil or nifedipine should be used.

Low molecular weight heparin, which prevents thromboembolic events, increases the risk of intracranial hemorrhage [78–80]. Therefore, pneumatic devices and/or compression stockings before occlusion of the aneurysm should be preferred [81–83]. If, in high-risk patients, low molecular weight heparin must be applied, it should be applied not earlier than 12 hours after surgical occlusion of the aneurysm and immediately after coiling [18].

Epileptic seizures occur at rates of 1–7% on initial onset, about 5% during hospitalization, and about 7% in the first year after SAH [84, 85]. Non-convulsive status epilepticus has been detected in about 8% of comatose patients [86–88]. However, continuous EEG monitoring is not recommended for various reasons, including lack of effectiveness [18, 89]. As routine use of phenytoin or fosphenytoin may worsen functional and cognitive outcome after SAH [90, 91], antiepileptic drugs should only be administered in apparent epileptic seizures and not as prophylaxis.

> Invasive neuromonitoring, including brain tissue oxygenation, microdialysis, cerebral perfusion, and electrocorticography (ECoG) are currently being investigated. These measurements may be recorded in operated patients, yet a general recommendation cannot be given, due to lack of valid data [92].

Specific prevention of rebleeding

After an aneurysm is detected via neuroimaging or angiography, the occlusion of this aneurysm should be aspired to as soon as technically and practically possible. This is due to the risk of rebleeding, which worsens massively the patient's outcome. The rebleeding rate during the first few hours, before the aneurysm can be occluded, is about 15%. The cumulative risk of rebleeding after the first day of the SAH is about 35–40% and after 4 weeks decreases to about 22% [93, 94]. A meta-analysis of 11 out of 268 studies with a total of 1814 patients revealed in a comparative evaluation of early versus late surgical clipping of ruptured aneurysms that early treatment (within 72 hours after SAH) of patients with a good clinical/neurological condition on admission (WFNS I–III) leads to a significantly better outcome [95].

The occlusion of the aneurysm can be done in two ways: neurosurgical clipping and endovascular coiling. The basic principle of the operation is the compression of the aneurysm neck, which is achieved with a clip. A craniotomy is needed. With the establishment of microsurgical techniques, the morbidity and mortality dropped to 5–15% [96–98]. Newer developments such as intra-operative indocyanine green angiography and Doppler sonography further improve the operation outcome [99]. If the clip is attached within 48–72 hours after onset of the SAH, the rate for obliteration is about 90%, depending on the localization of the aneurysm [100]. Operations at a later point of time have a significantly lower prognosis. The worst space of time is between the seventh and the tenth day, most likely because of the high vasospasm rate. The complication rate depends on the localization of the aneurysm, with the highest rate for the basilar artery [101] and comparable better rates in the MCA [102]. Older techniques such as trapping or wrapping are nowadays solely used as complementary measurements.

With the invention of Guglielmi detachable coils, endovascular treatments of intracranial aneurysms became possible as an alternative to craniotomy and clipping [103]. Here, electrolytic detachable platinum spirals (coils) are transferred via a small catheter in the aneurysm, filling it and triggering a thrombosis, thereby occluding the aneurysm. In small-necked aneurysms, an obliteration rate of 80–90% is achieved, with a complication rate about 9% [104].

The decision to coil or clip an aneurysm is complex and depends on multiple factors. The prospective, randomized, multicentric International Subarachnoid Aneurysm Trial (ISAT) study compared both procedures and included SAH patients, when it seemed that both measurements are possible [85, 105, 106]. Resulting from ISAT and other recent studies [107, 108], the decision on which method to apply should be made in a neurovascular center, including experienced vascular neurosurgeons and interventional neuroradiologists. If possible, the patient should be included in the decision.

Important factors in this discussion should be:

- the clinical status of the patient (age, comorbidity)
- the anticipated surgical ease or difficulty based on anatomical location and size,
- the competence, technical skills, and availability
- the anatomy of the access vessels (tortuosity, extent of arteriosclerotic change, collaterals)
- the width of aneurysm neck in comparison with the dome and the parent artery (wide-neck aneurysms are difficult to completely obliterate with coils, coils may migrate and be a source for emboli)
- presence of an intracerebral hematoma with mass effect.

If in this discussion both treatments are considered equally applicable, coiling should be preferred because of better long-term findings.

> The occlusion of the aneurysm can be done in two ways: neurosurgical clipping and endovascular coiling.

Hydrocephalus

The chance of developing hydrocephalus is about 20–30% in all patients with SAH, with a rate of 20% in the acute phase and about 10% in the chronic phase [109–112]. If a patient develops a symptomatic or neuroradiologically apparent hydrocephalus an external ventricular drainage (EVD) should be applied. Alternatively, lumbar puncture may be considered in patients when CT scan shows no blood in the third or fourth ventricle [18]. In the case of an early hydrocephalus, the EVD should be applied before performing the angiography. If done so, the treatment of the hydrocephalus is not delayed by the angiography.

Another advantage of the EVD is the possibility of recording and treating of ICP. The target value for ICP should be <25 mmHg, if possible <20 mmHg [113]. A sufficient cerebral perfusion pressure (CPP) between 50 and 70 mmHg should be targeted. If ICP values stay high for more than 7–10 days and after several attempts to remove the EVD, a permanent drain via ventriculo-peritoneal or ventriculo-atrial shunting should be executed.

If a patient develops hydrocephalus an external ventricular drainage (EVD) should be applied.

Delayed cerebral ischemia (DCI)

DCI is defined as the development of new focal neurological signs and/or deterioration in level of consciousness, lasting for more than one hour, or the appearance of new infarctions on CT or MRI [54, 114]. Vasospasm, hypovolemia, and spreading depolarizations cause DCI. DCI develops on day 3 after SAH onset, reaches its maximum at day 5–14 and resolves on day 21. Occurrence of DCI is a predictor of neurological outcome.

Measurements to detect and monitor DCI or hypovolemia include daily transcranial Doppler sonography, neurological examination (e.g. GCS every 6 hours), fluid balance and blood pressure monitoring.

Transcranial Doppler sonography can be done cheaply and fast, but should be performed by an experienced investigator. A mean flow velocity (Vm) of the MCA above 200 cm/s is highly correlated with an angiographic vasospasm of the artery. The same applies for an increase of Vm by more than 50 cm/s in 24 hours. Also, a Lindegaard Index (Vm of the MCA in relation to Vm in the extracranial ICA) above 6 is an indication for arterial vasospasm [115–118].

Further multimodal neuromonitoring can include partial brain tissue oxygen pressure, cerebral microdialysis to assess neurometabolites, cerebral perfusion, and continuous electroencephalography. Although some results are promising, especially in operated patients, there are insufficient data to give a general recommendation for these monitoring procedures [119].

If there is a reasonable suspicion for a vasospasm, further imaging studies should be applied. Appropriate techniques are CT angiography and CT perfusion, both highly correlating with conventional angiography [120, 121]. Alternatively, an MR with MR angiography can be performed.

To prevent DCI, recent studies provided evidence for the calcium-channel blocker nimodipine to be efficient in this respect [122–125]. Nimodipine (60 mg every 4 hours) should be administered orally (or via nasogastric tube) from day 1 to day 21 [126]. If an enteral administration is not possible, nimodipine should be applied intravenously. A decrease of the blood pressure must be compensated via volume infusion and, if need be, by sympathomimetics. The effect of nimodipine seems at least in part to be neuroprotective, as the actual vasospasm is not affected by intravenous administration.

If a DCI is proven, the treatment can be endovascular or hemodynamic. Hemodynamic measurements include hypertension and hypervolemia. As there are no randomized controlled trails available, the individual measurements cannot be assessed properly. Hypertension raises the CBF and the brain tissue oxygenation (ptiO$_2$) [127]. The risks of deliberately increasing arterial pressure and plasma volume include increased cerebral edema, and hemorrhagic transformation in areas of infarction [9, 128]. A normovolemia with a central nervous pressure over 4 mmHg, a MAP over 70 mmHg or a CPP over 60 mmHg should be aspired to [3]. A fluid restriction is accompanied with a higher risk for DCI and should therefore be avoided.

In endovascular treatment, a calcium-channel blocker such as nimodipine is administered via superselective angioplasty (Figure 12.3). It is indicated in focal-segmental vasospasm, proven in a prior CT or MR study [129–132].

Delayed cerebral ischemia (DCI) is defined as the development of new focal neurological signs and/or deterioration in the level of consciousness, or the appearance of new infarctions on CT or MRI. To prevent DCI, recent studies provided evidence for the calcium-channel blocker nimodipine to be efficient. If a DCI is proven, the treatment can be endovascular or hemodynamic.

A
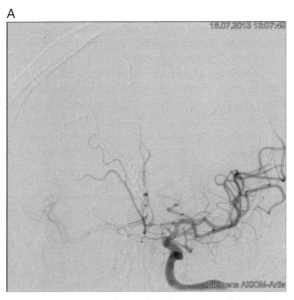

B
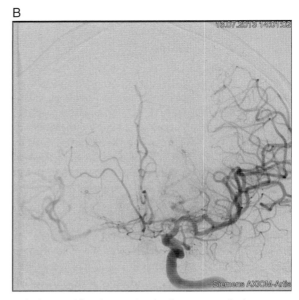

Figure 12.3. Angiographic display of vasospasm of the right anterior cerebral artery. After clipping the distal anterior cerebral artery aneurysm on the right side the pericallosal artery and the callosal marginal artery cannot be differentiated because of distinctive vasospasm of the anterior cerebral artery on both sides (A). Improvement is shown after superselective application of 2 mg nimodipine (B).

Electrolyte disturbances

Electrolyte disturbances are very common in patients with SAH. Especially hyponatremia occurs in about 20–40% of all cases [133]. There are two probable causes for hyponatremia, the renal salt-waste syndrome and the syndrome of inappropriate antidiuretic hormone secretion (SIADH) [73, 134]. Hyponatremia mostly begins at the end of the first week after SAH onset and last about 2 weeks. The treatment consists of administering isotonic crystalloids and volume therapy.

Perimesencephalic and prepontine SAH

In some cases with typical symptoms of SAH a circumscribed bleeding is found in the initial CT scan, but without evidence of an aneurysm, even in digital subtractive angiography (DSA). This is the case in about 15% of non-traumatic SAH [18] and is called perimesencephalic SAH (PMSAH). The blood is located within the midbrain cisterns, but not in the Sylvian fissure, the frontal hemispheric fissure, or the ventricles (with the exception of blood sedimentation in the ventricles) [135]. It is supposed that the PMSAH is more a venous than an arterial bleeding [136].

If the CT scan shows the typical blood pattern, a conventional angiography (DSA) should be performed,

as aneurysms are seldom, but do occur in 2.5–5%. Contrary to standard procedure, a repeated angiography after 2–3 weeks, which is recommended in all other non-traumatic SAH, is not necessary if the initial angiography could be performed technically sufficiently [137].

In PMSAH without evidence of aneurysms no intensive care therapy is strictly necessary, as the clinical progress is milder with less severe outcome than typical SAH [138]. The main complication is hydrocephalus, which should be treated as mentioned above. The development of DCI is much less common in PMSAH, and so the prophylactic administration of nimodipine in PMSAH cannot be recommended until prospective studies have demonstrated its effect. If DCI does occur, nimodipine should be used analogous to typical SAH.

The long-term prognosis is much better in PMSAH than in typical SAH. The risk of rebleeding is much lower. The survival of patients suffering a PMSAH is not decreased [139].

> In some cases with typical symptoms of SAH a circumscribed bleeding is found in the initial CT scan, but without evidence of an aneurysm. This is the case in about 15% of non-traumatic SAH and is called perimesencephalic SAH. The clinical progress is milder with less severe outcome than typical SAH.

Chapter summary

Subarachnoid hemorrhage (SAH) is a severe disease, where an arterial rupture mostly of one of the circle of Willis' arteries causes a bleeding in the subarachnoid space. The major symptom is a rapid-onset headache ("thunderclap headache"), often accompanied by vomiting and decrease of consciousness. The leading cause for a non-traumatic SAH is the rupture of an intracranial aneurysm.

Epidemiology: The incidence rate is 7 to 15 per 100 000 persons per year. The mean age lies at 50–60 years, the male:female ratio is 1:1.6. Major prognostic factors include the primary impairment due to the hemorrhage, secondary bleedings, hydrocephalus, and the delayed cerebral ischemia.

Risk factors: Risk factors can be divided into risk factors for aneurysm formation, aneurysm growth, and aneurysm rupture (SAH). Modifiable risk factors include arterial hypertension, cigarette smoking, and alcohol consumption. Non-modifiable risk factors include sex, age, size of the aneurysm, and family history.

Etiology: Eighty percent of all SAH result from intracranial aneurysm. Other causes include traumatic brain injuries and perimesencephalic SAH (PMSAH).

Clinical presentation: The major symptom is the sudden onset of thunderclap-like headache. Other typical symptoms include aberration of consciousness, vomiting, and epileptic seizures. Meningeal signs such as neck stiffness develop rapidly after the SAH onset. Depending on the localization of the aneurysm typical neurological signs can occur due to local compression.

Diagnosis: A CCT should be performed as soon as possible after admission to the hospital. If the neuroimaging is negative but the suspicion for a SAH persists, a lumbar puncture must be conducted. If the initial CCT or the spinal fluid detects a SAH, a CCT or MRI angiography should be initiated subsequently to demonstrate the aneurysm and for further therapeutic planning. If these imaging studies are negative or inconclusive digital subtraction angiography (DSA) must be performed. If no aneurysm is found in a non-traumatic SAH, a control angiography should be performed after 1–2 weeks.

Treatment: To prevent further bleedings an occlusion of the aneurysm must be realized probably within 24 hours. This can be done in two ways: either neurosurgically by clipping the aneurysm or endovascularly by coiling the aneurysm using catheter angiography. The decision which method is best for the patient depends on multiple factors and should be made in a neurovascular centre. To treat secondary complications, the patient must be assigned to an intensive care ward. Special attention must be given to the appearance of a hydrocephalus, the treatment of delayed cerebral ischemia (DCI), and the general intensive care management.

References

1. Suarez JI, Tarr RW, Selman WR. Aneurysmal subarachnoid hemorrhage. *N Engl J Med* 2006; **354**(4):387–96.

2. van Gijn J, Rinkel GJ. Subarachnoid haemorrhage: diagnosis, causes and management. *Brain* 2001; **124**:249–78.

3. Bederson JB, Connolly ES, Batjer HH, *et al.* Guidelines for the management of aneurysmal subarachnoid hemorrhage. *Stroke* 2009; **40**:994–1025.

4. Rabinstein AA, Lanzino G, Wijdicks EFM. Multidisciplinary management and emerging therapeutic strategies in aneurysmal subarachnoid haemorrhage. *Lancet Neurol* 2010; **9**:504–19.

5. Feigin VL, Lawes CM, Bennett DA, Anderson CS. Stroke epidemiology: a review of population-based studies of incidence, prevalence, and case-fatality in the late 20th century. *Lancet Neurol* 2003; **2**:43–53.

6. de Rooij NK, Linn FH, van der Plas JA, Algra A, Rinkel GJ. Incidence of subarachnoid haemorrhage: a systematic review with emphasis on region, age, gender and time trends. *J Neurol Neurosurg Psychiatry* 2007; **78**(12):1365–72.

7. Manno, EM. Subarachnoid hemorrhage. *Neurol Clin* 2004; **22**(2):347–66.

8. Fogelholm R, Hernesniemi J, Vapalahti M. Impact of early surgery on outcome after aneurysmal subarachnoid hemorrhage. A population-based study. *Stroke* 1993: **24**(11):1649–54.

9. Rinkel GJ, Djibuti M, Algra A, van Gijn J. Prevalence and risk of rupture of intracranial aneurysms: a systematic review. *Stroke* 1998; **29**(1):251–6.

10. Wartenberg KE. Update on the management of subarachnoid hemorrhage. *Fut Neurol* 2013; **8**(2):205–24.

11. Okamoto K, Horisawa R, Kawamura T, *et al.* Menstrual and reproductive factors for subarachnoid hemorrhage risk in women: a case–control study in nagoya, Japan. *Stroke* 2001; **32**(12):2841–4.

12. Qureshi AI, Suri MF, Yahia AM, *et al.* Risk factors for subarachnoid hemorrhage. *Neurosurgery* 2001; **49**(3):607–12; discussion 612–13.

13. Broderick JP, Brott T, Tomsick T, Huster G, Miller R. The risk of subarachnoid and intracerebral hemorrhages in blacks as compared with whites. *N Engl J Med* 1992; **326** (11):733–6.

14. Berlit P, Nahser H-C. Subarachnoidalblutung. In: Berlit P, ed. *Klinische Neurologie*. Berlin: Springer; 2011: 1175–84.

15. Neumann HP, Malinoc A, Bacher J, *et al.* Characteristics of intracranial aneurysms in the else kröner-fresenius registry of autosomal dominant polycystic kidney disease. *Cerebrovasc Dis Extra* 2012; **2**(1):71–9.

16. Brisman JL, Song JK, Newell DW. Cerebral aneurysms. *N Engl J Med* 2006; **355**(9):928–39.

17. Juvela S, Hillbom M, Numminen H, Koskinen P. Cigarette smoking and alcohol consumption as risk factors for aneurysmal subarachnoid hemorrhage. *Stroke* 1993; **24**(5):639–46.

18. Steiner T, Juvela S, Unterberg A, *et al.* European Stroke Organization guidelines for the management of intracranial aneurysms and subarachnoid haemorrhage. *Cerebrovasc Dis* 2013; **35**(2):93–112.

19. Nanda A, Vannemreddy PS, Polin RS, Willis BK. Intracranial aneurysms and cocaine abuse: analysis of prognostic indicators. *Neurosurgery* 2000; **46**(5):1063–7; discussion 1067–9.

20. Oyesiku NM, Colohan AR, Barrow DL, Reisner A. Cocaine-induced aneurysmal rupture: an emergent negative factor in the natural history of intracranial aneurysms? *Neurosurgery* 1993; **32**(4): 518–25; discussion 525–6.

21. Kernan WN, Viscoli CM, Brass LM, *et al.* Phenylpropanolamine and the risk of hemorrhagic stroke. *N Engl J Med* 2000; **343**(25):1826–32.

22. van Gijn J, Kerr RS, Rinkel GJ. Subarachnoid haemorrhage. *Lancet* 2007; **369**(9558):306–18.

23. Ghods AJ, Lopes D, Chen M. Gender differences in cerebral aneurysm location. *Front Neurol* 2012; **3**:78.

24. Nica DA, Rosca T, Dinca A, Stroi M. Multiple cerebral aneurysms of middle cerebral artery. Case report. *Rom Neurosurg* 2010; **17**(4):449–55.

25. Ingall TJ, Whisnant JP, Wiebers DO, O'Fallon WM. Has there been a decline in subarachnoid hemorrhage mortality? *Stroke* 1989; **20**(6):718–24.

26. Truelsen T, Bonita R, Duncan J, Anderson NE, Mee E. Changes in subarachnoid hemorrhage mortality, incidence, and case fatality in New Zealand between 1981–1983 and 1991–1993. *Stroke* 1998; **29**(11):2298–303.

27. Juvela S, Siironen J, Kuhmonen J. Hyperglycemia, excess weight, and history of hypertension as risk factors for poor outcome and cerebral infarction after aneurysmal subarachnoid hemorrhage. *J Neurosurg* 2005; **102**:998–1003.

28. Juvela S. Alcohol consumption as a risk factor for poor outcome after aneurysmal subarachnoid haemorrhage. *BMJ* 1992; **304**:1663–7.

29. Lichtman JH, Jones SB, Leifheit-Limson EC, Wang Y, Goldstein LB. 30-day mortality and readmission after hemorrhagic stroke among Medicare beneficiaries in Joint Commission primary stroke center-certified and noncertified hospitals. *Stroke* 2011; **42**(12):3387–91.

30. Pakarinen S. Incidence, aetiology, and prognosis of primary subarachnoid haemorrhage. A study based on 589 cases diagnosed in a defined urban population during a defined period. *Acta Neurol Scand* 1967; **43**(Suppl 29):1–28.

31. Mayer SA, Kreiter KT, Copeland D, *et al.* Global and domain-specific cognitive impairment and outcome after subarachnoid hemorrhage. *Neurology* 2002; **59**(11):1750–8.

32. Springer MV, Schmidt JM, Wartenberg KE, *et al.* Predictors of global cognitive impairment 1 year after subarachnoid hemorrhage. *Neurosurgery* 2009; **65**(6):1043–50; discussion 1050–1.

33. Huang AP, Arora S, Wintermark M, *et al.* Perfusion computed tomographic imaging and surgical selection with patients after poor-grade aneurysmal subarachnoid hemorrhage. *Neurosurgery* 2010; **67**(4):964–74; discussion 975.

34. Haug T, Sorteberg A, Finset A, *et al.* Cognitive functioning and health-related quality of life 1 year after aneurysmal subarachnoid hemorrhage in preoperative comatose patients (Hunt and Hess Grade V patients). *Neurosurgery* 2010; **66**(3):475–84; discussion 484–5.

35. Bailes JE, Spetzler RF, Hadley MN, Baldwin HZ. Management morbidity and mortality of poor-grade aneurysm patients. *J Neurosurg* 1990; **72**(4):559–66.

36. Shirao S, Yoneda H, Kunitsugu I, *et al.* Preoperative prediction of outcome in 283 poor-grade patients with subarachnoid hemorrhage: a project of the Chugoku-Shikoku Division of the Japan Neurosurgical Society. *Cerebrovasc Dis* 2010; **30**(2):105–13.

37. Nuno M, Patil CG, Lyden P, Drazin D. The effect of transfer and hospital volume in subarachnoid hemorrhage patients. *Neurocrit Care* 2012; **17**(3):312–23.

38. Ramrakha PS, Moore KP. *Oxford Handbook of Acute Medicine*, 2nd edn. Oxford: Oxford University Press; 2007: 466–70.

39. Linn FH, Rinkel GJ, Algra A, van Gijn J. Incidence of subarachnoid hemorrhage: role of region, year, and rate of computed tomography: a meta-analysis. *Stroke* 1996; **27**:625–9.

40. Hop JW, Brilstra EH, Rinkel GJ. Transient amnesia after perimesencephalic haemorrhage: the role of enlarged temporal horns. *J Neurol Neurosurg Psychiatry* 1998; **65**:590–3.

41. Poeck K, Hacke W. Neurologie: subarachnoidalblutung. *Neurologie.* Heidelberg: Springer; 2006: 264–87.

42. Linn FH, Rinkel GJ, Algra A, van Gijn J. The notion of "warning leaks" in subarachnoid haemorrhage: are such patients in fact admitted with a rebleed? *Neurol Neurosurg Psychiatry* 2000; **68**: 332–6.

43. Juvela. S. Minor leak before rupture of an intracranial aneurysm and subarachnoid hemorrhage of unknown etiology. *Neurosurgery* 1992; **30**(1):7–11.

44. Van Gjin J. Subarachnoid hemorrhage. In: Warrell DA, Cox TM, eds. *Oxford Textbook of Medicine*, 4th edn, vol 3. Oxford: Oxford University Press; 2003: 1032–4.

45. Sundaram MB, Chow F. Seizures associated with spontaneous subarachnoid hemorrhage. *Can J Neurol Sci* 1986; **13**(3):229–31.

46. Hamilton JC, Korn-Naveh L, Crago EA. Case studies in cardiac dysfunction after acute aneurysmal subarachnoid hemorrhage. *J Neurosci Nurs* 2008; **40**(5):269–74.

47. Kowalski RG, Claassen J, Kreiter KT, *et al.* Initial misdiagnosis and outcome after subarachnoid hemorrhage. *JAMA* 2004; **291**(7):866–9.

48. Teasdale G, Jennett B. Assessment of coma and impaired consciousness. A practical scale. *Lancet* 1974; **2**(7872):81–4.

49. Hunt WE, Hess RM. Surgical risk as related to time of intervention in the repair of intracranial aneurysms. *J Neurosurg* 1968; **28**(1):14–20.

50. Teasdale GM, Drake CG, Hunt W, *et al.* A universal subarachnoid hemorrhage scale: report of a committee of the World Federation of Neurosurgical Societies. *J Neurol Neurosurg Psychiatry* 1988; **51**(11):1457.

51. van Heuven AW, Dorhout Mees SM, Algra A, Rinkel GJ. Validation of a prognostic subarachnoid hemorrhage grading scale derived directly from the Glasgow Coma Scale. *Stroke* 2008; **39**:1347–8.

52. Perry JJ, Stiell IG, Sivilotti ML, *et al.* Sensitivity of computed tomography performed within six hours of onset of headache for diagnosis of subarachnoid haemorrhage: prospective cohort study. *BMJ* 2011; **343**:d4277.

53. Fisher CM, Kistler JP, Davis JM. Relation of cerebral vasospasm to subarachnoid hemorrhage visualized by computerized tomographic scanning. *Neurosurgery* 1980; **6**(1):1–9.

54. Frontera JA, Claassen J, Schmidt JM, *et al.* Prediction of symptomatic vasospasm after subarachnoid hemorrhage: the modified Fisher scale.

Neurosurgery 2006; **59**(1):21–7; discussion 21–7.

55. Claassen J, Bernardini GL, Kreiter K, *et al.* Effect of cisternal and ventricular blood on risk of delayed cerebral ischemia after subarachnoid hemorrhage; the Fisher scale revisited. *Stroke* 2001; **32**(9):2012–20.

56. Mitchell P, Wilkinson ID, Hoggard N, *et al.* Detection of subarachnoid haemorrhage with magnetic resonance imaging. *J Neurol Neurosurg Psychiatry* 2001; **70**(2):205–11.

57. Anzalone N, Triulzi F, Scotti G. Acute subarachnoid haemorrhage: 3D time-of-flight MR angiography versus intra-arterial digital angiography. *Neuroradiology* 1995; **37**(4):257–61.

58. Horikoshi T, Fukamachi A, Nishi H, Fukasawa I. Detection of intracranial aneurysms by three-dimensional time-of-flight magnetic resonance angiography. *Neuroradiology* 1994; **36**(3):203–7.

59. Huston J 3rd, Nichols DA, Luetmer PH, *et al.* Blinded prospective evaluation of sensitivity of MR angiography to known intracranial aneurysms: importance of aneurysm size. *AJNR Am J Neuroradiol* 1994; **15**(9):1607–14.

60. Schuierer G, Huk WJ, Laub G. Magnetic resonance angiography of intracranial aneurysms: comparison with intra-arterial digital subtraction angiography. *Neuroradiology* 1992; **35**(1):50–4.

61. Alberico RA, Ozsvath R, Casey S, Patel M. Helical CT angiography for the detection of intracranial aneurysms. *AJNR Am J Neuroradiol* 1996; **17**(5):1002–3.

62. Alberico RA, Patel M, Casey S, *et al.* Evaluation of the circle of Willis with three-dimensional CT angiography in patients with suspected intracranial aneurysms. *AJNR Am J Neuroradiol* 1995; **16**(8):1571–8; discussion 1579–80.

63. Ogawa T, Okudera T, Noguchi K, *et al.* Cerebral aneurysms:

evaluation with three-dimensional CT angiography. *AJNR Am J Neuroradiol* 1996; **17**(3):447–54.

64. Chao CY, Florkowski CM, Fink JN, Southby SJ, George PM. Prospective validation of cerebrospinal fluid bilirubin in suspected subarachnoid haemorrhage. *Ann Clin Biochem* 2007; **44**(Pt 2):140–4.

65. Perry JJ, Sivilotti ML, Stiell IG, *et al.* Should spectrophotometry be used to identify xanthochromia in the cerebrospinal fluid of alert patients suspected of having subarachnoid hemorrhage? *Stroke* 2006; **37**(10):2467–72.

66. Connolly ES Jr, Rabinstein AA, Carhuapoma JR, *et al.* Guidelines for the management of aneurysmal subarachnoid hemorrhage: a guideline for healthcare professionals from the American Heart Association/American Stroke Association. *Stroke* 2012; **43**(6):1711–37.

67. Forster DM, Steiner L, Hakanson S, Bergvall U. The value of repeat pan-angiography in cases of unexplained subarachnoid hemorrhage. *J Neurosurg* 1978; **48**(5):712–16.

68. Nguyen H, Zaroff JG. Neurogenic stunned myocardium. *Curr Neurol Neurosci Rep* 2009; **9**(6):486–91.

69. Cross DT 3rd, Tirschwell DL, Clark MA, *et al.* Mortality rates after subarachnoid hemorrhage: variations according to hospital case volume in 18 states. *J Neurosurg* 2003; **99**(5):810–17.

70. Berman MF, Solomon RA, Mayer SA, Johnston SC, Yung PP. Impact of hospital-related factors on outcome after treatment of cerebral aneurysms. *Stroke* 2003; **34**(9):2200–7.

71. Sarker SJ, Heuschmann PU, Burger I, *et al.* Predictors of survival after hemorrhagic stroke in a multi-ethnic population: the South London Stroke Register (SLSR). *J Neurol Neurosurg Psychiatry* 2008; **79**:260–5.

72. Lanzino G, Kassell NF, Germanson T, Truskowski L, Alves W. Plasma glucose levels and outcome after aneurysmal subarachnoid hemorrhage. *J Neurosurg* 1993; **79**: 885–91.

73. Wartenberg KE, Schmidt JM, Claassen J, *et al.* Impact of medical complications on outcome after subarachnoid hemorrhage. *Crit Care Med* 2006; **34**:617–23; quiz 624.

74. Dorhout Mees SM, van Dijk GW, Algra A, Kempink DR, Rinkel GJ. Glucose levels and outcome after subarachnoid hemorrhage. *Neurology* 2003; **61**:1132–3.

75. Dorhout Mees SM, Luitse MJ, van den Bergh WM, Rinkel GJ. Fever after aneurysmal subarachnoid hemorrhage. Relation with extent of hydrocephalus and amount of extravasated blood. *Stroke* 2008; **39**:2141–3.

76. Wijdicks EF, Vermeulen M, Murray GD, Hijdra A, van Gijn J. The effects of treating hypertension following aneurysmal subarachnoid hemorrhage. *Clin Neurol Neurosurg* 1990; **92**:111–17.

77. Diringer MN, Bleck TP, Claude Hemphill J 3rd, *et al.* Critical care management of patients following aneurysmal subarachnoid hemorrhage: recommendations from the Neurocritical Care Society's Multidisciplinary Consensus Conference. *Neurocrit Care* 2011; **15**(2):211–12.

78. Siironen J, Juvela S, Varis J, *et al.* No effect of enoxaparin on outcome of aneurysmal subarachnoid hemorrhage: a randomized, double-blind, placebo-controlled clinical trial. *J Neurosurg* 2003; **99**:953–9.

79. Juvela S, Siironen J, Varis J, Poussa K, Porras M. Risk factors for ischemic lesions following aneurysmal subarachnoid hemorrhage. *J Neurosurg* 2005; **102**:194–201.

80. Dickinson LD, Miller LD, Patel CP, Gupta SK. Enoxaparin

increases the incidence of postoperative intracranial hemorrhage when initiated preoperatively for deep venous thrombosis prophylaxis in patients with brain tumors. *Neurosurgery* 1998; **43**:1074–81.

81. Black PM, Baker MF, Snook CP. Experience with external pneumatic calf compression in neurology and neurosurgery. *Neurosurgery* 1986; **18**:440–4.

82. Naccarato M, Chiodo Grandi F, Dennis M, Sandercock PA. Physical methods for preventing deep vein thrombosis in stroke. *Cochrane Database Syst Rev* 2010; **4**:CD001922.

83. Lacut K, Bressollette L, Le Gal G, *et al.* Prevention of venous thrombosis in patients with acute intracerebral hemorrhage. *Neurology* 2005; **65**:865–9.

84. Claassen J, Peery S, Kreiter KT, *et al.* Predictors and clinical impact of epilepsy after subarachnoid hemorrhage. *Neurology* 2003; **60**(2):208–14.

85. Molyneux AJ, Kerr RS, Yu LM *et al.* International subarachnoid aneurysm trial (ISAT) of neurosurgical clipping versus endovascular coiling in 2143 patients with ruptured intracranial aneurysms: a randomised comparison of effects on survival, dependency, seizures, rebleeding, subgroups, and aneurysm occlusion. *Lancet* 2005; **366**(9488):809–17.

86. Little AS, Kerrigan JF, McDougall CG, *et al.* Nonconvulsive status epilepticus in patients suffering spontaneous subarachnoid hemorrhage. *J Neurosurg* 2007; **106**(5):805–11.

87. Claassen J, Mayer SA, Hirsch LJ. Continuous EEG monitoring in patients with subarachnoid hemorrhage. *J Clin Neurophysiol* 2005; **22**(2):92–8.

88. Dennis LJ, Claassen J, Hirsch LJ, *et al.* Nonconvulsive status epilepticus after subarachnoid

hemorrhage. *Neurosurgery* 2002; **51**:1136–43; discussion 1144.

89. Kull LL, Emerson RG. Continuous EEG monitoring in the intensive care unit: technical and staffing considerations. *J Clin Neurophysiol* 2005; **22**:107–18.

90. Naidech AM, Kreiter KT, Janjua N, *et al.* Phenytoin exposure is associated with functional and cognitive disability after subarachnoid hemorrhage. *Stroke* 2005; **36**(3):583–7.

91. Rosengart AJ, Huo JD, Tolentino J, *et al.* Outcome in patients with subarachnoid hemorrhage treated with antiepileptic drugs. *J Neurosurg* 2007; **107**(2):253–60.

92. Steinmetz H. Subarachnoidalblutung (SAB). In: Diener HC, Weimar C, ed. *Leitlinien für Diagnostik und Therapie in der Neurologie. 5. Auflage.* Stuttgart: Georg Thieme Verlag; 2012: 360–8.

93. Ohkuma H, Tsurutani H, Suzuki S. Incidence and significance of early aneurysmal rebleeding before neurosurgical or neurological management. *Stroke* 2001; **32**:1176–80.

94. Hijdra A, Vermeulen M, van Gijn J, van Crevel H. Rerupture of intracranial aneurysms: a clinicoanatomic study. *J Neurosurg* 1987; **67**:29–33.

95. de Gans K, Nieuwkamp DJ, Rinkel GJ, Algra A. Timing of aneurysm surgery in subarachnoid hemorrhage: a systematic review of the literature. *Neurosurgery* 2002; **50**:336–40; discussion 340–2.

96. David CA, Vishteh AG, Spetzler RF, *et al.* Late angiographic follow-up review of surgically treated aneurysms. *J Neurosurg* 1999; **91**(3):396–401.

97. Kassell NF, Torner JC, Haley EC Jr, *et al.* The International Cooperative Study on the Timing of Aneurysm Surgery. Part 1: overall management results. *J Neurosurg* 1990; **73**(1):18–36.

98. Raaymakers TW, Rinkel GJ, Ramos LM. Initial and follow-up screening for aneurysms in families with familial subarachnoid hemorrhage. *Neurology* 1998; **51**(4):1125–30.

99. Raabe A, Nakaji P, Beck J, *et al.* Prospective evaluation of surgical microscope integrated intraoperative near-infrared indocyanine green videoangiography during aneurysm surgery. *J Neurosurg* 2005; **103**:982–9.

100. Regli L, Dehdashti AR, Uske A, de Tribolet N. Endovascular coiling compared with surgical clipping for the treatment of unruptured middle cerebral artery aneurysms: an update. *Acta Neurochir Suppl* 2002; **82**:41–6.

101. Gruber DP, Zimmerman GA, Tomsick TA, *et al.* A comparison between endovascular and surgical management of basilar artery apex aneurysms. *J Neurosurg* 1999; **90**(5):868–74.

102. Regli L, Uske A, De Tribolet N. Endovascular coil placement compared with surgical clipping for the treatment of unruptured middle cerebral artery aneurysms: a consecutive series. *J Neurosurg* 1999; **90**(6):1025–30.

103. Guglielmi G, Vinuela F, Dion J, Duckwiler G. Electrothrombosis of saccular aneurysms via endovascular approach. Part 2: preliminary clinical experience. *J Neurosurg* 1991; **75**(1):8–14.

104. Brilstra EH, Rinkel GJ. Treatment of ruptured intracranial aneurysms by embolization with controlled detachable coils. *Neurologist* 2002; **8**(1):35–40.

105. Molyneux A, Kerr R, Stratton I, *et al.* International Subarachnoid Aneurysm Trial (ISAT) of neurosurgical clipping versus endovascular coiling in 2143 patients with ruptured intracranial aneurysms: a randomised trial. *Lancet* 2002; **360**(9342):1267–74.

106. Molyneux AJ, Kerr RSC, Birks J, *et al.*; ISAT Investigators. Risk of recurrent subarachnoid haemorrhage, death, or dependence and standardised mortality ratios after clipping or coiling of an intracranial aneurysm in the International Subarachnoid Aneurysm Trial (ISAT): long-term follow-up. *Lancet Neurol* 2009; **8**:427–33.

107. Scott RB, Eccles F, Molyneux AJ, *et al.* Improved cognitive outcomes with endovascular coiling or ruptured intracranial aneurysms. Neuropsychological outcomes from the International Subarachnoid Aneurysm Trial (ISAT). *Stroke* 2010; **41**:1743–7.

108. Johnston SC, Dowd CF, Higashida RT, *et al.* Predictors of rehemorrhage after treatment of ruptured intracranial aneurysms: the Cerebral Aneurysm Rerupture after Treatment (CARAT) study. *Stroke* 2008; **39**:120–5.

109. Mehta V, Holness RO, Connolly K, Walling S, Hall R. Acute hydrocephalus following aneurysmal subarachnoid hemorrhage. *Can J Neurol Sci* 1996; **23**(1):40–5.

110. Sheehan JP, Polin RS, Sheehan JM, Baskaya MK, Kassell NF. Factors associated with hydrocephalus after aneurysmal subarachnoid hemorrhage. *Neurosurgery* 1999; **45**(5):1120–7; discussion 1127–8.

111. Suarez-Rivera, O. Acute hydrocephalus after subarachnoid hemorrhage. *Surg Neurol* 1998; **49**(5):563–5.

112. Heros, RC. Acute hydrocephalus after subarachnoid hemorrhage. *Stroke* 1989; **20**:715–17.

113. Vatter H, Seifert V. Vasospasm pharmacology. *J Neurol Neurosurg Psychiatry* 2011; **82**:876–83.

114. Vergouwen MD, Vermeulen M, van Gijn J, *et al.* Definition of delayed cerebral ischemia after aneurysmal subarachnoid hemorrhage as an outcome event in clinical trials and observational studies: proposal of a multidisciplinary research group. *Stroke* 2010; **41**(10):2391–5.

115. Carrera E, Schmidt JM, Oddo M, *et al.* Transcranial Doppler for predicting delayed cerebral ischemia after subarachnoid hemorrhage. *Neurosurgery* 2009; **65**(2):316–23; discussion 323–4.

116. Lysakowski C, Walder B, Costanza MC, Tramer MR. Transcranial Doppler versus angiography in patients with vasospasm due to a ruptured cerebral aneurysm: a systematic review. *Stroke* 2001; **32**(10):2292–8.

117. Sloan MA, Alexandrov AV, Tegeler CH, *et al.* Assessment: transcranial Doppler ultrasonography: report of the Therapeutics and Technology Assessment Subcommittee of the American Academy of Neurology. *Neurology* 2004; **62**(9):1468–81.

118. Lindegaard KF, Nornes H, Bakke SJ, Sorteberg W, Nakstad P. Cerebral vasospasm after subarachnoid haemorrhage investigated by means of transcranial Doppler ultrasound. *Acta Neurochir Suppl (Wien)* 1988; **42**:81–4.

119. Unterberg AW, Sakowitz OW, Sarrafzadeh AS, Benndorf G, Lanksch WR. Role of bedside microdialysis in the diagnosis of cerebral vasospasm following aneurysmal subarachnoid hemorrhage. *J Neurosurg* 2001; **94**(5):740–9.

120. Wintermark M, Dillon WP, Smith WS, *et al.* Visual grading system for vasospasm based on perfusion CT imaging: comparisons with conventional angiography and quantitative perfusion CT. *Cerebrovasc Dis* 2008; **26**(2):163–70.

121. Chaudhary SR, Ko N, Dillon WP *et al.* Prospective evaluation of multidetector-row CT angiography for the diagnosis of vasospasm following subarachnoid hemorrhage: a comparison with digital subtraction angiography. *Cerebrovasc Dis* 2008; **25**(1–2):144–50.

122. Rinkel GJ, Feigin VL, Algra A, Vermeulen M, van Gijn J. Calcium antagonists for aneurysmal subarachnoid haemorrhage. *Cochrane Database Syst Rev* 2002; **4**:CD000277. Update in *Cochrane Database Syst Rev* 2005; **1**:CD000277.

123. Dorhout Mees SM, Rinkel GJ, Feigin VL, *et al.* Calcium antagonists for aneurysmal subarachnoid hemorrhage. *Cochrane Database Syst Rev* 2007; **3**:CD000277.

124. Pickard JD, Murray GD, Illingworth R, *et al.* Effect of oral nimodipine on cerebral infarction and outcome after subarachnoid haemorrhage: British aneurysm nimodipine trial. *BMJ* 1989; **298**(6674):636–42.

125. Unterberg AW. Subarachnoidalblutung/ Hirnarterienaneurysma. In: Piek J, Unterberg A, eds. *Grundlagen neurochirurgischer Intensivmedizin.* Munich: Zuckschwerdt Verlag GmbH; 2006: 331–47.

126. Allen GS, Ahn HS, Preziosi TJ, *et al.* Cerebral arterial spasm – a controlled trial of nimodipine in patients with subarachnoid hemorrhage. *N Engl J Med* 1983; **308**(11):619–24.

127. Raabe A, Beck J, Keller M, *et al.* Relative importance of hypertension compared with hypervolemia for increasing cerebral oxygenation in patients with cerebral vasospasm after subarachnoid hemorrhage. *J Neurosurg* 2005; **103**(6):974–81.

128. Dankbaar JW, Slooter AJC, Rinkel GJE, *et al.* Effect of different

components of triple-H therapy on cerebral perfusion in patients with aneurysmal subarachnoid haemorrhage: a systematic review. *Crit Care* 2010; **14**:R23.

129. Bejjani GK, Bank WO, Olan WJ, Sekhar LN. The efficacy and safety of angioplasty for cerebral vasospasm after subarachnoid hemorrhage. *Neurosurgery* 1998; **42**(5):979–86; discussion 986–7.

130. Hoh BL, Ogilvy CS. Endovascular treatment of cerebral vasospasm: transluminal balloon angioplasty, intra-arterial papaverine, and intra-arterial nicardipine. *Neurosurg Clin N Am* 2005; **16**(3):501–16.

131. Rosenwasser RH, Armonda RA, Thomas JE, *et al.* Therapeutic modalities for the management of cerebral vasospasm: timing of endovascular options. *Neurosurgery* 1999; **44**(5):975–9; discussion 979–80.

132. Feng L, Fitzsimmons BF, Young WL, *et al.* Intraarterially administered verapamil as adjunct therapy for cerebral vasospasm: safety and 2-year experience. *AJNR Am J Neuroradiol* 2002; **23**(8):1284–90.

133. Qureshi AI, Suri MF, Sung GY, *et al.* Prognostic significance of hypernatremia and hyponatremia among patients with aneurysmal subarachnoid hemorrhage. *Neurosurgery* 2002; **50**(4):749–55; discussion 755–6.

134. Audibert G, Steinmann G, de Talancé N, *et al.* Endocrine response after severe subarachnoid hemorrhage related to sodium and blood volume regulation. *Anesth Analg* 2009; **108**(6):1922–8.

135. Rinkel GJ, Wijdicks EF, Hasan D, *et al.* Outcome in patients with subarachnoid haemorrhage and negative angiography according to pattern of haemorrhage on computed tomography. *Lancet* 1991; **338**:964–8.

136. van der Schaaf IC, Velthuis BK, Gouw A, Rinkel GJ. Venous drainage in perimesencephalic hemorrhage. *Stroke* 2004; **35**(7):1614–18.

137. Huttner HB, Hartmann M, Kührmann M, *et al.* Repeated digital substraction angiography after perimesencephalic subarachnoid hemorrhage? *J Neuroradiol* 2006; **33**(2):87–9.

138. Hui FK, Tumialán LM, Tanaka T, Cawley CM, Zhang YJ. Clinical differences between angiographically negative, diffuse subarachnoid hemorrhage and perimesencephalic subarachnoid hemorrhage. *Neurocrit Care* 2009; **11**(1):64–70.

139. Greebe P, Rinkel GJ. Life expectancy after perimesencephalic subarachnoid hemorrhage. *Stroke* 2007; **38**(4):1222–4.

Further reading

Barth M, Capelle HH, Weidhauser S, *et al.* Effect of nicardipine prolonged-release implants on cerebral vasospasm and clinical outcome after severe aneurysmal subarachnoid hemorrhage: a prospective, randomized, double-blind phase IIa study. *Stroke* 2007; **38**(2):330–6.

Feigin VL, Lawes CM, Bennett DA, Barker-Collo SL, Parag V. Worldwide stroke incidence and early case fatality reported in 56 population-based studies: a systematic review. *Lancet Neurol* 2009; **8**(4):355–69.

Frontera JA, Fernandez A, Schmidt JM, *et al.* Defining vasospasm after subarachnoid hemorrhage: what is the most clinically relevant definition? *Stroke* 2009; **40**(6):1963–8.

Raabe A, Beck J, Berkefeld J, *et al.* Recommendations for the management of patients with aneurysmal subarachnoid hemorrhage. *Zentralbl Neurochir* 2005; **66**:79–91.

Report of World Federation of Neurological Surgeons Committee on a Universal Subarachnoid Hemorrhage Grading Scale. *J Neurosurg* 1988; **68**(6):985–6.

Rinkel GJE, Feigin VL, Algra A, *et al.* Circulatory volume expansion therapy for aneurysmal subarachnoid haemorrhage. *Cochrane Database Syst Rev* 2004; **4**: CD000483.

Rosengart AJ, Schultheiss KE, Tolentino J, Macdonald RL. Prognostic factors for outcome in patients with aneurysmal subarachnoid hemorrhage. *Stroke* 2007; **38**(8):2315–21.

Shea AM, Reed SD, Curtis LH, *et al.* Characteristics of nontraumatic subarachnoid hemorrhage in the United States in 2003. *Neurosurgery* 2007; **61**(6):1131–7; discussion 1137–8.

Whitfield PC, Kirkpatrick P. Timing of surgery for aneurysmal subarachnoid haemorrhage. *Cochrane Database Syst Rev* 2001; **2**: CD001697.

Chapter 13

Cerebral venous thrombosis

Jobst Rudolf

Introduction

Acute thrombosis of the cerebral sinuses and veins (cerebral venous thrombosis, CVT) is considered to be the cause of an acute stroke in approximately 1% of all stroke patients. However, the incidence of CVT is not known, as population-based studies are lacking. It has been estimated that annually about five to eight cases of CVT are identified among stroke patients of tertiary care hospitals [1]. Historically, CVT was considered a severe, almost inevitably fatal disease, as diagnosis in the pre-angiograph era was usually made post-mortem. However, modern neuroimaging techniques allow the diagnosis of CVT at an early stage and document that CVT is more frequent than was traditionally assumed, and that its prognosis is much better than is generally accepted, provided that the diagnosis is suspected, the respective neuroimaging examinations are performed in a timely manner, and therapy is initiated early, i.e. often with the diagnosis being clinically suspected only. The variety of clinical signs and symptoms renders the diagnosis of CVT a challenge to the physician. Diagnosis is still frequently overlooked or delayed due to the wide spectrum of clinical symptoms and the often subacute or lingering disease onset.

It is important to keep the diagnosis of CVT in mind in stroke cases that present with a fluctuating course, headache, epileptic seizures, or disturbances of the level of consciousness. With timely therapeutic intervention, CVT has a favorable prognosis, with an overall mortality rate of about 8% in recent studies [2]. However, thromboses of the inner cerebral veins as well as septic CVT remain severe diseases with high mortality rates.

Anatomy

The cerebral venous system consists of two distinct groups – the superficial and the deep cerebral veins – which eventually drain into the cerebral sinuses. The superficial veins of the brain that drain the cortex and the underlying white matter form a network of anastomoses that drain into the cortical sinuses, but number, diameter, and topography of these veins vary among individual patients. However, two major superficial veins can be identified in the majority of patients: the upper anastomotic vein of Trolard, which drains into the superior sagittal sinus, and the lower anastomotic vein of Labbé, which drains into the transverse sinus. Cerebral veins do not possess valves and therefore allow blood flow in both directions. This is the main reason why even larger thrombotic venous occlusions may remain clinically silent for a long time. In contrast, the deep veins that drain the basal ganglia and other deep subcortical structures do not possess the diversity of the superficial venous network. The basal veins of Rosenthal and the internal cerebral veins drain into the great cerebral vein of Galen and the straight sinus, and from there the transverse and sigmoid sinuses, finally reaching the vena cava via the jugular veins. Blood supply to the cerebellum and brainstem is drained from the posterior fossa by veins reaching the vein of Galen, the petrosal sinus or the lateral sinus. In contrast to veins, the cerebral sinuses are formed by duplication of the dura mater and are fixed to the osseous cranial structures. Thus, there is no possibility of influencing venous blood flow by means of vasoconstriction or vasodilatation.

Cerebral veins have a peculiar anatomy, as they do not follow the arteries as in other parts of the body.

Textbook of Stroke Medicine, Second Edition, ed. Michael Brainin and Wolf-Dieter Heiss. Published by Cambridge University Press. © Michael Brainin and Wolf-Dieter Heiss 2014.

Etiology

CVT may be due to infectious and non-infectious causes. Septic CVT is observed as a complication of bacterial infections of the visceral cranium, namely otitis, sinusitis, mastoiditis, and bacterial meningitis. The infectious agents reach the cerebral sinuses ascending via the draining veins of the face, the sinuses, or the ear, or following local inflammation that destroys osseous structures that separate the infectious focus from the brain. Clinical signs and symptoms of septic CVT comprise signs of systemic infection and of meningitis. Septic CVT remains a rare disease with high mortality in spite of modern therapeutic surgical and medical approaches (see below for details).

Aseptic CVT may stem from a variety of causes, all of them resembling those of extracranial thrombosis (Table 13.1). However, the cause of CVT remains unknown in approximately 15–20% of all patients, in spite of a thorough diagnostic workup [2–4].

> Septic CVT may be caused by bacterial infections of the visceral cranium, e.g. otitis, sinusitis, mastoiditis, and bacterial meningitis. Aseptic CVT may be caused by the same causes as extracranial thrombosis (see Table 13.1).

Pathophysiology

Venous thrombosis of the central nervous system (CNS) differs from arterial thromboses in many ways: venous thrombosis does not manifest acutely, as arterial thrombosis does, but is a subacute, often fluctuating process, in which endogenous prothrombotic and fibrinolytic processes occur concurrently. Regional cerebral blood flow (rCBF) is not significantly impaired, the autoregulation of cerebral perfusion is nearly fully maintained, and administration of acetazolamide induces – in contrast to arterial thrombosis – a significant increase of rCBF [5]. In venous congestion, disturbances of neuronal functional metabolism are tolerated for a much longer time than in arterial occlusion, and full recovery from severe focal and generalized neurological signs and symptoms may be observed in CVT even after weeks.

Intracranial hemorrhage is often observed in CVT, and its incidence may reach 40–50% [3, 6], a percentage significantly higher than in cerebral arterial thrombosis or embolism. The most common form of intracranial hematoma in CVT is intracerebral

Table 13.1. Potential causes of and risk factors associated with cerebral venous thrombosis [3, 4, 14, 16]

Genetic prothrombotic conditions
  Antithrombin III deficiency
  Protein C and protein S deficiency
  Factor V Leiden mutation and resistance to activated protein C
  Prothrombin G20210A mutation
  Mutations in the methylenetetrahydrofolate reductase (MTHFR) gene

Acquired prothrombotic states
  Nephrotic syndrome
  Antiphospholipid and anticardiolipin antibodies
  Homocysteinemia
  Pregnancy
  Puerperium

Infections
  Otitis, mastoiditis, sinusitis
  Meningitis
  Systemic infectious disease

Inflammatory disease
  Systemic lupus erythematosus
  Wegener's granulomatosis
  Sarcoidosis
  Inflammatory bowel disease (Crohn's disease, colitis ulcerosa)
  Adamantiades–Behçet disease

Hematological conditions
  Polycythemia, primary and secondary
  Thrombocythemia
  Leukemia
  Anemia, including paroxysmal nocturnal hemoglobinuria

Drugs
  Oral contraceptives
  Hormonal replacement therapy
  Steroids
  Cytotoxic drugs (e.g. asparaginase, tamoxifen)

Mechanical causes, trauma
  Head injury
  Injury to sinuses or jugular vein, jugular catheterization
  Neurosurgical procedures
  Lumbar puncture

Miscellaneous
  Dehydration, especially in children
  Cancer

bleeding, but subdural and – rarely – subarachnoid hemorrhage may be observed. In general, intracerebral hematoma in CVT is atypically localized in cortical and subcortical regions that do not correspond to territories of cerebral arteries. From a pathophysiological point of view, these bleedings are caused by the diapedesis of erythrocytes through the endothelial membrane, following the increase of the venous and capillary transmural pressure after venous thrombosis. The rationale for anticoagulant therapy with heparin or low molecular weight heparin (LMWH) is that preventing the re-occlusion of veins and sinuses reopened by endogenous fibrinolysis will result in a lowering of venous and capillary pressure. Thus, even in the presence of hemorrhage due to CVT, immediate anticoagulation results in clinical amelioration without increase in hematoma volume.

Hemorrhages are frequent in CVT.

Clinical features

Abrupt occlusion of a cerebral artery results in the acute manifestation of focal neurological symptoms due to ischemia of the brain tissue perfused by this artery. In contrast, CVT may remain clinically silent, as long as venous drainage is maintained by collateral veins or sinuses. Eventually, failure of collateral venous drainage will result in the gradual, fluctuating or progressive clinical manifestation of focal or generalized brain dysfunction. An exception to this rule is CVT in pregnancy and puerperium, where signs and symptoms of venous thrombosis may present within minutes or hours [7].

Clinical features of CVT differ according to the venous structures involved. Cortical CVT will present with signs and symptoms different from that of deep CVT, and septic CVT will show findings other than aseptic thrombosis.

In most prospective clinical series [2, 3, 6, 8], intense and diffuse headache was either the first (>70%) or the most common (75–90%) symptom of cortical venous thrombosis. Headache, as well as nausea, papilledema, visual loss, or sixth nerve palsy, is due to increased intracranial pressure. The onset of headache in CVT is subacute over hours and may precede the manifestation of other symptoms and signs by days or even weeks. Acute appearance of epileptic seizures is observed in 40–50% of all cases of CVT [2, 3, 6, 8], a percentage much higher than in arterial thrombosis of the brain. Seizures in CVT may present as simple partial seizures with post-ictal limb paresis or as complex partial seizures, and in both cases secondary generalization is often observed. Focal neurological signs may be observed in 30–50% of CVT patients [2, 3, 6, 8], but their localizing value is limited, due to the excellent collateralization of cerebral veins and the lack of venous valves that allows inversion of venous drainage in the case of localized thrombotic occlusion. Furthermore, the intensity of focal signs and symptoms may fluctuate over time. Motor symptoms may initially present as a monoparesis that gradually develops into a full-blown hemiparesis. With cortical CVT, higher cortical functions may be impaired, and aphasia or apraxia may be observed. Impairment of the level of consciousness (any degree from somnolence to deep coma) may be present in 30–50% of patients, and acute delirium or psychotic symptoms are observed in 20–25% [2, 3, 6, 8]. As a rule, extended thrombosis of cortical sinuses will result in symptoms and signs of generalized brain dysfunction (headache and other signs of increased intracranial pressure, impairment of the level of consciousness, generalized seizures), while isolated cortical venous thrombosis will result in focal neurological signs or focal seizures.

The rare thromboses of the inner cerebral veins (veins of Rosenthal, great vein of Galen, straight sinus, etc.) will result in a severe dysfunction of the diencephalon, reflected by coma and disturbances of eye movements and pupillary reflexes, a condition usually associated with poor outcome [9].

Thrombosis of the cavernous sinus may present with the characteristic combination of ocular chemosis, eye protrusion, painful ophthalmoplegia, trigeminal dysfunction, and – occasionally – papilledema. Cavernous sinus thrombosis may be unilateral, but the good collateralization between the cavernous sinuses, usually leads to bilateral symptoms, while extension of the thrombosis into the large sinuses is the exception. Most cases of cavernous sinus thrombosis are due to ascending infection from the orbita, the paranasal sinuses, or other structures of the viscerocranium and are accompanied by signs of local or systemic infection.

Symptoms of CVT are manifold: they may remain clinically silent as long as venous drainage is still maintained. Headache is the most common and frequently the first symptom of CVT. Epileptic seizures, focal neurological signs, impairment of the level of consciousness, and psychotic symptoms can occur.

Septic thrombosis of other sinuses is found as a complication of bacterial infection (e.g. otitis, mastoiditis, bacterial meningitis), and is always accompanied by symptoms and signs of systemic infection. Septic CVT accounts for about 5% of all cases of cerebral thrombosis, but its mortality remains extremely high.

> Septic CVT is accompanied by symptoms of systemic infection.

Diagnostic workup

Owing to the multitude of clinical manifestations as well as etiologies, the diagnosis of CVT presents a challenge to the clinical physician. The less distinct the clinical presentation is, the more difficult is the diagnosis of CVT. CVT may be suspected in the presence of headache and other signs of intracranial hypertension, alone or in combination with epileptic seizures and fluctuating neurological signs, especially if conditions are present that may favor thrombogenesis (e.g. bacterial infection, pregnancy and puerperium, malignancies, and known prothrombotic states; see Table 13.1). However, mono- or oligosymptomatic cases of CVT may be difficult to diagnose. In patients with signs and symptoms of systemic infection, CVT may be mistaken for meningo-encephalitis. The presence of CVT has to be suspected in young stroke patients, in painful stroke, in stroke with unusual presentation, and in patients with first-ever headache in combination with seizures of subtle focal signs.

The differential diagnosis of aseptic CVT comprises benign intracranial hypertension, but also all forms of intracranial hypertension due to neoplastic diseases. Aseptic thrombosis of the cavernous sinus leading to painful uni- or bilateral ophthalmoplegia has to be differentiated from the Tolosa–Hunt syndrome.

Computed tomography

Cerebral computed tomography (CCT) is widely available and is feasible in critically ill patients. Thus, CCT is often the first neuroimaging technique applied to patients with CVT and should be performed before and after the intravenous application of iodinated contrast media. However, CCT findings in CVT are often nonspecific and may consist of one or more of the following: localized or diffuse brain edema, focal hypodensities that do not comply with the boundaries of cerebral arterial territories, atypical hemorrhagic infarctions, or hematomas (Figure 13.1). Where available, CT venography may increase the

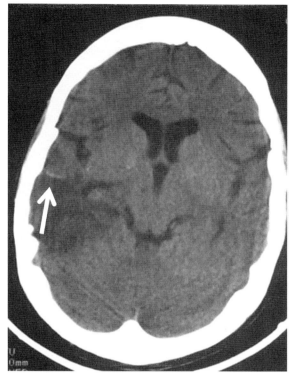

Figure 13.1. Unenhanced cranial computed tomography scan showing an atypical right temporal hemorrhagic venous infarction in a patient with isolated cortical venous thrombosis. Note the cord sign.

diagnostic yield of CCT in CVT [9]. CCT may be entirely normal in up to 25% of patients with angiographically proven CVT. Thus, the main indication of CCT in CVT is to rule out other conditions that may mimic or be confounded with CVT.

However, there are two CCT findings that – if present – are highly suggestive of CVT (Figures 13.1 and 13.2). The thrombotic occlusion of an isolated cortical vein may present as a thread-like hyperdense structure on non-contrast CCT ("cord sign"). After intravenous application of iodinated contrast media, the dura mater of the sinuses will show a distinct enhancement, and the non-enhancing intravenous thrombus may be discriminated as a triangle ("empty triangle" or "Delta-sign," in analogy to the design of the Greek capital letter Delta [Δ]). While the cord sign is found in up to 20% of CVT cases only, the Delta-sign has been described in 15–45% of CVT patients [10].

> A "cord sign," a thread-like hyperdense structure on non-contrast CCT, and a "Delta-sign," a triangle-shaped non-enhanced structure showing after application of

225

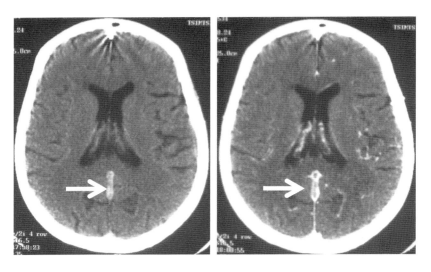

Figure 13.2. Cranial computed tomography in a patient with thrombosis of the straight sinus: the straight sinus presents as a hyperintense thread (cord sign) in non-enhanced CCT (left image), while after intravenous injection of iodinated contrast media the surrounding sinus structures show a distinct enhancement surrounding the thrombus (right image).

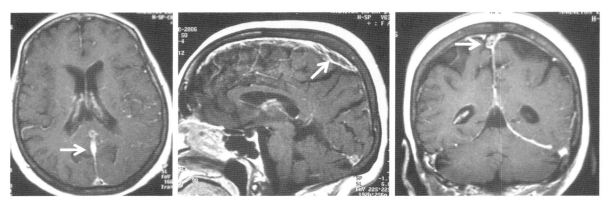

Figure 13.3. Magnetic resonance imaging (T1-weighted images after intravenous injection of paramagnetic contrast media) in a patient with thrombosis of the superior straight, sagittal, and right transverse sinus.

contrast media, are highly suggestive of CVT. Other findings are nonspecific, such as brain edema. The main indication of CCT in CVT is to rule out other conditions.

Magnetic resonance imaging

Cerebral magnetic resonance imaging (MRI, Figure 13.3) and magnetic resonance venography (MRV) are extremely sensitive in detecting CVT as well as the underlying parenchymal alterations. The ability of MRI and MRV to obtain images in various planes facilitates the visualization of the different cerebral sinuses. It is important to obtain – at least initially – tri-planar MRI in sagittal, axial, and coronal T1 and T2, T2*, and FLAIR sequences in combination with MRV, in order to minimize confusion of CVT

with sinus aplasia or hypoplasia and not to mistake the T2-weighted hypointense signal of deoxyhemoglobin and intracellular methemoglobin with flow voids [10, 11]. MRI and MRV allow direct imaging of the thrombus, whose signal intensity depends on clot age. Initially (days 1–5), thrombotic material gives an isointense signal on T1 images instead of the normal intraluminal flow void and a strongly hypointense signal on T2 images, indicating the presence of deoxyhemoglobin in erythrocytes of the thrombus. During the second week after clot formation, red blood cells are destroyed, and deoxyhemoglobin is metabolized into methemoglobin, and the thrombus yields a hyperintense signal on both T1- and T2-weighted images. After 2 weeks, the thrombus becomes hypointense on T1- and hyperintense on T2-weighted images, and recanalization may

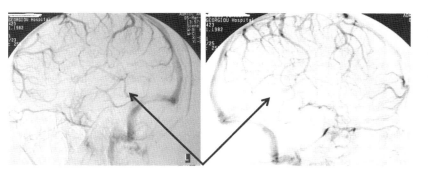

Figure 13.4. Digital subtraction angiography in a patient with isolated thrombosis of the right inferior anastomotic vein of Labbé (right), in contrast to physiological imaging of the cerebral vein findings of the contralateral hemisphere (left).

occur with the reappearance of flow void signaling. Partial or total recanalization is observed within 4–5 months after thrombosis [10–12]. MRI and MRV are non-invasive neuroimaging techniques and may easily be repeated for follow-up and reevaluation of the course of the disease. However, MRI and MRV are – in most cases – unable to detect isolated cortical venous thrombosis.

> MRI and MRV are highly sensitive in detecting CVT. They allow direct imaging of the thrombus; the signal intensity depends on clot age.

Digital subtraction angiography

Until recently, digital subtraction angiography (DSA) has been the gold standard for the diagnosis of CVT, documenting the partial filling of cerebral venous structures after intra-arterial injection of iodinated contrast media (Figure 13.4). However, DSA is an invasive diagnostic procedure, associated with a peri-procedural risk of death or stroke of about 1%. Furthermore, the interpretation of DSA (as of MRV or CT venography) may be complicated by the presence of anatomical variations, e.g. the hypoplasia of a transverse sinus [13]. Often, indirect signs of thrombosis, e.g. the dilatation of venous collaterals, or the regional prolongation of venous transition time, are the only findings that indicate the presence of CVT. Thus, the role of DSA in the diagnosis of CVT remains restricted to those patients where the clinical suspicion cannot be corroborated by other neuroimaging techniques.

> Owing to the high peri procedural risk, DSA is nowadays restricted to patients where other neuroimaging techniques are not feasible.

Other diagnostic findings

The diagnosis of CVT is based on the detection of venous thrombosis by the neuroimaging techniques described above. As differential diagnosis of CVT comprises a large number of diseases, diagnostic workup in patients with the final diagnosis of CVT requires extensive laboratory exams as well as other auxiliary testing: lumbar puncture, EEG, and transcranial duplex ultrasound are often performed, but most findings are nonspecific.

Most routine laboratory findings in the acute phase of aseptic CVT are nonspecific: mild leukocytosis, elevated erythrocyte sedimentation rate, and C-reactive protein (CRP) are the most common abnormalities. Acute thrombosis may be suspected if the D-dimers, a fibrinogen degradation product, are found to be elevated. However, elevated D-dimers just indicate active thrombosis (anywhere in the body), and normal values for D-dimers do not exclude acute CVT [14, 15].

Other laboratory markers for acute thrombosis include plasminogen activator inhibitor 1 (PAI-1), thrombin–antithrombin (TAT), and plasmin–antiplasmin (PAP) complexes. However, their diagnostic value in the acute phase of CVT is under debate, and testing is not widely available.

After the diagnosis of acute CVT, a thorough thrombophilia screening (Table 13.2) should be performed in all patients, but – if that is not feasible at a certain institution – at least patients with recurrent thromboembolic events or those with a positive family history of such disease should be referred to a specialized center for a hematological workup. Testing for protein C, protein S, and antithrombin deficiency should be performed 2 to 4 weeks after the completion of anticoagulation (see below), as there is only a very limited value of testing of these parameters in the acute setting or in patients under anticoagulation with vitamin K antagonists.

As the clinical features of CVT may be mistaken for those of meningo-encephalitis, lumbar puncture is

227

Table 13.2. Suggested thrombophilia screening in patients with cerebral venous thrombosis

Genetic prothrombotic conditions
    Antithrombin III
    Protein S
    Protein C
    Activated protein (APC) resistance
    Mutations in the MTHFR gene
    Prothrombin AG20210 mutation
    FV-Leiden mutation
    Factor VIII

Acquired prothrombotic conditions
    Homocysteine
    Vitamin B12
    Folic acid

Inflammatory diseases
    Lupus anticoagulant
    Anticardiolipin IgG and IgM antibodies
    Anti-beta2-glycoprotein IgG and IgM antibodies
    Anti-prothrombin IgG and IgM antibodies

often performed in these patients. Cerebrospinal fluid (CSF) findings in acute CVT include increased CSF pressure, a mild pleocytosis, and elevated CSF protein in about 50% of patients. However, these findings are nonspecific and do not allow the diagnosis of CVT. The diagnostic value of lumbar puncture in CVT patients is the exclusion of definite infectious meningo-encephalitis (or its diagnosis in septic CVT).

EEG in CVT patients may show focal or generalized slowing, or even focal or generalized epileptic discharges. However, EEG findings may be physiological in up to 25% of patients.

Transcranial duplex sonography may disclose an elevation in venous flow velocities in patients with severe CVT.

> Laboratory parameters and CSF findings in aseptic CVT are nonspecific. Normal values for D-dimers do not exclude acute CVT.
>
> Lumbar puncture is necessary to exclude or confirm infectious meningo-encephalitis in septic CVT. Thrombophilia screening should be performed especially in patients with recurrent thromboembolic events.

Therapy

Patients with acute CVT may present with signs and symptoms of acutely increased intracranial pressure or extended venous infarctions, and are in danger of dying within hours from cerebral herniation.

Impaired consciousness and cerebral hemorrhage on admission are associated with a poor outcome. The treatment priority in the acute phase is to stabilize the patient and to prevent herniation, followed by the initiation of anticoagulant treatment and the treatment of underlying causes, especially bacterial infections. As for all patients with acute stroke, patients with suspected CVT should be admitted to a stroke unit, in order to optimize care and minimize complications.

In 2010, the European Federation of Neurological Societies published the revision of its evidence-based guideline on the treatment of CVT [1], which is outlined in the following sections. In 2011, the management of CVT was also addressed in a statement for healthcare professionals issued by the Council on Stroke of the American Heart Association/American Stroke Association [16].

> Acute management:
>
> stabilization of the patient
> initiation of anticoagulant treatment
> prevention of herniation
> management of complications
> treatment of underlying causes, especially bacterial infections.

Anticoagulation

The rationale for immediate anticoagulation therapy in patients with definite and acute CVT is to stop prothrombotic processes and allow endogenous fibrinolysis to recanalize the occluded veins and sinuses. However, concern has been raised about the possible dangers of anticoagulation in the presence of hemorrhagic venous infarction, found in up to 40% of all CVT patients [2]. The issue has been addressed in two small randomized controlled trials [6, 8] that compared anticoagulant treatment with dose-adjusted unfractionated heparin (UFH [8]) or weight-adjusted LMWH (nadroparin 90 anti-Xa units/kg body weight bid) with placebo treatment [6]. The first study was terminated after inclusion of 10 patients in each group, as an interim analysis documented a beneficial effect of heparin treatment on morbidity and mortality. The second study documented a relative risk reduction for poor outcome of 38% with LMWH treatment, without reaching statistical significance. Both studies were criticized for inadequately small sample size [8] or baseline imbalance favoring the placebo group [6]. Patients with intracranial hemorrhage were included in both studies, and no new symptomatic cerebral hemorrhage occurred in either treatment group. A meta-analysis of the studies on immediate anticoagulation treatment for acute CVT showed a non-significant reduction in the pooled relative risk of death or dependency [17].

In the International Study on Cerebral Vein and Dural Sinus Thrombosis (ISCVT) study [2], more than 80% of the enrolled patients with CVT were treated with anticoagulation (two-thirds of patients received dose-adjusted UFH, one-third were treated with LMWH). A minority of patients received either low-dose LMWH antiplatelet treatment or no anticoagulants at all. There was a non-significant trend towards favorable outcome in patients under anticoagulation treatment compared with those not receiving anticoagulation, but no differences in treatment safety or efficacy were observed between patients on UFH or LMWH.

Based on the results of these studies, meta-analyses and observational data, both UFH and LMWH are considered safe and probably effective in CVT, and immediate anticoagulation is recommended even in the presence of hemorrhagic venous infarcts [1, 16]. When using intravenous UFH, the therapeutic goal is the doubling of activated partial thromboplastin time (aPTT), while LMWH is administered subcutaneously twice daily in a body-weight-adjusted total dose of 180 (2 × 90) anti-Xa units per day. Whether treatment with full-dose UFH or subcutaneously applied LMWH is equally effective for CVT is not clear, as direct comparisons are lacking. A meta-analysis which compared the efficacy of fixed-dose subcutaneous LMWH versus adjusted-dose UFH for extracerebral venous thromboembolism found superiority for LMWH and significantly fewer major bleeding complications [18]. Other advantages of LMWH include the subcutaneous instead of intravenous route of administration, which increases the mobility of patients, and the lack of a need for laboratory monitoring and subsequent dose adjustments. The advantage of dose-adjusted intravenous heparin therapy, particularly in critically ill patients, may be the fact that the aPTT normalizes within 1–2 hours after discontinuation of the infusion, if complications occur or surgical intervention becomes necessary. In addition, the anticoagulatory effect of heparin may be immediately antagonized with protamine, which is much less effective in LMWH treatment. Following current guidelines, and for the reasons mentioned above, LMWH should be preferred over heparin in uncomplicated CVT cases [1].

> Immediate anticoagulation is recommended, even in the presence of hemorrhagic venous infarcts.
> In critically ill patients, dose-adjusted intravenous heparin therapy (therapeutic goal: doubling of activated partial thromboplastin time [aPTT]) has the advantage of a short half-life and the possibility of antagonization with protamine. In uncomplicated CVT cases, LMWH should be preferred over heparin (dose: body-weight-adjusted 90 anti-Xa units twice daily).

Long-term treatment of CVT – as of other forms of venous thrombosis – with intravenous UFH or subcutaneous LMWH poses the question of patient compliance. Therefore, a switch to oral anticoagulation with vitamin K antagonists aiming at an international normalized ratio (INR) of 2.0–3.0 is recommended after the patient's condition has stabilized [1, 16]. There are insufficient data to determine the optimal duration of oral anticoagulation with vitamin K antagonists. As recanalization of occluded cerebral veins is observed until 5 months after diagnosis [12], it is suggested that effective anticoagulation should be performed for about 6 months after diagnosis of CVT. If no underlying disease is identified that justifies the continuation of oral anticoagulation, treatment with vitamin K antagonists should be stopped and antiplatelets (e.g. acetylsalicylic acid 100 mg qid) should be given for at least another 6 months [16]. Alternatively, and in analogy to patients with extracerebral venous thrombosis, oral anticoagulation may be given for 3 months if CVT was secondary to a transient risk factor, and for 6–12 months if it was idiopathic [19].

According to current guidelines [1, 16], oral anticoagulation is recommended for 6–12 months in patients with CVT and a "mild" hereditary thrombophilia such as protein C and S deficiency, or heterozygous factor V Leiden or prothrombin G20210A mutations. Long-term treatment should be considered for patients with a "severe" hereditary thrombophilia which carries a high risk of recurrence, such as antithrombin III deficiency, homozygous factor V Leiden mutation, or two or more thrombophilic conditions. "Indefinite" anticoagulation is recommended in patients with two or more episodes of idiopathic objectively documented extracerebral venous thrombosis [19]. In general, in the absence of controlled data, the decision on the duration of anticoagulant therapy must be based on individual hereditary and precipitating factors predisposing to CVT as well as on the potential bleeding risks of long-term oral anticoagulation. Regular follow-up visits should be performed after termination of anticoagulation and patients should be informed about early signs and symptoms (e.g. headache) indicating a possible relapse.

> For long-term treatment of CVT, a switch to oral anticoagulation with vitamin K antagonists (therapeutic goal: INR 2.0–3.0) is recommended. The duration of effective anticoagulation depends on CVT etiology.

Thrombolysis

Despite immediate anticoagulation, some patients show a distinct deterioration of their clinical condition, and this risk seems to be especially high in patients presenting with focal neurological signs and reduction of the level of consciousness. The recent ISCVT study identified coma on admission and thrombosis of the deep venous system apart from underlying causes as the most important predictors of a poor clinical outcome [2]. Thrombolytic therapy has the potential to provide faster restitution of venous outflow, and positive effects of both systemic and local thrombolytic treatment of CVT have been reported from case reports and small uncontrolled series. However, systematic reviews of thrombolysis in CVT do not show sufficient evidence to support the use of either systemic or local thrombolysis in this disorder [20, 21]. A potential publication bias in the current published work has been assumed, with possible under-reporting of cases with poor outcome and complications. In addition, treatment and assessment were non-blind, leading to a possible bias in outcome assessment [14].

Current guidelines [1, 16] state that there is insufficient evidence to support the use of either systemic or local thrombolysis in patients with CVT. If patients deteriorate despite adequate anticoagulation and other causes of deterioration have been ruled out, thrombolysis may be a therapeutic option in selected cases, possibly in those without hemorrhagic infarction or intracranial hemorrhage. However, optimal substance (urokinase or recombinant tissue plasminogen activator [rtPA]), dosage, route (systemic or local), and method of administration (repeated bolus or bolus plus infusion) are not known.

> Thrombolysis is not recommended in current guidelines.

Other therapeutic interventions

The use of direct intrasinus thrombolytic techniques and mechanical therapies (catheter thrombectomy, balloon-assisted thrombectomy) is only supported by case reports and small open case series. If clinical deterioration occurs despite the use of anticoagulation, or if the patient develops mass effect from a venous infarction or an intracerebral hemorrhage that causes intracranial hypertension resistant to standard therapies, these interventional techniques may be considered [16].There are no controlled trials or observational studies that address the role of aspirin in CVT management [16].

Symptomatic therapy

Symptomatic treatment of acute CVT comprises analgesia, sedation of agitated patients, management of epileptic seizures, and treatment of elevated intracranial pressure.

Pain, nausea, and agitation

Headache is the main symptom of CVT, may cause considerable agitation, and should be treated accordingly. Mild to moderate headache in CVT patients should be treated with paracetamol. Acetylsalicylic acid should be avoided, as the patient's bleeding risk may be increased due to the concomitant anticoagulation treatment. Severe headache may require treatment with opioids, but dose titration should be performed cautiously in order to avoid over-sedation.

Concomitant nausea requires parenteral antiemetic treatment with metoclopramide, minor neuroleptics (e.g. levopromazine, chlorpromazine) or HT_3 antagonists (e.g. ondansetron, granisetron).

If sedation of agitated patients is required, first-choice drugs are major neuroleptics (e.g. haloperidol), because they do not have a relevant impact on the patient's level of consciousness. It has to be kept in mind that other sedative drugs (e.g. benzodiazepines) impair the evaluation of the course of the disease and, therefore, their use should be restricted to necessary diagnostic or therapeutic interventions.

> For the treatment of headaches, paracetamol should be preferred over acetylsalicylic acid because of the patient's bleeding risk.

Epileptic seizures

All CVT patients presenting with seizures should receive antiepileptic treatment, as the risk of seizure recurrence and status epilepticus is extremely high.

For the same reason, effective drug plasma levels should be achieved as soon as possible. Therefore, first-line antiepileptic drugs (AEDs) in CVT patients are those that can be administered parenterally and allow a dosage that reaches therapeutic plasma drug levels within a short time, e.g. phenytoin, valproic acid, and levetiracetam.

There are insufficient data regarding the effectiveness of a prophylactic use of AEDs in patients with CVT. One study identified focal sensory deficits and the presence of focal edema or infarcts on admission CT/MRI as significant predictors of early symptomatic seizures [22]. These findings suggest that prophylactic treatment with AEDs may be a therapeutic option for those patients, whereas treatment is not warranted when there are no focal neurological deficits and no focal parenchymal lesions on brain scan (e.g. patients with isolated intracranial hypertension).

In spite of the high incidence of epileptic seizures in the acute phase of CVT, the risk of residual epilepsy is low, with reported incidence rates between 5% and 10.6% [2, 22] and the vast majority of late seizures occurring within the first year. A hemorrhagic lesion in the acute brain scan was the strongest predictor of post-acute seizures [22]. Late seizures are more common in patients with early symptomatic seizures than in those patients with none. Thus, prolonged treatment with AEDs for 1 year may be reasonable for patients with early seizures and a hemorrhagic lesion on admission CCT or MRI, whereas in patients without these risk factors, antiepileptic therapy may be tapered off gradually after the acute stage.

Current guidelines [1] state that prophylactic antiepileptic therapy may be an option in patients with focal neurological deficits and focal parenchymal lesions on admission CT/MRI, but that the optimal duration of treatment for patients with seizures remains unclear.

> Epileptic seizures should be treated with parenterally administered antiepileptic drugs (phenytoin, valproic acid, levetiracetam). Prophylactic treatment with antiepileptic drugs may be an option in patients with focal sensory deficits and focal edema or infarcts on admission CT/MRI.

Elevated intracranial pressure

Localized or diffuse brain edema is observed in about 50% of all patients with CVT. However, minor brain swelling (e.g. not resulting in midline shift or uncal herniation) needs no other treatment than anticoagulation, as anticoagulation improves venous drainage to a degree that effectively reduces intracranial pressure.

In patients with the clinical signs of isolated intracranial hypertension only, but threatened vision due to papilledema, lumbar puncture with sufficient CSF removal should be performed. In these patients, anticoagulation may be started 24 hours after CSF removal. This intervention is usually followed by a rapid improvement of headache and visual function. Although controlled data are lacking, acetazolamide should be considered in patients not responding to lumbar puncture. If visual function continues to deteriorate despite CSF removal and acetazolamide therapy, shunting procedures (lumbo-peritoneal shunting, optic nerve fenestration) are recommended [1, 16].

In the case of severe brain swelling, anti-edema treatment should follow the general rules for the treatment of raised intracranial pressure, i.e. head elevation to 30°, osmotic diuretics (e.g. glycerol or mannitol), and – after admission to an ICU – moderate controlled hyperventilation with a target pCO_2 of 30–35 mmHg. However, in CVT, osmodiuretic drugs are not as quickly eliminated from the intracerebral circulation as in other conditions of increased intracranial pressure. Osmodiuretics may thus reduce venous drainage and should therefore be used with caution only. Volume restriction should be avoided, as dehydration may further increase blood viscosity. Steroids cannot be generally recommended for treatment of elevated intracranial pressure, since their efficacy is unproven and their administration may be harmful, as steroids may promote the thrombotic process [1, 16, 23]. In single patients with impending herniation due to a unilateral hemispheric lesion, decompressive hemicraniectomy can be life-saving and even allow a good functional recovery, but evidence is anecdotal [24]. Decompressive hemicraniectomy may be needed as a live-saving measure, if large venous infarction leads to a critical increase in intracranial pressure. Likewise, large hematomas rarely may need to be considered for surgical evacuation, if associated with a progressive and severe neurological deficit [1, 16].

> Increased intracranial pressure in most cases responds to improved venous drainage after anticoagulation. In some patients with lumbar puncture with CSF removal, acetazolamide might be required.
> Steroids are not recommended, as they may promote the thrombotic process.

Infectious thrombosis

Infectious CVT requires immediate broad-spectrum antibiotic treatment and – often – surgical treatment of the underlying disease (e.g. otitis, sinusitis, mastoiditis). Until the results of microbiological cultures are available, third-generation cephalosporins (e.g. cefotaxime 2 g tid or ceftriaxone 2 g bid i.v.) should be given. As in aseptic CVT, anticoagulation should be initiated immediately and symptomatic therapy of septic CVT should adhere to the principles outlined for aseptic CVT, although controlled studies on the efficacy of these measures in septic CVT are lacking.

> Infectious CVT requires immediate broad-spectrum antibiotic treatment and often surgical treatment of the underlying disease.

Prognosis

The vital and functional prognosis of patients with acute CVT, as established in the ISCVT cohort, is astonishingly favorable, with an overall death or dependency rate of about 15% [2]. Long-term predictors of poor prognosis are the presence of CNS infection, malignancy, deep venous system thrombosis, intracranial hemorrhage, coma upon admission, age, and male sex.

In the acute phase of CVT, the case fatality is around 4–8% [2, 14]. The main causes of acute death are transtentorial herniation secondary to a large hemorrhagic lesion, multiple brain lesions, or diffuse brain edema. Other causes of acute death include status epilepticus, medical complications, and pulmonary embolism. Deterioration after admission occurs in about 23% of patients, with worsening of mental status, headache or focal deficits, or with new symptoms such as seizures. A new parenchymal lesion is present in one-third of patients who deteriorate. Fatalities after the acute phase are predominantly associated with the underlying disorder. The individual prognosis is difficult to predict, but the overall vital and functional prognosis of CVT is much better than that of arterial stroke, with about two-thirds of CVT patients recovering without sequelae [14].

> The overall death or dependency rate is about 15%.

Recurrence of cerebral venous thrombosis

After the acute phase of CVT, anticoagulation is continued not only to facilitate the recanalization of the occluded cerebral veins, but also in order to prevent the recurrence of intra- or extracerebral thrombosis. Recurrent CVT may be difficult to diagnose, if follow-up MRI or MRV examinations are not available. Therefore, it seems feasible to repeat MR venography in CVT patients after 4–6 months, as further recanalization cannot be expected after this point. This follow-up venography may serve as a reference in those cases where recurrent CVT is suspected.

However, recurrence of CVT is rarely observed, and the manifestation of other (extracerebral) thrombotic events is observed in about 5% of CVT patients [2]. This should be pointed out to patients recovering from CVT, who may need reassuring of the very low risk of further thrombotic events.

As pregnancy and puerperium are conditions that favor the manifestation of CVT, concern has been raised about the risk of future pregnancies in women with CVT. On the basis of available evidence, CVT and even pregnancy- or puerperium-related CVT are no contraindication for future pregnancies. Antithrombotic prophylaxis during pregnancy is probably unnecessary, unless a prothrombotic disorder has been diagnosed. However, women on vitamin K antagonists should be advised not to become pregnant because of the teratogenic effects of these drugs [14].

Special aspects
CVT in pregnancy and puerperium

Pregnancy induces changes in the coagulation system that persist into puerperium and result in a hypercoagulable state, which increases the risk of CVT. The greatest risk period includes the third trimester of pregnancy and the first post-partum weeks. Vitamin K antagonists as well as unfractionated heparin are associated with both the risk of fetal embryopathy and bleeding in the fetus and neonate and thus are generally conisdered to be contraindicated in pregnancy. Therefore, in the majority of women with CVT in pregnancy and puerperium, anticoagulation therapy will consist of LMWH until birth, and should be continued for at least 6 weeks post-partum, either with LMWH or vitamin K antagonists. As in non-pregnant women, fibrinolytic therapy is restricted to patients with deterioration in spite of systemic anticoagulation, and its use has been reported in pregnancy. On the basis of the available evidence, CVT is not a contraindication for further pregnancies.

However, considering the additional risk that pregnancy confers to women with a history of CVT, prophylaxis with LMWH during further pregnancies and puerperium should be considered beneficial (see Saposnik et al. [16] for details).

CVT in neonates

While the symptomatology, etiology, and therapy of CVT in older children resemble those of adult CVT in most respects, in neonates the causes, clinical presentation, outcome, and management are very different. Manifestation of CVT in neonates seems to be associated with maternal risk factors (hypertension, [pre-] eclampsia, gestational or chronic diabetes mellitus). The vast majority of neonates present with an acute illness at the time of diagnosis, most often dehydration, cardiac defects, sepsis, or meningitis. Leading clinical symptoms are epileptic seizures in two-thirds and respiratory distress or apnea in one-third of the neonates. There is a high incidence of intracranial hemorrhages (40–60% hemorrhagic infarctions, 20% intraventricular bleedings). A significant number of children are left with a considerable impairment (motor or cognitive deficits, epilepsy). Treatment is mostly symptomatic and comprises rehydration, antibiotics in the case of sepsis, and antiepileptic therapy. Heparin is rarely used in neonates, although a pilot study did not show any detrimental effect [25].

Taken together, the nonspecific presentation of neonatal CVT and its common association with an acute illness make the diagnosis even more difficult than in adults or older children. There is no consensus on heparin therapy in neonates, and the prognosis of CVT in neonates is more severe than in adults [14, 26].

CVT in elderly patients

Only recently, older patients were identified as a distinct subgroup of CVT patients. In ISCVT, about 8% of all patients were older than 65 years [27]. In general, these patients presented with clinical symptoms and signs different from those in younger patients: isolated intracranial hypertension was uncommon, whereas disturbances of mental status, alertness, and the level of consciousness were common. Carcinoma was found more often in older patients with CVT. The prognosis was worse, with half of the patients being dead or dependent at the end of follow-up.

Future developments

Many issues in the etiology, diagnosis, and management of CVT are still unresolved and controversially discussed. Epidemiological data on CVT are lacking from many parts of the world. Open questions concern many of our current management decisions, such as the role of local or systemic thrombolysis, decompressive hemicraniectomy, initiation and duration of antiepileptic prophylaxis, and the duration of anticoagulation treatment. It is mandatory to increase the level of evidence supporting our diagnostic or therapeutic decisions through prospective registries, case–control studies, and, whenever possible, randomized controlled trials. As CVT is a rare disease with few cases diagnosed annually even at large tertiary healthcare facilities, close cooperation between these centers is necessary to achieve progress in the diagnosis and treatment of CVT.

Chapter summary

Clinical features
The most common and frequently the first symptom of CVT is headache. The onset of headache in CVT is subacute over hours and is due to the increased intracranial pressure.
Epileptic seizures, focal neurological signs, impairment of the level of consciousness, and psychotic symptoms can occur.
Septic CVT is accompanied by symptoms of systemic infection.

Diagnostic workup
The main indication of CCT is to rule out other conditions.
MRI and MRV are highly sensitive in detecting CVT. They allow direct imaging of the thrombus; the signal intensity depends on clot age.
The diagnostic value of lumbar puncture in CVT patients is the exclusion or confirmation of infectious meningo-encephalitis in septic CVT.

Therapy
Stabilization of the patient.
Prevention of herniation.
Immediate initiation of anticoagulant treatment (LMWH with a body-weight-adjusted dose of 90 anti-Xa units twice daily or intravenous heparin with the therapeutic goal of doubling of aPTT).

Treatment of bacterial infections with broad antibiotics and surgery.

Switch to oral anticoagulation with vitamin K antagonists (therapeutic goal: INR 2.0–3.0) for long-term treatment.

Treatment of epileptic seizures with parenterally administered antiepileptic drugs (phenytoin, valproic acid, levetiracetam).

Acknowledgement

The author expresses his gratitude to Dr. Ioannis Tsitouridis, Director of the Department of Diagnostic Radiology at the General Hospital "Papageorgiou" (Thessaloniki, Greece), in whose department the neuroimaging procedures shown in this article were performed.

References

1. Einhäupl K, Stam J, Bousser MG, et al. EFNS guidelines on the treatment of cerebral venous and sinus thrombosis in adult patients. Eur J Neurol 2010; 17:1229–35.

2. Ferro JM, Canhao P, Stam J, et al. Prognosis of cerebral vein and dural sinus thrombosis. Results of the International Study on Cerebral Vein and Dural Sinus Thrombosis (ISCVT). Stroke 2004; 35:664–70.

3. Amery A, Bousser MG. Cerebral venous thrombosis. Clin Neurol 1992; 19:87–111.

4. Stam J. Thrombosis of the cerebral veins and sinuses. N Engl J Med 2005; 352:1791–8.

5. Schmiedek P, Einhaupl KM, Moser E. Cerebral blood flow in patients with sinus venous thrombosis. In: Einhaupl KM, Kempski O, Baethmann A, eds. Cerebral Sinus Thrombosis: Experimental and Clinical Aspects. New York: Plenum Press; 1990: 75–83.

6. De Bruijn SFTM, Stam J, for the Cerebral Venous Sinus Thrombosis Study Group. Randomized, placebo-controlled trial of anticoagulant treatment with low-molecular-weight heparin for cerebral sinus thrombosis. Stroke 1999; 30:484–8.

7. Cantu C, Barinagarrementiera F. Cerebral venous thrombosis associated with pregnancy and puerperium: a review of 67 cases. Stroke 1993; 24:1880–4.

8. Einhaupl K, Villringer A, Meister W, et al. Heparin treatment in sinus venous thrombosis. Lancet 1991; 338:597–600.

9. Van den Bergh WM, van der Schaaf I, van Gijn J. The spectrum of presentations of deep venous infarction caused by deep cerebral vein thrombosis. Neurology 2005; 65:192–6.

10. Renowden S. Cerebral venous sinus thrombosis. Eur Radiol 2004; 14:215–26.

11. Tsitouridis I, Papapostolou P, Rudolf J, et al. Non-neoplastic dural sinus thrombosis: an MRI and MRV evaluation. Riv Neuroradiol 2005; 18:581–8.

12. Baumgartner RW, Studer A, Arnold M, et al. Recanalization of cerebral venous thrombosis. J Neurol Neurosurgery Psychiatry 2003; 74:459–61.

13. Bono F, Lupo MR, Lavano A, et al. Cerebral MR venography of transverse sinuses in subjects with normal CSF pressure. Neurology 2003; 61:1267–70.

14. Bousser MG, Ferro J. Cerebral venous thrombosis: an update. Lancet Neurol 2007; 6:162–70.

15. Lalive PH, de Moerloose P, Lovblad K, et al. Is measurement of D-dimer useful in the diagnosis of cerebral venous thrombosis? Neurology 2003; 61:1057–60.

16. Saposnik G, Barinagarrementeria F, Brown HD, et al. Diagnosis and management of cerebral venous thrombosis: a statement for healthcare professionals from the American Heart Association/American Stroke Association. Stroke 2011; 42:1158–92.

17. Coutinho J, de Bruijn SF, Deveber G, Stam J. Anticoagulation for cerebral sinus thrombosis. Cochrane Database Syst Rev 2011; 8:CD002005.

18. Van Donden CJJ, van den Belt AGM, Prins HM, et al. Fixed dose subcutaneous low molecular weight heparins versus adjusted dose unfractionated heparin for venous thromboembolism. Cochrane Database Syst Rev 2004; 4:CD001100.

19. Buller HR, Agnelli G, Hull RH, et al. Antithrombotic therapy for venous thromboembolic disease. The seventh ACCP conference on antithrombotic and thrombolytic therapy. Chest 2004; 126:401–28.

20. Canhao P, Falcao F, Ferro JM. Thrombolytics for cerebral sinus thrombosis: a systematic review. Cerebrovasc Dis 2003; 15:159–66.

21. Ciccone A, Canhao P, Falcao F, Ferro JM, Sterzi R. Thrombolysis for cerebral vein and dural sinus thrombosis. Cochrane Database Syst.Rev 2004; 1:CD003693.

22. Ferro JM, Correia M, Rosas MJ, et al. Seizures in cerebral vein and dural sinus thrombosis. Cerebrovasc Dis 2003; 15:78–83.

23. Canhao P, Cortesao A, Cabral M, et al. Are steroids useful for the treatment of cerebral venous thrombosis? ISCVT results. Cerebrovasc Dis 2004; 17 (Suppl 5):16.

24. Rudolf J, Hilker R, Terstegge K, *et al.* Extended haemorrhagic infarction following isolated cortical venous thrombosis. *Eur Neurol* 1999; **41**:115–16.

25. deVeber G, Chan A, Monagle P, *et al.* Anticoagulation therapy in pediatric patients with sinovenous thrombosis: a cohort study. *Arch Neurol* 1998; **55**:1533–7.

26. Golomb MR. Sinovenous thrombosis in neonates. *Semin Cerebrovasc Dis Stroke* 2001; **1**:216–24.

27. Ferro JM, Canhao P, Bousser M-G, Barinagarrementeria F. Cerebral vein and dural sinus thrombosis in elderly patients. *Stroke* 2005; **36**:1927–32.

Chapter 1

Behavioral neurology of stroke

José M. Ferro, Isabel P. Martins, and Lara Caeiro

Introduction

Mental functions are the essence of mankind. The cognitive systems of the human brain allow us to build internal representations of the world that can be shared with our conspecifics, simulated, used to understand others' feelings and intentions, or to judge and plan actions into the future.

Mental representations are based on a large-scale neuronal network called the conceptual representation system or semantic system. It comprises modality specific and multimodal convergent regions [1] and is connected with more circumscribed and lateralized operational systems that allow us to translate thoughts into words (spoken or written), images, numbers, or other symbols, to store and retrieve information when necessary, and to make decisions or act upon them. Most of these operational abilities are subserved by distributed networks with areas of regional specialization, organized according to their specific processing capacities.

Cerebral lesions can produce different types of cognitive and behavioral dysfunction but the pattern of impairment observed after ischemic stroke is relatively stereotyped, since it follows the distribution of vascular territories. Yet, there are exceptions to this trend. In the very acute stage of stroke cognitive symptoms are likely to be amplified by additional regions of ischemic penumbra, mass effects, and diaschisis (impairment of intact regions that are functionally connected with the damaged area) while in the chronic stage, functional reorganization and brain plasticity mechanisms make neuroanatomical correlations loose and less predictable. Likewise, in certain pathological processes such as hemorrhagic stroke, vasculitis, and cerebral venous thrombosis the pattern of cognitive defects is less stereotyped due to the

variability of lesion topography or to particular pathogenic mechanisms that may cause diffuse impairment.

In this chapter we will present the most common cognitive and neurobehavioral deficits secondary to stroke, according to symptom presentation.

Language disorders

Aphasia is the main cognitive disturbance of left hemisphere stroke and has a marked impact on the individual's quality of life, autonomy, and ability to return to work or previous activities. It occurs after perisylvian lesions involving the branches of the middle cerebral artery. Since these lesions are circumscribed, the conceptual representation system is not extensively affected and those patients do not become demented. This is an important distinction that should be explained to the families and caregivers for it can be misunderstood. In fact, deficits in oral comprehension increase the likelihood of discharge to a setting other than home [2].

> Language disorders occur following left hemisphere stroke in the middle cerebral artery territory. They have a profound impact on the quality of life and autonomy of patients.

A brief bedside evaluation of language comprises four cardinal tests (naming, verbal comprehension, repetition, and speech fluency) that are useful for classifying aphasic syndromes and for inferring lesions' localization, since they have neuroanatomical correlates [3, 4]. Although these tests are also included in some brief tools for cognitive assessment, such as the "Mini Mental State Examination" (MMSE) or the "Montreal Cognitive Assessment," language evaluation should be performed beforehand, because aphasia may preclude the assessment of orientation, memory, or executive functions.

Bedside evaluation of aphasia includes at least four simple tests: (1) confrontation naming; (2) speech fluency; (3) auditory comprehension; and (4) repetition of words, pseudowords, and sentences. Language should be evaluated before cognitive assessment.

Confrontation naming, which relies on a large network around the left Sylvian fissure, is one of the most sensitive tasks for the diagnosis of aphasia and the degree of naming impairment (anomia) is a rough measure of aphasia severity. Assessment must be performed with common objects (coin, ring, spoon, pencil, wristwatch), to avoid the effect of cultural factors and aging upon naming. Patients' responses vary from word-finding difficulties (with pauses and tip-of-the-tongue phenomenon), paraphasias, use of supraordinal responses (fruit for apple), and descriptions of use (circumlocutions). Occasionally, patients present "category-specific impairments," a type of naming or recognition difficulty that affects predominantly a specific category of names: it may impair the names of living entities more than artifacts, actions but not objects, or proper names but not common names. These unusual cases are more common in lesions of the left temporal lobe and pole following posterior cerebral artery infarcts [5], suggesting that this region is a hub in the semantic system.

Speech fluency is analyzed during conversation and can be prompted by asking the patient to tell a personal event or a kitchen recipe or to describe a picture. Speech is usually classified as fluent or non-fluent (Table 14.1) [4], a distinction that is made easier if the listener concentrates on the effort, speech rate, and the number and duration of pauses and manages to ignore its content, as if listening to a foreign language. Fluent speech "sounds" normal as opposed to non-fluent speech that is interrupted by long pauses and hesitations and is produced with effort.

Verbal comprehension is tested by simple verbal commands ("close your eyes," "raise your arm," etc.). Speech comprehension relies upon a ventral language stream connecting the temporal lobe to the prefrontal cortex, which maps sound to meaning [6]. It can be disrupted either by cortical lesions or by the interruption of the subcortical fiber tracts connecting those areas. Poor lexical (words/nouns) comprehension is usually associated with temporal lobe lesions, while inferior frontal/opercular stroke tends to impair the understanding of sentences and syntax. The comprehension of discourse in real time, on the other hand, requires a much larger network that integrates

Table 14.1. Classification of speech fluency and anatomical correlates

Speech fluency

Fluent	Non-fluent
Normal output (words/minute)	Slow output
	Single words
Normal phrase length	Telegraphic sentences
Effortless	Effortful
No pauses	Hesitations, pauses, interruptions
Normal prosody	Loss of prosody
Sounds "normal"	Sounds "atypical"
Lesion localization:	
Temporo-parietal lesions	Pre-rolandic or subcortical lesions

incoming information with context, requiring working memory and top-down control [7]. It is easily broken in aphasia.

Finally, one should ask the patient to repeat words, pseudowords (pronounceable strings of syllables that do not belong to the lexicon), and sentences. Repetition evaluates the integrity of the dorsal language stream, which maps speech sounds to articulation (Table 14.2). Repetition is impaired in lesions of the posterior temporo-parietal region and the periventricular white matter fiber tracts [8]. Transcortical aphasias are characterized by a disproportionate capacity to repeat, compared to other language abilities and sometimes these patients repeat compulsively, a phenomenon called echolalia. In conduction aphasia, in contrast, patients have outstanding difficulty in repeating pseudowords or even words they can otherwise produce.

Difficulty in any of these four tasks may vary from mild (occasional difficulty) to severe, and the classification of aphasia varies accordingly (Table 14.3).

Effective language recovery, in adults, depends mostly upon the reorganization of the intact areas of the left hemisphere [9, 10].

The initial severity of language impairment is the main predictor of aphasia recovery.

Certain brain lesions may impair the ability to read (alexia or acquired dyslexia) or to write (agraphia/dysgraphia). Both conditions are commonly found

Table 14.2. Functional organization of language

Language processing pathways in the left hemisphere	Anatomy	Corresponding language functions	Lesion-induced language impairment
Dorsal stream	Premotor cortex, posterior insula, temporo-parietal region and periventricular white matter (superior longitudinal and arcuate fasciculus)	Mapping speech sounds to articulatory representations (motor programs): speech perception	Word repetition and speech production
Ventral stream	Anterior and middle temporal lobe, ventrolateral prefrontal cortex, and ventral extreme capsule between the insula and putamen	Mapping speech sounds to meaning: speech recognition	Word/sentence (lexical/ semantic) comprehension

Adapted from Hickok and Poeppel [6] and Kümmerer et al. [8].

Table 14.3. Language profile of different aphasic syndromes

Taxonomic classification of aphasia

Speech fluency	Lexical comprehension	Word-pseudoword repetition	Aphasia type
Non-fluent	Normal	Normal	Transcortical motor
Non-fluent	Normal	Poor	Broca's
Non-fluent	Poor	Normal	Isolation of speech areas
Non-fluent	Poor	Poor	Global
Fluent	Normal	Normal	Anomic
Fluent	Normal	Poor	Conduction
Fluent	Poor	Normal	Transcortical sensory
Fluent	Poor	Poor	Wernicke's

in aphasia but may occur in isolation following lesions of the left hemisphere.

The study of patients with reading or writing disorders has contributed to the understanding of the cognitive processes subserving those abilities and to the building of theoretical models of written language processing. They have shown that there are separate pathways to process particular categories of words (regular vs. irregular; meaningful words vs. functional words, such as "to," "if," "so"), nonwords, or specific tasks (copying vs. writing spontaneously). This information has been incorporated into the assessment and classification of these disorders [11].

Alexia and agraphia can be classified as central or peripheral, depending on whether the impairment affects the central processing or its afferent or efferent pathways.

The best-known peripheral alexia is "pure alexia" (also called "alexia without agraphia" or "letter-by-letter reading"). This is a rather counterintuitive syndrome, whereby patients are unable to read but can write to dictation or spontaneously. There is an inability to associate visually presented written words with their sound or meaning but this difficulty is overcome through the tactile and auditory modalities (patients can read words spelled aloud), showing that the central reading processing is intact. Patients may be able to read single letters or small words but reading becomes rather difficult, laborious, or impossible as word size increases, as they try

Table 14.4. Acquired alexias

Type of alexia	Reading by auditory (spelling) or tactile modality	Writing	Word length effect (worse with polysyllabic words)	Ability to read pseudowords	Ability to read irregular words
1. Peripheral	Normal	Normal	Yes	Impaired	Impaired
2. Central:	Impaired	Impaired	No		
2.a. Deep dyslexia				Impaired	Relatively preserved with semantic errors
2.b. Surface dyslexia				Preserved reading of regular words and pseudowords	Impaired with regularization errors

to read letter by letter. This syndrome results from a disconnection between the primary visual areas and the "word form area" in the left fusiform gyrus due to left temporo-occipital infarcts involving the posterior splenium.

In central dyslexias, the impairment is independent of the presentation modality (visual, auditory, or tactile) and involves writing and spelling. There are two main types of central dyslexia (Table 14.4). In "deep dyslexia" patients may grasp the meaning of some written words, including irregular words, producing semantic paraphasias (*orange* for *lemon*) when reading aloud, but are unable to read function words or nonwords, which are deprived of meaning. In contrast, in "surface dyslexia" patients can read aloud regular words and pseudowords (because they can convert letters to their corresponding sound), but have difficulty reading irregular words or accessing their meaning. These opposite types of impairment have shown the existence of two pathways for reading: a fast whole-word recognition with access to meaning (used when one reads frequent and meaningful words) and a step-by-step conversion that is useful for reading new or infrequent words.

When alexia occurs in the context of aphasia, reading impairment for words is more often associated with frontal lesions while alexia for nonwords is more likely to occur in posterior lesions [12].

Acquired writing disorders are also classified as central and peripheral. In "central agraphias" writing impairment is similar across different output modalities (handwriting, spelling, or typing) and can be of a "deep type" (phonological dysgraphia) with preserved

access to meaning, or a "surface type" (or "lexical agraphia," whereby sound-to-grapheme conversion is preserved and there is a particular difficulty writing irregular words). There are also patients with a predominant defect of the "graphemic buffer." This is a short-term memory "device" that enables the writer to keep the word "on line" as it is being written in real time. Those cases are characterized by a particular difficulty in writing long words. In contrast, peripheral agraphia is a selective damage in the selection of letters or letter drawing that can be overcome by typing or the use of anagrams and is associated with normal spelling.

Deep forms of dyslexia and dysgraphia are associated with large left hemisphere strokes, while surface types result from more limited lesions. It is possible that reading and writing/spelling rely on identical cognitive processes, but in reverse order (the "shared components hypothesis") and share the same neural network that includes the angular, supramarginal, and fusiform gyrus (BA 37) and BA 22 and 44/45, as suggested in a study performed in acute stroke patients [13].

Neglect

Neglect is an inability to attend to, orient, or explore the hemispace contralateral to a brain lesion. Since the right hemisphere is dominant for spatial attention, this syndrome is usually observed following right hemisphere stroke (affecting some 36–80% of acute stroke patients) [14] and in the left-hand side of space. Neglect has a negative impact on daily living activities and on functional recovery, because patients

Table 14.5. Cortical networks underlying attention

	Function	Anatomy	Type of defect
Ventral attentional network	Non-spatial attention: Arousal and vigilance, detection of relevant stimuli and reorienting attention; visual working memory	Lateralized to the right hemisphere: Temporo-parietal junction, inferior parietal lobule, ventral frontal cortex, superior temporal gyrus	Left hemispatial neglect
Dorsal attentional network	Hemispatial attention: Saliency mapping, shift of attention to salient stimulus, and control of eye saccades to stimuli, in an egocentric framed contralateral space	Bilateral Frontal eye fields, intraparietal sulcus, superior parietal lobe, precuneus	Visuomotor ataxia

Adapted from Corbetta and Shulman [15].

cannot be expected to focus on a symptom that consists exactly of lack of awareness.

> Neglect is an inability to attend to, orient, or explore the hemispace contralateral to a brain lesion, usually of the right hemisphere.

Attention relies on a large network with two main processing pathways (Table 14.5) [15]: a ventral network, clearly lateralized to the right hemisphere, is responsible for stimulus detection, reorientation, and arousal, while a bilateral dorsal pathway controls spatial attention and eye movements to the contralateral space, within an egocentric frame. Although the ventral system does not map spatial representation its damage causes hemispatial neglect, possibly because it induces a dysfunction and imbalance of the dorsal system [15]. Since there are many anatomical regions that participate in those systems neglect may occur with lesions at different sites: anterior cingulate gyrus (responsible for its motivational aspects), frontal-parietal and superior temporal regions (mapping the perception of space and intentional/exploratory aspects of attention) as well as subcortical structures, such as the thalamus and the striatum. Extensive lesions, advanced age, defective arousal, and associated leukoaraiosis increase the severity of neglect.

Neglect can produce different symptoms that must be looked for to be detected. It can affect different compartments of space: personal space (forgetting to dress, groom the left side of the body), peri-personal or "hand reach" space (failing to detect or orient to surrounding objects or persons), the distant space ("at eye reach"), leading to spatial disorientation, or the representational space (mental imagery). It may occur spontaneously or only during competing sensory stimulation (extinction phenomena) and in any sensory modality (visual, tactile, auditory). In its most severe form it comprises anosognosia or denial of illness.

The most common tests used to diagnose neglect are performed in the peri-personal space and require the patient to draw, copy, or cross out lines or other stimuli (cancellation tasks) or to read or write. A qualitative analysis of the defect allows us to further classify the defect as viewer-centered or "egocentric neglect" (involving the angular gyrus) whereby the patient ignores all stimuli on the contralateral half of the space, and stimulus-centered or "alocentric neglect" (right superior temporal cortex) characterized by poor attention to the contralateral side of individual stimuli [16]. Viewer-centered neglect is much more common, easily noticed, and diagnosed than stimulus-centered neglect. The latter may go unrecognized because the defects are much more subtle and require a careful comparison of both sides of a stimulus. Neglect symptoms that occur following left hemisphere lesions (on the right side of the space) are object-centered type.

Memory disturbances

Memory is not a unitary function. It consists of five independent systems and involves three processes (encoding, storing/consolidation, and retrieval). Both depend on specific neural networks that may dissociate following a brain lesion.

Classification of memory systems (Table 14.6) [16] depends upon three main vectors: duration of memory traces (fractions of seconds, seconds, or "for life"), content (explicit knowledge or motor routines), and access to consciousness (explicit or implicit).

According to the processes affected amnesia is further subdivided in reference to a specific time event into anterograde (patients cannot encode/consolidate new information) and retrograde (the difficulty lies in retrieving information that was already stored).

Amnesic strokes, i.e. infarcts presenting amnesia for recent events as the main clinical feature, can result from posterior cerebral artery, posterior communicating artery, anterior and posterior choroidal artery, anterior cerebral and anterior communicating artery thrombosis or embolism. Infarcts in the territories of the two last arteries can also be secondary to subarachnoid hemorrhage and its complications and to the surgical and less often to the endovascular treatment of aneurysms located in these arteries. Single case reports or small case series of amnestic stroke have been reported following infarcts of the inferior genu of the internal capsule inferior, the mammillothalamic tract, the fornix, or the retrosplenium [10]. Anterolateral and medial thalamic hemorrhages, caudate and intraventricular hemorrhages, and venous infarcts due to thrombosis of the deep venous system also produce memory defects.

A quarter of posterior cerebral artery infarcts result in memory defects (Table 14.7) [11]. These amnestic strokes usually have mesial temporal involvement and the damage extends beyond the hippocampus to the entorhinal cortex, perirhinal cortex, collateral isthmus, or parahippocampal gyrus. The memory defect is more frequent and severe after left-sided and especially after bilateral infarcts. Left posterior cerebral artery infarcts cause either a verbal amnesia or a global amnesia, while right lesions produce visuospatial memory defects, including deficits in the memory for familiar faces or locations and topographical amnesia. Confabulations appear to be more likely if there is a dual lesion (temporo-occipital and thalamic).

Infarcts restricted to the hippocampus due to occlusion of the middle or the posterior hippocampal arteries, either complete, lateral, or dorsal, also produce persisting memory defects, affecting mostly learning. Small, dot- or comma-shaped infarcts cause a syndrome of transient global amnesia [17].

In thalamic infarcts [18], memory defects (Table 14.7) are also a distinct feature of anterior,

Table 14.6. Memory systems

Primary (short term)

Declarative

    Semantic
    Episodic

Implicit

    Procedural
    Priming – facilitation from a previous exposure
    Classic conditioning
    Sensory recording systems

Table 14.7. Summary of main features of major amnestic stroke syndromes

Characteristic stroke type	Hippocampal PCA infarct	Thalamic anterior or mesial thalamic infarct	Basal forebrain rupture of ACoA aneurysm
Anterograde amnesia	Severe	Severe	Severe
Retrograde amnesia	None or mild	None or mild	Moderate
Encoding defect	Severe	Severe	Severe
Consolidation defect	Severe	Severe	Severe
Retrieval defect	None or mild	Severe	Severe
Recognition defect	None or mild	None or mild	False recognitions
Working memory	Normal	None or mild defect	Normal
Procedural memory	Normal	Normal	Normal
Meta-memory	Normal or mild defect	Normal or mild defect	Impaired
Confabulations	Occasional	Frequent	Very frequent

PCA = posterior cerebral artery, ACoA = anterior communicating artery.

dorsomedial, and, in the variant types, anteromedian and central infarcts. Combined polar and paramedian infarcts also cause a severe and persistent amnesia. Left thalamic infarcts can produce "pure amnesia" in the form of a verbal or global amnesia. Memory disturbances are more frequent and severe after left than after right thalamic infarcts. Right thalamic infarcts cause visual and/or visuospatial amnesia. Following unilateral infarcts (left or right) a complete or partial recovery of memory disturbances can be expected. Bilateral infarcts produce global and severe amnesia and a persistent deficit, with slow and limited improvement. In thalamic amnesia confabulations, intrusions, and perseveration are frequent. Distractibility, alternating good and poor performance, and better performance on first attempts are also characteristic.

Memory defects are a frequent clinical feature of subarachnoid hemorrhage due to ruptured anterior communicating artery aneurysms and may also follow posterior communicating artery aneurysm rupture. They are a frequent and disabling long-term sequela: the Australian Cooperative Research on Subarachnoid Haemorrhage Group (2000) [19] found problems with memory in 50% of survivors. Recently, hippocampal atrophy was found on neuroimaging studies in subarachnoid hemorrhage survivors [20].

Amnesia following rupture of anterior communicating artery aneurysms is characterized by a severe anterograde and a moderate retrograde amnesia (Table 14.7). There is a high susceptibility to interference, false recognitions, confabulations, and anosognosia. Amnesia is related to damage to the anterior cingulum, subcalosal area, and basal forebrain. Temporal error contexts are associated with ventromedial prefrontal cortex damage, but for spontaneous confabulations to occur there must be additional orbitofrontal deficit [21]. The brain has a mechanism to distinguish mental activity representing ongoing perception of reality from memories and ideas. Confabulations can be traced to fragments of previous actual experiences. Confabulators confuse ongoing reality with the past because they fail to suppress evoked memories that do not pertain to the current reality. The role of the anterior limbic system is the suppression of currently irrelevant mental associations. It represents "now" in human thinking.

> Classification of memory systems depends upon duration of memory traces, content, and access to consciousness.

> Amnesia can be further subdivided into anterograde and retrograde.

> Amnesia can result from lesions in the hippocampus, thalamus, or basal forebrain.

Executive deficits

Executive functions are classically assigned to the prefrontal lobes. Three types of prefrontal lobe functions are usually considered: (1) dorsolateral (executive/cognitive), including working memory, programming/planning, concept formation, monitoring of actions and external cues and metacognition; (2) orbital (emotional/self-regulatory), consisting of inhibition of impulses and of non-relevant sensorial information and motor activity; and (3) mesial (action regulation), including motivation. These functions are served by three prefrontal–subcortical loops: dorsolateral, lateral orbital, and anterior cingulate, whose dysfunction produces three distinct clinical syndromes composed respectively of executive deficits, uninhibited behavior, and apathy. Executive difficulties manifest as difficulty deciding, leaving decisions to proxy, and being stubborn or rigid. Examples of uninhibited behavior include inappropriate familiarity, being distractible and shouting when constrained, and manipulation or utilization behavior. Recent models propose four main executive functions: dual task coordination, switch retrieval, selective attention and holding, and manipulation of information stored in long-term memory, so-called working memory; and three executive processes: updating, shifting, and inhibition [22]. Table 14.8 lists instruments that can be used to evaluate executive functions.

There are few systematic studies of executive functioning and other "frontal" syndromes in stroke patients. About one-third of acute stroke patients show either disinhibition or indifference and 30–40% display executive deficits in formal testing [23, 24]. Among patients with subarachnoid hemorrhage one-half to two-thirds have executive deficits [25]. Stroke in some specific locations can cause executive deficits, disinhibition, or apathy. Examples are middle cerebral artery infarcts with frontal lobe or striatocapsular involvement; uni- or bilateral anterior cerebral artery infarcts; anterior or paramedian thalamic infarcts; striatocapsular, thalamic, intraventricular, or frontal intracerebral hemorrhages; subarachnoid hemorrhage due to rupture of anterior communicating artery aneurysms; and thrombosis of the sagittal sinus or of the deep venous system.

Table 14.8. Neuropsychological evaluation of "frontal lobe" functions

Interview

> Frontal Behavioral Inventory
> EXIT-25 – Executive Interview
> Neuropsychiatric Inventory (NPI)

Bedside evaluation

> Frontal Assessment Battery at bedside

Specific tests

> Speed and motor control – tapping test, reaction times, Pordue Pegboard
> Sustained attention – letter or other cancellation test, Trail Making A
> Speed and shifting – Digit-Symbol or Symbol-Digit, Trail Making B
> Inhibition – Stroop Test B
> Initiative – phonological and semantic verbal fluency tasks
> Concept formation and set shifting – Wisconsin Card Sorting Test, mazes
> Problem solving – mazes, Towers (Hanoi, London), gambling task

Table 14.9. Classification of visual agnosias

According to the type of visual stimuli

Visual agnosia for

> Letters and words
> Other symbols
> Colors
> Objects
> Specific classes of objects
> Faces
> Locations

According to the functional processes involved

> Apperceptive visual agnosia
> > Form agnosia
> > Integrative agnosia
> Associative visual agnosia
> > Disconnection or loss of semantic access
> > Loss of semantic knowledge

Executive deficits due to lesions in the prefrontal lobe occur in about one-third of stroke patients and can be divided into three distinct clinical syndromes:

- executive deficits – corresponding to the dorsolateral prefrontal lobe
- uninhibited behavior – corresponding to the lateral orbital prefrontal lobe
- apathy – corresponding to the anterior cingulate prefrontal lobe.

Visual agnosia

The human brain has two parallel visual systems: a ventral occipito-temporal stream, whose main function is the recognition of visual stimuli (the "what" system), and a dorsal occipito-parietal stream, whose main function is the spatial localization of visual stimuli (the "where" system) [26]. The paradigm of human dysfunction of the ventral system is visual agnosia while that of the dorsal system is Balint's syndrome.

Visual agnosias are disorders of visual recognition and are one of the clinical manifestations of posterior cerebral artery infarcts and occipito-temporal hemorrhages. Agnosias can be seen in patients improving from cortical blindness. Visual agnosias can be classified following the type of stimuli that is defectively recognized or following the impaired functional step

in the processing of information from the visual system to the semantic and the language systems (Table 14.9).

Apperceptive visual object agnosia is characterized by the presence of perceptual defects in visuoperceptive tasks and a defective perception of elementary perceptual features (color, shape, contour, brightness). The most distinctive feature of patients with apperceptive visual agnosia is visual matching errors when trying to match identical visual stimuli. Their naming errors are morphological, based on visual similarity. They perform better with real objects than with drawings. There are two varieties of apperceptive visual agnosia: form and integrative agnosia. Patients with form agnosia cannot perceive contours, although they can perceive brightness, color, or luster. They have a better recognition of moving than of static objects. In contrast, patients with integrative agnosia perceive single contours but cannot integrate them in a coherent structure of the object, and produce predominantly visual similarity errors. Apperceptive visual agnosia is due to bilateral occipital or occipito-temporal lesions.

In associative visual object agnosia the distinctive feature is the intact perception. Although minor errors can be detected in complex perceptual tasks, the perception of elementary perceptual features (color, shape, contour, brightness) is correct, as is the matching of visual stimuli. Naming errors are semantic-related, perseverations, or confabulatory. A variety of associative visual agnosia is semantic access agnosia (visuo-verbal or visuo-semantic disconnection). Patients with this type of agnosia show not only intact

243

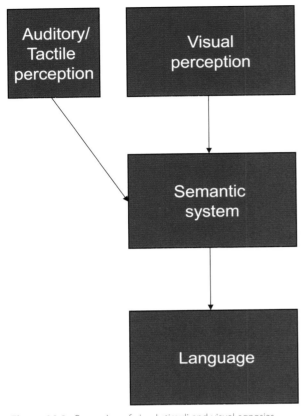

Apperceptive visual
agnosia

Semantic access
agnosia

Agnosia due to loss of
semantic knowledge

"Optic"
aphasia

Aphasia

Figure 14.1. Processing of visual stimuli and visual agnosias.

naming in other modalities (tactile, auditory) but also a correct use of objects. They may be able to select the correct name of an object in multiple-choice tasks and can sort objects by semantic categories. They may also be able to describe or pantomime the use of visually presented objects and have a superior naming of actions than of objects. Associative visual agnosia results from left or bilateral occipito-temporal lesions. In the literature the term optic aphasia is also found. It refers to a syndrome closely linked to visual agnosia and to transcortical sensory aphasia, and is often found during recovery from those. Patients have a disproportionate difficulty in naming stimuli presented visually, but otherwise do not display other features of visual agnosia (Figure 14.1).

Testing for color agnosia deserves a note. A careful check for achromatopsia in the whole or part of the visual field should precede other tasks. Color perception is checked by asking the patient to match identical colors. To test the visual–verbal connection we ask the patient to name colors and to point to named colors. To evaluate whether there is color anomia and to ensure that

language is intact we ask for color names in responsive naming (e.g. "Tell me the names of the colors of the national flag"). Finally, we can test visual–semantic connections by showing the patient drawings of stimuli which are painted in the correct and the wrong colors (e.g. blue banana) and asking the patient whether the colors are correct. Functional and lesion localization studies found that the V4v, V8, and V4a areas and the lingual gyrus are the human brain "color areas" [27]. Strokes causing color agnosia are left posterior cerebral infarcts with inferior temporal involvement. Color agnosia is more frequent than object agnosia.

Prosopagnosia is defined as an inability to recognize visually familiar faces, i.e. faces known by the patient, despite preserved visual perception. Recent studies using functional imaging indicate that the human brain areas activated by personally familiar faces (family, friends, etc.), famous familiar faces (media, politicians, sports people, etc.), and even of one's own child vs. familiar unrelated children are in part distinct. Current cognitive models consider a core system necessary for the recognition of visual appearance (the system which is disturbed in proso-pagnosia), and an extended system relative to person knowledge and to emotion related to or triggered by the perception of a face [28]. Prosopagnosia should not be confused with visuoperceptive deficits in tests using unknown faces, nor with the common complaint of prosopanomia (difficulty in recalling the names of known persons). Patients with prosopagnosia retain their ability to recognize people through other cues, such as voice, gait, size, and clothes. They may also be able to recognize faces by facial features, e.g. moustache, scar, or accessories, e.g. spectacles, rings. They may be able to identify gender, ethnicity, age, and emotional expression. They have a normal semantic knowledge about people. Functional and anatomical studies identified the occipital face area, the fusiform face area, and the superior temporal sulcus as the areas crucial in processing information relative to human faces [29]. Prosopagnosia can be found in 4–7% of posterior cerebral artery infarcts, either bilateral inferomedial or less commonly right inferomedial [30].

Hyperfamiliarity for unknown faces has also been reported.

> Visual agnosias are disorders of visual recognition and are one of the clinical manifestations of posterior cerebral artery infarcts and occipito-temporal hemorrhages. Special testing can identify apperceptive and associative visual object agnosia (apperceptive visual object agnosia: perceptive defects of the contours of objects or defect integration of the contour in a coherent structure of the object; associative visual object agnosia: intact perception with naming errors), color agnosia, and prosopagnosia (an inability to recognize visually familiar faces).

Delirium

Delirium is a disturbance of consciousness, with a change in cognition or development of a perceptual disturbance, which develops over a short period, fluctuates during the course of the day, and cannot be explained by pre-existing dementia (Table 14.10). Stroke is a rare cause of delirium. On the other hand, delirium often (10–48%) complicates acute stroke [31–36]. Delirium must be differentiated clinically from disorientation in time, topographical disorientation, delusions and hallucinations, amnesia, fluent aphasia, mania, psychosis, and even severe depression. Strokes in strategic locations (e.g. posterior cerebral artery, dorsomedial thalamic, caudate infarcts and hemorrhages, right middle cerebral artery, intraventricular hemorrhage, subarachnoid hemorrhage) [31, 32, 37] can cause acute agitated confusional states,

with a variable combination of declarative episodic memory defect, hyperactive motor behavior, apathy and other personality changes, delusions or hallucinations, and disturbed sleep cycle.

Delirium can be detected by the routine testing of mental status or with a specific simple instrument such as the Confusion Assessment Method. The severity of the delirium can be graded using scales such as the Delirium Rating Scale or the Clinical Institute Withdrawal Assessment of Alcohol Scale, Revised (CIWA-Ar) scale (if delirium is related to alcohol withdrawal).

Predictors of the development of delirium in stroke patients can be grouped as (1) vulnerable

Table 14.10. Main clinical features of delirium

Acute onset
  Occurs abruptly, over a period of hours or days

Fluctuating course
  Symptoms come and go and fluctuate in severity over a 24-hour period
  Lucid intervals

Inattention
  Difficulty focusing, sustaining and shifting attention
  Difficulty maintaining conversation or following commands

Disorganized thinking
  Disorganized or incoherent speech
  Rambling or irrelevant conversation or an unclear or illogical flow of ideas

Altered level of consciousness
  Clouding of consciousness, with reduced clarity of awareness of environment

Cognitive deficits
  Global or multiple: orientation, memory, language

Perceptual disturbances
  Illusions, hallucinations

Psychomotor disturbances
  Hyperactive type: agitated, hyper-vigilant
  Hypoactive type: decreased motor activity, lethargy

Altered sleep–wake cycle
  Daytime drowsiness, nighttime insomnia, fragmented sleep, reversed sleep cycle

Emotional disturbances
  Intermittent or labile fear, paranoia, anxiety, depression, apathy, irritability, anger, or euphoria

patients, (2) stroke type, and (3) precipitating factors. Older patients and those with previous dementia or cognitive decline, previous delirium, or vision impairment are more prone to become delirious. Supratentorial strokes, total anterior circulation infarct (TACI) type, cardioembolic strokes, intracerebral hemorrhage as well as strokes causing severe paresis or neglect or a decrease in alertness are more likely to be complicated by delirium. Precipitating factors of delirium in stroke patients include intake of drugs with anticholinergic activity (even subtle anticholinergic activity, such as selective serotonin reuptake inhibitors (SSRIs), antiemetics, baclofen, or ipratropium bromide) before or during hospitalization, high blood urea nitrogen/creatinine, infections, and metabolic complications [34, 37]. A checklist for the precipitants of delirium is given in Table 14.11.

The pathogenesis of delirium is incompletely understood (Figure 14.2). There is reduced oxidative

Table 14.11. Checklist for precipitants of delirium in stroke patients

- Previous dementia, mild cognitive impairment, or cognitive decline
- Previous delirium
- Medication side-effect
- Medication with anticholinergic activity
- Medication intoxication or withdrawal
- Alcohol or illicit drug intoxication or withdrawal
- Fever; infection
- Pain: shoulder, bed sores, visceral, immobility
- Fall with bone fracture
- Subdural hematoma
- Full bladder
- Respiratory distress
- Metabolic disturbance
- Sleep apnea
- Non-convulsive epileptic status
- Sensory deprivation

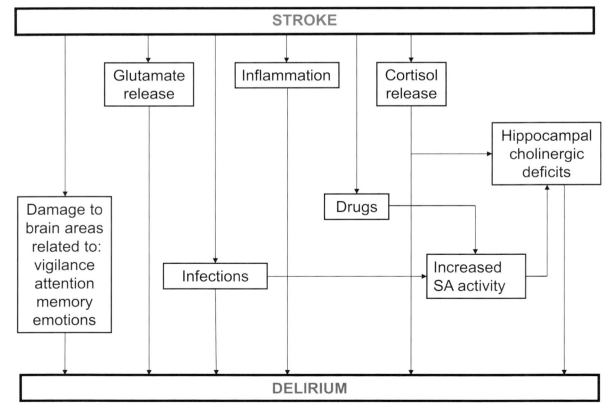

Figure 14.2. Proposed schematic pathophysiological model of post-stroke delirium (SA = serum anticholinergy).

metabolism and cerebral blood flow, mainly in the frontal lobes and parietal lobes. There is evidence of a cholinergic deficit and of increased serum anticholinergic activity. However, other neurotransmitters such as serotonin, gamma-aminobutyric acid (GABA), dopamine, and glutamate are probably also involved. A role of inflammation and of cytokines (interleukin-1, -2, -6, tumor necrosis factor-α (TNF-α)) has been recently proposed. The stress–hypercortisolemia hypothesis of delirium is based on the finding of increased adrenocorticotropic hormone (ACTH) levels in the first hours of delirium and of higher post-dexamethasone cortisol levels in delirious patients.

Delirium is an ominous prognostic sign: acute stroke patients with delirium have a higher risk of longer hospital stay, in-hospital death, death and dependency at 6–12 months, being admitted to a nursing home or other long-term care facility, recurrent delirium, and dementia [31, 32, 38].

> Delirium often complicates acute stroke and is a bad prognostic sign.

> Delirium is related to
> - vulnerable patients
> - stroke type and
> - precipitating factors.

Anger and aggressiveness

Anger and aggression are complex human emotions and behaviors depending on several anatomical structures, including the frontal lobes, the amygdala, the hypothalamus, lenticulo-capsular-pontine areas [39], and the brainstem. Anger is a primary emotion with three components: the emotional (anger), the cognitive (hostility), and the behavioral (aggression). The State-Trait Anger Expression Inventory-2™ (STAXI-2™) is a validated scale to measure the expression of anger, comprising a state-trait anger scale and an anger expression scale [40].

A few studies [41–44] have evaluated anger and its components systematically in stroke patients and found a frequency ranging from 17% to 34%. In acute stroke, state-anger can be detected in 20% of the patients and trait-anger in 24% [45]. Anger in stroke patients was associated with younger age, depression, anxiety, lower MMSE, and with hemorrhagic strokes with the proximity of the lesion to the frontal pole. Kim *et al.* [39] described an association with motor dysfunction, dysarthria, emotional incontinence, and higher frequency of anger in strokes involving the frontal, lenticulo-capsular, and basal pontine areas, but other studies found no association with a specific stroke localization.

An interesting aspect is the dissociations that were found in acute stroke patients between the emotional, cognitive, and behavioral components of anger and between the subjective experience of anger and what could be observed [43]. Patients may behave aggressively without feeling angry or experience only hostility.

In acute stroke, aggressive behavior appears to be mainly due to a failure of regulatory inhibitory control. On the other hand, the hospital environment may be or may be perceived as hostile or humiliating. Premorbid personality traits of neuroticism were associated with post-stroke agitation and irritability in one study [46].

Post-stroke anger is less studied but is commonly reported and increases the caregiver's burden [47]. Some studies suggested a possible relationship between serotonergic neurotransmitters and aggression or impulsivity. Post-stroke anger can be improved by SSRIs such as fluoxetine [48].

> In acute stroke, aggressive behavior appears to be mainly due to a failure of regulatory inhibitory control.

Psychotic disorders, hallucinations, and delusions

Psychotic disorders due to stroke are rare. They are classified according to the predominant symptom, with prominent hallucinations or with delusions. Delusions are of two main types: delusional misidentification syndromes and delusional ideation. This can be observed in patients with Wernicke's aphasia and severe comprehension defect. Kumral and Oztürk [49] found that delusions started 0–3 days after stroke, and the predominant types were mixed, persecutory, jealousy, and suspicion. Delusional ideation was transient, with a mean duration of 13 days. The prevalence of psychosis and of delusional ideation (1–5%) in stroke survivors is also low. It is predominantly associated with right hemispheric strokes. There is no association between delusion type and infarct site.

The delusional misidentification syndromes include Capgras syndrome, where the patient believes a familiar person is not the real person but has been replaced by a similar one; Fregoli syndrome, where the patient believes it is the same person but with different features; and intermetamorphosis, where the familiar person has been transformed into another one. Somatoparaphrenia is associated with hemiassomatognosia and denial of hemiplegia. In spatial delirium the patient believes he/she is in a different place than the actual one, even in the face of compelling counter-evidence. Spatial delirium can have three grades of severity or stages of evolution: (1) confabulatory mislocation: "I am not in hospital X but in hospital Y"; (2) reduplication: "I am not in the real hospital X but in an identical building"; (3) chimeric assimilation: "I am not in the real hospital X but in my house which was transformed into a hospital." Spatial delirium is in some cases associated with delirium, neglect, memory or visuospatial disturbances and is seen predominantly after right hemispheric lesions.

Hallucinations in stroke patients are predominantly visual and can be due to: (1) sensory deprivation: poor vision (Charles Bonnet syndrome), darkness, deafness; (2) delirium and substance withdrawal (alcohol, drugs); (3) rostral brainstem and thalamic lesions (peduncular hallucinosis) (subcortical hallucinations); (4) partial occipital lesions ("release" hallucinations) (cortical hallucinations). Functional imagery studies showed that in subjects with visual hallucinations there was activation of the ventral extrastriate visual cortex and that the type of hallucinations reflected the functional specialization of the activated region.

In rostral brainstem and thalamic strokes, hallucinations are vivid, complex, visual, naturalist, and scenic. Less frequently they are auditory or combined. They appear during the day or night, and last for minutes. Patients have variable insight and reactive behavior, but sometimes there is a strong emotional reaction of anxiety and fear. Peduncular hallucinosis can recur in a stereotyped manner over weeks. In posterior cerebral artery infarcts, hallucinations are more common after partial occipital lesions. Hallucinations are complex, colored, stereotyped, featuring animal or human figures. They are apparent in the abnormal visual field. They appear in general with a delay of days after the vascular event. The phenomenology of hallucinations does not always reflect the localization of the lesion, because the damaged area may serve as the focus of an abnormally activated neuronal network. Visual hallucinations can be associated with seizures and the EEG may show epileptiform activity. Visual hallucinations usually resolve spontaneously, but are resistant to treatment with neuroleptics or antiepileptic drugs.

Auditory hallucinations are much rarer than visual hallucinations and have been reported following right temporal and left dorsomedial thalamic strokes. These auditory hallucinations are transient [50].

> Psychotic disorders due to stroke are rare. Most frequent are visual hallucinations related to rostral brainstem, thalamic, and partial occipital lesions.

Disturbances of emotional expression control

The prevalence of crying in acute stroke patients has been estimated at between 12% and 27%, but disorders of emotional expression control are more frequent (11–40%) and often appear delayed after stroke onset [51]. This disorder consists of uncontrollable outbursts of laughing, crying, or both, with paroxysmal onset, transient duration of seconds or minutes, stereotyped, precipitated by nonspecific or inappropriate stimuli but also by appropriate stimuli in an inappropriate context. Patients cannot control the extent or duration of the episode. The outbursts are incongruent or exaggerated in comparison with the emotional feelings. There is no mood change during the episode and no sense of relief when it ends. There are many crying situations and many content areas of crying situations. The crying frequency is very high. It is more frequent in men and in the presence of others.

Disorders of emotional expression control are sometimes associated with depression but more often they can be dissociated. Other behavioral and cognitive correlates include irritability and ideas of reference, decreased sexual activity, and lower MMSE scores. Disorders of emotional expression control have an adverse impact on the quality of life of stroke survivors. They can disrupt communication, cause embarrassment, and therefore curtail social activities.

Disorders of emotional expression control have been classically associated with bilateral subcortical strokes. More recent systematic studies have shown that they can follow not only bilateral subcortical strokes, but also bilateral pontine and unilateral strokes, including large anterior, cortico-subcortical lesions, lenticulo-capsular or thalamocapsular lesions, and also basal pontine strokes.

The pathophysiology of the uncontrolled outbursts of laughing and crying is poorly understood. Wilson [52] proposed a patho-anatomical model consisting of a putative fasciorespiratory control center for emotional expression located in the brainstem with a dual route of control from the motor cortex: a voluntary pathway through the pyramidal and geniculate tracts, which initiates voluntary laughter and crying and inhibits involuntary initiated laughter or crying, and an involuntary pathway consisting of a frontal/temporal–basal ganglia–ventral brainstem circuitry, which initiates and also terminates involuntary laughter or crying. Uncontrolled laughing and crying could result from release of the fasciorespiratory control center from the motor cortex or from disruption of the involuntary pathway. There is recent evidence of disruption of ascending serotoninergic pathways in disorders of emotional expression control.

Uncontrolled laughing and crying can improve significantly with treatment with several classes of antidepressants (SSRIs, tricyclic antidepressants [TCAs], baclofen, and levodopa).

An uncontrollable prolonged burst of laughing, called after Féré *fou rire prodromique*, can exceptionally anticipate by seconds to days the onset of the focal deficit in acute stroke [53].

> Disorders of emotional expression control (outbursts of laughing, crying, or both) are frequent and are often associated with bilateral subcortical strokes.

Anxiety disorders

Post-stroke anxiety disorders have received comparatively less attention than post-stroke depression although 20–25% of stroke patients experience anxiety [54].

The core symptoms of generalized anxiety disorder are being anxious or worried and having difficulty in controlling worries. Diagnostic and Statistical Manual (DSM-IV-TR) criteria require in addition three or more symptoms such as restlessness, decreased energy, poor concentration, irritation, nervous tension, and insomnia. In the acute stage restlessness, decreased energy, poor concentration, irritation, nervous tension, and insomnia are more common in "anxious or worried" stroke patients, while during follow-up restlessness and nervous tension are more consistently associated with anxiety, while decreased energy is a nonspecific complaint.

The prevalence of post-stroke anxiety, with or without depression, is higher in hospital settings (acute stroke patients: 28%, 15–17%, and 3–13%, respectively; stroke survivors: 24%, 6–17%, and 3–11%, respectively) than in community studies (11%, 8%, and 1–2%,

respectively). The prevalence of agoraphobia is estimated to be 17%. Anxiety disorders are often associated with depression. About a third of the patients with initial anxiety remain anxious months after stroke.

Besides depression, there are other consistent clinical and psychiatric correlates of anxiety such as previous depression or anxiety and alcohol abuse. Less consistent correlates include younger age, female gender, aphasia, history of insomnia, and cognitive impairment. Functional and social correlates of anxiety include impairment in activities of daily living, impairment in social functioning, being single, living alone, or having no social contacts outside the family [55]. The most consistent anatomical association of post-stroke anxiety was with anterior circulation strokes. Anxiety in the acute phase of stroke may be due to previous substance use or withdrawal (alcohol, benzodiazepines, and illicit drugs).

Concerning the outcome of post-stroke anxiety, a sizeable proportion, ranging from one-quarter to one-half, does not recover. Post-stroke anxiety with associated depression has an unfavorable prognosis and usually lasts longer and remains stable all over a period of 3 years [56]. Post-stroke anxiety without depression does not influence functional or cognitive recovery but is associated with worse social functioning and quality of life.

Pharmacological treatments are useful in the treatment of post-stroke anxiety. In a recent systematic review [57] of stroke patients presenting anxiety and comorbid depression, pharmacological therapy including paroxetine and buspirone was effective in reducing anxiety. In another systematic review and meta-analyses [58] SSRIs also appeared to improve anxiety.

> About 20% of stroke patients experience anxiety. Post-stroke anxiety disorders are often associated with depression, previous psychiatric disorders, and alcohol abuse.

Post-traumatic stress disorder

Stroke and transient ischemic attack can be experienced as a traumatic event and it may be re-experienced as an unpleasant and uncontrollable intrusion. Post-traumatic stress disorder is estimated to affect 10% to 31% [59, 60] of stroke survivors and is associated with depression and anxiety. Post-traumatic stress disorder after stroke is more common in women, in patients with low educational

249

level, and in those with premorbid neuroticism or with a negative affect or appraisal of the stroke experience.

Post-stroke mania

Post-stroke mania is an infrequent complication of stroke (1–2%). It is a prominent and persistent disturbance in mood characterized by elevated, expansive, or irritable mood. Clinical features of post-stroke mania also include increased rate or amount of speech; talkativeness; language thought and content disturbance, such as flights of ideas, racing thoughts, grandiose ideation, and lack of insight; hyperactivity and social disinhibition, and decreased need for sleep. In severe cases distractibility, confusion, delusions, and hallucinations may be also present. To distinguish between true post-stroke mania and a reactivation of previous undiagnosed primary mania, it is crucial to obtain a careful history of previous manic or hypomanic episodes or symptoms.

Post-stroke mania can be related to predisposing genetic (family/personal history of mood disorder) factors, subcortical brain atrophy, and damage to the right corticolimbic (fronto-basal ganglia-thalamic-cortical) pathways. However, mania can be detected in stroke patients without personal or familial predisposing factors, after lesions in both hemispheres, and also after subarachnoid hemorrhage [61]. Patients with post-stroke mania can experience recurrent episodes.

Post-stroke depression

Post-stroke depression is a prominent and persistent mood disturbance characterized by depressed mood and/or anhedonia (lack of interest or lack of pleasure) in all or almost all activities. These symptoms define the DSM-IV-TR criteria of "Mood Disorder Due to Stroke," which included the subtypes "with depressive features" or "similar to a major depressive episode." Loss of energy, decreased concentration, and psychomotor retardation are also frequent, as well as the somatic symptoms of decreased appetite and insomnia. Guilt is less common. The risk of suicide after stroke is low. However, 15% of acute stroke patients had suicidal thoughts, 22% of them with explicit plans to complete suicide. The most important risk factors for suicidal thoughts are lower educational level, younger age, female gender, a previous mood disorder, and depression [62, 63].

Reports on the incidence and prevalence of post-stroke depression give highly variable figures, depending on the setting of the study, the time since stroke, the case mix, and the criteria/method used to diagnose depression. Post-stroke depression incidence ranges from 7% to 21% and remains stable up to 10 years after stroke [64]. A recent systematic review reported a mean prevalence of 33% (29–36%) [65]. The prevalence of post-stroke depression ranges from 5% to 67% among all types of stroke patients. Severe depression has a frequency ranging from 9% to 26%, while in the acute phase depression is present in 16–52% of the patients [66]. At 2 years, 18–55% of stroke survivors are depressed. The rate of recovery from depression after stroke is moderate (range 15% to 57%).

Concerning the features of stroke which increase the risk of post-stroke depression, all stroke types are similarly prone to depression. The hemispheric side is also not relevant, although in some studies the frequency and severity of depression were higher after left-sided lesions, in particular during the first months after stroke. Higher lesion volumes, cerebral atrophy, silent infarcts, and white matter lesions are all associated with a higher risk of post-stroke depression.

Predictors of post-stroke depression are pre-stroke depression, cognitive impairment, stroke severity, and anxiety [64]. The relationship between depression and disability depends on several factors: the personality of the patients, their subjectivity (i.e. the subjective experience of the stroke), their lifestyle, the severity of neurological impairment, and social isolation. Acute depressive symptoms mainly have a biological determinism, while post-stroke depression at 1–2 years has an additional psychosocial determinism.

> Post-stroke depression has a high prevalence and may remain stable up to 10 years after stroke. Pharmacotherapy for post-stroke depression is recommended. Antidepressants lead to an improvement of symptoms and complete remission of depressive episodes. The selection of the most appropriate antidepressant for the individual patient has to consider not only efficacy but also the side-effects that must be avoided in each patient.

Personality changes

Persistent personality disturbances, defined as a change from the previous characteristic personality, are one of the most frustrating behavioral disturbances found after stroke. For the caregiver these changes are hard to cope with and they are difficult to control pharmacologically. There are several types of personality changes in stroke patients: aggressive, disinhibited, paranoid, labile, and apathetic types. In the apathetic type the predominant feature is marked apathy and indifference. Apathy is a disorder of motivation. In severe forms, there is lack of feeling, emotion, interest, and concern; flat affect; indifference; no initiative or decisions; and little spontaneous speech or actions. Responses are either absent, delayed, or slow. A key feature is the dissociation between impaired self-activation and preserved hetero-activation. Subtle symptoms of apathetic personality change include lack of interest in previous activities and hobbies, preference for passive activities (sitting, watching TV), no "zapping" of TV channels, paucity in starting a conversation, speaking mainly in response to other people, and lack of complaining. Apathetic patients look depressed, but they deny "low" mood. Relatives are more worried than the patient. Stroke in anatomical locations that interrupt the cingulate-subcortical thalamo-striate loop can produce apathy. These include anterior or medial thalamic nuclei, caudate, inferior capsular genu, bilateral palidal, uni- or bilateral anterior cerebral artery, and baso-frontal strokes.

The rate of apathy after stroke (in acute and post-acute phases) ranges between 34.6% and 36.3% [67, 68]. Apathy is associated with older age and cognitive impairment (mostly executive functions). About half of the apathetic patients remained apathetic in the long range. Apathy is associated with depression, most probably because the two share symptoms such as diminishing interest in daily activities and decrease in activity. The rate of apathy without concomitant depression decreases to 21.4% while depression without concomitant apathy decreases even more to a rate of 12.1%, proving that the two are distinct entities. No particular stroke lesion location or lateralization is associated with apathy.

In acute stroke, 15.2–71% (rate of 39.5%) of the patients present with apathy, which is associated with older age, cognitive impairment, and denial.

Systematic studies investigating post-stroke apathy in stroke survivors detected apathy in 20.1–55.2% (rate of 34.3%) of the patients 1–15 months after stroke. Patients with recurrence of stroke have higher rate of apathy, compared with first-ever stroke [67]. Apathy was associated with cognitive impairment (defects in attention, concentration, working memory, and reasoning) with deficits in activities of daily living. Apathy was associated with right-sided lesions involving subcortical circuits, which comprised the ipsilateral frontal white matter, anterior capsule, basal ganglia, and thalamus.

There is insufficient evidence to support routine pharmacological treatment of post-stroke apathy. Nevertheless, nefiracetam and donepezil have some beneficial effects on post-stroke apathy [68].

> Persistent personality changes are frequent and for the caregiver one of the most annoying behavioral disturbances found after stroke. Apathetic personality change is present in one of every three stroke patients. About half of the apathetic patients remain apathetic long after stroke onset.

Chapter summary

- **Aphasia** occurs following middle cerebral artery territory lesions of the left hemisphere. Cardinal tests: (1) confrontation naming; (2) analysis of speech (fluent and non-fluent); (3) verbal auditory comprehension; (4) repetition of words, pseudowords, and sentences.
- **Alexia and agraphia** are commonly found in aphasia, but may occur in isolation following lesions of the left hemisphere. They can be classified as central and peripheral, and as "deep" and "surface" types.
- **Neglect** is an inability to attend to, orient, or explore the hemispace contralateral to a brain lesion, usually of the right hemisphere.
- **Amnesia** can be classified according to the affection of the memory system (duration of memory traces, content, and access to consciousness) and further subdivided into anterograde and retrograde. Amnesia can result from thrombosis or embolism of the posterior cerebral artery, posterior communicating artery, anterior and posterior choroidal artery, and anterior cerebral and anterior communicating arteries.
- **Prefrontal lobe deficits:**
  - executive deficits (showing difficulty deciding, leaving decisions to proxy, and being stubborn or rigid), corresponding to the dorsolateral prefrontal lobe;
  - uninhibited behavior (inappropriate familiarity, being distractible, and manipulation or utilization behavior), corresponding to the lateral orbital prefrontal lobe;

- apathy, corresponding to the anterior cingulate prefrontal lobe.
- **Visual agnosias** are disorders of visual recognition (for classification see Table 14.9) and are one of the clinical manifestations of posterior cerebral artery infarcts and occipito-temporal hemorrhages.
- **Delirium** often complicates acute stroke and is a bad prognostic sign. Predictors are a vulnerable patient, the type of stroke, and precipitating factors (e.g. drugs or infections).
- **Hallucinations** in stroke patients are predominantly visual. Lesion: rostral brainstem

and thalamic and partial occipital. Other reasons: sensory deprivation or delirium or substance withdrawal.
- **Depression** has a high prevalence after stroke. All stroke types are similarly prone to depression, but higher lesion volumes, cerebral atrophy, silent infarcts, and white matter lesions are associated with a higher risk.
- **Persistent personality changes** such as apathetic type are rather frequent and are disturbing for caregivers of patients after stroke.

References

1. Binder JR, Desai RH. The neurobiology of semantic memory. *Trends Cogn Sci* 2011; **15**:527–36.

2. González-Fernández M, Christian AB, Davis C, Hillis AE. Role of aphasia in discharge location after stroke. *Arch Phys Med Rehabil* 2013; **94**:851–5.

3. Kümmerer D, Hartwigsen G, Kellmeyer P, *et al.* Damage to ventral and dorsal language pathways in acute aphasia. *Brain* 2013; **136**:619–29.

4. Kreisler A, Godefroy O, Delmaire C, *et al.* The anatomy of aphasia revisited. *Neurology* 2000; **4**:1117–23.

5. Capitani E, Laiacona M, Pagani R, *et al.* Posterior cerebral artery infarcts and semantic category dissociations: a study of 28 patients. *Brain* 2009; **132**:965–81.

6. Hickok G, Poeppel D. The cortical organization of speech processing. *Nat Rev Neurosci* 2007; **8**:393–402.

7. Egidi G, Caramazza A. Cortical systems for local and global integration in discourse comprehension. *Neuroimage* 2013; **71**:59–74.

8. Kümmerer D, Hartwigsen G, Kellmeyer P, *et al.* Damage to ventral and dorsal language pathways in acute aphasia. *Brain* 2013; **136**:619–29.

9. Saur D, Lange R, Baumgaertner A, *et al.* Dynamics of language reorganization after stroke. *Brain* 2006; **129**:1371–84.

10. Fridriksson J, Richardson JD, Fillmore P, Cai B. Left hemisphere plasticity and aphasia recovery. *Neuroimage* 2012; **60**:854–63.

11. Plaut D, McClelland J, Seidenberg M, Patterson K. Understanding normal and impaired word reading. *Psychol Rev* 1996; **103**:56–115.

12. Cloutman LL, Newhart M, Davis CL, Heidler-Gary J, Hillis AE. Neuroanatomical correlates of oral reading in acute left hemispheric stroke. *Brain Lang* 2011; **116**:14–21.

13. Philipose LE, Gottesman RF, Newhart M, *et al.* Neural regions essential for reading and spelling of words and pseudowords. *Ann Neurol* 2007; **62**:481–92.

14. Azouvi P, Samuel C, Louis-Dreyfus A, *et al.* French Collaborative Study Group on Assessment of Unilateral Neglect (GEREN/GRECO). Sensitivity of clinical and behavioural tests of spatial neglect after right hemisphere stroke. *J Neurol Neurosurg Psychiatry* 2002; **73**:160–6.

15. Corbetta M, Shulman GL. Spatial neglect and attention networks. *Annu Rev Neurosci* 2011; **34**:569–99.

16. Shirani P, Thorn J, Davis C, *et al.* Severity of hypoperfusion in distinct brain regions predicts severity of hemispatial neglect in different reference frames. *Stroke* 2009; **40**:3563–6.

17. Szabo K, Förster A, Jäger T, *et al.* Hippocampal lesion patterns in acute posterior cerebral artery stroke: clinical and MRI findings. *Stroke* 2009; **40**:2042–5.

18. Graff-Radford NR, Damasio H, Yamada T, Eslinger PJ, Damasio AR. Nonhaemorrhagic thalamic infarction. Clinical, neuropsychological and electrophysiological findings in four anatomical groups defined by computerized tomography. *Brain* 1985; **108**:485–516.

19. Hackett ML, Anderson CS. Health outcomes 1 year after subarachnoid hemorrhage: an international population-based study. The Australian Cooperative Research on Subarachnoid Hemorrhage Study Group. *Neurology* 2000; **55**:658–62.

20. Bendel P, Koivisto T, Hänninen T, *et al.* Subarachnoid hemorrhage is followed by temporomesial

volume loss: MRI volumetric study. *Neurology* 2006; **67**:575–82.

21. Gilboa A, Alain C, Stuss DT, *et al*. Mechanisms of spontaneous confabulations: a strategic retrieval account. *Brain* 2006; **129**:1399–414.

22. Collette F, Hogge M, Salmon E, Van der Linden M. Exploration of the neural substrates of executive functioning by functional neuroimaging. *Neuroscience* 2006; **139**:209–21.

23. Nys GM, van Zandvoort MJ, de Kort PL, *et al*. Cognitive disorders in acute stroke: prevalence and clinical determinants. *Cerebrovasc Dis* 2007; **23**:408–16.

24. Zinn S, Bosworth HB, Hoenig HM, Swartzwelder HS. Executive function deficits in acute stroke. *Arch Phys Med Rehabil* 2007; **88**:173–80.

25. Keiter KT, Copeland D, Bernardini GL, *et al*. Predictors of cognitive dysfunction after subarachnoid hemorrhage. *Stroke* 2002; **33**:200–8.

26. James TW, Culham J, Humphrey GK, Milner AD, Goodale MA. Ventral occipital lesions impair object recognition but not object-directed grasping: an fMRI study. *Brain* 2003; **126**:2463–75.

27. Bouvier SE, Engel SA. Behavioral deficits and cortical damage loci in cerebral achromatopsia. *Cereb Cortex* 2006; **16**:183–91.

28. Gobbini MI, Haxby JV. Neural systems for recognition of familiar faces. *Neuropsychologia* 2007; **45**:32–41.

29. Sorger B, Goebel R, Schiltz C, Rossion B. Understanding the functional neuroanatomy of acquired prosopagnosia. *Neuroimage* 2007; **35**:836–52.

30. Brandt T, Steinke W, Thie A, Pessin MS, Caplan LR. Posterior cerebral artery territory infarcts: clinical features, infarct topography, causes and outcome.

Multicenter results and a review of the literature. *Cerebrovasc Dis* 2000; **10**:170–82.

31. Dahl MH, Rønning OM, Thommessen B. Delirium in acute stroke–prevalence and risk factors. *Acta Neurol Scand Suppl* 2010; **190**:39–43.

32. Dostović Z, Smajlović D, Sinanović O, Vidović M. Duration of delirium in the acute stage of stroke. *Acta Clin Croat* 2009; **48**:13–17.

33. Hénon H, Lebert F, Durieu I, *et al*. Confusional state in stroke: relation to preexisting dementia, patient characteristics, and outcome. *Stroke* 1999; **30**:773–9.

34. Caeiro L, Ferro JM, Albuquerque R, Figueira ML. Delirium in the first days of acute stroke. *J Neurol* 2004; **251**:171–8.

35. Gustafson Y, Olsson T, Eriksson S, Asplund K, Bucht G. Acute confusional states (delirium) in stroke patients. *Cerebrovasc Dis* 1991; **1**:257–64.

36. Sheng AZ, Shen Q, Cordato D, Zhang YY, Yin Chan DK. Delirium within three days of stroke in a cohort of elderly patients. *J Am Geriatr Soc* 2006; **54**:1192–8.

37. Caeiro L, Menger C, Ferro JM, Albuquerque R, Figueira ML. Delirium in acute subarachnoid haemorrhage. *Cerebrovasc Dis* 2005; **19**:31–8.

38. Shi Q, Presutti R, Selchen D, Saposnik G. Delirium in acute stroke: a systematic review and meta-analysis. *Stroke* 2012; **43**:645–9.

39. Kim JS, Choi S, Kwon SU, Seo YS. Inability to control anger or aggression after stroke. *Neurology* 2002; **58**:1106–8.

40. Borteyrou X, Bruchon-Schweitzer M, Spielberger CD. The French adaptation of the STAXI-2, C.D. Spielberger's State-trait anger expression

inventory. *Encephale* 2008; **34**:249–55.

41. Ghika-Schmid F, van Melle G, Guex P, Bogousslavsky L. Subjective experience and behaviour in acute stroke: the Lausanne Emotion in Acute Stroke Study. *Neurology* 1999; **52**:22–8.

42. Paradiso S, Robinson RG, Arndt S. Self-reported aggressive behavior in patients with stroke. *J Nerv Ment Dis* 1996; **184**:746–53.

43. Santos CO, Caeiro L, Ferro JM, Albuquerque R, Luísa Figueira M. Anger, hostility and aggression in the first days of acute stroke. *Eur J Neurol* 2006; **13**:351–8.

44. Chan KL, Campayo A, Moser DJ, Arndt S, Robinson RG. Aggressive behavior in patients with stroke: association with psychopathology and results of antidepressant treatment on aggression. *Arch Phys Med Rehabil* 2006; **87**:793–8.

45. Santos AC. Anger in acute stroke. Determinants and impact on treatment compliance and well-being of caregivers. Unpublished PhD thesis, University of Liboa, 2014.

46. Greenop KR, Almeida OP, Hankey GJ, van Bockxmeer F, Lautenschlager NT. Premorbid personality traits are associated with post-stroke behavioral and psychological symptoms: a three-month follow-up study in Perth, Western Australia. *Int Psychogeriatr* 2009; **21**:1063–71.

47. Choi-Kwon S, Mitchell PH, Veith R, *et al*. Comparing perceived burden for Korean and American informal caregivers of stroke survivors. *Rehabil Nurs* 2009; **34**:141–50.

48. Choi-Kwon S, Han SW, Kwon SU, *et al*. Fluoxetine treatment in poststroke depression, emotional incontinence, and anger proneness: a double-blind, placebo-controlled study. *Stroke* 2006; **37**:156–61.

49. Kumral E, Oztürk O. Delusional state following acute stroke. *Neurology* 2004; **62**:110–13.

50. Lampl Y, Lorberboym M, Gilad R, Boaz M, Sadeh M. Auditory hallucinations in acute stroke. *Behav Neurol* 2005; **16**:211–16.

51. House A, Dennis M, Molyneux A, Warlow C, Hawton K. Emotionalism after stroke. *BMJ* 1989; **298**:991–4.

52. Wilson SAK. Some problems in neurology. II. Pathological laughing and crying. *J Neurol Psychopathol* 1923; **4**:299–333.

53. Coelho M, Ferro JM. Fou rire prodromique. Case report and systematic review of literature. *Cerebrovasc Dis* 2003; **16**:101–4.

54. Campbell Burton CA, Murray J, Holmes J, *et al.* Frequency of anxiety after stroke: a systematic review and meta-analysis of observational studies. *Int J Stroke* 2013; **8**:545–59.

55. Robinson RG. Poststroke anxiety disorders. Clinical and lesion correlates. In: Robinson RG, ed. *The Clinical Neuropsychiatry of Stroke. Cognitive, Behavioral, and Emotional Disorders Following Vascular Brain Injury*, 2nd edn. Cambridge: Cambridge University Press; 2006: 326–33.

56. Morrison V, Pollard B, Johnston M, MacWalter R. Anxiety and depression 3 years following stroke: demographic, clinical, and psychological predictors. *J Psychosom Res* 2005; **59**:209–13.

57. Campbell Burton CA, Holmes J, Murray J, *et al.* Interventions for treating anxiety after stroke. *Cochrane Database Syst Rev* 2011; **12**: CD008860.

58. Mead GE, Hsieh CF, Lee R, *et al.* Selective serotonin reuptake inhibitors (SSRIs) for stroke recovery. *Cochrane Database Syst Rev* 2012; **11**: CD009286.

59. Favrole P, Jehel L, Levy P, *et al.* Frequency and predictors of post-traumatic stress disorder after stroke: a pilot study. *J Neurol Sci* 2013; **327**:35–40.

60. Bruggimann L, Annoni JM, Staub F, *et al.* Chronic posttraumatic stress symptoms after nonsevere stroke. *Neurology* 2006; **66**:513–16.

61. Santos CO, Caeiro L, Ferro JM, Figueira ML. Mania and stroke: a systematic review. *Cerebrovasc Dis* 2011; **32**:11–21.

62. Santos CO, Caeiro L, Ferro JM, Figueira ML. A study of suicidal thoughts in acute stroke patients. *J Stroke Cerebrovasc Dis* 2012; **21**:749–54.

63. Pompili M, Venturini P, Campi S, *et al.* Do stroke patients have an increased risk of developing suicidal ideation or dying by suicide? An overview of the current literature. *CNS Neurosci Ther* 2012; **18**:711–21.

64. Ayerbe L, Ayis S, Wolfe CD, Rudd AG. Natural history, predictors and outcomes of depression after stroke: systematic review and meta-analysis. *Br J Psychiatry* 2013; **202**:14–21.

65. Hackett ML, Yapa C, Parag V, Anderson CS. Frequency of depression after stroke: a systematic review of observational studies. *Stroke* 2005; **36**:1330–40.

66. Caeiro L, Ferro JM, Santos CO, Figueira ML. Depression in acute stroke. *J Psychiatry Neurosci* 2006; **31**:377–83.

67. Caeiro L, Ferro JM, Costa J. Apathy secondary to stroke: a systematic review and meta-analysis. *Cerebrovasc Dis* 2013; **35**:23–39.

68. van Dalen JW, Moll van Charante EP, Nederkoorn PJ, van Gool WA, Richard E. Poststroke apathy. *Stroke* 2013; **44**:851–60.

Stroke and dementia

Barbara Casolla and Didier Leys

Introduction

Stroke and dementia are tightly related. About 1 patient in 10 already has dementia when stroke occurs, 1 in 10 will develop dementia after a first-ever stroke, and this percentage increases dramatically to 1 in 3 in patients with stroke recurrence [1]. In the population currently living in Western countries, of three persons at least one will develop dementia, stroke, or both [2]. Stroke is the leading cause of physical disability in adults: of 1 million inhabitants, 2400 patients have a stroke every year, of whom more than 50% will die or become dependent 1 year later [3]. Dependency after stroke is often due to dementia [4]. Even in stroke survivors who are independent, mild cognitive or behavioral changes may have consequences on familial and professional activities [5]. In the EU, 6.3 million people are affected by dementia [6]. The prevalence of dementia increases with advancing age and is estimated to affect more than 30% of people over 80 years of age. Cerebrovascular diseases account for most cases of older-onset dementia [7–9] and the pathological correlates are more likely to be found when compared to the neurofibrillary tangle and cortical beta amyloid plaques together [10]. The cognitive consequences of stroke carry an associated burden of increased mortality [11, 12], recurrence [13], institutionalization [4], dependency [14], and delayed discharge [15]. Moreover, dementia is one of the largest contributors to all causes of morbidity in Europe, as measured by disability adjusted life years [6].

The relationship between stroke and dementia is more complex than being just a coexistence of two frequent disorders. Besides being a potential cause of dementia, stroke negatively influences the time course of Alzheimer's disease (AD). Post-stroke dementia (PSD) is a significant independent predictor of stroke recurrence [13] and is associated with impaired survival after stroke [16]. Moreover, stroke and AD share many risk factors, such as increasing age, arterial hypertension, and ApoE4 [5]. Reciprocally, dementia may increase stroke risk [17]. The prevalence of stroke and of dementia are likely to increase in the next years, because of the decline in mortality after stroke and aging of Western populations [18, 19]. Therefore, the burden of stroke-related dementia is also likely to increase in the future [5].

Definitions

PSD includes any dementia that occurs after stroke, irrespective of its cause, i.e. vascular, degenerative, or mixed [5]. The concept of PSD is useful for patients who are followed up after a stroke, before an extensive diagnostic workup makes possible a classification into vascular dementia (VaD), degenerative dementia (especially AD), and mixed dementia, i.e. dementia due to the coexistence of vascular lesions of the brain and neurodegenerative lesions, usually of Alzheimer type, both types of lesions being not necessarily severe enough to induce dementia when isolated.

VaD refers to the spectrum of cognitive decline causally associated with brain lesions of vascular origin. The term VaD cannot be used for all patients who have had a stroke and are demented, because many of them have AD.

Limits of this review

This chapter will not cover: (i) cognitive impairment no dementia, but we should bear in mind that the cognitive burden of stroke is severely underestimated, cognitive impairment no dementia being three times

Textbook of Stroke Medicine, Second Edition, ed. Michael Brainin and Wolf-Dieter Heiss. Published by Cambridge University Press. © Michael Brainin and Wolf-Dieter Heiss 2014.

more frequent in patients who have had a stroke than in stroke-free controls [20]; and (ii) dementia associated with apparently purely "silent" vascular lesions of the brain (silent infarcts, microbleeds, and leukoaraiosis), i.e. brain lesions presumably of vascular origin that occur in the absence of clinical symptoms of stroke or transient ischemic attacks. Therefore, our review will focus only on dementia that occurs – or was already present – in patients who have had clinical symptoms of stroke.

Search strategy

References for this review were identified by searches of Medline between 1970 and March 20, 2013 and references cited by relevant articles. Manuscripts were selected on the basis of the presence of the following key words in the title: (i) dementia or cognition or cognitive decline or cognitive impairment or cognitive dysfunction or Alzheimer; plus (ii) stroke or cerebrovascular or infarct or haemorrhage or hemorrhage or ischaemia or ischemia or white matter or leucoaraiosis or leukoaraiosis or microbleed. We reviewed only manuscripts, with abstracts published in English, French, German, Italian, or Dutch. Abstracts and reports from meetings were not included. The final reference list was generated based on originality and relevance to the topics covered in the review (dementia in patients who have clinical signs of stroke). Due to the limitation of 50 references for this chapter, we finally gave priority to the most recent references, and we used a previous review written by one of us [5] anytime it was possible, especially in the section on factors influencing the occurrence of dementia after stroke. Therefore, many relevant references published before can be found in our previous review [5], and are not cited in this chapter.

Descriptive epidemiology of dementia occurring after stroke

Prevalence of dementia in stroke survivors

The prevalence of dementia among people who have had a stroke is similar to that observed in patients who have never had a stroke but are 10 years older [21]. Similarly, dementia is 3.5 to 5.8-fold more frequent in patients who have had a stroke than in stroke-free controls, after adjustment on age [22].

Pendlebury and Rothwell showed that 90% of the heterogeneity on the prevalence rate of PSD could be explained by differences in methodology [1]. Among patients who have experienced a stroke the prevalence rate of PSD varies depending on time of assessment, the study setting (hospital or population-based studies), and whether the patients have a pre-existing cognitive decline or recurrent strokes. The criteria used for the diagnosis of PSD contribute to the heterogeneity [5, 23]. The prevalence of dementia in the first year after stroke ranges from 7% in population-based studies when patients with pre-existing cognitive decline are excluded, up to 40% in hospital-based studies when patients with pre-existing cognitive decline and recurrent stroke are included [1]. In hospital-based studies including first-ever or recurrent stroke and excluding pre-existing dementia, the prevalence rate is about 20% [1]. Details on studies evaluating the prevalence of PSD are provided in Table 15.1.

Incidence of new-onset dementia in stroke survivors

Incidence studies are limited by similar methodological issues [5]. Many so-called PSD are actually not "new-onset" dementia, but undiagnosed pre-existing dementia revealed after stroke. Although many studies lacked a systematic approach for the screening of pre-existing dementia, Pendlebury and Rothwell found a pooled prevalence rate of 9–14%[1]. In a recent study on a large cohort of patients with hemorrhagic strokes, the prevalence of pre-existing dementia reached 16%, amounting up to 37% in recurrent strokes [24]. Moreover, a lobar location of hemorrhage is strongly associated with a higher rate of pre-existing dementia and with clinical correlates that suggest an underlying neurodegenerative process [24]. Again, differences in incidence rates of dementia depend on the study setting [1]. When pre-stroke dementia patients are excluded, in hospital-based studies the incidence of PSD is about 20% at 3–6 months and linearly increases by 3% per year [1]. The incidence rate of dementia is lower when considering population-based studies and higher when recurrent strokes are included [1]. After recurrences, the rate of dementia doubles if compared to first-ever stroke, probably the rate being dependent on the exact number of recurrences. The incidence rate steeply

Table 15.1. Prevalence of post-stroke dementia. Studies are classified by increasing duration of follow-up. The same study may appear several times if several assessments were performed at different time intervals after stroke. References of the studies cited in this table can be found in Leys *et al.* [5].

First author, year	Follow-up (months)	Number of patients	Population characteristics	Criteria for dementia	Prevalence (%)
Tatemichi, 1990	7–10 days	726	Ischemic stroke Age ≥60 years	Clinician's opinion	16.3
Andersen, 1996	1	220	First-ever stroke Age: 60–80 years	Mattis Dementia Rating Scale	32.0
Tatemichi, 1992	3	251	Ischemic stroke Age ≥60 years	DSM III R	26.3
Censori, 1996	3	110	First-ever ischemic stroke	NINDS-AIREN	13.6
Pohjasvaara, 1998	3	337	Ischemic stroke Age: 55–85 years	DSM III	31.8
Barba, 2000	3	251	Stroke Age ≥18 years	DSM IV	22.1
Desmond, 2000	3	453	Ischemic stroke Age ≥60 years	DSM III R	26.3
Madureira, 2001	3	237	Stroke patients with no previous functional deficit	NINDS-AIREN	5.9
Lin, 2003	3	283	Ischemic stroke, no patient with previous TIA	ICD-10	9.2
Mok, 2004	3	75	Ischemic stroke associated with small-vessel disease	Clinical dementia rating scale ≥ 1	13.3
Tang, 2004	3	280	Stroke Age ≥ 60 years	DSM IV	15.5
Zhou, 2004	3	434	Ischemic stroke Age ≥55 years	DSM IV	27.2
Rasquin, 2004	6	146	First-ever ischemic stroke Age ≥40 years MMS ≥15 (acute stage)	DSM IV	8.5
Andersen, 1996	6	220	First-ever stroke Age: 60–80 years	Mattis Dementia Rating Scale	26.0
Hénon, 2001	6	202	Stroke Age ≥40 years	ICD-10	22.8
Inzitari, 1998	12	339	Stroke	Proxy-informant interview based on ICD-10	16.8
Hénon, 2001	12	202	Stroke Age ≥40 years	ICD-10	21.4
Rasquin, 2004	12	196	First-ever ischemic stroke Age ≥40 years MMS ≥15 (acute stage)	DSM IV	10.0

Table 15.1. (cont.)

First author, year	Follow-up (months)	Number of patients	Population characteristics	Criteria for dementia	Prevalence (%)
Linden, 2004	18	149	Stroke Age ≥70 years	DSM III R	28.0
Hénon, 2001	24	202	Stroke Age ≥40 years	ICD-10	21.6
Hénon, 2001	36	202	Stroke Age ≥40 years	ICD-10	19.2

DSM = Diagnostic and Statistical Manual of Mental Disorders; NINDS = National Institute of Neurological Disorders and Stroke; AIREN = Association Internationale pour la Recherche et l'Enseignement en Neurosciences; ICD = International Classification of Disease.

increases in the first year and progressively keeps a slower linear increase over subsequent time [1].

Relative risk of dementia after stroke

A history of stroke approximately doubles the risk of dementia incidence in the population aged >65 years but people who survived without dementia to 85 years are not at increased risk of dementia incidence compared with their stroke-free age-matched subjects [25]. The excess risk of dementia increases in studies on incidence compared to studies on prevalence of PSD. This likely reflects both the higher risk of dementia within the first few months after stroke and the higher rate of mortality in individuals with stroke and dementia. In the first year after stroke, patients have a 9-fold increased risk of incident dementia when compared with controls. The excess rate of incident dementia in stroke patients vs. controls persists in the following years, but after the first year, it decreases to 2–4 times the background risk. In the Framingham study, the results were similar 10 years after stroke, after adjustment for age, sex, education level, and exposure to individual risk factors for stroke [26]. In the Rochester study, the risk of AD was doubled after 25 years. A study where stroke was not associated with an increased risk of dementia [27] was actually conducted in non-aphasic patients, with mild first-ever strokes, and only 1 year of follow-up, i.e. the best conditions to minimize the incidence of new-onset dementia. Finally, the results of hospital- and community-based studies can be summarized as follows: (i) stroke doubles the risk

of dementia, (ii) the attributable risk is highest during the first year after stroke, then declines and the relative risk of dementia remains stable around 2–4, (iii) the risk of delayed dementia (including AD) remains also doubled 10 years and more after stroke.

Factors influencing the occurrence of dementia after stroke

Determinants of PSD that have been found in at least two independent studies, or have been identified recently, are listed in Table 15.2.

Demographic and medical characteristics of the patient

The most important demographic predictors of dementia after stroke, shared with pre-stroke dementia, are older age (weighted mean difference = 5.1, 4.6–5.7 years, p< 0.0001), low educational level, prior cognitive decline, and premorbid disability [28]. Being White as opposed to being Black or Hispanic is protective. Female sex was not generally a significant independent predictor of PSD when multivariate adjustment was done for age and other risk factors.

Among vascular risk factors, diabetes mellitus and atrial fibrillation are independent predictor factors of PSD [1]. Myocardial infarction was found to be an independent risk factor for dementia after stroke in several studies [5] but a recent meta-analysis [1] did not confirm the result. Arterial hypertension, ischemic heart disease, cholesterol, prior TIA, and

Table 15.2. Determinants of dementia after stroke. This table includes only determinants of dementia after stroke that have been found in at least two independent studies or identified recently. A few determinants may not have been confirmed in other studies, often because of lack of statistical power. References of the studies cited in this table and published before April 30, 2005 can be found in Leys *et al.* [5].

Demographic and medical characteristics of the patient

Demographic variables
Increasing age
Low education level

Pre-stroke dependency
Dependency

Pre-stroke cognitive decline
Pre-stroke cognitive decline without dementia

Vascular risk factors
Diabetes mellitus
Atrial fibrillation
Myocardial infarction
ApoE4 genotype

Hypoxic-ischemic disorders
Epileptic seizures
Sepsis
Cardiac arrhythmias
Congestive heart failure

Silent brain lesions
Silent infarcts
Global cerebral atrophy
Medial temporal lobe atrophy
Leukoaraiosis

Stroke characteristics

Stroke severity
More severe clinical deficit at onset
Stroke recurrence
Stroke volume

Location of the cerebral lesions
Supratentorial lesions
Left hemispheric lesions
Anterior and posterior cerebral artery territory infarcts
Strategic infarcts
Multiple lesions

smoking were not associated with PSD [1]. The influence of alcohol consumption on PSD remains unproven [5]. All these vascular factors were associated with pre-stroke dementia, but not with PSD, suggesting that the development of PSD is more dependent on stroke-related factors. Nonetheless,

the results concerning the vascular risk factors should be interpreted with caution because they could still be confounded with stroke-related factors, including severity of stroke, mortality, and recurrence. Results on ApoE4 genotype are inconsistent. ApoE4 genotype is independently associated with an increased risk of dementia after stroke in some studies [29], but not all.

Pre-existing silent brain lesions in stroke patients

Silent infarcts, i.e. cerebral infarcts seen on CT- or MRI-scans that have never been associated with a relevant neurological deficit, are associated with an increased risk of dementia after stroke [5]. Their influence is more important when the follow-up is longer: in the Lille study, silent infarcts were associated with dementia after stroke at year 3 but not at year 2 and in the Maastricht study silent infarcts were independently related with dementia after 12 months, but not after 1 and 6 months [30, 31]. Stroke patients with associated silent infarcts seem to have steeper decline in cognitive function than those without, but this decline might be confined to those with additional silent infarcts after baseline.

Patients with small-vessel disease (SVD) have various degrees of brain atrophy that is considered part of the SVD spectrum. The underlying cause is the coexistence of the aging process, degenerative mechanism, and subcortical vascular changes. Global cerebral atrophy is associated with a higher risk of dementia after stroke [5].

Medial temporal lobe atrophy (MTLA) represents a stronger predictor of pre-stroke dementia than PSD, suggesting a primary role in primary degenerative brain pathology. MTLA clearly differentiates demented from non-demented patients after a first-ever ischemic stroke, even after exclusion of patients who had pre-stroke cognitive impairment [5]. Stroke patients with MTLA may have pre-clinical AD that is clinically revealed by stroke [32]. However, MTLA is not specific to AD, as it has also been observed in VaD [5].

The presence and severity of leukoaraiosis are independent predictors of both pre-stroke and post-stroke dementia [33]. In multivariate models, leukoaraiosis remained predictive of PSD. Nonetheless, potential confounding factors are higher stroke severity and recurrence, associated with leukoaraiosis and the coexistence with neuroimaging correlates of SVD (cerebral atrophy, lacunar infarcts) [34, 35].

Brain microbleeds (BMBs) are related to cerebral amyloid angiopathy, hypertension, and atherosclerosis [36]. They are frequent in ischemic stroke patients, especially those with intracerebral arteriolopathies and in patients with VaD, and a lower degree of AD [36, 37]. BMBs are generally considered clinically silent, although recent evidence suggests that they may contribute to such clinical deficits as emotional lability in stroke [38]. Moreover, BMBs are also indicators of underlying brain vascular pathology, with consequences on executive dysfunction and cognitive decline after stroke [39, 40]. In a recent study the authors showed that the absence of BMBs may be associated with a higher likelihood of reversion from cognitive impairment no dementia phenotype after stroke [38]. However, the question of their influence on the risk of PSD has never been systematically addressed and further study with large sample size are required to explore the effect of BMB location on cognitive functions after stroke.

Stroke characteristics

Most factors associated with PSD are related to the stroke itself. Most studies found that a more severe clinical deficit at onset is associated with a higher risk of dementia after stroke [5]. Besides, a study where stroke volumes were evaluated showed a relationship between a higher stroke volume and the risk of dementia [41].

Multiple infarcts in multiple locations impact the cognitive performances more than a single infarct or multiple infarcts in a single location [42]. We could expect that having infarcts in more than one location may result in different risk of having PSD.

Differences in survival rates between stroke subtypes (ischemic or hemorrhagic) make it difficult to state that the risk of dementia is influenced by the type of stroke. Nevertheless, hemorrhagic stroke was predictive for PSD in the meta-analysis [1].

In the Framingham study large artery infarcts, lacunar infarcts, and infarcts of unknown origin were associated with a higher risk of dementia after stroke [26]. In other studies, the risk of dementia after stroke was lower in patients with SVD [5]. These results are influenced by the higher mortality rate in stroke subtypes associated with more severe deficits, i.e. in stroke survivors who are the most likely to develop

dementia [5]. The presence of multiple strokes distributed in time and location (previous stroke, multiple infarcts, and recurrent stroke) are also associated with a higher risk of dementia after stroke [5].

Supratentorial lesions, left hemispheric lesions, and strokes presenting with aphasia are predictors of PSD [1]. Anterior and posterior cerebral artery territory infarcts and so-called "strategic infarcts" i.e. single cerebral infarcts that may lead to dementia by their own in the absence of any other lesion, have been found to be associated with an increased risk of dementia after stroke in at least two independent studies [5]. Strategic locations (left angular gyrus, inferomesial temporal and mesiofrontal locations, thalami, left capsular genu, caudate nuclei) have been described more than 20 years ago in single case reports, or in small series, usually without MRI, and without follow-up. Therefore, other vascular brain lesions or coexisting AD cannot be excluded in most cases. This concept should be revisited in large prospective studies, with MRI and long follow-up to exclude associated AD [5].

Several complications of stroke such as early epileptic seizures, incontinence, sepsis, delirium, cardiac arrhythmias, congestive heart failure, hypoxic ischemic episodes, and hypotension are also independently associated with an increased risk of dementia after stroke [1, 5]. However, these statistical associations do not mean a causal relationship: it is also possible that dementia increases the risk of such events [5].

Causes of post-stroke dementia

The most frequent causes of dementia after stroke are VaD, AD, and mixed AD-VaD [5]. AD and mixed AD-VaD account for up to 61% of patients with dementia after stroke (Table 15.3). Two Asian studies did not confirm this high proportion of AD patients, but in one the study population was at least 10 years younger than in all other studies, and patients who were lost to follow-up at the 3-month evaluation were more cognitively impaired at the acute stage, and in the other the diagnosis of VaD was based on the DSM IV criteria, which are less specific [43, 44, 45].

In the following circumstances vascular lesions are the most prominent or even the only determinants of dementia after stroke: (i) in stroke patients who are too young to have Alzheimer lesions, and became demented just after stroke; (ii) when cognitive functions were normal before stroke, impaired

Table 15.3. Causes of new-onset dementia after stroke. Studies are classified by increasing duration of follow-up. The same study may appear more than once in this table if assessments were performed at different time intervals. References of the studies cited in this table can be found in Leys *et al.* [5].

Author, year	Follow-up after stroke*	Number of patients[†]	Study population	VaD (%)	AD (%)	AD+VaD (%)
Tatemichi, 1990	7–10 days	726	Hospital	39	36	25
Tatemichi, 1992	3	251	Hospital	56	36	–
Pohjasvaara, 1998	3	337	Hospital	81	19	–
Barba, 2000	3	251	Hospital	75	25	–
Desmond, 2000	3	453	Hospital	57	39	–
Tang, 2004	3	280	Hospital	98	–	2
Kokmen, 1996	12	–	Community		41	–
Zhu, 2000	36	–	Community	100	–	–
Hénon, 2001	36	202	Hospital	67	33	–
Ivan, 2004	120	–	Community	51	–	37

* In months unless specified.
[†] Available only for hospital-based studies. VaD = vascular dementia; AD = Alzheimer's disease.

immediately after, and did not worsen – or even slightly improved – over time; (iii) when a specific vascular condition known to cause stroke and dementia (e.g. CADASIL [Cerebral autosomal dominant arteriopathy with subcortical infarcts and leukoencephalopathy]) is proven by a specific marker; or (iv) when the lesion is located in a strategic area. In many other circumstances dementia is the consequence of the coexistence of Alzheimer and vascular lesions.

Even when vascular lesions or Alzheimer pathology do not lead to dementia by themselves, their association may reach the threshold of brain lesions required to induce dementia [32]: when a stroke occurs in a patient with asymptomatic Alzheimer pathology, the period of pre-clinical AD may be shortened and the clinical onset of AD may therefore be anticipated [32]. Patients usually have a clinical presentation of AD that appears several months or years after stroke. Vascular risk factors exacerbate post-stroke brain damage and there is evidence that they are associated with reduced recovery of cognitive function after stroke. These concepts of mixed dementia emphasize the fact that those patients have two disorders and should be treated for AD and receive appropriate stroke prevention. Considering those patients as having pure AD may lead to an underestimation of the need for secondary stroke

prevention measures. The hypothesis of a possible summation of lesions is supported by the results of the Optima and of the Nun studies, showing that among patients who met neuropathological criteria for AD, those with brain infarcts had poorer cognitive functions before death and a higher prevalence of dementia [46]. This hypothesis was also supported by the results of the Syst-Eur dementia substudy showing that nitrendipine decreases the incidence rate of AD [47], suggesting that stroke prevention reduces the risk of new-onset AD.

Influence of dementia on stroke outcome

Mortality

Both population- and hospital-based studies have shown that stroke patients with dementia after stroke have higher mortality rates than non-demented stroke patients, independently of age and comorbidities. The long-term mortality rate after stroke is 2- to 6-fold higher in patients with dementia, after adjustment for demographic factors, associated cardiac diseases, stroke severity, and stroke recurrence [11, 34]. This increase in mortality rate in stroke patients with dementia may be due to increased overall mortality rate in patients with dementia, a more severe underlying vascular disease, or a higher risk of any nonspecific complication in patients with dementia [5]. It is also possible that, in the presence of dementia, patients receive less appropriate stroke prevention [5]. Stroke patients with dementia may also be less compliant for stroke prevention.

Stroke recurrence

Dementia diagnosed 3 months after stroke is associated with a 3-fold increased risk of stroke recurrence [48]. Dementia may be a marker for a more severe vascular disease leading to an increased risk of recurrence [5]. Less intensive stroke prevention and lack of compliance may contribute to the increased risk of recurrence [48]. Leukoaraiosis could also be a confounding factor, as it is associated with an increased risk of stroke recurrence [30].

Functional outcome

Although mild cognitive impairment (MCI) is out of the scope of this chapter, the recent Secondary Prevention of Small Subcortical Strokes (SPS3) trial on lacunar stroke identified MCI in a half of the study population [49]. Cognitive impairment, often overlooked, represents a clinical sequela more prevalent than physical disability and affecting more than 40% of patients with no significant disability in lacunar strokes. Interestingly, the authors showed that MCI may occur in patients without physical disability, especially in younger patients [49]. Therefore, cognitive effects of lacunar stroke should be considered at least as important as disability related to motor or sensory deficits [49].

Moreover, the few available data on the influence of dementia on functional outcome after stroke suggest that stroke patients with dementia are more impaired and more dependent in daily living activities than stroke patients without dementia [5].

Treatments of stroke in patients with dementia

There are no conclusive data in randomized clinical trials that may help to determine how acute stroke therapy and stroke prevention should be conducted in patients who are demented before or develop dementia after stroke [5].

In the absence of studies specifically designed for stroke patients with dementia, current guidelines for stroke prevention should be applied, but we should bear in mind that the specific issue of secondary prevention of stroke in patients with dementia (either pre-existing or new-onset dementia) is not addressed in any guidelines. Therefore, an effective primary stroke prevention, specific treatment in the acute phase, and optimal secondary prevention strategies should be settled up by the stroke specialist to prevent PSD. Moreover, in a recent trial with citicoline, also known as cytidine diphosphate-choline, the authors showed that a long-term treatment (12 months) improved some cognitive performances in patients with acute stroke [50].

Accordingly, a symptomatic approach of the dementia syndrome is necessary, depending on the presumed cause (AD, VaD, or mixed AD-VaD). Both AD and VaD share a cholinergic deficit, and both conditions show improvement under cholinesterase inhibitors [5].

Conclusions

Recognition of dementia in stroke patients is important because it indicates a worse outcome with higher mortality rates, more recurrences, and more functional impairment. Research should now focus on a delineation of the concept of post-stroke cognitive decline without dementia, which may be a preliminary stage of dementia after stroke, be much more frequent in practice, and be a better target for therapeutic approaches. Moreover, it could be relevant to outline the relationship between stroke subtype and cognition. Other epidemiological studies are also necessary to evaluate the evolution over time of the burden of dementia after stroke at the community level, in order to have a better knowledge of the need in term of resources and its evolution over time.

Chapter summary

> Post-stroke dementia (PSD) includes any dementia that occurs after stroke, irrespective of its cause, i.e. vascular, degenerative, or mixed.
>
> The prevalence of dementia among people who have had a stroke is similar to that observed in patients who have never had a stroke but are 10 years older.

The incidence of PSD (with pre-stroke dementia patients excluded) is about 20% at 3–6 months and linearly increases by 3% per year. After recurrences, the rate of dementia doubles if compared to first-ever stroke.

The results of hospital- and community-based studies can be summarized as follows: (i) stroke doubles the risk of dementia, (ii) the attributable risk is the highest within the first year after stroke, then declines and the relative risk of dementia remains stable around 2–4, (iii) the risk of delayed dementia (including Alzheimer's disease [AD]) remains also doubled 10 years and more after stroke.

Factors influencing the occurrence of dementia after stroke are: older age, low educational level, prior cognitive decline and premorbid disability, diabetes mellitus, and atrial fibrillation. Results on the influence of ApoE4 genotype and myocardial infarction on the risk of dementia after stroke are inconsistent.

Most factors associated with PSD are related to the stroke itself. A more severe clinical deficit at onset is associated with a higher risk of dementia after stroke. And there is a relationship between the risk of dementia and the stroke volume, and the number and the location of infarcts.

The most frequent causes of dementia after stroke are vascular dementia, AD, and mixed dementia.

Patients with dementia after stroke have 2- to 6-fold higher mortality than non-demented stroke patients and a 3-fold increased risk of stroke recurrence.

An effective primary stroke prevention, specific treatment in the acute phase, and optimal secondary prevention strategies should be settled up by the stroke specialist to prevent PSD.

References

1. Pendlebury ST, Rothwell PM. Prevalence, incidence, and factors associated with pre-stroke and post-stroke dementia: a systematic review and meta-analysis. *Lancet Neurol* 2009; **8**:1006–18.

2. Seshadri S, Wolf PA. Lifetime risk of stroke and dementia: current concepts, and estimates from the Framingham Study. *Lancet Neurol* 2007; **6**:1106–14.

3. Hankey GJ, Warlow CP. Treatment and secondary prevention of stroke: evidence, costs, and effects on individuals and populations. *Lancet* 1999; **354**:1457–63.

4. Pasquini M, Leys D, Rousseaux M, Pasquier F, Henon H. Influence of cognitive impairment on the institutionalisation rate 3 years after a stroke. *J Neurol Neurosurg Psychiatry* 2007; **78**:56–9.

5. Leys D, Henon H, Mackowiak-Cordoliani MA, Pasquier F. Poststroke dementia. *Lancet Neurol* 2005; **4**:752–9.

6. Wittchen HU, Jacobi F, Rehm J, *et al.* The size and burden of mental disorders and other disorders of the brain in Europe 2010. *Eur Neuropsychopharmacol* 2011; **21**:655–79.

7. Schneider JA, Arvanitakis Z, Bang W, Bennett DA. Mixed brain pathologies account for most dementia cases in community-dwelling older persons. *Neurology* 2007; **69**:2197–204.

8. Sonnen JA, Larson EB, Crane PK, *et al.* Pathological correlates of dementia in a longitudinal, population-based sample of aging. *Ann Neurol* 2007; **62**:406–13.

9. Savva GM, Wharton SB, Ince PG, *et al.* Age, neuropathology, and dementia. *N Engl J Med* 2009; **360**:2302–9.

10. Matthews FE, Brayne C, Lowe J, *et al.* Epidemiological pathology of dementia: attributable-risks at death in the Medical Research Council Cognitive Function and Ageing Study. *PLoS Med* 2009; **6**:e1000180.

11. Barba R, Morin MD, Cemillan C, *et al.* Previous and incident dementia as risk factors for mortality in stroke patients. *Stroke* 2002; **33**:1993–8.

12. Henon H, Durieu I, Lebert F, Pasquier F, Leys D. Influence of prestroke dementia on early and delayed mortality in stroke patients. *J Neurol* 2003; **250**:10–16.

13. Sibolt G, Curtze S, Melkas S, *et al.* Poststroke dementia is associated with recurrent ischemic stroke. *J Neurol Neurosurg Psychiatry* 2013; **84**:722–6.

14. Narasimhalu K, Ang S, De Silva DA, *et al.* The prognostic effects of poststroke cognitive impairment no dementia and domain-specific cognitive impairments in nondisabled ischemic stroke patients. *Stroke* 2011; **42**:883–8.

15. Appelros P. Prediction of length of stay for stroke patients. *Acta Neurol Scand* 2007; **116**:15–19.

16. Melkas S, Oksala NK, Jokinen H, *et al.* Poststroke dementia predicts poor survival in long-term follow-up: influence of prestroke cognitive decline and previous stroke. *J Neurol Neurosurg Psychiatry* 2009; **80**:865–70.

17. Chi NF, Chien LN, Ku HL, Hu CJ, Chiou HY. Alzheimer disease and risk of stroke: a population-based cohort study. *Neurology* 2013; **80**:705–11.

18. Ukraintseva S, Sloan F, Arbeev K, Yashin A. Increasing rates of dementia at time of declining mortality from stroke. *Stroke* 2006; **37**:1155–9.

19. Rothwell PM, Coull AJ, Giles MF, *et al.* Change in stroke incidence, mortality, case-fatality, severity, and risk factors in Oxfordshire, UK from 1981 to 2004 (Oxford Vascular Study). *Lancet* 2004; **363**:1925–33.

20. Linden T, Skoog I, Fagerberg B, Steen B, Blomstrand C. Cognitive impairment and dementia 20 months after stroke. *Neuroepidemiology* 2004; **23**:45–52.

21. De Ronchi D, Palmer K, Pioggiosi P, *et al.* The combined effect of age, education, and stroke on dementia and cognitive impairment no dementia in the elderly. *Dement Geriatr Cogn Disord* 2007; **24**:266–73.

22. Prencipe M, Ferretti C, Casini AR, *et al.* Stroke, disability, and dementia: results of a population survey. *Stroke* 1997; **28**:531–6.

23. Erkinjuntti T, Ostbye T, Steenhuis R, Hachinski V. The effect of different diagnostic criteria on the prevalence of dementia. *N Engl J Med* 1997; **337**:1667–74.

24. Cordonnier C, Leys D, Dumont F, *et al.* What are the causes of pre-existing dementia in patients with intracerebral haemorrhages? *Brain* 2010; **133**:3281–9.

25. Savva GM, Stephan BC. Epidemiological studies of the effect of stroke on incident dementia: a systematic review. *Stroke* 2010; **41**:e41–6.

26. Ivan CS, Seshadri S, Beiser A, *et al.* Dementia after stroke: the Framingham Study. *Stroke* 2004; **35**:1264–8.

27. Srikanth VK, Anderson JF, Donnan GA, *et al.* Progressive dementia after first-ever stroke: a community-based follow-up study. *Neurology* 2004; **63**:785–92.

28. Ojala-Oksala J, Jokinen H, Kopsi V, *et al.* Educational history is an independent predictor of cognitive deficits and long-term survival in postacute patients with mild to moderate ischemic stroke. *Stroke* 2012; **43**:2931–5.

29. Jin YP, Ostbye T, Feightner JW, Di Legge S, Hachinski V. Joint effect of stroke and APOE 4 on dementia risk: the Canadian Study of Health and Aging. *Neurology* 2008; **70**:9–16.

30. Henon H, Durieu I, Guerouaou D, *et al.* Poststroke dementia: incidence and relationship to prestroke cognitive decline. *Neurology* 2001; **57**:1216–22.

31. Rasquin SM, Verhey FR, van Oostenbrugge RJ, Lousberg R, Lodder J. Demographic and CT scan features related to cognitive impairment in the first year after stroke. *J Neurol Neurosurg Psychiatry* 2004; **75**:1562–7.

32. Pasquier F, Leys D. Why are stroke patients prone to develop dementia? *J Neurol* 1997; **244**:135–42.

33. Pasquier F, Henon H, Leys D. Relevance of white matter changes to pre- and poststroke dementia. *Ann N Y Acad Sci.* 2000; **903**:466–9.

34. Henon H, Vroylandt P, Durieu I, Pasquier F, Leys D. Leukoaraiosis more than dementia is a predictor of stroke recurrence. *Stroke* 2003; **34**:2935–40.

35. Jokinen H, Kalska H, Mantyla R, *et al.* White matter hyperintensities as a predictor of neuropsychological deficits post-stroke. *J Neurol Neurosurg Psychiatr.* 2005; **76**:1229–33.

36. Cordonnier C, Al-Shahi Salman R, Wardlaw J. Spontaneous brain microbleeds: systematic review, subgroup analyses and standards for study design and reporting. *Brain* 2007; **130**:1988–2003.

37. Cordonnier C, van der Flier WM, Sluimer JD, *et al.* Prevalence and severity of microbleeds in a memory clinic setting. *Neurology* 2006; **66**:1356–60.

38. Tang WK, Chen YK, Lu JY, *et al.* Microbleeds and post-stroke emotional lability. *J Neurol Neurosurg Psychiatry* 2009; **80**:1082–6.

39. Werring DJ, Frazer DW, Coward LJ, *et al.* Cognitive dysfunction in patients with cerebral microbleeds on T2*-weighted gradient-echo MRI. *Brain* 2004; **127**:2265–75.

40. Greenberg SM, Eng JA, Ning M, Smith EE, Rosand J. Hemorrhage burden predicts recurrent intracerebral hemorrhage after lobar hemorrhage. *Stroke* 2004; **35**:1415–20.

41. Sachdev P, Brodaty H. Vascular dementia: an Australian perspective. *Alzheimer Dis Assoc Disord* 1999; **13** (Suppl 3): S206–12.

42. Saczynski JS, Sigurdsson S, Jonsdottir MK, *et al.* Cerebral infarcts and cognitive performance: importance of location and number of infarcts. *Stroke* 2009; **40**:677–82.

43. Lin JH, Lin RT, Tai CT, *et al.* Prediction of poststroke dementia. *Neurology* 2003; **61**:343–8.

44. Tang WK, Chan SS, Chiu HF, *et al.* Frequency and determinants of poststroke dementia in Chinese. *Stroke* 2004; **35**:930–5.

45. Gold G, Bouras C, Canuto A, *et al.* Clinicopathological validation study of four sets of clinical criteria for vascular dementia. *Am J Psychiatry* 2002; **159**:82–7.

46. Snowdon DA, Greiner LH, Mortimer JA, *et al.* Brain infarction and the clinical expression of Alzheimer disease.

The Nun Study. *JAMA* 1997; **277**:813–17.

47. Forette F, Seux ML, Staessen JA, *et al.* Prevention of dementia in randomised double-blind placebo-controlled Systolic Hypertension in Europe (Syst-Eur) trial. *Lancet* 1998; **352**:1347–51.

48. Moroney JT, Bagiella E, Tatemichi TK, *et al.* Dementia after stroke increases the risk of long-term stroke recurrence. *Neurology* 1997; **48**:1317–25.

49. Jacova C, Pearce LA, Costello R, *et al.* Cognitive impairment in lacunar strokes: the SPS3 trial. *Ann Neurol* 2012; **72**:351–62.

50. Alvarez-Sabin J, Ortega G, Jacas C, *et al.* Long-term treatment with citicoline may improve poststroke vascular cognitive impairment. *Cerebrovasc Dis* 2013; **35**:146–54.

Chapter

16

Ischemic stroke in the young and in children

Valeria Caso and Didier Leys

Introduction

Stroke is a major public health issue because of its frequency, risk of death and residual physical cognitive and/or behavioral changes, along with risk of recurrent cardiac or cerebral vascular event [1–3]. Although strokes occur at a mean age of 75 years in Western countries, [4–6] they also occur in young patients, and even in children [4–7]. Most strokes occurring in young patients are ischemic in origin, accounting for 2% and 12% of all strokes, according to community- and hospital-based data, respectively [8, 9].

In this chapter, we will focus on ischemic strokes in young adults, specifically their epidemiology, causes, treatments, and outcomes.

Epidemiology

Currently, "young" is defined in the literature as under 45 years of age. Most young people having stroke are between 40 and 45 years of age [7].

Overall incidence rates under the age of 45 range from 7 to 15 in 100 000 people/year for all stroke (ischemic and hemorrhagic) [10–14], with higher rates reported in some countries [15]. A few studies reporting similar incidence rates have examined all stroke in the 15- to 44-year-old age group [16, 17] or ischemic stroke only in the 15- to 49-year-old age group (6.6 to 11.4 in 100 000 people/year) [9, 18, 19]. Under the age of 35, rates have been reported to be less than 10 in 100 000 people/year; ranging from 0 to 9. There may be a greater incidence of stroke in developing countries, such as Libya, which has a reported rate of 47 in 100 000 people/year for all strokes under the age of 45 [15]. High rates of 70 in 100 000 have also been reported for Japanese

35 to 44 years of age [20], whereas the Northern Manhattan Stroke Study reported a rate of 26 in 100 000 for Hispanics aged 22 to 44 [21]. The Greater Cincinnati/Northern Kentucky Stroke Study reported rates on 35- to 44-year-old American Blacks, with a relative stroke risk of 5 compared to Whites of the same age, equal to 96 in 100 000 and 19 in 100 000, respectively. In the 0- to 34-year-old Black group, a relative risk (RR) of 2.2 was observed [22, 23]. This trend is supported by the results of the Northern Manhattan Stroke Study, which reported a non-significant trend of increased risk among Blacks aged 22 to 44 years old [21]. Interestingly, two studies of Caribbean Blacks have demonstrated similar stroke rates to those reported in other young stroke populations [24, 25], suggesting that the increased risk among young Blacks in the United States is related to socioeconomic variables, although high rates have been observed in South African Blacks of all ages [26]. Very high young stroke rates have also been observed in a rural population from Northern Portugal [27]. With regard to sex differences in the incidence of young stroke, rates are higher in males than females in the 35- to 44-year-old age group [4, 11]. Regarding young women, the incidence of ischemic stroke during pregnancy is around 43 per million deliveries, which is similar to that observed in non-pregnant women of the same age [28]. Population-based estimates of the incidence of stroke in children, including hemorrhagic stroke, range from 2.3 to 13.0 per 100 000 children [29]. About 50% of incident strokes in children are ischemic, with a higher incidence reported for boys [29].

> Overall incidence rates under the age of 45 range from 7 to 15 in 100 000 people/year for all stroke (ischemic and hemorrhagic), with higher rates reported in some countries.

Diagnostic workup

Diagnostic workup for young stroke patients does not generally differ from that of older patients except for the protocol in determining cause. In fact, recommendations from the European Stroke Organisation are not age specific [30]. Cervical and transcranial ultrasounds, magnetic resonance angiography of cervical and intracranial arteries, continuous ECG monitoring, and transthoracic and transesophageal echocardiography need to be performed according to the same recommendations specified for older stroke patients, and will therefore not be detailed in this chapter.

Cerebral ischemia occurring during pregnancy requires the same diagnostic workup as that for non-pregnant women. Specifically, magnetic resonance imaging (MRI) is the investigation of choice over both CT and percutaneous angiography, although its safety profile for the fetus has never been evaluated. Gadolinium enhancement is, however, not recommended as its effects on the fetus remain unknown.

The patient interview

Interviews of the patient and close relatives can provide information on the cause of cerebral ischemia. Therefore, they need to be carried out repeatedly focusing on the following checklist:

- any presence of cervical pain or headache occurring before stroke (in favor of a dissection)
- any presence of pulsatile tinnitus before stroke (in favor of a dissection)
- recent intake of illicit substances (in favor of toxic angiopathies)
- recent intake of vasoconstrictive drugs (in favor of toxic angiopathies)
- history of migraine with aura (in favor of migrainous infarct)
- history of definite systemic inflammatory disorder, or suggestive clinical features such as photosensitivity, arthritis, pericarditis, pleuritis, repetitive spontaneous miscarriage, oral or genital aphtosis, unexplained fever, anemia, thrombopenia, proteinuria (in favor of cerebral vasculitis)
- family history of ischemic stroke occurring in young patients (in favor of genetic causes, such as CADASIL [cerebral autosomal dominant arteriopathy with subcortical infarcts and leukoencephalopathy])

- family history of migraine with aura, severe depression or dementia occurring in young patients (in favor of CADASIL)
- personal history of irradiation (in favor of post-irradiation arteriopathy)
- any personal medical history that may orientate towards a specific etiology of cerebral ischemia.

Skin examination

A thorough skin examination needs to be performed focusing on:

- features of abnormal skin elasticity, varicose veins, spontaneous ecchymosis, abnormal scars (in favor of Ehlers–Danlos disease)
- papulosis (in favor of malignant atrophic papulosis, so-called Degos disease)
- livedo racemosa (in favor of Sneddon disease)
- neurofibromas and *"taches café au lait"* (in favor of von Recklinghausen disease)
- angiokeratomas (in favor of Fabry disease)
- facial lentiginosis (possibly associated with cardiac myxoma).

Fundoscopic examination

Fundoscopic examination needs to be performed to identify signs of:

- hypertensive retinopathy
- cholesterol emboli
- perivascular retinitis (in favor of Eales syndrome)
- multiple retinal ischemia (in favor of Susac syndrome).

The biological workup

The biological workup needs to include:

- the same biological workup as in older patients: blood cell count, glucose level, cholesterol and triglyceride levels, erythrocyte sedimentation rate, fibrinogen, and C-reactive protein
- in selected patients, in the absence of a clearly identified cause of cerebral ischemia the following should be investigated for:
  - activated cephalin time (when increased, lupus anticoagulant needs to be excluded)
  - serology for syphilis and human immune deficiency virus (HIV)
  - electrophoresis of proteins

- dosage of antiphospholipid antibodies in case of multiple spontaneous miscarriages, deep venous thrombosis, false positivity of syphilitic serology, or systemic disorder
- the exclusion of congenital thrombophilia in the presence of personal or family history of multiple venous thrombosis (proteins C and S, antithrombin III, resistance to activated protein C, mutation of factor V Leiden, mutation of thrombin gene), but these causes of thrombophilia are rare causes for cerebral ischemia except in the case of cerebral venous thrombosis.

Diagnostic workup must include a large variety of symptoms and careful examination of other systems (skin, retina) as well as a search for systemic diseases.

Causes of ischemic stroke in the young

There are huge differences in the breakdown of etiologies depending on the centers and countries where the data are collected [7, 8, 17, 31–40]. Despite an extensive diagnostic workup, the cause of cerebral ischemia remains undetermined in up to 45% of young patients [7, 8, 17, 31–33, 37, 38, 41, 42]. To this regard, even at specialized centers, diagnostic workup can be negative because it was performed too late after stroke onset [41]. The most frequent cause in western countries is cervical artery dissection, whereas, in non-industrialized countries, valvulopathies are the most frequent causes. In this chapter we will describe etiologies according to the TOAST classification [43], although the first three categories (large-vessel atherosclerosis, cardioembolism, and small-vessel occlusion) are rare in young patients.

Large-vessel atherosclerosis

Large-vessel atherosclerosis accounts for less than 10% of cerebral ischemia before the age of 45 years, and is found mainly in males between 40 and 45 years. Atherosclerosis has no known specificity concerning the clinical presentation, diagnosis, and predisposing factors. Smoking is a major risk factor in this age category, and a family history is frequent, suggesting a genetic predisposition [44]. Recently, the prevalence of both extracranial and intracranial atherosclerotic stenoses and occlusions in both transient ischemic attack (TIA) and ischemic stroke patients aged 18–55 years in the large European,

multicenter database of the Stroke in Young Fabry Patients 1 (SIFAP1) study have been reported. In these patients with ischemic stroke, the overall prevalence of carotid artery stenoses and occlusions was 8.9%, of which 81% were symptomatic. Non-stenotic carotid plaques were more common in males compared to females (15.8% vs. 7.7%; p = 0.001), and in middle-aged patients compared to young patients (17.0% vs. 4.9%; p = 0.001). Supratentorial intracranial artery stenoses and occlusions were reported to be 11.8%. Diversely, supratentorial stenoses occurred more frequently in middle-aged patients (13.0% vs. 7.8%; p = 0.001), whereas occlusions were equally present at non-significant rates of 3.2% for each [45].

Cardioembolism

The main causes of cardioembolism in young patients are listed in Table 16.1. A few of them deserve more details.

Atrial fibrillation

Atrial fibrillation is associated with a very low risk of cerebral emboli in young people when occurring in the absence of either underlying cardiopathy (lone atrial fibrillation) and of vascular risk factors. However, it confers a high risk of cerebral emboli when there are risk factors for stroke, especially high blood pressure, or an underlying cardiopathy, such as mitral stenosis or cardiomyopathy. In the absence of any evidence of atrial fibrillation on ECG, the search for paroxysmal atrial fibrillation by endovascular stimulation can provide results that are difficult to interpret in the absence of reliable controls. Most studies on endovascular stimulation have been conducted in too-small cohorts, and have therefore lacked statistical power. The efficacy of endovascular stimulation remains debatable even in subgroups that may be at risk, such as patients with interatrioseptal abnormalities [46].

Infectious endocarditis

Infectious endocarditis is not always associated with fever. In the early stage, transthoracic echocardiography (TTE) and transesophageal echocardiography (TEE) may reveal vegetations. When negative, these investigations should be repeated.

Patent foramen ovale (PFO)

Patent foramen ovale (PFO) is present in 10–20% of young patients with cerebral ischemia [47, 48], which has been suggested to be familial, especially for females [49]. PFO is characterized by a communication between the right and left atriums which becomes functional when the pressure in the right atrium becomes higher than that in the left one (e.g. pulmonary embolism, Valsalva maneuver). PFO is diagnosed by TTE or TEE with contrast, or transcranial Doppler with contrast. When there is a causal relationship, possible mechanisms of cerebral ischemia include paradoxical emboli (requiring deep venous thrombosis, pulmonary embolism, and cerebral ischemia without other potential causes), local thrombosis in the PFO (most likely hypothesis but almost never proven), or paroxysmal atrial fibrillation [46]. The risk of recurrence after a first ischemic stroke in the presence of an isolated PFO has been reported to be the same as that for ischemic stroke patients of similar age who have no PFO [50].

Table 16.1. Main cardiac sources of cerebral ischemia in young adults

High-risk cardiopathies

- atrial fibrillation associated with cardiopathy, or vascular risk factors or previous systemic emboli
- mitral stenosis
- mechanical prosthetic valve
- infectious endocarditis
- marastic endocarditis
- intracardiac thrombus
- acute myocardial infarction
- ventricular akinesia
- dilated cardiomyopathy
- intracardiac tumor (myxoma, papillary fibroelastoma)
- paradoxical emboli through a PFO or interatrial communication
- congenital cardiopathies with cyanosis
- IASA plus PFO
- complication of catheterism and cardiac surgery

Low-risk cardiopathies

- lone atrial fibrillation
- mitral valve prolapse
- mitral calcification
- bioprosthesis
- aortic stenosis
- bicuspid aortic valve
- Lambl excrescence
- isolated IASA
- isolated PFO

IASA = interatrioseptal aneurysm; PFO = patent foramen ovale.

Transcranial Doppler with contrast enhancement best evidences a right-to-left shunt, which is a marker of PFO in most cases. However, though very rarely, a pulmonary arteriovenous malformation disease can be the cause of right-to-left shunt and when so Rendu–Osler is present. Therefore, the presence of a shunt without evidence of a PFO should lead to a suspicion of pulmonary arteriovenous malformation.

Interatrioseptal aneurysm (IASA)

Interatrioseptal aneurysm (IASA) is defined as a protrusion of the interatrial septum in either atrium and is rare in the absence of PFO [50]. Diagnostic criteria are, on TEE, an excursion of 10 mm or more during cardiac contraction, having a base of at least 15 mm [50]. Presence of IASA is more frequent in young patients who have had an ischemic stroke of unknown cause [48], but in the absence of associated PFO, the presence of an IASA is not to be considered a marker of increased risk of recurrence [50]. Paroxysmal atrial fibrillation and local thrombosis in the IASA are the most likely mechanisms of cerebral ischemia when a causal relationship exists.

Associated PFO and IASA

The association of PFO and IASA (Figure 16.1) in patients aged 55 years or less, who have had an ischemic stroke of unknown cause, is a marker of increased risk of recurrence [50]. Furthermore, the FOP-ASIA study [50], after 4 years of follow-up, reported a rate of recurrent strokes equal to 15.2% (95% confidence

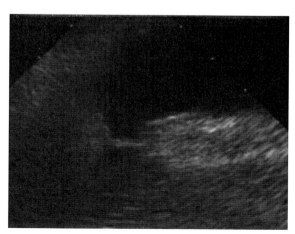

Figure 16.1. Transesophageal echocardiography showing a patent foramen ovale and an interatrioseptal aneurysm.

interval [CI] 1.8–28.6%) in patients with PFO and IASA, whereas it was only 2.3% (95% CI 0.3–4.3%) in those with isolated PFO, 4.2% (95% CI 1.8–6.6%) in those without PFO and IASA, and 0.0% in those with isolated IASA. Therefore, the coexistence of PFO and IASA seems to be associated with a 4.2-fold increased risk of recurrence (95% CI 1.5–11.8). However, the recently published Closure trial (Evaluation of the STARFlex Septal Closure System in Patients with a Stroke and/or Transient Ischemic Attack due to Presumed Paradoxical Embolism through a Patent Foramen Ovale) reported that, in patients with cryptogenic stroke or TIA who had a PFO, closure with a device did not lead to a greater benefit than medical therapy alone for the prevention of either recurrent stroke or TIA [51]. Moreover, recurrences have been reported to be due to causes other than paradoxical embolism [51].

These results were supported by the RESPECT trial (Randomized Evaluation of Recurrent Stroke Comparing PFO Closure to Established Current Standard of Care Treatment) [52]. The primary analysis of this trial did not demonstrate that endovascular PFO closure was superior to medical therapy alone in the prevention of stroke (1.33% vs. 1.73% at 1 year, 1.60% vs. 3.02% at 2 years, and 2.21% vs. 6.40% at 3 years, hazard ratio [HR] 0.492, 95% CI 0.217–1.114, p = 0.0830). However, the per-protocol analysis of 20 events suggested benefit from PFO closure, HR 0.366, 95% CI 0.141–0.955, p = 0.032. Additionally, subset analyses suggested equal benefit in the presence of a substantial shunt or atrial septal aneurysm. This benefit should be better defined upon the results from the ongoing REDUCE trial (GORE® HELEX® Septal Occluder/GORE® Septal Occluder and Antiplatelet Medical Management for Reduction of Recurrent Stroke or Imaging-Confirmed TIA in Patients With Patent Foramen Ovale).

Mitral valve prolapse

Mitral valve prolapse is defined as a protrusion of one or two mitral valves in the left atrium and has been found in 2–6% of the general population [53]. However, its diagnostic criteria often lacked precision in studies and its role in cerebral ischemia remains unclear and controversial. The risk of cerebral emboli in patients with mitral valve prolapse is very low except in cases of either associated atrial fibrillation or endocarditis.

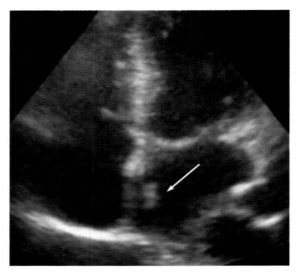

Figure 16.2. Transesophageal echocardiography showing a left atrial myxoma (arrow).

Intracardiac myxoma

Intracardiac myxoma (Figure 16.2) is the most frequent intracardiac tumor. Its prevalence is 10 per million inhabitants and is usually located in the left atrium. In less than 50% of cases, it leads to systemic emboli associated with fatigue, weight loss, fever, and sometimes cardiac signs such as dyspnea, murmur, or variations in blood pressure. Most myxomas remain asymptomatic and are revealed after an ischemic stroke. The presence of facial lentiginosis (rare autosomal dominant disorder) may be associated with a myxoma.

Papillary fibroelastoma

Papillary fibroelastoma is a benign tumor which is usually located on a cardiac valve, making it difficult to distinguish from vegetation.

Peripartum cardiomyopathies

Peripartum cardiomyopathies are multifactorial and associated with a high mortality rate. They are very rare in Western countries, but are reported rather frequently in sub-Saharan countries during the last month of pregnancy and during the post-partum period [54]. The clinical presentation is that of a cardiac failure [55], often associated with cerebral emboli [55].

Small-vessel occlusion

Lacunar infarcts are small infarcts of less than 15 mm located in the deep white matter, basal ganglia, and brainstem and are the consequence of an occlusion of a single deep perforating intracerebral artery less than 400 μm in diameter. These perforators have no collaterals and their occlusions more than often lead to an infarct. Short-term outcome is usually good, but the risk of cognitive decline and dementia is great following multiple recurrences.

Lipohyalinosis

Lipohyalinosis is a disorder leading to occlusions of the deep perforators. Arterial hypertension is the most important risk factor, but such hypertensive arteriolopathies are very rare before the age of 45 years.

CADASIL

CADASIL is a genetic disorder of small deep perforating arteries identified on the basis of clinical, MRI (Figure 16.3), and genetic criteria [56, 57]. CADASIL is due to a mutation of the *Notch3* gene on chromosome 19 [57], leading to an accumulation within the walls of small perforators and this leads to progressive occlusions. CADASIL is associated with migraine with aura, depression, multiple subcortical infarcts, and, at the final stage, dementia with pseudobulbar palsy [56, 57]. White matter changes are always already severe on MRI when the first symptoms manifest, which is usually during the third decade of life [57]; leading to death within 20 years after the first symptoms.

Other definite causes of cerebral ischemia

These other causes include the following.

Diseases of large arteries

- *Cervical artery dissections* are the leading cause of cerebral ischemia in the young in Western countries when a cause can be clearly identified [7, 58]. In most cases, no trauma can be identified, or the trauma is mild and a causal relationship between a trivial trauma and dissection is even disputable [58, 59]. The most likely hypothesis to explain most cases is that of a trivial trauma [7] involving an artery prone to dissection for genetic [60, 61] or infectious reasons [62]. Inherited elastic tissue disorders, especially Ehler–Danlos type IV, predispose to dissections but are rarely diagnosed.
- *Dissections associated with intracranial aneurysms* as well as familial cases are rare. But, when they do occur, they are usually due to an underlying elastic tissue disorder. Recurrences of stroke and of dissections are rare [58, 59], and their overall outcomes can be considered as excellent except when stroke is severe at the acute stage [58, 59]. Currently, diagnosis is achieved utilizing reliable non-invasive investigations, such as Doppler ultrasonography and MRI. Both of these techniques are able to evidence the mural hematoma (Figure 16.4) [58, 59].
- *Post-irradiation cervical arteriopathies* in young patients are often due to irradiation for hematological disorders, and less frequently for throat cancers. Radiodermatitis is always present in the area of irradiation, which can lead to local atheroma. Outcome is primarily dependent on the underlying disorder rather than on

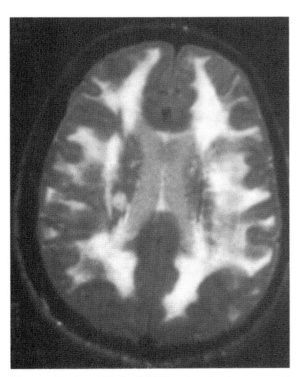

Figure 16.3. Brain MRI of a CADASIL patient showing severe white matter abnormalities and lacunas.

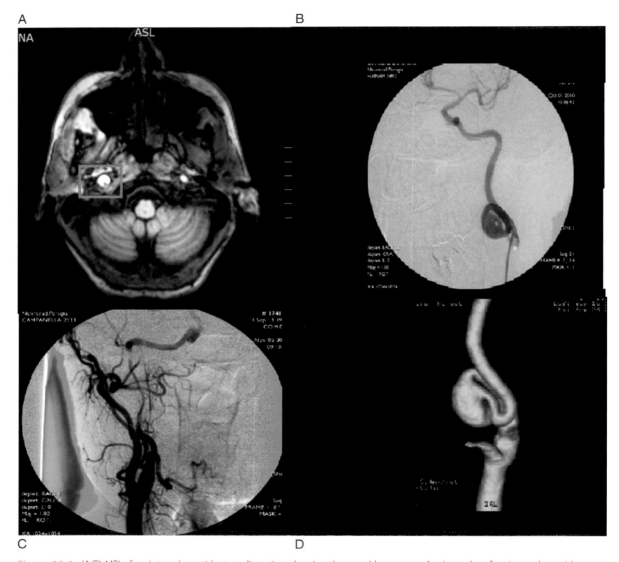

Figure 16.4. (A/B) MRI of an internal carotid artery dissection, showing the mural hematoma. Angiography of an internal carotid artery dissection with distal occlusion. (C/D) Angiography and CT angiography of pseudoaneurysm.

irradiation arteriopathy, especially in asymptomatic cases [63].

- *Cervical fibromuscular dysplasia of cervical arteries* is associated with a low risk of ischemic stroke, except in cases of dissection, and can be either isolated or associated with other locations such as renal arteries. Recklinghausen disease or elastic tissue disorders are often found in these patients.

- *Intracranial dissections* are very rare and difficult to diagnose. They mainly occur in children, and are often revealed after a cerebral ischemia. They can trigger a subarachnoid hemorrhage especially when located in the vertebrobasilar territory. Their prognosis is usually poor. Regarding the undiagnosed asymptomatic cases there are no data concerning prevalence.

- *Moyamoya disease* is a progressive intracranial vasculopathy that usually becomes symptomatic in children or young adults and may lead to ischemia, hemorrhage, or both. Angiography shows a tight stenosis or occlusion of the intracranial carotid arteries associated with

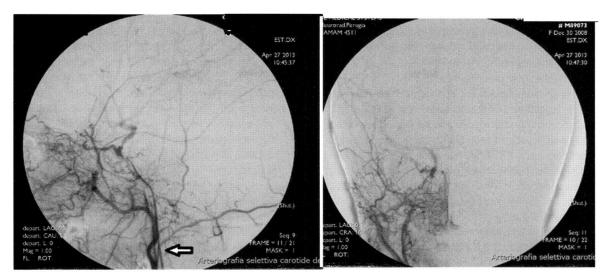

Figure 16.5. Conventional angiography of moyamoya (arrow) with distal occlusion of the right internal carotid artery with collaterals with the reperfusion of the ophthalmic artery and carotid syphon.

intracerebral neo-vessels (Figure 16.5). Any disorder that leads to progressive stenosis or occlusion of intracranial carotid arteries in children or in young adults may be a cause of moyamoya.

- *Secondary vasculitis occurring during a systemic disorder* or as a first-ever manifestation.
  - Systemic disorders where cerebral vasculitis is minor (panarteritis nodosa, Churg–Strauss syndrome, systemic lupus erythematosus, Sjögren syndrome, Behçet syndrome, sarcoidosis, Crohn's disease, ulcerative rectocolitis) are usually diagnosed on the basis of other manifestations of the disease and depending on the type of systemic disorder. Sarcoidosis can be diagnosed by neuropathological biopsy whereas systemic lupus erythematosus can be diagnosed according to diagnostic criteria.
  - Takayasu disease is a chronic inflammatory disease that progressively involves the aorta and the brachiocephalic arteries occurring prevalently in females before 45 years of age. In these patients cerebral ischemia is most often due to progressive stenoses or occlusion of the cervical artery when arising from the aortic arch.
  - Buerger disease, better known as thromboangiitis obliterans, is a segmental inflammatory vasculitis involving arteries of intermediate and small calibers as well as superficial veins. Moreover, this disorder generally involves peripheral arteries but only seldom cerebral arteries.
  - Eales disease is an inflammatory vasculitis that mostly involves retinal arteries though very rarely does it involve cerebral arteries. Its causal relationship with cerebral ischemia is uncertain.
  - Acute multifocal placoid pigment epitheliopathy is a bilateral primary disorder that is characterized by permanent visual deficits and rarely is it associated with cerebral vasculitis [64]. Its clinical picture is that of a decreased visual acuity and fever. Diagnosis is based upon evidence of specific lesions at fundoscopy and inflammatory cerebrospinal fluid (CSF). Standard treatment includes intravenous corticosteroids and immunosuppressant therapy [64].
  - Köhlmeier–Degos disease or malignant atrophic papulosis is a systemic vasculitis that involves for the most part the skin. When either the brain or the bowel is involved, the disease is defined as severe.
- *Secondary vasculitis occurring in the context of an infectious disorder.* This type of vasculitis has been reported to manifest in patients with bacterial infections including syphilis, tuberculosis, Lyme

disease; viral infections including ophthalmic herpes zoster, HIV; parasites including malaria, cysticercosis, etc.; and mycotic infections including aspergillosis, candidosis, and cryptococcosis.

- *Primary vasculitis of the central nervous system* is a non-infectious, non-sarcoidosic inflammatory granulomatous disorder having giant cells which are restricted to the leptomeningeal and cerebral arteries [65]. Its incidence is reported to be 2.4 new cases per year per million inhabitants [65], and it occurs in both genders around 40 years of age. The first symptom is usually headache, followed by subacute focal neurological deficits, sometimes transient, and seizures [65]. Cerebral infarcts are usually multiple, cortical, and sometimes associated with hemorrhages. There is no systemic biological sign of inflammation and fever is rarely observed. Furthermore, CSF may be normal, but is usually characterized by an increased number of lymphocytes with or without oligoclonal bands. Neuroradiological features include the following: (i) on CT or MRI scans multiple infarcts of small size in cortical areas, with or without associated hemorrhages, and (ii) on conventional angiography or MRA multiple beadings in intracranial arteries in various territories [65]. These findings are not specific whereas a biopsy of the leptomeningeal arteries is. In the absence of treatment (corticosteroids sometimes associated with cyclophosphamide for at least 1 year) or in the case of failure of treatment, the outcome is poor, with occurrence of cognitive decline, dementia, and a high mortality rate [65]. It is possible that primary vasculitis of the central nervous system is a heterogeneous entity that actually consists of several subsets of diseases [65].
- *Sneddon syndrome* is a potential cause of recurrent cerebral ischemia. Each episode is usually of mild severity but repeated recurrence can lead to dementia. Prior to ischemia, patients generally have livedo racemosa, which is a purple livedo, involving the trunk and the most proximal part of the limbs, that does not disappear with cutaneous warming, unlike the innocuous livedo reticularis. Here, antiphospholipid antibodies are revealed. Although there is not a high level of evidence, oral anticoagulation is recommended by experts.

- *Acute reversible cerebral angiopathies* have been reported. Despite severe clinical presentations, their outcomes are usually excellent. Clinical presentation most often consists of a combination of severe headache, vomiting, epileptic seizures, and focal neurological deficits. Possible etiologies include the use of a vasoconstrictive drug, cocaine, or amphetamines; reversible hypertensive encephalopathies; pheochromocytoma; carcinoid tumors; or vasospasm after subarachnoid hemorrhage.
- *Post-partum cerebral angiopathy* is a rare entity that usually occurs in the first 2 weeks after delivery. This angiopathy is believed to belong to the group of toxic angiopathies. Its clinical presentation is similar to that of the above discussed *acute reversible cerebral angiopathies*. Also here, outcome is usually excellent [66, 67]. Angiography, either conventional or preferably MRA, shows multiple beadings in large intracranial arteries that disappear spontaneously within a few weeks (Figure 16.6) [66, 67]. This angiopathy is favored by estrogen withdrawal, the use of vasoconstrictive drugs, and possibly bromocriptine [66, 67].
- *Eclampsia* is the main cause of maternal mortality and preterm birth in Western countries [68]. Clinical presentation generally consists of headache, visual impairment, confusion or coma, epileptic seizures, and focal neurological deficits [68, 69]. The HELLP syndrome (Hemolysis, Elevated Liver

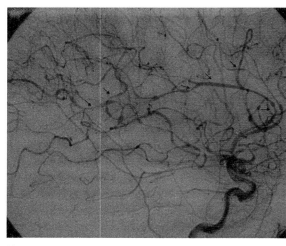

Figure 16.6. Post-partum angiopathy: beading (arrows) of cerebral arteries.

274

enzymes, Low Platelets) is a subtype of eclampsia [70]. MRI can reveal in either FLAIR or T2 sequences, multiple hyperintense signals, which are: isolated or more frequently confluent, more prominent in posterior areas, bilateral, and located at the junction between the cortex and the subcortical white matter [71, 72]. These abnormalities completely disappear after a few days or weeks. Cerebral infarcts may lead to residual deficits, but in most patients who survive the acute stage, long-term outcome is favorable [28].

- *Unruptured aneurysms of intracranial arteries* may be a cause of cerebral ischemia secondary to a local intra-saccular thrombosis and subsequent distal emboli.

Hematological diseases

- *Thrombotic thrombocytopenic purpura (Moschcowitz syndrome)* is a systemic disorder characterized by fever, renal failure, thrombocytopenia, and hemolytic anemia with a negative Coombs test [73]. Cerebral infarcts are present in most cases [73]. The neurological manifestations may be the first manifestations of the disease [73]. Diagnosis is easily achieved from a low platelet count and the presence of schizocytes.

- *Hemoglobinopathies*

  . Sickle-cell disease is a cause of ischemic stroke in children and young adults as well as pregnant women [29].

  . Beta thalassemia is also a possible cause of cerebral ischemia.

- *Nocturnal paroxysmal hemoglobinuria (Marchiafava–Micheli disease)*

- *Congenital thrombophilia* is characterized by deficits in proteins C and S or antithrombin III, resistance to activated protein C, mutation of factor V Leiden, or mutation of the thrombin gene. These have been proven to be causes of cerebral venous thrombosis, but their roles in arterial ischemia remain disputable [74]. Indeed, in a recent meta-analysis, the role of factor V Leiden was analyzed in 18 case–control studies of ischemic stroke in adults ≤50 years of age. The authors reported that in those patients where stroke was likely to be related to a prothrombotic genetic condition ("selected" ischemic stroke studies) factor V Leiden was more strongly associated with stroke (odds ratio [OR] 2.73; 95%

CI 1.98 –3.75), whereas among the eight "unselected" ischemic stroke studies, the association between factor V Leiden and stroke was substantially weaker (OR 1.40; 95% CI 0.998–1.95) [75]. Another case–control study reported an increased incidence of prothrombin gene mutation, as well as more than one thrombophilic defect among young stroke patients with a PFO compared to those with stroke without evidence of PFO [76].

- *Acquired thrombophilia includes antiphospholipid antibody syndrome* and is known to cause arterial and venous occlusions, recurrent spontaneous miscarriages, as well as biological changes such as thrombocytopenia, false positivity of syphilis serology, and activated cephalin time increase. It may be either associated with a systemic disorder such as systemic lupus erythematosus or primary. Various mechanisms can lead to cerebral ischemia: prothrombotic state, Libman–Sacks endocarditis, or early atheroma.

- *Other hematological causes* of cerebral ischemia in young people can include polycythemia, iron-deficiency anemia, leukemia, thrombocytemia, hypereosinophilic syndrome, endovascular lymphoma, disseminated intravascular coagulation, and hyperviscosity syndromes.

Metabolic disorders

- *Fabry disease* is an X-linked recessive lysosomal storage disease resulting from deficient alpha-galactosidase which can cause an endothelial vasculopathy followed by cerebral ischemia [77]. Few female cases have been reported [77], while various types of mutations have been identified. The typical clinical picture is made up of episodes of unexplained fever, cutaneous angiokeratomas located in the trunk and proximal part of limbs, crisis of painful acroparesthesia of feet and hands, corneal opacities, hypohydrosis, and ultimately cardiac and renal failure. Ischemic strokes occurring during the fourth decade of life are often associated with headache and more than often located in the vertebrobasilar territory. Ischemic strokes are generally triggered by dolichomega intracranial arteries, occlusions of the deep perforating arteries due to the accumulation of sphingolipids, cardiopathies, and a prothrombotic state. The frequency of Fabry disease has been reported to be 1.2% in young

275

ischemic stroke patients with a negative diagnostic workup in a large German study [77]. Despite its rarity, it is important that physicians consider it as a possible diagnosis because of possible therapeutic consequences with infusion of alpha-galactosidase [77]. Diagnosis is performed on the basis of a low plasma alpha-galactosidase activity or mutation in the *alpha-GAL* gene in males, and only by identification of the mutation in females [77].

- *Homocystinuria* has a reported prevalence of 3 per million inhabitants. One-third of these patients will have a venous or arterial event during their lives. In patients with increased homocysteine a mutation in the gene of the methyltetrahydrofolate reductase (MTHFR) is often found. However, it is more frequent to observe a slight increase in plasma homocysteine (>15 μmol/l), which is thought to be more a concomitant factor than a real cause. Folic acid supplementations reduce the serum level of homocysteine, but whether they also reduce the rate of vascular events remains to be proven.
- *MELAS syndrome (Mitochondrial Encephalopathy with Lactic Acidosis and Stroke-like episodes)* is a mitochondriopathy due to several types of mutation in the mitochondrial DNA. The major clinical features are, in a patient around 30 years of age, progressive deafness, stroke-like episodes (usually transient and located in posterior territories), seizures, cognitive impairment as well as recurrent episodes of both headache and vomiting. Other manifestations of the disease can include: progressive external ophthalmoplegia with ptosis, muscular pain at exercise, lactic acidosis after exercise, presence of ragged red fibers on muscular biopsy, cataracts, hypogonadism, diabetes mellitus, hypothyroidism, and cardiomyopathy.

Non-cruoric emboli

- *Gas emboli* can occur during cesarean sections, traumatic deliveries, subclavian catheter accidents, gynecological and cardiac surgeries, and diving accidents [78]. The clinical picture typically consists of acute respiratory failure and acute diffuse encephalopathy, preceded by severe anxiety and dyspnea [78]. In a few minutes, tachycardia, seizures, and coma can develop, leading to death [78]. When gas embolism is suspected, patients should be placed in a left lateral decubitus position.

- *Amniotic emboli* can occur after difficult deliveries in the presence of vaginal lesions. This embolism can lead to acute pulmonary edema and seizures [28, 79].
- *Fat emboli* generally occur in long bones' fractures or after liposuction surgery [80].

Choriocarcinoma

Choriocarcinoma is a malignant trophoblastic tumor that has been revealed in 1 pregnancy out of 40 000. Lesions of the arterial wall may occur and lead to cerebral ischemia in the absence of metastasis [81].

Rare causes of cerebral ischemia of undetermined mechanism in young people

- *Sweet syndrome (acute febrile neutrophilic dermatosis)* is a dermatological disorder characterized by multiple pustules and painful purple skin lesions due to a neutrophilic infiltration [82]. This disorder usually has concomitant features of systemic inflammation such as fever, conjunctivitis or other types of ocular inflammation, and arthritis [82]. *Sweet syndrome* mainly occurs around the age of 40 and may be associated with cancer [82]. Cerebral ischemia is often associated, but a causal relationship is not proven.
- *Kawasaki syndrome* is a panarteritis of arteries of intermediate and small caliber that may lead to coronary or cerebral artery occlusions [83].
- *Susac syndrome* (or SICRET syndrome) is a rare disease occurring in young women of unknown pathogenesis, consisting of a triad with retinal arterial occlusion, hearing loss by cochlear ischemia, and diffuse vascular encephalopathy [84].
- *HERNS syndrome (hereditary endotheliopathy with retinopathy and stroke)* is an autosomal dominant hereditary syndrome characterized by retinopathy, nephropathy, and ischemic stroke. Fundoscopic examination reveals a typical vasculopathy [85].

Cerebral ischemia of undetermined and unknown causes

Before classifying a patient in this category it is important to be sure that the diagnostic workup has been extensive enough and repeated over time. In fact, often the etiology is found during the follow-up.

Risk factors for stroke in the young

Conventional risk factors

Conventional risk factors for stroke (arterial hypertension, smoking, and hypercholesterolemia) are also risk factors in the young, but their attributable risks are lower than in older patients. These risk factors are more frequent in young patients with a negative diagnostic workup [7]. Data from "Get with the Guidelines–Stroke database" from 2005 through 2010 reported a high rate of conventional vascular risk factors in consecutive inpatients aged 18–45 years with ischemic stroke/transient ischemic attack [86], while data from the Nationwide Inpatient Sample (NIS), including 20% of all US community hospitals, reported that the prevalence of hypertension, diabetes, obesity, lipid disorders, and tobacco use increased from 1995 to 2008 among adolescents and young adults (aged 15–44 years) hospitalized with acute ischemic stroke. These increases in coexisting traditional stroke risk factors were associated with an increase in ischemic strokes for young adults [87].

More specific risk factors in the young

Oral contraceptive therapy

Oral contraception (OC), even progesterone-only formulations, as well as high estrogen dosage, has been reported to increase stroke risk in young women [88]. The third generation of low-dose OCs is associated with a 2-fold increased risk of stroke [89]. Characteristics of OC agents, such as higher hormonal dosages and higher percentages of estrogens, increase stroke risks; other conventional factors that increase stroke risks, in combination with OC, include hypertension, hyperlipidemia, obesity, age (>35), and smoking, all of which have a dose-responsive risk effect [90]. However, their annual absolute risk is low; 1 in 5880 females without vascular risk factors treated [91]. For this, oral contraceptive therapy is contraindicated only for high-risk females defined as those who have already had a stroke or have another vascular risk factor.

Migraines

Migraines, mostly with aura, are reported to be associated with both hemorrhagic and ischemic strokes [92–96], coronary events [97], and all-cause mortality. A recent meta-analysis has reported an increased risk of ischemic stroke in females with any migraine, versus females with no migraine (pooled RR 2.08;

95% CI 1.13–3.84), but not in males with any migraine versus no migraine (1.37, 0.89–2.11) [98].

The relationship between migraine with aura and ischemic stroke appears to be independent of conventional cardiovascular risk factors, except for smoking and oral contraceptive use [98]. Females with migraine have been reported to have an increased frequency of deep white matter lesions on imaging, which may indicate silent subclinical infarcts [99]. However, the specific role of migraine is not understood in determining stroke. The concept of migrainous infarct is not proven: it requires the exclusion of other causes and a typical temporal relationship, the neurological deficit being a prolongation of a typical aura.

HIV infection

HIV infection is also associated with an increased risk of ischemic stroke. The mechanisms of stroke are multiple in HIV-infected patients, with important roles played by both vasculitis and hypercoagulability state [100].

Pregnancy

Pregnancy is associated with an increased risk of ischemic stroke [6, 28, 101]. Stroke during pregnancy is one of the leading causes of maternal death [102–104]. The peri/post-partum period is the period of the highest vascular risk, generally due to: hormonal alterations, hemodynamic changes, hypercoagulability, and blood pressure fluctuation that may interact at a systemic level in susceptible subjects and cause stroke. There may be other local effects such as vascular stasis (especially third trimester) and trauma during labor and delivery that may result in paradoxical thromboembolism or cerebral artery dissection (mainly vertebral artery) in vulnerable subjects. Nonetheless, stroke during pregnancy is more than often attributable to the pregnancy itself, whereas other specific causes only are rarely responsible. However, a study conducted on females who already had had an ischemic stroke showed no significant increase in the incidence of recurrent stroke during subsequent pregnancies.

> Risk factors for stroke in the young consist of conventional risk factors (arterial hypertension, smoking, hypercholesterolemia), oral contraception (the third generation of low-dose OCs is associated with a 2-fold increased risk of stroke), migraines, HIV, and pregnancy.

Outcome

Studies to date that have evaluated the long-term outcome of young stroke patients have been heterogeneous and thus cannot be reliably compared. This is because these studies have included all types of stroke including intracerebral ischemia [14, 17, 31, 37, 105], subarachnoid hemorrhages [14, 17, 31, 37], as well as TIAs. These studies have used different thresholds for both age and recruitment methods, which more than likely produced bias [7, 31, 42, 106]. Moreover, most of these studies have been conducted on small samples, have been retrospective, and have included only a partial follow-up [14, 17, 33, 37, 40, 106, 107], have excluded recurrent cases [14, 31, 37, 108], or have included only patients who survived the acute stage. All of these realities favor bias for less severe cases and better outcomes.

Mortality

Reported mortality rates are low at short and intermediate terms [7, 8, 17, 31, 33–40, 42, 106]. In the Lille cohort of 287 patients, aged between 15 and 45 years, with a mean follow-up of 3 years, with none lost to follow-up, the mortality rate was 4.5% after 1 year and 0.8% per year for the next 2 years [7]. The FUTURE (Follow-Up of Transient Ischemic Attack and Stroke Patients and Unelucidated Risk Factor Evaluation) study was a prospective cohort study of prognosis after TIA and stroke in adults aged 18 through 50 years admitted to Radboud University Nijmegen Medical Centre between January 1, 1980, and November 1, 2010. At the end of follow-up, 20% of patients had died. For each stroke type, observed 20-year mortality among 30-day survivors exceeded expected mortality in the general population. Concerning ischemic stroke, the cumulative 20-year mortality among 30-day survivors was higher in males than in females (33.7% [95% CI, 26.1%–41.3%] vs. 19.8% [95% CI, 13.8%–25.9%]). The standardized mortality ratio was reported to be 4.3 (95% CI, 3.2–5.6) for females and 3.6 (95% CI, 2.8–4.6) for males. For all etiological subtypes of ischemic stroke, observed mortality exceeded expected mortality [109].

Recurrent vascular events (stroke or coronary syndromes)

The risk of recurrent vascular events is low in young stroke patients, but it can be high depending on the cause of cerebral ischemia. In the Lille cohort, the risk of recurrent stroke was 1.4% during the first year and then 1.0% per year during the next 2 years, while the risk of myocardial infarction was 0.2% per year [7]. Likewise, risk of recurrent stroke has been reported to be very low in cervical artery dissection [2, 58, 59, 110, 111].

Furthermore, a negative diagnostic workup is also associated with a low risk of new events [7, 50]. Children are known to have a higher recurrence rate compared to young adults.

Epilepsy

Epilepsy is a more frequent complication after an ischemic stroke in young patients than stroke recurrence, with a reported risk at 3 years being between 5% and 7% [7, 112]. Most young patients with post-stroke epilepsy have their first seizure during the first year after stroke [7, 112].

Quality of life

Even if most patients remain independent, many lose their jobs or divorce over the 3 years following their ischemic strokes [7]. Likely explanations for these events are: depression, fatigue, mild cognitive or behavioral changes, or alteration in social cognition. In a western Norway population-based cohort of patients <50 years with ischemic stroke compared to healthy controls, pain, sleeping problems, and social isolation were higher among patients than controls [16].

Therefore, ischemic strokes in young patients are frequently associated with a decline in quality of life that is not explained by handicap [5, 7, 35].

> The **outcome** is overall good. Reported mortality rates are low at short and intermediate terms. The risk of recurrent vascular events is low. But ischemic strokes in young patients are frequently associated with a decline in quality of life that is not explained by handicap.

Pregnancy after an ischemic stroke

A multicenter French study [113] was conducted on 373 consecutive women who had had an ischemic stroke between 18 and 40 years of age and were followed-up over a 5-year period. An overall risk of recurrent stroke of 0.5% at year 5 (95% CI 0.3–0.95) was observed in periods without pregnancy, and 1.8% (95% CI 0.5–7.5) with pregnancy. These findings suggest that young women who have had an ischemic stroke have an overall low risk of recurrence during a subsequent pregnancy and the risk does not significantly increase during pregnancy [113].

Specificities of children

Besides a higher recurrence rate, children are also more prone to have seizures, altered mental status, as well as dystonia and dyskinesia compared to adults [29].

Secondary prevention after ischemic stroke in young adults

The three main characteristics of ischemic stroke present in young patients are their causes, overall good outcome, and regarding women their fertility status (contraception, pregnancy, and future menopause), and these influence secondary prevention after stroke. As for elderly subjects, secondary prevention measures mainly depend on the presumed cause. For this reason, an extensive and early diagnostic workup is required, as well as an extensive evaluation of risk factors. For young patients secondary prevention requires an optimal management of vascular risk factors, an appropriate antithrombotic therapy (oral anticoagulation and antithrombotic agents depending on the cause), and removal of the source in specific cases (severe internal artery stenoses, cardiac myxoma, etc.). The specificities of stroke prevention in young adults are the following: (i) oral contraceptive therapy should be avoided in most cases; (ii) in the absence of evidence-based data, cervical artery dissections may be treated either by antiplatelet therapy or by anticoagulation [114], but, because of the low rate of recurrence after the fourth week, there is no reason to prescribe oral anticoagulation for more than a few weeks or in patients at increased risk for bleeding; (iii) patients who have a negative diagnostic workup but a PFO at risk (large PFO, or PFO associated with an inter atrioseptal aneurysm) have a 4-fold increased risk of recurrence under aspirin, and should preferably be randomized in trials comparing oral anticoagulation and closure; (iv) the combination of aspirin plus dipyridamole is the standard therapy for patients who can tolerate aspirin, have no clear cardiac indication for clopidogrel, and do not develop headache; (v) as randomized controlled trials have suggested that estrogens increase the severity of ischemic strokes, patients should be informed that hormonal replacement therapy will not be recommended

after menopause unless new data indicate otherwise; (vi) young pregnant women should be informed on secondary prevention measures (continue aspirin up until the last 6 weeks and replace oral anticoagulation with subcutaneous heparin).

When diagnostic workup results are negative, the length of antiplatelet therapy after an ischemic stroke is left to the discretion of the treating physician. However, it must be remembered that patients without any risk factors generally have low risk of recurrence. Thus, in this subgroup it seems to be best that these patients be treated not more than a few years.

> Secondary prevention requires an optimal management of vascular risk factors, an appropriate antithrombotic therapy for a few weeks to a few years, removal of the source in specific cases, and avoidance of oral contraceptive or hormonal replacement therapy.

Conclusion

The etiologies of ischemic stroke in the young are multiple; however, outcome is good in most patients.

Chapter summary

Diagnostic workup

Follow the recommendations from the European Stroke Organisation **plus** a special protocol for determining the cause:
- Intensive patient interview about the presence of headache, tinnitus, drug abuse, history of migraine, history or clinical features of systemic inflammatory disorder, genetic causes, history of irradiation.
- Careful skin examination, fundoscopy, biological workup.
- In selected patients: activated cephalin time, serology for syphilis and HIV, protein electrophoresis, antiphospholipid antibodies, testing for thrombophilia.

Causes

Large-vessel atherosclerosis (less than 10%)
Small-vessel occlusion such as CADASIL
Cardioembolism
Atrial fibrillation
Infectious endocarditis
Patent foramen ovale
Interatrioseptal aneurysm
Mitral valve prolapse
Intracardiac myxoma

279

Diseases of large arteries
Cervical artery dissections
Post-irradiation cervical arteriopathies
Cervical fibromuscular dysplasia
Intracranial dissections
Moyamoya
Secondary vasculitis (panarteritis nodosa, systemic lupus erythematosus, sarcoidosis, Takayasu disease, thrombangitis obliterans)
Primary vasculitis of the central nervous system
Sneddon syndrome
Post-partum cerebral angiopathy and eclampsia
Unruptured aneurysms of intracranial arteries
Hematological disorders
Thrombotic thrombocytopenic purpura
Sickle-cell disease
Nocturnal paroxysomal hemoglobinuria
Congenital thrombophilia
Metabolic disorders such as Fabry disease, homocystinuria, MELAS syndrome
Gas emboli, amniotic emboli, fat emboli
Choriocarcinoma

The first three categories (large-vessel atherosclerosis, cardioembolism, and small-vessel occlusion) are rare in young patients. Cervical artery dissections are the leading cause of cerebral ischemia in the young in Western countries, and in non-industrialized countries, valvulopathies.

Risk factors

Conventional risk factors (arterial hypertension, smoking, hypercholesterolemia)
Oral contraception (the third generation of low-dose oral contraceptives is associated with a 2-fold increased risk of stroke)
Migraines

HIV
Pregnancy

The **outcome** is overall good. Reported mortality rates are low at short and intermediate terms. The risk of recurrent vascular events is low. But ischemic strokes in young patients are frequently associated with a decline in quality of life that is not explained by handicap.

Secondary prevention

Optimal management of vascular risk factors, an appropriate antithrombotic therapy (oral anticoagulation and antithrombotic agents depending on the cause), and removal of the source in specific cases (severe internal artery stenoses, cardiac myxoma, etc.)

The specificities of secondary stroke prevention in young adults are the following:

- oral contraceptive therapy and hormonal replacement therapy after menopause should be avoided in most cases;
- cervical artery dissections may be treated either by antiplatelet therapy or by anticoagulation for a few weeks;
- patients who have a negative diagnostic workup but a patent foramen ovale (PFO) should preferably be randomized in trials comparing oral anticoagulation and closure;
- aspirin plus dipyridamole is the standard therapy for patients who can tolerate aspirin, have no clear cardiac indication for clopidogrel, and do not develop headache;
- young pregnant women should continue aspirin up until the last 6 weeks and replace oral anticoagulation with subcutaneous heparin.

References

1. Bamford J, Sandercock P, Dennis M, Burn J, Warlow C. Classification and natural history of clinically identifiable subtypes of cerebral infarction. *Lancet* 1991; 337(8756):1521–6.

2. Hankey GJ, Warlow CP. Treatment and secondary prevention of stroke: evidence, costs, and effects on individuals and populations. *Lancet* 1999; 354(9188):1457–63.

3. Murray CJ, Lopez AD. Global mortality, disability, and the contribution of risk factors: Global Burden of Disease Study. *Lancet* 1997; 349(9063):1436–42.

4. Bonita R. Epidemiology of stroke. *Lancet* 1992; 339(8789):342–4.

5. Carolei A, Marini C, Di Napoli M, et al. High stroke incidence in the prospective community-based L'Aquila registry (1994–1998). First year's results. *Stroke* 1997; 28(12):2500–6.

6. Giroud M, Milan C, Beuriat P, et al. Incidence and survival rates during a two-year period of intracerebral and subarachnoid haemorrhages, cortical infarcts, lacunes and transient ischaemic attacks. The Stroke Registry of Dijon: 1985–1989. *Int J Epidemiol* 1991; 20(4):892–9.

7. Leys D, Bandu L, Henon H, et al. Clinical outcome in 287 consecutive young adults (15 to 45 years) with ischemic stroke. *Neurology* 2002; 59(1):26–33.

8. Bogousslavsky J, Pierre P. Ischemic stroke in patients under age 45. *Neurol Clin* 1992; **10**(1):113–24.

9. Naess H, Nyland HI, Thomassen L, *et al.* Incidence and short-term outcome of cerebral infarction in young adults in western Norway. *Stroke* 2002; **33**(8):2105–8.

10. Wolfe CD, Giroud M, Kolominsky-Rabas P, *et al.* Variations in stroke incidence and survival in 3 areas of Europe. European Registries of Stroke (EROS) Collaboration. *Stroke* 2000; **31**(9):2074–9.

11. Vibo R, Korv J, Roose M. The Third Stroke Registry in Tartu, Estonia: decline of stroke incidence and 28-day case-fatality rate since 1991. *Stroke* 2005; **36**(12):2544–8.

12. Jerntorp P, Berglund G. Stroke registry in Malmo, Sweden. *Stroke* 1992; **23**(3):357–61.

13. Minelli C, Fen LF, Minelli DP. Stroke incidence, prognosis, 30-day, and 1-year case fatality rates in Matao, Brazil: a population-based prospective study. *Stroke* 2007; **38**(11):2906–11.

14. Marini C, Totaro R, De Santis F, *et al.* Stroke in young adults in the community-based L'Aquila registry: incidence and prognosis. *Stroke* 2001; **32**(1):52–6.

15. Radhakrishnan K, Ashok PP, Sridharan R, Mousa ME. Stroke in the young: incidence and pattern in Benghazi, Libya. *Acta Neurol Scand* 1986; **73**(4):434–8.

16. Ellekjaer H, Holmen J, Indredavik B, Terent A. Epidemiology of stroke in Innherred, Norway, 1994 to 1996. Incidence and 30-day case-fatality rate. *Stroke* 1997; **28**(11):2180–4.

17. Nencini P, Inzitari D, Baruffi MC, *et al.* Incidence of stroke in young adults in Florence, Italy. *Stroke* 1988; **19**(8):977–81.

18. Putaala J, Metso AJ, Metso TM, *et al.* Analysis of 1008 consecutive patients aged 15 to 49 with first-ever ischemic stroke: the Helsinki young stroke registry. *Stroke* 2009; **40**(4):1195–203.

19. Kristensen B, Malm J, Carlberg B, *et al.* Epidemiology and etiology of ischemic stroke in young adults aged 18 to 44 years in northern Sweden. *Stroke* 1997; **28**(9):1702–9.

20. Morikawa Y, Nakagawa H, Naruse Y, *et al.* Trends in stroke incidence and acute case fatality in a Japanese rural area: the Oyabe study. *Stroke* 2000; **31**(7):1583–7.

21. Jacobs BS, Boden-Albala B, Lin IF, Sacco RL. Stroke in the young in the northern Manhattan stroke study. *Stroke* 2002; **33**(12):2789–93.

22. Broderick J, Brott T, Kothari R, *et al.* The Greater Cincinnati/Northern Kentucky Stroke Study: preliminary first-ever and total incidence rates of stroke among blacks. *Stroke* 1998; **29**(2):415–21.

23. Kissela B, Schneider A, Kleindorfer D, *et al.* Stroke in a biracial population: the excess burden of stroke among blacks. *Stroke* 2004; **35**(2):426–31.

24. Smadja D, Cabre P, May F, *et al.* ERMANCIA: Epidemiology of Stroke in Martinique, French West Indies: Part I: methodology, incidence, and 30-day case fatality rate. *Stroke* 2001; **32**(12):2741–7.

25. Corbin DO, Poddar V, Hennis A, *et al.* Incidence and case fatality rates of first-ever stroke in a black Caribbean population: the Barbados Register of Strokes. *Stroke* 2004; **35**(6):1254–8.

26. Osuntokun BO, Bademosi O, Akinkugbe OO, Oyediran AB, Carlisle R. Incidence of stroke in an African City: results from the Stroke Registry at Ibadan, Nigeria, 1973–1975. *Stroke* 1979; **10**(2):205–7.

27. Correia M, Silva MR, Matos I, *et al.* Prospective community-based study of stroke in Northern Portugal: incidence and case fatality in rural and urban populations. *Stroke* 2004; **35**(9):2048–53.

28. Sharshar T, Lamy C, Mas JL. Incidence and causes of strokes associated with pregnancy and puerperium. A study in public hospitals of Ile de France. Stroke in Pregnancy Study Group. *Stroke* 1995; **26**(6):930–6.

29. Amlie-Lefond C, Sebire G, Fullerton HJ. Recent developments in childhood arterial ischaemic stroke. *Lancet Neurol* 2008; **7**(5):425–35.

30. European Stroke Organisation (ESO) Executive Committee; ESO Writing Committee Guidelines for management of ischaemic stroke and transient ischaemic attack 2008. *Cerebrovasc Dis* 2008; **25**(5):457–507.

31. Marini C, Totaro R, Carolei A. Long-term prognosis of cerebral ischemia in young adults. National Research Council Study Group on Stroke in the Young. *Stroke* 1999; **30**(11):2320–5.

32. Adams HP Jr, Kappelle LJ, Biller J, *et al.* Ischemic stroke in young adults. Experience in 329 patients enrolled in the Iowa Registry of stroke in young adults. *Arch Neurol* 1995; **52**(5):491–5.

33. Bogousslavsky J, Regli F. Ischemic stroke in adults younger than 30 years of age. Cause and prognosis. *Arch Neurol* 1987; **44**(5):479–82.

34. Hoffmann M. Stroke in the young in South Africa–an analysis of 320 patients. *S Afr Med J* 2000; **90**(12):1226–37.

35. Kappelle LJ, Adams HP Jr, Heffner ML, *et al.* Prognosis of young adults with ischemic stroke. A long-term follow-up study assessing recurrent vascular events and functional outcome in the Iowa Registry of Stroke in Young Adults. *Stroke* 1994; **25**(7):1360–5.

281

36. Kwon SU, Kim JS, Lee JH, Lee MC. Ischemic stroke in Korean young adults. *Acta Neurol Scand* 2000; **101**(1):19–24.

37. Leno C, Berciano J, Combarros O, *et al.* A prospective study of stroke in young adults in Cantabria, Spain. *Stroke* 1993; **24**(6):792–5.

38. Lisovoski F, Rousseaux P. Cerebral infarction in young people. A study of 148 patients with early cerebral angiography. *J Neurol Neurosurg Psychiatry* 1991; **54**(7):576–9.

39. Nayak SD, Nair M, Radhakrishnan K, Sarma PS. Ischaemic stroke in the young adult: clinical features, risk factors and outcome. *Natl Med J India* 1997; **10**(3):107–12.

40. Neau JP, Ingrand P, Mouille-Brachet C, *et al.* Functional recovery and social outcome after cerebral infarction in young adults. *Cerebrovasc Dis* 1998; **8**(5):296–302.

41. Chan MT, Nadareishvili ZG, Norris JW. Diagnostic strategies in young patients with ischemic stroke in Canada. *Can J Neurol Sci* 2000; **27**(2):120–4.

42. Ferro JM, Crespo M. Prognosis after transient ischemic attack and ischemic stroke in young adults. *Stroke* 1994; **25**(8):1611–16.

43. Adams HP Jr, Bendixen BH, Kappelle LJ, *et al.* Classification of subtype of acute ischemic stroke. Definitions for use in a multicenter clinical trial. TOAST. Trial of Org 10172 in Acute Stroke Treatment. *Stroke* 1993; **24**(1):35–41.

44. Oliviero U, Orefice G, Coppola G, *et al.* Carotid atherosclerosis and ischemic stroke in young patients. *Int Angiol* 2002; **21**(2):117–22.

45. von Sarnowski B, Schminke U, Tatlisumak T, *et al.* Prevalence of stenoses and occlusions of brain-supplying arteries in young stroke patients. *Neurology* 2013; **80**(14):1287–94.

46. Berthet K, Lavergne T, Cohen A, *et al.* Significant association of atrial vulnerability with atrial septal abnormalities in young patients with ischemic stroke of unknown cause. *Stroke* 2000; **31**(2):398–403.

47. Lechat P, Mas JL, Lascault G, *et al.* Prevalence of patent foramen ovale in patients with stroke. *N Engl J Med* 1988; **318**(18):1148–52.

48. Lucas C, Goullard L, Marchau M Jr, *et al.* Higher prevalence of atrial septal aneurysms in patients with ischemic stroke of unknown cause. *Acta Neurol Scand* 1994; **89**(3):210–13.

49. Arquizan C, Coste J, Touboul PJ, Mas JL. Is patent foramen ovale a family trait? A transcranial Doppler sonographic study. *Stroke* 2001; **32**(7):1563–6.

50. Mas J, Arquizan C, Lamy C, *et al.* Recurrent cerebrovascular events in young adults with patent foramen ovale, atrial septal aneurysm or both. *N Engl J Med* 2001; **345**(8579):1740–6.

51. Furlan AJ, Reisman M, Massaro J, *et al.* Closure or medical therapy for cryptogenic stroke with patent foramen ovale. *N Engl J Med* 2012; **366**(11):991–9.

52. Carroll JD, Saver JL, Thaler DE, *et al.* Closure of patent foramen ovale versus medical therapy after cryptogenic stroke. *N Engl J Med* 2013; **368**(12):1092–100.

53. Procacci PM, Savran SV, Schreiter SL, Bryson AL. Prevalence of clinical mitral-valve prolapse in 1169 young women. *N Engl J Med* 1976; **294**(20):1086–8.

54. Demakis JG, Rahimtoola SH, Sutton GC, *et al.* Natural course of peripartum cardiomyopathy. *Circulation* 1971; **44**(6):1053–61.

55. Homans DC. Peripartum cardiomyopathy. *N Engl J Med* 1985; **312**(22):1432–7.

56. Chabriat H, Vahedi K, Iba-Zizen MT, *et al.* Clinical spectrum of CADASIL: a study of 7 families. Cerebral autosomal dominant arteriopathy with subcortical infarcts and leukoencephalopathy. *Lancet* 1995; **346**(8980):934–9.

57. Joutel A, Corpechot C, Ducros A, *et al.* Notch3 mutations in CADASIL, a hereditary adult-onset condition causing stroke and dementia. *Nature* 1996; **383**(6602):707–10.

58. Leys D, Moulin T, Stojkovic T, Begey S, Chavot D. Follow-up of patients with history of cervical-artery dissection. *Cerebrovasc Dis* 1995; **5**:337–40.

59. Touze E, Gauvrit JY, Moulin T, *et al.* Risk of stroke and recurrent dissection after a cervical artery dissection: a multicenter study. *Neurology* 2003; **61**(10):1347–51.

60. Gallai V, Caso V, Paciaroni M, *et al.* Mild hyperhomocyst(e)inemia: a possible risk factor for cervical artery dissection. *Stroke* 2001; **32**(3):714–18.

61. Pezzini A, Del Zotto E, Archetti S, *et al.* Plasma homocysteine concentration, C677T MTHFR genotype, and 844ins68bp CBS genotype in young adults with spontaneous cervical artery dissection and atherothrombotic stroke. *Stroke* 2002; **33**(3):664–9.

62. Guillon B, Berthet K, Benslamia L, *et al.* Infection and the risk of spontaneous cervical artery dissection: a case-control study. *Stroke* 2003; **34**(7):e79–81.

63. Marcel M, Leys D, Mounier-Vehier F, *et al.* Clinical outcome in patients with high-grade internal carotid artery stenosis after irradiation. *Neurology* 2005; **65**(6):959–61.

64. O'Halloran HS, Berger JR, Lee WB, *et al.* Acute multifocal placoid pigment epitheliopathy and central nervous system involvement: nine new cases and a review of the literature. *Ophthalmology* 2001; **108**(5):861–8.

65. Salvarani C, Brown RD Jr, Calamia KT, *et al.* Primary central nervous system vasculitis: analysis of 101 patients. *Ann Neurol* 2007; **62**(5):442–51.

66. Janssens E, Hommel M, Mounier-Vehier F, *et al.* Postpartum cerebral angiopathy possibly due to bromocriptine therapy. *Stroke* 1995; **26**(1):128–30.

67. Rascol A, Guiraud B, Manelfe C, Clanet M. *Accidents vasculaires cérébraux de la grossesse et du post-partum.* 2nd edn. Conférence de la salpêtrière sur les maladies vasculaires cérébrales. Paris: J. B. Ballière; 1979: 84–127.

68. Goldenberg RL, Culhane JF, Iams JD, Romero R. Epidemiology and causes of preterm birth. *Lancet* 2008; **371**(9606):75–84.

69. Sibai B, Dekker G, Kupferminc M. Pre-eclampsia. *Lancet* 2005; **365** (9461):785–99.

70. Barton JR, Sibai BM. Care of the pregnancy complicated by HELLP syndrome. *Obstet Gynecol Clin North Am* 1991; **18**(2):165–79.

71. Fredriksson K, Lindvall O, Ingemarsson I, *et al.* Repeated cranial computed tomographic and magnetic resonance imaging scans in two cases of eclampsia. *Stroke* 1989; **20**(4):547–53.

72. Digre KB, Varner MW, Osborn AG, Crawford S. Cranial magnetic resonance imaging in severe preeclampsia vs eclampsia. *Arch Neurol* 1993; **50**(4):399–406.

73. Garg AX, Suri RS, Barrowman N, *et al.* Long-term renal prognosis of diarrhea-associated hemolytic uremic syndrome: a systematic review, meta-analysis, and meta-regression. *JAMA* 2003; **290** (10):1360–70.

74. Douay X, Lucas C, Caron C, Goudemand J, Leys D. Antithrombin, protein C and protein S levels in 127 consecutive young adults with ischemic stroke. *Acta Neurol Scand* 1998; **98** (2):124–7.

75. Hamedani AG, Cole JW, Mitchell BD, Kittner SJ. Meta-analysis of factor V Leiden and ischemic stroke in young adults: the importance of case ascertainment. *Stroke* 2010; **41**(8):1599–603.

76. Pezzini A, Del Zotto E, Magoni M, *et al.* Inherited thrombophilic disorders in young adults with ischemic stroke and patent foramen ovale. *Stroke* 2003; **34**(1):28–33.

77. Rolfs A, Bottcher T, Zschiesche M, *et al.* Prevalence of Fabry disease in patients with cryptogenic stroke: a prospective study. *Lancet* 2005; **366** (9499):1794–6.

78. Corson SL. Venous air and gas emboli in operative hysteroscopy. *J Am Assoc Gynecol Laparosc* 2002; **9**(1):106; author reply 106.

79. Levy R, Furman B, Hagay ZJ. Fetal bradycardia and disseminated coagulopathy: atypical presentation of amniotic fluid emboli. *Acta Anaesthesiol Scand* 2004; **48**(9):1214–15.

80. Mentz HA. Fat emboli syndromes following liposuction. *Aesthetic Plast Surg* 2008; **32**(5): 737–8.

81. Weir B, MacDonald N, Mielke B. Intracranial vascular complications of choriocarcinoma. *Neurosurgery* 1978; **2**(2):138–42.

82. Cohen PR. Sweet's syndrome–a comprehensive review of an acute febrile neutrophilic dermatosis. *Orphanet J Rare Dis* 2007; **2**:34.

83. De Rosa G, Pardeo M, Rigante D. Current recommendations for the pharmacologic therapy in Kawasaki syndrome and management of its cardiovascular complications. *Eur Rev Med Pharmacol Sci* 2007; **11**(5):301–8.

84. Reiniger IW, Thurau S, Haritoglou C, *et al.* Susac-Syndrom: Fallberichte und Literaturübersicht. *Klin Monatsbl Augenheilkd* 2006; **223**(2):161–7.

85. Jen J, Cohen AH, Yue Q, *et al.* Hereditary endotheliopathy with retinopathy, nephropathy, and stroke (HERNS). *Neurology* 1997; **49**(5):1322–30.

86. Ji R, Schwamm LH, Pervez MA, Singhal AB. Ischemic stroke and transient ischemic attack in young adults: risk factors, diagnostic yield, neuroimaging, and thrombolysis. *JAMA Neurol* 2013; **70**(1):51–7.

87. George MG, Tong X, Kuklina EV, Labarthe DR. Trends in stroke hospitalizations and associated risk factors among children and young adults, 1995–2008. *Ann Neurol* 2011; **70**(5):713–21.

88. Allais G, Gabellari IC, Mana O, *et al.* Migraine and stroke: the role of oral contraceptives. *Neurol Sci* 2008; **29**(Suppl 1): S12–14.

89. Baillargeon JP, McClish DK, Essah PA, Nestler JE. Association between the current use of low-dose oral contraceptives and cardiovascular arterial disease: a meta-analysis. *J Clin Endocrinol Metab* 2005; **90**(7):3863–70.

90. Bhat VM, Cole JW, Sorkin JD, *et al.* Dose-response relationship between cigarette smoking and risk of ischemic stroke in young women. *Stroke* 2008; **39**(9):2439–43.

91. Mant J, Painter R, Vessey M. Risk of myocardial infarction, angina and stroke in users of oral contraceptives: an updated analysis of a cohort study. *Br J Obstet Gynaecol* 1998; **105**(8):890–6.

92. Tzourio C, Iglesias S, Hubert JB, *et al.* Migraine and risk of ischaemic stroke: a case-control study. *BMJ* 1993; **307** (6899):289–92.

93. Kurth T, Slomke MA, Kase CS, *et al.* Migraine, headache, and the risk of stroke in women: a prospective study. *Neurology* 2005; **64**(6):1020–6.

94. Stang PE, Carson AP, Rose KM, *et al.* Headache, cerebrovascular symptoms, and stroke: the Atherosclerosis Risk in Communities Study. *Neurology* 2005; **64**(9):1573–7.

95. Chang CL, Donaghy M, Poulter N. Migraine and stroke in young women: case-control study. The World Health Organization Collaborative Study of Cardiovascular Disease and Steroid Hormone Contraception. *BMJ* 1999; **318**(7175):13–18.

96. Kurth T, Kase CS, Schurks M, Tzourio C, Buring JE. Migraine and risk of haemorrhagic stroke in women: prospective cohort study. *BMJ* 2010; **341**:c3659.

97. Bigal ME, Kurth T, Santanello N, *et al.* Migraine and cardiovascular disease: a population-based study. *Neurology* 2010; **74**(8):628–35.

98. Schurks M, Rist PM, Bigal ME, *et al.* Migraine and cardiovascular disease: systematic review and meta-analysis. *BMJ* 2009; **339**:b3914.

99. Kruit MC, van Buchem MA, Hofman PA, *et al.* Migraine as a risk factor for subclinical brain lesions. *JAMA* 2004; **291**(4):427–34.

100. Ortiz G, Koch S, Romano JG, Forteza AM, Rabinstein AA. Mechanisms of ischemic stroke in HIV-infected patients. *Neurology* 2007; **68**(16):1257–61.

101. Stirling Y, Woolf L, North WR, Seghatchian MJ, Meade TW. Haemostasis in normal pregnancy. *Thromb Haemost* 1984; **52**(2):176–82.

102. Bouvier-Colle MH, Varnoux N, Costes P, Hatton F, et le groupe d'experts sur la mortalité maternelle. Mortalité maternelle en France. Fréquence et raisons de sa sous-estimation dans la statistique des causes médicales de décès. *J Gynecol Obstet Biol Reprod (Paris)* 1991; **20**(7):885–91.

103. Gibbs CE. Maternal death due to stroke. *Am J Obstet Gynecol* 1974; **119**(1):69–75.

104. Kaunitz AM, Hughes JM, Grimes DA, *et al.* Causes of maternal mortality in the United States. *Obstet Gynecol* 1985; **65**(5):605–12.

105. Qureshi AI, Safdar K, Patel M, Janssen RS, Frankel MR. Stroke in young black patients. Risk factors, subtypes, and prognosis. *Stroke* 1995; **26**(11):1995–8.

106. Chancellor AM, Glasgow GL, Ockelford PA, Johns A, Smith J. Etiology, prognosis, and hemostatic function after cerebral infarction in young adults. *Stroke* 1989; **20**(4):477–82.

107. Johnson DM, Kramer DC, Cohen E, *et al.* Thrombolytic therapy for acute stroke in late pregnancy with intra-arterial recombinant tissue plasminogen activator. *Stroke* 2005; **36**(6):e53–5.

108. Camerlingo M, Casto L, Censori B, *et al.* Recurrence after first cerebral infarction in young adults. *Acta Neurol Scand* 2000; **102**(2):87–93.

109. Rutten-Jacobs LC, Arntz RM, Maaijwee NA, *et al.* Long-term mortality after stroke among adults aged 18 to 50 years. *JAMA* 2013; **309**(11):1136–44.

110. Pozzati E, Giuliani G, Acciarri N, Nuzzo G. Long-term follow-up of occlusive cervical carotid dissection. *Stroke* 1990; **21**(4):528–31.

111. Schievink WI, Mokri B, O'Fallon WM. Recurrent spontaneous cervical-artery dissection. *N Engl J Med* 1994; **330**(6):393–7.

112. Lamy C, Domigo V, Semah F, *et al.* Early and late seizures after cryptogenic ischemic stroke in young adults. *Neurology* 2003; **60**(3):400–4.

113. Lamy C, Hamon JB, Coste J, Mas JL. Ischemic stroke in young women: risk of recurrence during subsequent pregnancies. French Study Group on Stroke in Pregnancy. *Neurology* 2000; **55**(2):269–74.

114. Engelter ST, Brandt T, Debette S, *et al.* Antiplatelets versus anticoagulation in cervical artery dissection. *Stroke* 2007; **38**(9):2605–11.

Stroke units and clinical assessment

Danilo Toni and Ángel Chamorro

Introduction

There is convincing evidence from a large number of randomized controlled trials that the outcomes of stroke patients managed in dedicated stroke units are better than those of patients managed in general medical or neurological wards [1–3]. Stroke units are the essential part of the chain of recovery and form the backbone of prehospital, in-hospital, and posthospital care, that is, from home back to home.

In addition to stroke unit care, thus far only thrombolytic therapy and hemicraniectomy have been shown to improve the outcome of stroke patients. The acute therapies and interventions in stroke are described in Chapters 18 and 19. The basic functions of the stroke unit, mainly covered in other chapters of this book, are etiological diagnostic workup (Chapters 2–5 and 8–15), general management and proactive prevention of complications (Chapters 20 and 21), secondary prevention of stroke and other vascular endpoints (Chapter 22), and early rehabilitation (Chapter 23).

The purpose of this chapter is to characterize the chain of recovery of acute stroke patients from emergency phone call to acute stroke unit, including clinical evaluation of the patient and aspects of general stroke management that can be optimally delivered in stroke units, in light of current guidelines.

Prehospital care and referral

According to the European Stroke Organisation (ESO) [4], emergency care of the acute stroke victim depends on a 4-step chain: (1) rapid recognition of, and reaction to, stroke signs and transient ischemic attacks (TIAs), (2) immediate emergency medical service (EMS) contact and priority EMS dispatch, (3)

priority transport with prenotification to the receiving hospital, and (4) timely and competent in-hospital treatment at the emergency department.

The general emergency phone number (112 in most European countries, 911 in the United States) is the first link in the chain of survival and recovery for acute stroke patients. National stroke-awareness campaigns always emphasize the importance of recognizing the symptoms of acute stroke and calling the emergency number immediately before doing anything else. This is usually done by a family member, since the stroke patient is not able to make the call himself/herself. There is class II level B evidence that educational programs to increase awareness of stroke at the population level are beneficial, and the same holds true for EMS professionals, both paramedics and physicians [5].

EMS transport to and arrival at the emergency department (ED) increase the likelihood of a patient presenting within the 4.5-hour time window allowing thrombolysis to be considered, compared to private physician referral and self-transport, and significantly reduce the time from symptom onset to CT evaluation [6, 7]. Failure to use the emergency number is the most common and most devastating error, with respect to the possibility of timely recanalization therapy. Delays during acute stroke management have been identified at the population level (due to failure to recognize the symptoms of stroke and calling the emergency number), at the level of the emergency services and emergency physicians (due to a failure to implement stroke code), and at the hospital level (due to delays in in-hospital logistics and neuroimaging) [8, 9].

To optimize stroke identification, prehospital professionals should use a prehospital stroke screening instrument that has been prospectively evaluated for sensitivity, specificity, reproducibility, and validity. Such instruments include the Los Angeles Prehospital Stroke Screen (LAPSS), the Cincinnati Prehospital Stroke Scale (CPSS, or Face-Arm-Speech-Test [FAST]), and the Melbourne Ambulance Stroke Screen (MASS), which all have been reported to have a sensitivity exceeding 90% [10–14]. The electronic validated algorithm of questions should be used during the emergency phone call.

The stroke code is activated immediately when stroke is suspected [7]. Using a predefined protocol, the patient will be transported to the stroke center, which will be notified in advance. Prehospital notification of an inbound stroke patient has been demonstrated to shorten the delay from ED arrival to initial neurological assessment and initial brain imaging, and to increase the proportion of patients treated with recombinant tissue plasminogen activator (rtPA). Physicians, nurses, CT/MR technologists, and pharmacists are able to utilize early notification to mobilize necessary resources for the patient. This is called the Stroke Alarm at the ED. Stroke alarm also means that the patient has a priority for CT and emergency laboratory evaluation. The ESO Guidelines include a class II level B recommendation for immediate EMS contact, priority EMS dispatch and priority transport with prenotification of the receiving hospital, and a class III level B recommendation that suspected stroke victims should be transported without delay to the nearest medical center with a stroke unit that can provide ultra-early treatment [5]. In current guidelines, there is also a class III level B recommendation for immediate ED triage; clinical, laboratory, and imaging evaluation; accurate diagnosis; therapeutic decision and administration of appropriate treatments at the receiving hospital [5].

In-hospital delays may account for at least 16% of total time lost between stroke onset and recanalization therapy. Reasons for in-hospital delays are a failure to identify stroke as emergency, inefficient in-hospital transport, delayed medical assessment and imaging, and uncertainty in administering thrombolysis [15, 16]. In Helsinki, the ED reorganization of acute stroke care has been shown to result in reduced delays in acute stroke treatment, i.e. shorter door-to-rtPA times. The present mean door-to-needle time is 20 minutes, which is based on almost 2000 patients treated [16]. The main components of the reorganization were:

- Triage
- ED with written protocols for stroke patients
- ED prenotification by the EMS
- ED rebuild with easy-access CT
- digital patient records, including digital imaging system (PACS) [16].

In remote and rural areas helicopter transfer should be considered to improve access to treatment (class III level C) [5]. Telemedicine is also a feasible, valid, and reliable means of facilitating thrombolysis for patients in distant or rural hospitals, where timely air or ground transportation is not feasible (class II level B). The quality of treatment, complication rates, and short- and long-term outcomes are similar for acute stroke patients treated with rtPA via a telemedicine consultation at local hospitals and those treated in academic centers [17–19].

As an alternative, stroke treatment in a specialized ambulance, staffed with a neurologist, paramedic, and radiographer and equipped with a CT scanner, point-of-care laboratory, and a teleradiology system, appears to be feasible and without safety concerns [20]. Its effectiveness in reducing call-to-needle times needs to be scrutinized in a prospective controlled study. Further, the cost-effectiveness of this approach and its utility in different urban scenarios should also be addressed in further studies.

> To ensure that a stroke patient presents within the time window allowing thrombolysis to be considered, several pre-admission conditions have to be guaranteed:
>
> - awareness of stroke at the population level with rapid recognition of and reaction to stroke signs and TIAs
> - emergency medical service transport to the emergency department
> - prehospital notification of the stroke patient
> - emergency department reorganization with easy-access CT.

Stroke unit care

Striking discrepancies in infrastructure and quality of stroke care, but also in costs and outcome, have been identified in Europe [21], indicating the urgent need for a common and agreed concept of well-organized evidence-based stroke care in European countries, and for standardized, methodologically sound regional or national audits of stroke care [4]. Three basic principles of organized stroke unit care have been proven to be highly effective in terms of improved outcome (fewer deaths, less dependency). They include (1) a dedicated stroke ward, (2) a multiprofessional team approach, and (3) a system of comprehensive stroke unit care. All three principles are based on evidence level I [5].

Dedicated stroke ward care means that acute stroke patients are treated in a geographically defined area of the hospital admitting exclusively stroke and TIA patients and not patients with other disorders. The outcomes of stroke and TIA patients managed in dedicated stroke units are better than those of patients managed in general medical or neurological wards [3], and the benefit of organized stroke unit care covers all groups of stroke patients, including ischemic [5] and hemorrhagic stroke [22]. There is also no indication that age or sex limits the benefits of organized stroke unit care. Indeed, elderly patients and those with severe stroke benefit most from stroke unit care [1,23]. The benefits of stroke unit care may decline over time elapsed since stroke onset, and preferably acute stroke patients should be admitted acutely, but patients should not be excluded from stroke unit care simply because of delayed presentation, particularly if the patient requires a closer attention that cannot be provided in general wards. There is also sufficient evidence that the benefits seen in stroke unit trials are replicated in routine practice, as long as these evidence-based principles of organized stroke unit care are considered in daily routine [24].

The multiprofessional team approach implicates that stroke units must be staffed with physicians, nurses, physiotherapists, occupational therapists, speech and swallowing therapists, neuropsychologists where available, and social workers (including a case manager) with special interest, training, and expertise in stroke care. The physicians are neurologists or internists provided that their focus is stroke care and that they are specifically trained in stroke medicine. Likewise, comprehensive stroke unit care means that acute stroke management, that is, diagnostic workup and treatment, is seamlessly combined with early mobilization and rehabilitation and secondary prevention, according to the needs of the patient (out of bed within 24-hour principle).

There are many types of stroke units including acute stroke units, combined acute and rehabilitation stroke units, and rehabilitation stroke units admitting patients after a delay of 1–2 weeks [1, 2]. The ESO has recently defined the essential components and facilities for ESO Stroke Units [4], which are shown in Table 17.1. Accordingly, the Stroke Unit criteria

are organized (1) to ensure vital functions, (2) to provide early diagnostic investigations, (3) to allow basic surveillance and (4) stroke-specific therapeutic interventions, (5) to perform general therapeutic and diagnostic interventions, (6) to start secondary prevention, and (7) to combine this with multiprofessional early mobilization and rehabilitation procedures. Both the First [24] and Second Helsingborg Declaration [2], and the guidelines by the ESO [5], recommend that all stroke patients should have access to care in specialized stroke units. However, currently only one of seven stroke patients in Europe has admission to stroke unit care, and 42% of them are treated in hospitals that have no facilities nor expertise to provide good care for stroke patients [21].

Stroke care organization at the receiving hospital makes a difference in the rate of successfully thrombolysed patients. A randomized controlled trial compared the time from emergency call to therapy decision between mobile stroke unit and regular hospital interventions. The study was stopped early because the mobile stroke unit reduced the median time from alarm to therapy decision from 76 to 35 minutes [25]. This treatment approach showed similar benefits in reducing the delay from alarm to end of CT, alarm to end of laboratory analysis, and to intravenous thrombolysis for eligible ischemic stroke patients.

> According to the ESO, the Stroke Unit criteria are organized (1) to ensure vital functions, (2) to provide early diagnostic investigations, (3) to allow basic surveillance and (4) stroke-specific therapeutic interventions, (5) to perform general therapeutic and diagnostic interventions, (6) to start secondary prevention, and (7) to combine this with multiprofessional early mobilization and rehabilitation procedures.

Early activities at a stroke unit

The time window for treatment of patients with acute stroke is narrow and requires well-organized services at the ED and acute stroke unit. The points which must be kept in mind include:

- acute emergency management of stroke requires parallel processes at different levels of patient management
- acute assessment of neurological and vital functions parallels treatment of acutely life-threatening conditions

Table 17.1. Facilities necessary for European Stroke Organisation Stroke Units

Departments and clinics	Multiprofessional stroke unit Inpatient rehabilitation (in-house) Outpatient rehabilitation available Collaboration with outside rehabilitation center Stroke outpatient clinic
Staff available	Stroke-trained physician Multiprofessional team Stroke-trained nurses Social worker
Investigations available	Brain CT scan 24/7 CT priority for stroke patients Extracranial duplex sonography Transthoracic echocardiography Transesophageal echocardiography
Hyperacute interventions	Intravenous rtPA protocols Respiratory support Access to hemicraniectomy* Access to surgery for hematoma Access to intra-arterial interventions*
Stroke unit interventions	Agreed written protocols for common problems
Stroke unit monitoring	Monitoring of heart rate Monitoring of oxygen saturation Monitoring of blood pressure Monitoring of breathing Monitoring of temperature
Stroke unit assessment	Early rehabilitation assessment** Food and fluid management Speech therapy start <2 days Physiotherapy start <2 days Dysphagia management (swallowing screened on admission) Physiological management Early mobilization Skilled stroke nursing
Stroke unit multiprofessional team care	Coordinated multiprofessional stroke unit care (care in a discrete area in the hospital, staffed by a specialist stroke multiprofessional team with regular multiprofessional meetings for planning care) Early discharge planning
Interventions: other	Access to surgery for aneurysms Access to carotid surgery

* Access means not necessarily on-site, but defined partnership with a providing institution.
** By an appropriately trained professional.

- the selection of special treatment strategies does not need that the subtype of acute ischemic stroke has been defined.

Time is the most important factor, especially the first minutes and hours after stroke onset. During those hours the following tasks need to be performed:

- differentiate between different types of stroke (either ischemic or hemorrhagic)
- assess the underlying cause of brain ischemia
- provide a basis for physiological monitoring of the stroke patient
- identify concurrent diseases or complications associated with stroke
- rule out other brain diseases
- assess prognosis.

Clinical assessment

There is general agreement that stroke severity should be assessed by trained staff using the National Institutes of Health Stroke Scale (NIHSS). In addition, the initial examination should include:

- observation of breathing and pulmonary function
- evaluation of concomitant heart disease
- assessment of blood pressure (BP) and heart rate
- determination of arterial oxygen saturation using infrared pulse oximetry
- detection of dysphagia, preferably using a validated scale.

Close monitoring is essential (see Chapter 19) to ascertain stable vital functions (airway, breathing, and cardiovascular function). If they are compromised, intensive care may be necessary until the clinical situation is stable.

Diagnostic workup

Table 17.2 lists the diagnostic procedures recommended by the ESO. Neurovascular diagnosis based on predominantly non-invasive angiographic tests should become the standard, and is already applied in many stroke centers [4]. In-depth discussion of diagnostic workup can be found in Chapters 2–5.

In addition to imaging, early evaluation of physiological parameters, routine blood tests, and 12-channel electrocardiography (ECG) followed by continuous ECG recording should be performed according to the ESO recommendations. When arrhythmias are suspected and no other cause of stroke is found, a 24-hour Holter ECG monitoring should also be performed, although modern patient-monitoring systems may have the same functionality built in. Diagnostic cardiac ultrasound is recommended in selected patients. Systematic use of these methods may result in an increased proportion of cardioembolic stroke [5, 26].

Table 17.2. Diagnostic tests at the acute stroke unit recommended by ESO [5]

In all patients

1   Brain imaging: CT or MRI
2   ECG
3   Laboratory tests
     Complete blood count and platelet count, prothrombin time or INR, PTT, serum electrolytes, blood glucose, CRP or sedimentation rate, hepatic and renal chemical analysis

When indicated

4   Extracranial and transcranial duplex/Doppler ultrasound
5   MRA or CTA
6   Diffusion and perfusion MR or perfusion CT
7   Echocardiography (transthoracic and/or transesophageal)
8   Chest X-ray
9   Pulse oximetry and arterial blood gas analysis
10   Lumbar puncture
11   EEG
12   Toxicology screen

CRP = C-reactive protein; INR = international normalized ratio; PTT = partial thrombin time.

General management, monitoring, and complications

The success of stroke unit care is believed to depend on general management, careful monitoring, and normalization of physiological parameters, as well as proactive prevention and treatment of medical complications. No randomized controlled trials (RCTs) address this, therefore level I class A recommendations do not exist. The recommendations are based on consensus statements of experts, such as Guidelines for Management of Ischemic Stroke and Transient Ischemic Attack by the ESO [5]. The cornerstones of this approach, as recommended by the ESO, are summarized in Tables 17.3 and 17.4 and will be discussed in more detail in Chapter 20.

Acute treatment

Acute treatments and interventions for stroke including thrombolytic therapy and endovascular procedures are discussed in Chapters 18 and 19. From the organizational point of view, intravenous thrombolytic therapy is most often administered in the ED instead of the stroke unit, where rescue therapies after unsuccessful intravenous thrombolysis may still be considered, provided that the time window is still open and depending on the indications and possible contraindications for the therapy. Stroke unit administration of i.v. rtPA requires immediate transfer of the patient, bypassing the ED. The specific treatments at a stroke unit are shown in Table 17.5 [5].

Elevated intracranial pressure

The most common cause of death in the acute stage of a major stroke is increased intracranial pressure and herniation due to brain edema. Decompressive craniectomy has now a class I level A recommendation in malignant ischemic middle cerebral artery (MCA) stroke patients younger than 60 years of age, and it is currently the only treatment shown in RCTs to be able to reduce mortality in this patient group [27]. The recent ESO Guidelines give practical advice on how to treat stroke patients with increased intracranial pressure (Table 17.6) [5].

Secondary prevention

Secondary prevention, discussed in detail in Chapter 22, should start as early as possible, i.e. at

289

Table 17.3. ESO Guidelines for general monitoring and treatment [5]

- Intermittent monitoring of neurological status, pulse, blood pressure, temperature, and oxygen saturation is recommended for 72 hours in patients with significant persisting neurological deficits
- It is recommended that oxygen should be administered if the oxygen saturation falls below 95%
- Regular monitoring of fluid balance and electrolytes is recommended in patients with severe stroke or swallowing problems (class IV, GCP)
- Normal saline (0.9%) is recommended for fluid replacement during the first 24 hours after stroke
- Routine blood pressure lowering is not recommended following acute stroke
- Cautious blood pressure lowering is recommended in patients with extremely high blood pressures (>220/120 mmHg) on repeated measurements, or with severe cardiac failure, aortic dissection, or hypertensive encephalopathy
- It is recommended that abrupt blood pressure lowering be avoided
  - It is recommended that low blood pressure secondary to hypovolemia or associated with neurological deterioration in acute stroke should be treated with volume expanders
- Monitoring serum glucose levels is recommended
- Treatment of serum glucose levels >180 mg/dl (>10 mmol/l) with insulin titration is recommended
- It is recommended that severe hypoglycemia (<50 mg/dl [<2.8 mmol/l]) should be treated with intravenous dextrose or infusion of 10–20% glucose
- It is recommended that the presence of pyrexia (temperature >37.5 °C) should prompt a search for concurrent infection
  - Treatment of pyrexia (temperature >37.5 °C) with paracetamol and fanning is recommended
- Antibiotic prophylaxis is not recommended in immunocompetent patients
- Swallowing assessment is recommended but there are insufficient data to recommend a specific approach for treatment
- Oral dietary supplements are only recommended for non-dysphagic stroke patients who are malnourished
- Early commencement of nasogastric (NG) feeding (within 48 hours) is recommended in stroke patients with impaired swallowing
- It is recommended that percutaneous enteral gastrostomy (PEG) feeding should not be considered in stroke patients in the first 2 weeks

Table 17.4. ESO Guidelines for management of complications [5]

- It is recommended that infections after stroke should be treated with appropriate antibiotics
- Prophylactic administration of antibiotics is not recommended, and levofloxacin can be detrimental in acute stroke patients
- Early rehydration and graded compression stocking are recommended to reduce the incidence of venous thromboembolism
- Early mobilization is recommended to prevent complications such as aspiration pneumonia, deep vein thrombosis (DVT), and pressure ulcers
- It is recommended that low-dose subcutaneous heparin or low molecular weight heparins should be considered for patients at high risk of DVT or pulmonary embolism

the ED or in the stroke unit at the latest. It is recommended that aspirin (160–325 mg loading dose) should be given within 48 hours after ischemic stroke if thrombolysis is not administered, or 24 hours after thrombolysis. Selection of treatment is based on the most likely etiology of the stroke and all the patient's risk factors. Secondary prevention strategies should be planned and initiated at the stroke unit and continued in community health care by a primary care physician or family doctor as soon as the patient has been discharged from the hospital [5].

Early rehabilitation

Rehabilitation of stroke patients is discussed in Chapter 23. All patients need to be assessed at the stroke unit by a physiotherapist, occupational therapist, speech therapist, and neurophysiologist of the multidisciplinary stroke team within the first week after the onset of stroke [5]. There is great variability in rehabilitation resources and staff between geographical regions and hospitals, but in general all available therapists should be involved in the early assessment and design of the rehabilitation plan of every acute stroke patient. The rehabilitation plan is much like a tailor-made suit, which is started at the stroke unit and continued and modified based on the progress of the patient at a rehabilitation hospital, outpatient clinic, and at home. For all stroke patients follow-up by community health care is crucial to ensure that the functional outcome reached during rehabilitation will

Table 17.5. ESO Guidelines for specific treatments [5]

- Intravenous rtPA (0.9 mg/kg body weight, maximum 90 mg), with 10% of the dose given as a bolus followed by a 60-minute infusion, is recommended within 4.5 hours

  - It is recommended that intravenous rtPA should be offered to patients over the age of 18 years, with no upper age limit
  - Multimodal imaging may be used to select patients who might benefit from thrombolysis beyond 4.5 hours or to enhance efficacy in RCTs, but is not recommended for routine clinical practice
  - It is recommended that blood pressures of 185/110 mmHg or higher is lowered before thrombolysis
  - It is recommended that intravenous rtPA may be used in patients with seizures at stroke onset, if the neurological deficit is related to acute cerebral ischemia

- Intra-arterial treatment of acute middle cerebral artery (MCA) occlusion within a 6-hour time window is recommended as an option

  - Intra-arterial thrombolysis or mechanical thrombectomy is recommended for acute basilar occlusion in selected patients, when available. Intravenous thrombolysis for basilar occlusion is recommended up to at least 4.5 hours
  - It is recommended that if thrombolytic therapy is planned or given, aspirin or other antithrombotic therapy should not be initiated within 24 hours

- It is recommended that aspirin (160–325 mg loading dose) be given within 48 hours after ischemic stroke (authors' note: in patients not receiving intravenous thrombolysis)

Table 17.6. ESO Guidelines for elevated intracranial pressure [5]

- Surgical decompressive therapy within 48 hours after symptom onset is recommended in patients up to 60 years of age with evolving malignant MCA infarcts
- It is recommended that osmotherapy can be used to treat elevated intracranial pressure prior to surgery if this is considered
- No recommendation can be given regarding hypothermic therapy in patients with space-occupying infarctions
- It is recommended that ventriculostomy or surgical decompression be considered for treatment of large cerebellar infarctions that compress the brainstem

endure. Many patients need the rehabilitation services of the community from time to time to be able to keep their independence in daily life and to be able to live in their own homes, knowing that such late rehabilitation is not supported by RCTs [5].

Conclusions

According to the frequently cited ESO 2008 Guidelines, it is now recommended (class I level A) that all stroke patients irrespective of age, sex, or severity of stroke should be treated in a stroke unit. The health-care system should ensure that acute stroke patients can access high-technology medical and surgical stroke care when required (class III level B). The development of clinical networks, including telemedicine, is recommended to expand the access to high-technology specialist stroke care (class II level B) [5].

Is this the recipe for the future? It is easy to predict that among the key elements for future success in acute stroke care will be centralized acute care, shortening delays at every step, increasing stroke awareness, identification of barriers that may prevent direct and immediate access to a stroke center, ERC, EMS and ED involvement in prehospital management, in-hospital pathways and protocols as well as well-organized systematic routines for fast implementation of evidence-based medicine, including tele-stroke in selected hospitals.

Chapter summary

Emergency medical service (EMS) transport of a stroke patient to the emergency department (ED) increases the likelihood of a patient presenting within the 4.5-hour time window allowing thrombolysis to be considered. To reduce delays, awareness of stroke at the population level is pivotal. Prehospital professionals should use a prehospital stroke screening instrument that has been prospectively evaluated for sensitivity, specificity, reproducibility, and validity. Prehospital notification of inbound stroke patients has been demonstrated to shorten the delay from ED arrival to initial neurological assessment and initial brain imaging, and to increase the proportion of patients treated with rtPA. Reorganization of acute stroke care has been shown to result in reduced delays in acute stroke treatment, i.e. shorter door-to-rtPA times.

A stroke unit is defined as an organized inpatient area that exclusively or nearly exclusively takes care of stroke patients and is managed by a multidisciplinary team of specialists who are knowledgeable about stroke care. Acute stroke patients are more likely to survive, return home, and regain independence if they receive stroke unit care. Five principles are relevant for the beneficial effect of stroke units:

- a dedicated stroke unit confined only to acute stroke patients
- a multidisciplinary team approach
- a stroke unit concept delivering both hyper-acute treatment and early mobilization and rehabilitation by the same multidisciplinary team, including diagnostics and secondary prevention
- automated monitoring of vital functions within the first 72 hours
- thrombolysis for selected patients.
- Activities at a stroke unit:

- early assessment, including type of stroke, the underlying cause of brain ischemia, and other brain diseases
- clinical assessment of stroke severity, breathing and pulmonary function, dysphagia, concomitant heart disease, blood pressure, heart rate, and arterial oxygen saturation
- diagnostic workup
- general management, careful monitoring, and normalization of physiological parameters, as well as proactive prevention and treatment of medical complications
- acute treatments and interventions of stroke, including thrombolytic therapy and endovascular procedures
- management of elevated intracranial pressure (e.g. decompressive craniectomy)
- start of secondary prevention measures, e.g. aspirin
- design of the rehabilitation plan.

References

1. Stroke Unit Trialists' Collaboration. Organised inpatient (stroke unit) care for stroke. *Cochrane Database Syst Rev* 2007; **4**:CD000197.

2. Kjellström T, Norrving B, Shatchkute A. Helsingborg Declaration 2006 on European stroke strategies. *Cerebrovasc Dis* 2007; **23**(2–3):231–41.

3. Terént A, Asplund K, Farahmand B, *et al.*; Riks-Stroke Collaboration. Stroke unit care revisited: who benefits the most? A cohort study of 105,043 patients in Riks-Stroke, the Swedish Stroke Register. *J Neurol Neurosurg Psychiatr* 2009; **80**(8):881–7.

4. Ringelstein EB, Chamorro A, Kaste M, *et al.*; ESO Stroke Unit Certification Committee. European Stroke Organisation recommendations to establish a stroke unit and stroke center. *Stroke* 2013; **44**(3):828–40.

5. European Stroke Organisation (ESO) Executive Committee; ESO Writing Committee. Guidelines for management of ischemic stroke and transient ischemic attack 2008. *Cerebrovasc Dis* 2008; **25**(5):457–507.

6. Berglund A, Svensson L, Sjöstrand C, *et al.* Higher prehospital priority level of stroke improves thrombolysis frequency and time to stroke unit the Hyper Acute STroke Alarm (HASTA) Study. *Stroke* 2012; **43**(10):2666–70.

7. Baldereschi M, Piccardi B, Di Carlo A, *et al.*; for the Promotion and Implementation of Stroke Care in Italy Project – Working Group. Relevance of prehospital stroke code activation for acute treatment measures in stroke care: a review. *Cerebrovasc Dis* 2012; **34**(3):182–90.

8. El Khoury R, Jung R, Nanda A, *et al.* Overview of key factors in improving access to acute stroke care. *Neurology* 2012; **79**(13 Suppl 1):S26–34.

9. Meretoja A, Kaste M. Pre- and in-hospital intersection of stroke care *Ann N Y Acad Sci* 2012; **1268**:145–51.

10. Kothari R, Barsan W, Brott T, *et al.* Frequency and accuracy of prehospital diagnosis of acute stroke. *Stroke* 1995; **26**(6):937–41.

11. Kothari RU, Pancioli A, Liu T, *et al.* Cincinnati prehospital stroke scale: reproducibility and validity. *Ann Emerg Med* 1999; **33**(4):373–8.

12. Nor A, McAllister C, Louw S, *et al.* Agreement between ambulance paramedic- and physician-recorded neurological signs using the Face Arm Speech Test (FAST) in acute stroke patients. *Stroke* 2004; **35**(6):1355–9.

13. Kidwell CS, Starkman S, Eckstein M, *et al.* Identifying stroke in the field. Prospective validation of the Los Angeles prehospital stroke screen (LAPSS). *Stroke* 2000; **31**(1):71–6.

14. Bray JE, Martin J, Cooper G, *et al.* Paramedic identification of stroke: community validation of the Melbourne ambulance stroke screen. *Cerebrovasc Dis* 2005; **20**(1):28–33.

15. Lindsberg PJ, Happola O, Kallela M, *et al.* Door to thrombolysis: ER reorganization and reduced delays

to acute stroke treatment. *Neurology* 2006; **67**(2):334–6.

16. Meretoja A, Strbian D, Mustanoja S, *et al.* Reducing in-hospital delay to 20 minutes in stroke thrombolysis. *Neurology* 2012; **79**(4);306–12.

17. Audebert H, Schenkel J, Heuschmann P, *et al.* Effects of the implementation of a telemedical stroke network: the Telemedic Pilot Project for Integrative Stroke Care (TEMPiS) in Bavaria, Germany. *Lancet Neurol* 2006; **5**(9):742–8.

18. Hess DC, Wang S, Gross H, *et al.* Telestroke: extending stroke expertise into underserved areas. *Lancet Neurol* 2006; **5**(3):275–8.

19. Zaidi SF, Jumma MA, Urra XN, *et al.* Telestroke-guided intravenous tissue-type plasminogen activator treatment achieves a similar clinical outcome as thrombolysis at a comprehensive stroke center. *Stroke* 2011; **42**(11):3291–3.

20. Weber JE, Ebinger M, Rozanski M, *et al.*; STEMO-Consortium. Prehospital thrombolysis in acute stroke: results of the PHANTOM-S pilot study. *Neurology* 2013; **80**(2):163–8.

21. Leys D, Ringelstein EB, Kaste M, Hacke W; Executive Committee of the European Stroke Initiative. Facilities available in European hospitals treating stroke patients. *Stroke* 2007; **38**(11):2985–91.

22. Steiner T, Kaste M, Forsting M, *et al.* Recommendations for the management of intracranial haemorrhage – part I: spontaneous intracerebral haemorrhage. The European Stroke Initiative Writing Committee and the Writing Committee for the EUSI Executive Committee. *Cerebrovasc Dis* 2006; **22**(4):294–316.

23. Langhorne P, Dennis M. *Stroke Units: An Evidence Based Approach.* London: BMJ Books; 1999.

24. Aboderin I, Venables G. Stroke management in Europe. Pan European Consensus Meeting on Stroke Management. *J Intern Med* 1996; **240**(4):173–80.

25. Walter S, Kostopoulos P, Haass A, *et al.* Diagnosis and treatment of patients with stroke in a mobile stroke unit versus in hospital: a randomised controlled trial. *Lancet Neurol* 2012; **11**(5):397–404.

26. De Castro S, Papetti F, Di Angelantonio E, *et al.* Feasibility and clinical utility of transesophageal echocardiography in the acute phase of cerebral ischemia. *Am J Cardiol* 2010; **106**(9):1339–44.

27. Vahedi K, Hofmeijer J, Juettler E, *et al.* for DECIMAL, DESTINY, and HAMLET investigators. Early decompressive surgery in malignant infarction of the middle cerebral artery: a pooled analysis of three randomised controlled trials. *Lancet Neurol* 2007; **6**(3):215–22.

293

Acute therapies for stroke

18

Richard E. O'Brien and Kennedy R. Lees

Introduction

Acute stroke is a medical emergency, and this is now recognized by healthcare systems around the world. The acute management of stroke can be complex and reflects the number and variety of potential interventions that are now available within the immediate aftermath of symptom onset. The aim of any intervention is to improve patient outcome and reduce or prevent disability. Over several decades research studies have contributed valuable information to our knowledge of acute stroke management. With advances in pharmacotherapeutics and other interventions clinical practice has changed dramatically in recent times and research studies continue to inform and develop clinical practice.

This chapter will present the evidence and best practice guidance for interventions during the first 24–48 hours following stroke, based upon the European Stroke Organisation Guidelines 2008 and the European Stroke Initiative recommendations for the management of intracranial hemorrhage and their relevant updates [1–4]. For the purposes of this chapter, the interventions discussed will generally be limited to the initial 48 hours following ictus. Access to some of these therapies may not be universal and may be dictated by local availability at individual stroke units. As with other aspects of stroke care, however, close cooperation and interdisciplinary communication are essential.

Thrombolysis

In respect of acute interventions, one of the most significant advances during the last two decades has been the widespread introduction of intravenous thrombolysis as a standard therapy for a well-selected

population of patients with acute ischemic stroke. At present, the only thrombolytic agent licensed in Europe for the treatment of ischemic stroke is recombinant tissue plasminogen activator (rtPA), alteplase. The evidence for its use has evolved over the last 20 years and originated from six landmark clinical trials: the Alteplase Thrombolysis for Acute Noninterventional Therapy in Ischemic Stroke (ATLANTIS) trials A and B; the European Cooperative Acute Stroke Study (ECASS) and ECASS II; and the two-part National Institute of Neurological Disorders and Stroke (NINDS) rtPA study [1, 5–8]. These studies varied in timing and dose of rtPA, which may account for some of the differences in outcomes reported in each of the trials. The NINDS rtPA study demonstrated an odds ratio of 1.7 (95% confidence interval 1.2–2.6) for a favorable outcome at 3 months with rtPA treatment when administered within 3 hours of ischemic stroke onset, with the number needed to treat to achieve a favorable outcome of 7 [6]. In contrast, the ECASS studies (I and II) did not confirm significant benefit of rtPA although this was when administration occurred within 6 hours of ictus [5, 7]. However, analysis of the pooled data from the ATLANTIS, ECASS, and NINDS rtPA trials later confirmed the beneficial effect of timely intervention with intravenous thrombolysis [9]. This analysis included 2775 patients in whom thrombolysis was initiated within 6 hours of ischemic stroke onset. The odds of a favorable outcome were inversely associated with delay from stroke onset to treatment, with those patients treated earliest following their stroke having the most favorable outcome. Favorable outcome at 3 months was defined as a modified Rankin Score (mRS) of 0 or 1, a Barthel Index between 95 and 100, and National Institutes of Health Stroke Scale

(NIHSS) score of 0 or 1. More specifically, the analysis identified an adjusted odds ratio for favorable outcome at 3 months of 2.81 (95% confidence interval 1.75–4.50) for patients treated within the first 90 minutes of stroke, 1.55 (1.12–2.15) when treatment was commenced 91–180 minutes following onset, falling to 1.40 (1.05–1.85) and 1.15 (0.90–1.47) when thrombolytic treatment was commenced within 181–270 and 271–360 minutes from stroke onset, respectively [9]. The benefits of thrombolysis are therefore largest when treatment is initiated early and minimizing delays to treatment is imperative in improving patient outcome. These benefits have been demonstrated without a significantly increased risk of death, but the proportion of patients with significant parenchymal hemorrhage, defined as dense blood clot exceeding 30% infarct volume with significant space-occupying effect, was larger in rtPA-treated patients (5.6% versus 1.0% in those who received treatment between 91 and 180 minutes following stroke onset). Of clinical importance, the proportion of patients suffering secondary parenchymal hemorrhage was associated with increasing age, but not with time from onset to treatment or baseline NIHSS score.

Based upon these clinical trial data, the provisional European licence for alteplase in acute ischemic stroke was for use within 3 hours of stroke onset. A request associated with the European licence was that outcome data should be collected prospectively for the first 3 years or 1000 patients on patients in whom alteplase was used for acute ischemic stroke thrombolysis. The Safe Implementation of Thrombolysis in Stroke – Monitoring Study (SITS-MOST) collected data on 6483 patients [10]. Reassuringly, it provided evidence that the use of intravenous thrombolysis in routine clinical practice resulted in outcomes comparable to those observed in clinical trials. The proportions of patients achieving independence (mRS <3) at 3 months in the SITS-MOST group were similar to those in the pooled randomized controlled trials, with lower rates of symptomatic intracerebral hemorrhage (ICH) and mortality observed in the SITS-MOST data. This confirmed the safety and efficacy of using rtPA for acute ischemic stroke in well-selected patients with acute ischemic stroke.

Initially, regulatory authorities placed an upper limit of 3 hours for routine use of alteplase after stroke although the evidence showed benefit extending beyond 3 hours. The SITS register demonstrated that treatment at an average of 3 hours 15 minutes and until 4.5 hours after stroke onset remains as safe as earlier treatment in routine clinical practice [11]. This suggested that whilst early treatment remains desirable, patients in whom treatment cannot start within 3 hours should not be deprived of therapy for the sake of a few minutes delay. More compelling were the results of the third ECASS trial, which found an odds ratio for achieving favorable outcome of 1.34 (95% confidence interval 1.02–1.76) with treatment in the 3.0–4.5-hour window [12], effectively confirming the estimate of 1.4 that derived from meta-analysis [9].

Updated analysis of observational data from the Safe Implementation of Treatments in Stroke – International Stroke Thrombolysis Registry (SITS-ISTR) reported on the outcomes of 23 942 patients treated with thrombolysis between 2002 and 2010, 2376 of whom were treated between 3 and 4.5 hours of stroke onset [13]. The efficacy of treatment within 4.5 hours was confirmed, with minor increases in the rates of symptomatic ICH and mortality in those treated between 3 and 4.5 hours being offset by the benefits of treatment. These SITS-ISTR data showed an increase in the overall number of patients receiving thrombolysis beyond 3 hours following the publication of ECASS III, but this was not at the expense of timely treatment with the numbers of patients receiving treatment within 3 hours remaining constant, reinforcing the need to administer thrombolytic therapy without undue delay. Indeed, pooled data have clearly demonstrated the effects of diminishing outcomes with treatment delays, as shown in Figures 18.1 and 18.2 [14].

The third International Stroke Trial (IST-3) sought to determine whether a greater range of patients may benefit from intravenous thrombolysis [15]. Investigators randomized patients to receive intravenous rtPA or control up to 6 hours from stroke onset with no upper age limit to recruitment. More than 3000 patients were included, across 12 countries. The trial was neutral on its primary endpoint but on secondary outcomes, thrombolysis was associated with functional benefit despite significant increases in early symptomatic intracranial hemorrhage (7% versus 1%) and death (11% versus 7%) within the first 7 days of stroke. By 6 months, mortality was similar in each group, however. Fifty-three percent of patients in IST-3 were older than 80 years. Benefits of thrombolysis were confirmed in these patients,

295

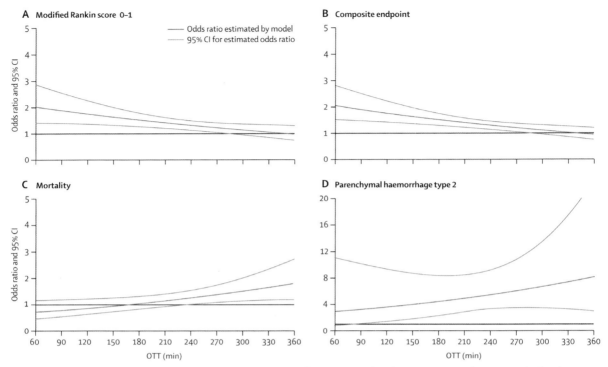

Figure 18.1. Relation of onset to treatment delay with treatment effect. Relation of stroke onset to start of treatment (OTT) with treatment effect after adjustment for prognostic variables assessed by (A) day 90 modified Rankin score 0–1 versus 2–6 (interaction p=0·0269, n=3530 [excluding EPITHET[7] data p=0·0116, n=3431]); (B) global test that incorporates modified Rankin score 0–1 versus 2–6, Barthel Index score 95–100 versus 90 or lower and NIHSS score 0–1 versus 2 or more (interaction p=0·0111, n=3535 [excluding EPITHET[7] data p=0·0049, n=3436]); (C) mortality (interaction p=0·0444, n=3530 [excluding EPITHET[7] data p=0·0582, n=3431]); and (D) parenchymal haemorrhage type 2 (interaction p=0·4140, n=3531 [excluding EPITHET[7] data p=0·4578, n=3431]). Thus, for parenchymal haemorrhage type 2, the fitted line is not statistically distinguishable from a horizontal line. For each graph, the adjusted odds ratio is shown with the 95% CIs. CIs from the models will differ from those shown in the tables because the model uses data from all patients treated within 0–360 min whereas the categorised analyses in the tables are based on subsets of patients: the modelled CIs are deemed to be more reliable. Reprinted from reference [14] with permission from Elsevier.

which is an important factor in clinical practice when considering whether to offer thrombolysis to older patients.

Data from IST-3 underline the need for rapid initiation of treatment and offer some reassurance around the robustness of treatment safety and efficacy in borderline cases. Beyond the elderly subgroup, for whom substantial randomized data are now available to support the recommendations to treat irrespective of age (at time of writing, marketing authorization for alteplase in Europe has not been extended to patients aged over 80 years), so far no new relaxation of the selection criteria for use of thrombolysis have been advanced [16]. However, evidence can be gathered from other sources.

Post-hoc analyses of thrombolysis data have identified factors associated with a poor outcome following intravenous thrombolysis, and these results have helped to inform clinical practice. Elevated serum glucose, increasing age, and increasing stroke severity are among the poor prognostic factors that have been identified [17]. Appropriate patient selection is therefore important when considering whether a patient may be suitable for thrombolysis treatment. However, some of these factors, such as age, may also be identifying a subgroup in whom benefits of treatment could be substantial. A non-randomized, controlled comparison of outcomes among patients with a variety of common contraindications or warnings to use of intravenous alteplase has suggested that many of these factors have limited influence on the effect of treatment, at least when patients have been selected by experienced clinicians [18]. It is good practice to discuss the risks and benefits of treatment with

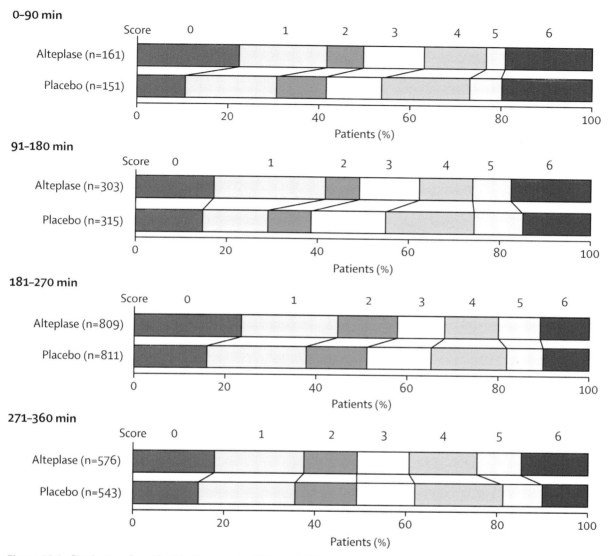

Figure 18.2. Distribution of modified Rankin scores by OTT interval. OTT = onset to start of treatment. Definitions of scores: 0 = no symptoms at all. 1 = no significant disability despite symptoms; able to carry out all usual duties and activities. 2 = slight disability; unable to carry out all previous activities but able to look after own affairs without assistance. 3 = moderate disability; requiring some help, but able to walk without assistance. 4 = moderately severe disability; unable to walk without assistance and unable to attend to own bodily needs without assistance. 5 = severe disability; bedridden, incontinent, and requiring constant nursing and attention. 6 = dead. The alteplase versus placebo distributions were compared within each interval by Cochran-Mantel-Haenszel test without adjustment for prognostic factors: (A) 0–90 min, p = 0.354; (B) 91–180 min, p = 0.0522; (C) 181–270 min, p = 0.0308; (D) 271–360 min, p = 0.4537. Reprinted from reference [14] with permission from Elsevier.

patients or their family before treatment is commenced, and data are available to support clinicians in this. It is important to emphasize that the aim of thrombolytic treatment is to improve the likelihood of the patient being independent several months after their stroke.

Thrombolysis is contraindicated in patients with seizure at stroke onset due to the possibility of confusion with Todd's paresis, which may be present as a stroke mimic, although its use can be considered if the neurological deficit is due to acute cerebral ischemia [4]. Patients with severe hypertension at the time of

Table 18.1. Indications and contraindications for intravenous thrombolysis in acute ischemic stroke

Indication	Contraindication
Stroke onset within 4.5 hours	Previous intracranial hemorrhage
CT/MRI exclusion of hemorrhage and extensive infarct (>1/3 of MCA territory)	Ischemic stroke within 3 months
Serum glucose >2.7 and <22.2 mmol/l	Seizure at stroke onset
BP <185 mmHg systolic and/or 110 mmHg diastolic	Recent major surgery
NIHSS >3 and <25	Unexplained hemorrhage
Age >18 years	INR >1.4 Platelets <150 × 10⁹/l Rapid neurological recovery

INR = international normalized ratio; MCA = middle cerebral artery.

admission were excluded from the trials of thrombolysis and therefore blood pressure (BP) is recommended to be below 185/110 mmHg before, and for the first 24 hours after, thrombolytic therapy. Severe hypertension increases the risks of hemorrhagic transformation following thrombolysis [17].

Intravenous rtPA is therefore recommended for use in appropriately selected individuals within 4.5 hours of stroke onset and should be offered to patients over the age of 18 years with no upper age limit [3, 4]. Indications and contraindications are listed in Table 18.1. The dose of alteplase is weight-dependent at 0.9 mg/kg up to a maximum dose of 90 mg. Ten percent of the total dose is administered as an intravenous bolus with the remaining 90% delivered over 1 hour.

> Intravenous thrombolysis is a standard therapy for a well-selected population of patients with acute ischemic stroke within 4.5 hours of stroke onset.

Prior antiplatelet treatment is associated with an increased risk of intracranial hemorrhage, although not overall clinical outcome, as is aspirin administration within 90 minutes of rtPA administration [15, 19]. Aspirin and other antiplatelets or anticoagulants should therefore be avoided for 24 hours

following thrombolysis, as should arterial puncture at a non-compressible site.

Various techniques have been employed to help facilitate effective thrombolysis and vessel recanalization, including transcranial Doppler "sonothrombolysis" and microbubble administration, but these are not currently in routine clinical use [3, 20]. Multimodal imaging technologies, such as perfusion CT and diffusion-weighted MRI, are being studied in the hope of improving patient selection for thrombolysis and extending the time window for intervention, but such procedures are not currently in routine use and are beyond the scope of this chapter.

> The approved agent is recombinant tissue plasminogen activator (rtPA), alteplase, in a dose of 0.9 mg/kg up to a maximum dose of 90 mg (10% administered as a bolus, 90% over 1 hour). Patients with a delay >4.5 hours, BP >185/110 mmHg, or severe stroke (NIHSS >24) should be excluded.

Having identified patients who are potential candidates for intravenous thrombolysis, systems must be in place to ensure their timely transfer to an appropriate medical facility and rapid access to assessment and imaging once admitted. The exact structure of a stroke service will vary depending on local factors. Structuring thrombolysis services in places where patient populations are spread over large rural areas can be particularly challenging. The structure of such a service will differ depending on local needs and no single model can be claimed to be superior to another. Novel technologies such as telemedicine have been employed in some rural areas. The important common factors which ensure a safe and effective service are that patients should be assessed and diagnosed by physicians experienced in stroke care [1, 10]. Brain imaging should also be reviewed by a physician with the appropriate experience and training, although this does not necessarily need to be a radiologist. In practice, due to the time constraint of initiating therapy within 4.5 hours of stroke onset, consideration needs to be given to the geographical location of the acute stroke unit in comparison to radiology and other acute services.

Although some evidence exists to support the use of intra-arterial thrombolysis for proximal occlusions of the middle cerebral artery (MCA) within 6 hours of onset, it is not currently established as a routine treatment option in the majority of centers [1]. The studies investigating intra-arterial thrombolysis used pro-urokinase, which is currently not available in

Europe, and large-scale studies using rtPA as an intra-arterial agent are lacking. Clinical trials investigating the efficacy of the combination of intravenous and intra-arterial rtPA compared to intravenous thrombolysis alone are ongoing but published data comparing endovascular intervention following intravenous rtPA to intravenous rtPA alone have not demonstrated beneficial outcomes [1, 21]. No significant difference between intravenous and intra-arterial thrombolysis has been demonstrated for patients with basilar artery occlusion in non-randomized comparisons [1].

> Intra-arterial thrombolysis is used in selected cases up to 6 hours after MCA and basilar artery occlusion, but is not established as a routine treatment option.

Patients who meet the criteria for intravenous thrombolysis remain in the minority, with rates for intravenous thrombolysis varying, but relatively low, throughout Europe. Whilst strategies are being developed to improve the rapid recognition and assessment of patients who may be suitable for intravenous thrombolysis, the majority of patients remain ineligible. For those who are ineligible for intravenous thrombolysis as part of routine clinical care, and in whom participating in a clinical research trial is either inappropriate or impossible, best supportive care is offered and other alternative interventions should be considered.

Mechanical embolus removal

The Mechanical Embolectomy Removal in Cerebral Ischemia (MERCI) trial, published in 2005, reported vessel recanalization in 68 of the 141 (48%) patients ineligible for conventional intravenous thrombolysis and in whom the embolectomy device was deployed within 8 hours of stroke onset [22]. This exceeds the proportion expected from a historical control population (18%) and favorable neurological outcomes were observed in those patients who achieved successful recanalization. Subsequent randomized trial and other cohort study data have shown that alternative devices, including the Trevo and Solitaire Retrievers, have better revascularization rates and improved clinical outcomes than the MERCI device [23–25]. Intra-arterial thrombolysis has not been shown to be superior to intravenous thrombolysis and its use is not part of standard clinical practice currently, although further studies are underway.

More recent data in 656 patients randomized to receive intravenous rtPA with endovascular intervention (intra-arterial thrombolysis or clot retrieval) or intravenous rtPA alone has failed to demonstrate a significant benefit with endovascular intervention [21]. Endovascular intervention is not, therefore, currently part of routine clinical practice although it may be useful in carefully selected individuals in whom there are contraindications to intravenous thrombolysis.

> Endovascular intervention is not yet routine clinical practice but clinical trials are still underway.

Aspirin

The benefits of low-dose aspirin in preventing recurrent serious vascular events in patients with transient ischemic attack (TIA), ischemic stroke, or myocardial infarction have been established for more than 10 years [26]. The potential benefits of commencing aspirin therapy in patients early after the onset of ischemic stroke were not realized until the publication of two large randomized controlled trials, the Chinese Acute Stroke Trial (CAST) and the International Stroke Trial (IST) [27, 28]. With a combined study population of more than 40 000 patients, these two landmark studies provide strong evidence supporting the early introduction of aspirin following ischemic stroke. Aspirin was commenced within 48 hours of stroke onset in both studies, and continued for up to 14 days in the IST and up to 4 weeks in the CAST. In the CAST aspirin treatment was associated with a slight increase in hemorrhagic stroke (1.1% vs. 0.9%), offset by a significant 14% reduction in mortality (3.3% vs. 3.9%) and early recurrent ischemic stroke (1.6% vs. 2.1%). This corresponded to 11 fewer patients per 1000 treated with aspirin who were dead or dependent at the time of discharge [28]. Similar results were observed in the IST with a significant reduction in early recurrent ischemic stroke observed in the aspirin-treated group (2.8% vs. 3.9%) without an associated excess of ICH, although the number of early deaths was similar between groups [27]. Early aspirin use (within 48 hours of stroke onset) was associated with a significant reduction in death or non-fatal recurrent stroke. In absolute terms, 13 fewer patients per 1000 treated with aspirin were dead or dependent at 6 months following their stroke. In both studies, a CT scan to exclude ICH was mandatory only in comatose patients, although it was considered preferable prior to randomization. Given that access to brain imaging, either by CT or MRI, is now generally universally available within the first 24 hours of admission to an acute stroke unit, aspirin can justifiably be withheld until intracerebral bleeding has been excluded. CT readily distinguishes between ischemic and hemorrhagic stroke within the first 5–7 days and is most cost-effective when performed immediately [1, 29]. The dose of aspirin prescribed varied between the CAST and IST (160 mg daily and 300 mg daily respectively) and other doses have been used in other studies. Once intracranial hemorrhage has been excluded aspirin should be administered at the earliest opportunity at a dose of 300 mg either orally or rectally depending on the patient's ability to swallow safely. Subsequent doses can be lower (75–300 mg), with the evidence suggesting that the same benefit can be conferred with 75 mg daily whilst avoiding the potential side-effects which are more commonly observed at higher doses [30]. Although the absolute benefits provided by early aspirin use are small, this intervention is available to the majority of patients who have suffered ischemic strokes. Therefore, on a population level, initiating early aspirin treatment has the potential to reduce the number of recurrent vascular events by several thousand worldwide.

> A dose of 300 mg aspirin should be administered within 48 hours of stroke onset after exclusion of intracranial hemorrhage through a CT scan. Subsequent doses can be lower (75–300 mg).

Other antiplatelets

Whether or not other antiplatelet agents, with or without aspirin, confer additional vascular risk reduction has been extensively investigated. Evidence exists to support the use of the combination of aspirin and dipyridamole in secondary prevention [31], and also that the antiplatelet agent clopidogrel is at least equivalent to aspirin and dipyridamole combined [32].

The combination of aspirin and clopidogrel has been shown to be of some value in patients with significant internal carotid artery stenosis with distal emboli [33], although the same combination has also been shown to be associated with increased hemorrhagic risk in patients with completed stroke [34]. Short-term dual antiplatelet use with aspirin and clopidogrel has been evaluated in high-risk patients presenting within 24 hours of non-disabling stroke or TIA [35]. Preliminary results from the Clopidogrel

in High-risk patients with Acute Non-disabling Cerebrovascular Events (CHANCE) trial have reported significant improvements in 3-month stroke-free survival in the study population of 5170 individuals who were randomized to receive either clopidogrel 300 mg loading dose, followed by 75 mg daily, or placebo for 21 days in addition to aspirin (hazard ratio 0.68; 95% confidence interval 0.57–0.81, p < 0.001) [36]. The rates of ICH and severe bleeding appeared to be low and were similar between the groups, although minor bleeding was more common in the dual antiplatelet group. CHANCE was conducted in an exclusively Chinese population. Confirmation in a European or North American population may be desirable.

Despite encouraging early clinical trial data use of combined antiplatelet agents in the acute setting is not presently routine. It is, however, good practice to commence appropriate secondary prevention antiplatelet therapy at the earliest opportunity in appropriate patients with a safe swallow.

The glycoprotein-IIa-IIIb inhibitor abciximab has been studied in acute stroke patients but showed an increased risk of symptomatic or fatal intracranial hemorrhage without an associated benefit and therefore its use is not advised [1].

> Current evidence supports the use of aspirin in the context of acute ischemic stroke with further evaluation of combination antiplatelet agents being required.

Heparin for cardioembolic stroke

The IST investigated the use of aspirin and subcutaneous unfractionated heparin in a two-by-two factorial design. The beneficial effects of aspirin have already been discussed but the study also identified three fewer deaths within 14 days per 1000 patients treated with heparin (non-significant) and significantly fewer early recurrent strokes (2.9% vs. 3.8%) and pulmonary emboli (0.5% vs. 0.8%) [27]. After 6 months, however, the mortality rate was identical in those patients treated with heparin compared to those who were not. Unfortunately, heparin use was associated with more hemorrhagic strokes (1.2% vs. 0.4%) and resulted in a significant excess of nine transfused or fatal extracranial hemorrhages per 1000 patients treated. The risk of hemorrhagic complications was greater in the group which received a higher dose of subcutaneous heparin. Studies of other unfractionated heparin preparations have also failed to show significant benefit when commenced early following ischemic stroke, with the increased risk of hemorrhagic complications outweighing any potential benefit [1]. In a meta-analysis of early anticoagulant therapy, the reduction in recurrent ischemic stroke observed was almost identical to the risk excess for symptomatic intracranial hemorrhage [37]. There is therefore currently no evidence to support the routine use of anticoagulants in all patients in the early aftermath of ischemic stroke.

For patients in whom stroke is due to a cardioembolic etiology, in a meta-analysis of seven trials involving 4624 patients within 48 hours of stroke onset, anticoagulation was associated with a non-significant reduction in early recurrent ischemic stroke (odds ratio 0.68; 95% confidence interval 0.44–1.06) without any significant change in death or disability at final follow-up (odds ratio 1.01; 95% confidence interval 0.82–1.24) [38]. A significant and almost 3-fold risk (odds ratio 2.89; 95% confidence interval 1.19–7.01) of symptomatic intracranial hemorrhage was identified with number needed to harm being 55. Despite the lack of supporting evidence, some authorities would advocate early anticoagulation with full-dose heparin in selected patients at high risk of re-embolization [1]. Evidence of a large infarction on brain imaging (e.g. >50% of the MCA territory) or extensive microvascular disease and uncontrolled arterial hypertension are contraindications to full anticoagulation in the early post-stroke period.

> There is currently no evidence to support the routine use of anticoagulants in all patients in the early aftermath of ischemic stroke.

Neuroprotection

Neuronal injury progresses rapidly following the onset of cerebral ischemia and therefore a substance which attenuates this process may potentially reduce the extent of cerebral damage. The free-radical-trapping agent NXY-059 showed initial promise as a potential neuroprotective agent when introduced within 6 hours of ischemic stroke onset, but a larger randomized controlled trial involving more than 3000 patients did not demonstrate any benefit of NXY-059 over placebo [39]. The agent was also ineffective in those patients who had been treated with intravenous thrombolysis. Furthermore there was also no effect in patients with primary ICH. Whilst other studies of novel neuroprotective agents are ongoing, there is currently no evidence to support their routine clinical use.

> Up to now all neuroprotective therapies have been without clinical efficacy.

Blood pressure – see Chapter 20

Hypertension is a well-recognized risk factor for first-ever and recurrent stroke [40, 41] and is commonly observed in the immediate post-stroke period. In the IST, 82% of patients had systolic BPs measured in excess of 140 mmHg during the first 48 hours following admission, with 28% having a systolic BP ≥80 mmHg [42]. Similarly, in the CAST three-quarters had systolic BP ≥140 mmHg, with one-quarter of patients having systolic BP ≥180 mmHg within 48 hours of admission [28]. Of the 624 patients who were included in the NINDS rtPA Stroke Trial, 19% had admission systolic BP > 185 mmHg and diastolic BP >110 mmHg. Within the first 24 hours of randomization, 60% had BP in excess of 180 mmHg systolic or 105 mmHg diastolic [43]. Despite high BP being very common following stroke, the early management of BP following ischemic stroke remains controversial and is the subject of ongoing research.

Although hypertension in the immediate post-stroke period is frequently observed, BP tends to spontaneously fall within the first hours and days following the acute event, with the pattern of blood pressure change varying with stroke subtype [41, 44]. Precipitous falls in BP have, however, been associated with poor outcome and should be avoided [45]. A 'U-shaped' association between admission BP and stroke outcome has been identified, with very high and very low BP being associated with poor post-stroke outcome. Analysis of the IST revealed a 3.8% increased risk of death and 4.2% increased risk of early recurrent stroke within 14 days with each 10 mmHg rise in systolic BP above 150 mmHg. For every 10 mmHg admission systolic BP was below 150 mmHg, the risk of early death rose by 17.9%, and the risk of death or dependency was increased by 3.6% at 6 months [42]. Further analyses have confirmed the association between elevated systolic, diastolic, and mean arterial BP in the acute stroke period and poor outcome following ischemic stroke. Early recurrent stroke has been suggested as one possible mechanism by which elevated BP may be associated with poor outcome [46]. Cerebral perfusion becomes dependent upon systemic arterial BP following stroke due to impairment of cerebral autoregulation, and therefore changes in systemic BP can directly influence cerebral perfusion [41]. Hypertension may sustain cerebral perfusion to the ischemic penumbra, with BP having been shown to fall spontaneously in response to successful recanalization of cerebral vessels following thrombolytic treatment, perhaps suggesting the restoration of cerebral autoregulation [47]. High pre-thrombolysis BP has also been shown to be associated with poor recanalization [48] and sustained hypertension may contribute to worsening cerebral edema and hemorrhagic transformation following acute ischemic stroke. Cardiovascular complications as well as early stroke recurrence in patients with elevated post-stroke BPs have been proposed as possible mechanisms for poor outcome [46].

There is therefore evidence that high (and low) post-stroke BP is associated with a poor outcome, although the relationship is not a straightforward one. The true relationship may depend on a combination of absolute BP level and the variability in BP following stroke and also upon stroke subtype and comorbidities. The optimum post-stroke BP, and how to achieve it, is therefore yet to be identified. Indeed, it is also unclear as to whether pre-existing antihypertensive medication should be continued or withdrawn following stroke [49].

> A U-shaped relationship between baseline systolic BP and both early and late death or dependency after ischemic stroke has been demonstrated in clinical trials.

A Cochrane systematic review of published and unpublished studies examining various interventions aimed at deliberately altering blood pressure within 2 weeks of acute stroke concluded that there was insufficient evidence to evaluate the effects of altering BP on outcome during the acute phase of stroke [50]. Numerous clinical trials are currently ongoing and each hopes to provide valuable knowledge and insight into how this common clinical situation is best managed.

This lack of certainty is reflected in clinical guidance, with clinicians avoiding the active reduction of BP in the early post-stroke period [51]. Until evidence is available to the contrary, current clinical guidelines do not advocate the active reduction of hypertension in the immediate post-stroke period unless there is a concurrent indication to do so [1]. Such indications include hypertensive encephalopathy, myocardial infarction, aortic dissection, and

pre-eclampsia. Similarly, there is no conclusive evidence that low BP should be actively elevated following acute ischemic stroke [1]. Until strong evidence becomes available, some centers have developed local protocols for cautiously lowering BP when systolic BP exceeds the threshold required for thrombolysis (185/110 mmHg), although these are based on clinical experience rather than specific evidence. If elevated BP is to be lowered in the acute post-stroke period, the reduction should be cautious (North American guidelines suggest a maximum reduction of 15–25% in the first 24 hours) [52], and by means of a short-acting agent. The optimum agent to lower BP, including to allow thrombolytic therapy to be administered, is also unclear. A short-acting intravenous beta-blocker such as labetalol or intravenous nitrates may be useful in this situation as the effects are readily reversed on withdrawal of the agent. Sublingual calcium-channel blockers should be avoided.

> The optimum post-stroke BP, and how to achieve it, is yet to be identified. Current clinical guidelines do not advocate the active reduction of hypertension in the immediate post-stroke period unless there is a concurrent indication to do so. If elevated BP is to be lowered in the acute post-stroke period, the reduction should be cautious.

Blood glucose – see Chapter 20

Measurement of blood glucose is mandatory for all patients with suspected stroke. Hypoglycemia (serum glucose <2.8 mmol/l) with consequent neuroglycopenia is an important stroke mimic and is readily corrected by the intravenous infusion of 10–20% dextrose [1]. Hyperglycemia has a reported prevalence of up to 68% of acute stroke admission, and is not restricted to those patients with previously diagnosed diabetes mellitus [53]. The prevalence of previously unrecognized diabetes mellitus or impaired glucose tolerance may be between 20% and 30% [54]. There is evidence of a positive association between elevated admission plasma glucose and poor post-stroke outcome, with increasing stroke severity, higher mortality, and reduced functional recovery observed in those with hyperglycemia [53]. Control of hyperglycemia following myocardial infarction and in critically ill patients being managed in intensive care units was thought to confer a beneficial outcome, and so it was suggested that the same may be true in the context of acute stroke [55–57]. Currently, however, there is no evidence to support the routine active lowering of hyperglycemia following acute stroke. A large randomized controlled trial of an active intervention aimed at achieving and maintaining euglycemia following stroke (ischemic and hemorrhagic) recruited 933 patients and randomized them to glucose-potassium-insulin (GKI) infusion versus 0.9% saline (control group) [58]. Only small reductions in plasma glucose were achieved, with the mean difference between the active treatment and control groups being 0.57 mmol/l, which probably reflects the median glucose at admission, which was only modestly elevated at 7.8 mmol/l and 7.6 mmol/l in the active treatment and control groups respectively. The 90-day mortality did not differ significantly between the groups although this study was limited by slow recruitment and therefore underpowered. A post-hoc analysis identified an increase in the proportion of patients with a poor outcome where a reduction in glucose of ≥2 mmol/l was achieved using GKI, which raises the possibility that large reductions in post-stroke hyperglycemia may not be well tolerated. Until additional evidence becomes available, the routine use of insulin infusion regimes to control moderate post-stroke hyperglycemia cannot be recommended. Based upon clinical opinion, some acute stroke units may intervene to control post-stroke hyperglycemia in patients with blood glucose >10 mmol/l, although this decision must be made on an individual patient basis [1]. Further research is required in order to determine the optimum method of achieving and maintaining post-stroke euglycemia.

> Measurement of blood glucose is mandatory for all patients with suspected stroke. Hypoglycemia should be corrected by an intravenous dextrose infusion. The routine use of insulin regimes to control post-stroke hyperglycemia cannot be recommended.

Body temperature – see Chapter 20

Increased body temperature following stroke has been shown to be associated with poor outcome. Studies of antipyretic medication and thermal cooling devices have not provided conclusive evidence of efficacy but it is good practice to monitor and treat pyrexia in the immediate post-stroke period. A rise in body temperature can be centrally mediated following stroke, but more commonly it suggests the presence of intercurrent infection. Its occurrence should alert the clinician to this possibility and, if clinically appropriate, such infections should be treated. Raised body temperature following stroke is commonly treated with antipyretic medication [1]. Paracetamol 1 g can be administered every 4–6 hours, to a total dose of 4 g/24 hours in adult patients, via the oral, rectal, or intravenous routes. For patients who have suffered severe MCA infarction, induced mild hypothermia (brain temperature 32–33 °C) reduces mortality, but increases the risks of severe side-effects during re-warming, including recurrent intracranial pressure crisis [1]. Mild hypothermia in combination with decompressive surgery may be of benefit in patients with severe MCA infarction, although the evidence for temperature reduction is limited [1].

> Raised body temperature following stroke is commonly treated with antipyretic medication.

Brain edema and surgical intervention

For patients suffering from large MCA territory infarctions mortality is as high as 80% [59]. Early deterioration and death are often due to cerebral edema and rising intracranial pressure, which can occur within 24 hours of stroke, but usually becomes evident between days 2 and 5 following stroke onset [1]. Medical therapy includes airway management, oxygenation, pain control, and control of body temperature. Intracranial pressure should be maintained at ~70 mmHg and can be lowered by using intravenous mannitol (25–50 g every 3–6 hours), glycerol (4 × 250 ml 10% glycerol over 30–60 minutes), or hypertonic saline, although the evidence for such interventions comes from mainly observational data [1]. Dexamethasone and corticosteroids are not indicated and hypotonic and dextrose-containing solutions should be avoided [1].

Surgical decompression of evolving malignant MCA infarction should be considered in certain selected patients. Evidence for this comes from the pooled analysis of three European studies of decompressive craniotomy: the DECIMAL (decompressive surgery in malignant middle cerebral artery infarcts) study; the DESTINY (decompressive surgery for the treatment of malignant infarction of the middle cerebral artery) study; and the HAMLET trial (hemicraniectomy after middle cerebral artery infarction with life-threatening edema trial) [59]. The effects of surgery in the three trials were consistent and, based upon the 93 patients included in the pooled analysis, showed a significant improvement in the proportion of patients with mRS ≤4 at 1 year, mRS ≤3 at 1 year, and survivors at 1 year irrespective of function. The numbers needed to treat were 2, 4, and 2 respectively. Importantly, there was no increase in the numbers of survivors left with severe disability (mRS ≤5). Whether older patients may gain similar benefit from such an intervention has been investigated in the multicenter DESTINY II study, which was stopped prematurely when planned interim analysis of the data suggested efficacy [60]. Final results are awaited but early analysis suggests that a significantly greater proportion of patients >60 years old undergoing hemicraniectomy had mRS 0–4 at 6 months compared to those who did not receive surgery [61].

Until further evidence becomes available patients who should be considered for decompressive hemicraniectomy are those up to 60 years old with evolving MCA infarction and NIHSS >15 in whom consciousness is impaired (score of 1 or greater on item 1a of the NIHSS) and who have evidence of infarct in >50% of the MCA territory on CT [1]. Neurosurgical opinion should be sought at an early opportunity, with the aim of performing surgery within 48 hours of stroke onset.

> Intracranial pressure should be maintained at ~70 mmHg and can be lowered by using intravenous mannitol (25–50 g every 3–6 hours), glycerol (4 × 250 ml 10% glycerol over 30–60 minutes), or hypertonic saline. Surgical decompression of evolving malignant MCA infarction should be considered in certain selected patients.

Cerebellar infarction

Neurosurgical opinion should also be sought in patients with space-occupying posterior fossa infarctions. Although randomized controlled trial evidence is not available, expert opinion advises that decompressive surgery and ventriculostomy can be considered in cases of cerebellar infarction as prognosis can be favorable [1].

Intracerebral hemorrhage

ICH is not an isolated clinical entity, but a term used to describe the consequences of a variety of pathologies. It accounts for around 20% of strokes and includes primary ICH, secondary ICH, and subarachnoid hemorrhage (SAH) [2]. Primary ICH is commonly associated with hypertension or cerebral amyloid angiopathy, while secondary ICH results from a number of pathologies including, but not limited to, aneurysms, arteriovenous malformation (AVM), neoplastic disease, cerebral vasculitis, and venous sinus thrombosis [2]. Whilst a detailed description of the management of all ICH is discussed in Chapter 11, an outline of the principles of the initial management of ICH will be discussed here.

Once ICH has been confirmed on brain imaging, some aspects of the patients' immediate management differ from that following ischemic stroke. Clearly, thrombolysis is contraindicated! Coagulopathy should be identified and treated as quickly as possible, although ICH associated with oral anticoagulation will be discussed separately.

Early BP manipulation is also controversial in patients with ICH. Patients with ICH are frequently chronically hypertensive and may therefore tolerate, and perhaps require, higher cerebral perfusion pressures in order to maintain adequate cerebral perfusion. Conversely, hypertension may be associated with hematoma expansion [2]. Limited data are available to guide clinical practice, but the current European Stroke Initiative recommendations advise that in patients following ICH in whom there is a history of chronic hypertension, BP should be gradually lowered to below a mean arterial pressure (MAP) of 120 mmHg, whilst avoiding reductions of >20%, and MAP should not be lowered below 84 mmHg. A target BP of 160/100 mmHg is used for such patients. In patients without a history or clinical evidence of previously sustained hypertension, upper limits of 160/95 mmHg are accepted before BP lowering is advocated, with a target BP of 150/90 mmHg (MAP 110 mmHg) [2]. In support of active BP reduction following ICH, the Intensive Blood Pressure Reduction in Acute Cerebral Haemorrhage Trial (INTERACT) reported reductions in mean hematoma growth in patients following ICH without intraventricular hemorrhage who had intensive BP lowering (target systolic BP of 140 mmHg) compared to those patients who received standard-guideline-based BP control (target systolic BP of 180 mmHg) commenced within 6 hours of onset and continued for 7 days (13.7% vs. 36.3% proportional increase, p = 0.04) [62]. Although the difference in proportional mean hematoma growth within 6 hours was no longer significant (p = 0.06) after adjustment for initial hematoma volume and time from onset to CT, the data would suggest that intensive lowering of BP appears to reduce hematoma expansion. No difference in death, neurological deterioration, or disability was identified between the groups at 90-day follow-up in this study of 404 patients, although a larger study to determine the effects on clinical outcomes is under way. Furthermore, results from the Antihypertensive Treatment of Acute Cerebral Hemorrhage (ATACH) study provide additional data to support the association between active BP lowering and reduced hematoma expansion, although the efficacy trial continues to recruit [63]. A number of oral and intravenous agents have been studied and no single agent has been shown to be superior. Titration and revision of these thresholds may be required in order to maintain an adequate cerebral perfusion pressure.

Avoiding venous thromboembolism is as important in patients following ICH as it is in post-ischemic stroke patients. Graduated compression stockings have not yet been confirmed to be effective in patients following ICH, although their use is widespread [2]. Anticoagulants in the form of subcutaneous heparins may cause hematoma expansion and are therefore best avoided within the initial days following ICH [2]. The advice of the Seventh ACCP Conference on Antithrombotic and Thrombolytic Therapy recommends that low doses of unfractionated or low molecular weight heparin can be started on the second day following ICH in patients who are neurologically stable, although evidence of the efficacy of doing so is not available [64].

Raised intracranial pressure can be lowered if necessary by using medical methods previously discussed. Where this is unsuccessful, therapeutic hyperventilation can be utilized in order that adequate cerebral perfusion pressures are achieved [2]. Seizure is more commonly encountered in patients with ICH compared to ischemic stroke and non-convulsive status has been described, which will require anticonvulsant therapy [2].

Surgical intervention for ICH depends on a number of factors, including size, location, and the presence of intraventricular expansion of the hemorrhage (IVH). In the Surgical Trial in Intracerebral Haemorrhage (STICH) study, there was no difference in outcome between those patients who received early surgical intervention (<24 hours) and those who were managed conservatively [65]. However, a trend towards a significant benefit was observed in patients who suffered a deterioration in conscious level, from a Glasgow Coma Score of between 9 and 12, and in

whom the ICH was superficial (≤1 cm from the surface) and no IVH compared to patients with deep hematomas who do not benefit from surgical intervention. This particular subset of patients warrants further investigation, which is currently ongoing. Although not confirmed by randomized controlled trials, surgical intervention for cerebellar hematoma should be considered, as outcomes are favorable [2]. In particular, ventricular drainage for subsequent hydrocephalus should be considered depending on the individual patient. For patients with intraventricular hemorrhage, there is some evidence to support the use of intraventricular drainage with thrombolytic agents administered via the catheter to prevent catheter obstruction, though trials on this continue [2].

The use of recombinant factor VIIa (rFVIIa) has been studied in patients with spontaneous ICH [2]. Recombinant factor VIIa initiates coagulation and therefore may be associated with increased thrombotic tendency. Consequently, trials of its use have been limited to patients without a history of previous ischemic events. In the first clinical trial with rFVIIa, the use of rFVIIa within 4 hours of ICH limited hematoma expansion, decreased mortality, and improved 3-month outcome, although arterial thromboembolic events were significantly increased in the highest-dose group (160 μg/kg). A further trial involving more than 800 patients also found reduced hematoma expansion and significantly improved NIHSS scores compared to placebo when rFVIIa was used within 4 hours of ICH at a dose of 80 μg/kg, but no sustained advantage in terms of functional outcome was identified [66]. Until more data are available, use of rFVIIa cannot be regarded as part of standard clinical care.

ICH whilst anticoagulated is associated with more severe hemorrhage, larger rebleeds, and a worse outcome, with an increased risk of death [2]. For patients who suffer ICH whilst anticoagulated, the priority is to reverse the anticoagulation. This can usually be effectively achieved by using a combination of intravenous vitamin K and prothrombin complex concentrate, or fresh frozen plasma.

> With intracerebral hemorrhage (ICH), thrombolysis is contraindicated. Hypertension should be gradually lowered. Raised intracranial pressure can be lowered if necessary. Surgical intervention for ICH depends on a number of factors, including size, location, and the presence of intraventricular expansion of the hemorrhage.

Summary

In order that patients obtain the full potential benefit of acute stroke therapies, significant changes in the way stroke services are configured have been required. Patient education and early recognition of symptoms and an appreciation that patients with suspected stroke should be transported to an appropriate medical facility in a time-efficient manner have been essential. Additionally, the recognition by medical and nursing staff of stroke as a medical emergency necessitating rapid clinical assessment, diagnosis, and treatment has been essential in maximizing the potential benefit from the array of established and evolving acute stroke interventions.

Chapter summary

Intravenous thrombolysis is a standard therapy for a well-selected population of patients with acute ischemic stroke. The only thrombolytic agent licensed in Europe for the treatment of ischemic stroke is recombinant tissue plasminogen activator (rtPA), alteplase. It should be offered to patients aged >18 years presenting within 4.5 hours of stroke onset. There is no upper age limit. Intracranial hemorrhage needs to be excluded on brain imaging.

At present European regulatory agencies do not support the routine use of intravenous rtPA in patients beyond 4.5 hours, or in those with severe stroke (NIHSS >24) or where there is extensive early ischemic changes on CT. Factors associated with a poor outcome following intravenous thrombolysis are elevated serum glucose, increasing age, and increasing stroke severity. Thrombolysis is not usually given to patients with seizure at stroke onset, although it can be considered if the neurological deficit is due to cerebral ischemia. Blood pressure (BP) is recommended to be below 185/110 mmHg, and consideration can be given to actively lowering it to this threshold to allow thrombolysis if necessary.

The dose of alteplase is weight-dependent at 0.9 mg/kg up to a maximum dose of 90 mg. Ten percent of the total dose is administered as an intravenous bolus with the remaining 90% delivered over 1 hour. Aspirin and other antiplatelets or anticoagulants should be avoided for 24 hours following thrombolysis.

Transcranial Doppler "sonothrombolysis," microbubble and intra-arterial thrombolysis administration are currently not in routine clinical use.

Strong evidence supports the early introduction of **aspirin** following ischemic stroke. A dose of 300 mg (orally or rectally) should be administered within 48 hours of stroke onset, but after exclusion of intracerebral hemorrhage (ICH) through a CT scan. Subsequent doses can be lower (75–300 mg).

The efficacy of either dipyridamole, clopidogrel, or a combination of antiplatelet agents has not been investigated in the context of acute stroke and therefore there is no evidence to support their routine use in the acute setting. It is, however, good practice to commence appropriate secondary prevention antiplatelet therapy at the earliest opportunity in appropriate patients.

There is currently no evidence to support the routine use of **anticoagulants** in all patients in the early aftermath of cardioembolic ischemic stroke. Despite the lack of supporting evidence, some authorities would advocate early anticoagulation with full-dose heparin in selected patients at high risk of re-embolization. Evidence of a large infarction on brain imaging (e.g. >50% of the MCA territory) or extensive microvascular disease and uncontrolled arterial hypertension are contraindications to full anticoagulation in the early post-stroke period.

Despite **high blood pressure** being very common following stroke, the early management of BP following ischemic stroke remains controversial. A 'U-shaped' association between admission BP and stroke outcome has been identified, with very high and very low BP being associated with poor post-stroke outcome. Hypertension may sustain cerebral perfusion to the ischemic penumbra, but sustained hypertension may contribute to worsening cerebral edema and hemorrhagic transformation, as well as leading to cardiovascular complications. The optimum post-stroke BP, and how to achieve it, is therefore yet to be identified. Current clinical guidelines do not advocate the active reduction of hypertension in the immediate post-stroke period unless there is a concurrent indication to do so. Active lowering of BP to below thrombolysis thresholds can be considered if thrombolysis is being considered. If elevated BP is to be lowered in the acute post-stroke period, the reduction should be cautious (North American guidelines suggest a maximum reduction of 15–25% in the first 24 hours), and by means of a short-acting agent.

Measurement of **blood glucose** is mandatory for all patients with suspected stroke. Hypoglycemia should be corrected by an intravenous dextrose infusion. There is evidence of a positive association between elevated admission plasma glucose and poor post-stroke outcome, with increasing stroke severity, higher mortality, and reduced functional recovery observed in those with hyperglycemia. Currently, however, there is no evidence to support the routine active lowering of hyperglycemia following acute stroke. The routine use of insulin infusion regimens to control moderate post-stroke hyperglycemia cannot be recommended. On an individual patient basis, extreme hyperglycemia can be corrected.

Raised body temperature following stroke is commonly treated with antipyretic medication. Induced mild hypothermia (brain temperature 32–33 °C) reduces mortality, but increases the risk of severe side-effects.

Intracranial pressure should be maintained at ~70 mmHg and can be lowered by using intravenous mannitol (25–50 g every 3–6 hours), glycerol (4 × 250 ml 10% glycerol over 30–60 minutes), or hypertonic saline. Surgical decompression of evolving malignant MCA infarction should be considered in certain selected patients.

With **intracerebral hemorrhage**, thrombolysis is contraindicated. Hypertension should be gradually lowered (target BP 160/100 mmHg in patients with, and 150/100 mmHg in patients without chronic hypertension). No single antihypertensive agent has been shown to be superior. Low doses of unfractionated or low molecular weight heparin may be started on the second day following ICH in patients who are neurologically stable. Raised intracranial pressure can be lowered if necessary. Surgical intervention for ICH depends on a number of factors, including size, location, and the presence of intraventricular expansion of the hemorrhage. The use of recombinant factor VIIa (rFVIIa) cannot be recommended.

References

1. European Stroke Organisation (ESO) Executive Committee; ESO Writing Committee. Guidelines for the management of ischaemic stroke and transient ischaemic attack 2008. *Cerebrovasc Dis* 2008; **25**:457–507.

2. Steiner T, Kaste M, Forsting M, *et al.* Recommendations for the management of intracranial haemorrhage - part 1: spontaneous intracerebral haemorrhage. The European Stroke Initiative Writing Committee and the Writing Committee for the EUSI Executive Committee. *Cerebrovasc Dis* 2006; **22**:294–316.

3. European Stroke Organisation. *Guidelines for Stroke Management.* Available from: http://www.eso-stroke.org/recommendations.php?cid=9&sid=1 (accessed April 28, 2013).

4. Karolinska Stroke Update. *Consensus Statements 2012.* Available from: http://www.strokeupdate.org/ Cons_Reperf_IVT_2012.aspx (accessed April 28, 2013).

5. Hacke W, Kaste M, Fieschi C, *et al.* Intravenous thrombolysis with recombinant tissue plasminogen activator for acute hemispheric stroke. The European Cooperative Acute Stroke Study (ECASS). *JAMA* 1995; **274**(13): 1017–25.

6. The National Institute of Neurological Disorders and Stroke rt-PA Stroke Study Group. Tissue plasminogen activator for

acute ischaemic stroke. *N Engl J Med* 1995; **333**:1581–7.

7. Hacke W, Kaste M, Fieschi C, *et al.* Randomised double-blind placebo controlled trial of thrombolytic therapy with intravenous alteplase in acute ischaemic stroke (ECASS II). Second European-Australasian Acute Stroke Study Investigators. *Lancet* 1998; **352**:1245–51.

8. Clark WM, Wissman S, Albers GW, *et al.* Recombinant tissue-type plasminogen activator (Alteplase) for ischemic stroke 3 to 5 hours after symptom onset: The ATLANTIS Study: a randomized controlled trial. Alteplase Thrombolysis for Acute Noninterventional Therapy in Ischemic Stroke. *JAMA* 1999; **282**(21):2019–26.

9. Hacke W, Donnan G, Fieschi C, *et al.* Association of outcome with early stroke treatment: pooled analysis of ATLANTIS, ECASS and NINDS rt-PA stroke trials. *Lancet* 2004; **363**:768–74.

10. Wahlgren N, Ahmed N, Davalos A, *et al.* Thrombolysis with alteplase for acute ischaemic stroke in the Safe Implementation of Thrombolysis in Stroke-Monitoring Study (SITS-MOST): an observational study. *Lancet* 2007; **369**:275–82.

11. Wahlgren N, Ahmed N, Davalos A, *et al.* Thrombolysis with alteplase 3–4.5h after acute ischaemic stroke (SITS-ISTR): an observational study. *Lancet* 2008; **372**:1303–9.

12. Hacke W, Kaste M, Bluhmki E, *et al.* Thrombolysis with alteplase 3 to 4.5 hours after acute ischemic stroke. *N Engl J Med* 2008; **359**(13):1317–29.

13. Ahmed N, Wahlgren N, Grond M, *et al.* Implementation and outcome of thrombolysis with alteplase 3–4.5 h after an acute stroke: an updated analysis from

SITS-ISTR. *Lancet Neurol* 2010; **9**(9):866–74.

14. Lees KR, Bluhmki E, von Kummer RD, *et al.* Time to treatment with intravenous alteplase and outcome in stroke: an updated pooled analysis of ECASS, ATLANTIS, NINDS, and EPITHET trials. *Lancet* 2010; **375** (9727):1695–703.

15. IST-3 collaborative group, Sandercock P, Wardlaw JM, *et al.* The benefits and harms of intravenous thrombolysis with recombinant tissue plasminogen activator within 6 h of acute ischaemic stroke (the third International Stroke Trial [IST-3]): a randomised controlled trial. *Lancet* 2012; **379**(9834): 2352–63.

16. Wardlaw JM, Murray V, Berge E, *et al.* Recombinant tissue plasminogen activator for acute ischaemic stroke: an updated systematic review and meta-analysis. *Lancet* 2012; **379** (9834):2364–72.

17. Lansberg MG, Thijs VN, Bammer R, *et al.* Risk factors of symptomatic intracerebral hemorrhage after tPA therapy for acute stroke. *Stroke* 2007; **38**(8): 2275–8.

18. Frank B, Grotta JC, Alexandrov AV, *et al.* Thrombolysis in stroke despite contraindications or warnings? *Stroke* 2013; **44**(3):727–33.

19. Zinkstok SM, Roos YB. Early administration of aspirin in patients treated with alteplase for acute ischaemic stroke: a randomised controlled trial. *Lancet* 2012; **380**(9843):731–7.

20. Molina CA, Ribo M, Rubiera M, *et al.* Microbubble administration accelerates clot lysis during continuous 2-MHz ultrasound monitoring in stroke patients treated with intravenous tissue plasminogen activator. *Stroke* 2006; **37**(2):425–9.

21. Broderick JP, Palesch YY, Demchuk AM, *et al.* Endovascular therapy after intravenous t-PA versus t-PA alone for stroke. *N Engl J Med* 2013; **368**(10): 893–903.

22. Smith WS, Sung G, Starkman S, *et al.* Safety and efficacy of mechanical embolectomy in acute ischemic stroke: results of the MERCI trial. *Stroke* 2005; **36**(7): 1432–8.

23. Nogueira RG, Lutsep HL, Gupta R, *et al.* Trevo versus Merci retrievers for thrombectomy revascularisation of large vessel occlusions in acute ischaemic stroke (TREVO 2): a randomised trial. *Lancet* 2012; **380**(9849): 1231–40.

24. Broussalis E, Trinka E, Hitzl W, *et al.* Comparison of stent-retriever devices versus the Merci retriever for endovascular treatment of acute stroke. *Am J Neuroradiol* 2013; **34**(2):366–72.

25. Saver JL, Jahan R, Levy EI, *et al.* Solitaire flow restoration device versus the Merci Retriever in patients with acute ischaemic stroke (SWIFT): a randomised, parallel-group, non-inferiority trial. *Lancet* 2012; **380**(9849): 1241–9.

26. Collaborative overview of randomised trials of antiplatelet therapy-I: Prevention of death, myocardial infarction, and stroke by prolonged antiplatelet therapy in various categories of patients. Antiplatelet Trialists' Collaboration. *BMJ* 1994; **308** (6921):81–106.

27. The International Stroke Trial (IST): a randomised trial of aspirin, subcutaneous heparin, both, or neither among 19,435 patients with acute ischaemic stroke. International Stroke Trial Collaborative Group. *Lancet* 1997; **349**:1569–81.

28. CAST: randomised placebo-controlled trial of early aspirin use in 20,000 patients with acute

ischaemic stroke. CAST (Chinese Acute Stroke Trial) Collaborative Group. *Lancet* 1997; **349**:1641–9.

29. Wardlaw JM, Keir SL, Seymour J, *et al.* What is the best imaging strategy for acute stroke? *Health Technol Assess* 2004; **8**:1–180.

30. Antithrombotic Trialists' Collaboration. Collaborative meta-analysis of randomised trials of antiplatelet therapy for prevention of death, myocardial infarction, and stroke in high risk patients. *BMJ* 2002; **324**(7329): 71–86.

31. ESPRIT Study Group, Halkes PH, van Gijn J, *et al.* Aspirin plus dipyridamole versus aspirin alone after cerebral ischaemia of arterial origin (ESPRIT): randomised controlled trial. *Lancet* 2006; **367**:1665–73.

32. Sacco RL, Diener H-C, Yusuf S, *et al.* Aspirin and extended-release dipyridamole versus clopidogrel for recurrent stroke. *N Engl J Med* 2008; **359**(12):1238–51.

33. Markus HS, Droste DW, Kaps M, *et al.* Dual antiplatelet therapy with clopidogrel and aspirin in symptomatic carotid stenosis evaluated using doppler embolic signal detection: the Clopidogrel and Aspirin for Reduction of Emboli in Symptomatic Carotid Stenosis (CARESS) trial. *Circulation* 2005; **111** (17):2233–40.

34. Diener H-C, Bogousslavsky J, Brass LM, *et al.* Aspirin and clopidogrel compared with clopidogrel alone after recent ischaemic stroke or transient ischaemic attack in high-risk patients (MATCH): randomised, double-blind, placebo-controlled trial. *Lancet* 2004; **364**:331–7.

35. Fau WY, Johnston SC. Rationale and design of a randomized, double-blind trial comparing the effects of a 3-month clopidogrel-aspirin regimen versus aspirin alone for the treatment of high-risk patients with acute

nondisabling cerebrovascular event. *Am Heart J* 2010; **160** (3):380–6.e1.

36. Wang Y, Wang Y, Zhao X, *et al.* Clopidogrel and aspirin versus aspirin alone for the treatment of high-risk patients with acute non-disabling cerebrovascular event (CHANCE): a randomized, double-blind, placebo-controlled multicenter trial. *International Stroke Conference 2013.* 2013: Honolulu, Hawaii, USA.

37. Gubitz G, Sandercock P, Counsell C. Anticoagulants for acute ischaemic stroke. *Cochrane Database Syst Rev* 2004; 3:CD000024.

38. Paciaroni M, Agnelli G, Micheli S, Caso V. Efficacy and safety of anticoagulant treatment in acute cardioembolic stroke: a meta-analysis of randomized controlled trials. *Stroke* 2007; **38**(2):423–30.

39. Shuaib A, Lees KR, Lyden P, *et al.* NXY-059 for the treatment of acute ischaemic stroke. *N Engl J Med* 2007; **357**:562–71.

40. Friday G, Alter M, Lai S-M. Control of hypertension and risk of stroke recurrence. *Stroke* 2002; **33**(11):2652–7.

41. Robinson TG, Potter JF. Blood pressure in acute stroke. *Age Ageing* 2004; **33**:6–12.

42. Leonardi-Bee J, Bath PM, Phillips SJ, Sandercock PA; IST Collaborative Group. Blood pressure and clinical outcomes in the International Stroke Trial. *Stroke* 2002; **33**:1315–20.

43. Brott T, Lu M, Kothari R, *et al.* Hypertension and its treatment in the NINDS rt-PA Stroke Trial. *Stroke* 1998; **29**:1504–9.

44. Bath P, Chalmers J, Powers W, *et al.* International Society of Hypertension (ISH): statement on the management of blood pressure in acute stroke. *J Hypertens* 2003; **21**(4):665–72.

45. Castillo J, Leira R, Garcia MM, *et al.* Blood pressure decrease

during the acute phase of ischaemic stroke is associated with brain injury and poor stroke outcome. *Stroke* 2004; **35**:520–7.

46. Willmot, M, Leonardi-Bee J, Bath PM. High blood pressure in acute stroke and subsequent outcome. A systemic review. *Hypertension* 2004; **43**:18–24.

47. Mattle HP, Kappeler L, Arnold M, *et al.* Blood pressure and vessel recanalization in the first hours after ischemic stroke. *Stroke* 2005; **36**:264–9.

48. Tsivgoulis G, Saqqur M, Sharma VK, *et al.* Association of pretreatment blood pressure with tissue plasminogen activator-induced arterial recanalization in acute ischemic stroke. *Stroke* 2007; **38**:961–6.

49. Robinson TG, Potter JF, Ford GA, *et al.* Effects of antihypertensive treatment after acute stroke in the Continue or Stop Post-Stroke Antihypertensives Collaborative Study (COSSACS): a prospective, randomised, open, blinded-endpoint trial. *Lancet Neurol* 2010; **9**(8):767–75.

50. Blood Pressure in Acute Stroke Collaboration (BASC). Interventions for deliberately altering blood pressure in acute stroke. *Cochrane Database Syst Rev* 2001; 3:CD000039. DOI 10.1002/114651858.CD000039.

51. O'Brien RE, Lees KR. Management of acute poststroke blood pressure and detection of atrial fibrillation: a postal questionnaire of UK stroke physicians' current clinical practice. *Scott Med J* 2012; **57** (4):204–8.

52. Adams HP, Jr., del Zoppo G, Alberts MJ, *et al.* Guidelines for the early management of adults with ischemic stroke: a guideline from the American Heart Association/American Stroke Association Stroke Council, Clinical Cardiology Council, Cardiovascular Radiology and

Intervention Council, and the Atherosclerotic Peripheral Vascular Disease and Quality of Care Outcomes in Research Interdisciplinary Working Groups: the American Academy of Neurology affirms the value of this guideline as an educational tool for neurologists. *Stroke* 2007; **38**(5):1655–711.

53. Capes SE, Hunt D, Malmberg K, Pathak P, Gerstein HC. Stress hyperglycaemia and prognosis of stroke in nondiabetic and diabetic patients: a systematic overview. *Stroke* 2001; **32**:2426–32.

54. Scott J, Gray C, O'Connell J, Alberti K. Glucose and insulin therapy in acute stroke; why delay further? *QJM* 1998; **91**:511–15.

55. Malmberg K, Ryden L, Effendic S, *et al.* Randomised trial of insulin glucose infusion followed by subcutaneous insulin treatment in diabetic patients with acute myocardial infarction. The DIGAMI Study. *J Am Coll Cardiol* 1995; **26**:57–65.

56. Van den Berghe G, Wouters P, Weekers F, *et al.* Intensive insulin therapy in critically ill patients. *N Engl J Med* 2001; **345**:1359–67.

57. The NICE-SUGAR Study Investigators. Intensive versus conventional glucose control in critically ill patients. *N Engl J Med* 2009; **360**(13):1283–97.

58. Gray CS, Hildreth AJ, Sandercock PA, *et al.* Glucose-potassium-insulin infusions in the management of post-stroke hyperglycaemia: the UK Glucose Insulin in Stroke Trial (GIST-UK). *Lancet Neurol* 2007; **6**:397–406.

59. Vahedi K, Hofmeijer J, Juettler E, *et al.* Early decompressive surgery in malignant infarction of the middle cerebral artery: a pooled analysis of three randomised controlled trials. *Lancet Neurol* 2007; **6**:215–22.

60. Juttler E, Bosel J, Amiri H, *et al.* DESTINY II: DEcompressive Surgery for the Treatment of malignant INfarction of the middle cerebral arter Y II. *Int J Stroke* 2011; **6**(1):79–86.

61. Hacke W, Bosel J, Amiri H, *et al.*; DESTINY II Study Group. DESTINY II (DEcompressive Surgery for the Treatment of malignant INfarction of the middle cerebral arter Y II): primary endpoint results. *8th World Stroke Congress.* 2012: Brasilia, Brazil.

62. Anderson CS, Huang Y, Wang JG, *et al.* Intensive blood pressure reduction in acute cerebral haemorrhage trial (INTERACT): a randomised pilot trial. *Lancet Neurol* 2008; **7**(5):391–9.

63. Qureshi A I, Palesch YY. Antihypertensive Treatment of Acute Cerebral Hemorrhage (ATACH) II: design, methods, and rationale. *Neurocrit Care* 2011; **15**:559–76.

64. Albers GW, Amarenco P, Easton JD, Sacco RL, Teal P. Antithrombotic and antithrombolytic therapy for ischaemic stroke: the Seventh ACCP Conference on Antithrombotic and Thrombolytic Therapy. *Chest* 2004; **126**:483S–512S.

65. Mendelow AD, Gregson BA, Fernandes HM, *et al.* Early surgery versus initial conservative treatment in patients with spontaneous supratentorial intracerebral haematomas in the International Surgical Trial in Intracerebral Haemorrhage (STICH): a randomised trial. *Lancet* 2005; **365**(9457):387–97.

66. Mayer SA, Brun NC, Begtrup K, *et al.* Efficacy and safety of recombinant activated factor VII for acute intracerebral hemorrhage. *N Engl J Med* 2008; **358**(20):2127–37.

19

Interventional intravascular therapies for stroke

Pasquale Mordasini, Jan Gralla, and Gerhard Schroth

Introduction

Acute ischemic stroke is a major cause of death and disability in industrialized countries. The management, diagnosis, and treatment approaches for acute ischemic stroke have changed enormously in the past decades. Initially, stoke management consisted solely of prevention, treatment of medical complications and symptoms, and rehabilitation, whereas nowadays various different thrombolytic drugs and endovascular treatment approaches are available. The most significant modifiable factors influencing the clinical outcome are time span between symptom onset and revascularization, recanalization and reperfusion rate, and the occurrence of secondary complications such as symptomatic intracranial hemorrhage [1]. Of those, recanalization has been shown to be the most crucial modifiable prognostic factor for favorable patient outcome. Successful recanalization overall increases the chance of favorable outcome 4-fold compared to patients without recanalization and reduces mortality rate 4-fold [1]. The importance of recanalization is even more pronounced in basilar artery occlusion, where the chance of an independent life is only 2% in patients without recanalization [2]. Therefore, the current treatment options for acute stroke aim at fast and effective flow restoration to the cerebral tissue. This chapter summarizes current aspects of cerebral digital subtraction angiography (DSA) in the context of endovascular stroke treatment, the working principle, and results of the major trials of existing endovascular catheter-based treatment approaches, including intra-arterial thrombolysis using thrombolytic agents and various mechanical recanalization techniques.

Cerebral digital subtraction angiography

Cerebral catheter angiography is still considered the gold standard for imaging of the cerebral vasculature. Indications include diagnostic imaging of primary neurovascular diseases, such as intracranial aneurysms, arteriovenous malformations (AVMs), dural arteriovenous fistulas (dAVFs), atherosclerotic stenosis, vasculopathy (e.g. vasculitis, vasospasm), and acute ischemic stroke, as well as imaging follow-up after treatment (e.g. after aneurysm coiling/clipping, treatment of AVMs or dAVFs). Diagnostic angiography is performed as the first step prior to endovascular procedures. Vascular access is usually gained by femoral puncture, alternatively by radial, brachial, axillary, or rarely by direct carotid or aortic puncture. Endovascular catheters of various sizes and shapes depending on the vascular anatomy and target vessel are navigated under fluoroscopic control within the arterial system using steerable wires. Imaging acquisition is based on the use of X-ray technology and intra-arterial application of iodinated contrast material. The established technical principle for image acquisition is DSA. Using DSA a plain X-ray image is acquired as a so-called "mask image," which is then after contrast injection subtracted from the subsequently acquired contrasted X-ray images. The resulting run of subtracted images consequently depicts only the vasculature without the surrounding bony or soft-tissue anatomy. The advantage of DSA is the combination of high spatial resolution of up to $100–150\,\mu m$ and the high temporal resolution of up to 7.5 frames per second, which has not been reached yet by other non-invasive imaging modalities.

Disadvantages are mainly due to the invasiveness of the procedure. Neurological complications due to thromboembolism from catheters and wires, disruption of atherosclerotic plaques, and dissections overall occur in around 1.3%, where approximately 0.9% account for transient or reversible and 0.5% for permanent neurological deficits [3]. Less common neurological complications include transient cortical blindness and amnesia. Non-neurological complications of cerebral angiography include hematoma and pseudoaneurysm formation at the puncture site, including retroperitoneal hematoma, allergic reactions and nephropathy due to the application of iodinated contrast media, and pulmonary thromboembolism or thromboembolism to the lower extremity. The rate of complications is strongly related to the underlying disease process and patient condition, such as atherosclerotic disease, recent cerebral ischemic event, advanced age, procedure time, hypertension, diabetes, and renal insufficiency [4–6]. DSA in the context of endovascular acute stroke treatment is able to differentiate between occlusion and pseudo-occlusion of a brain-supplying vessel (e.g. internal carotid artery [ICA]) and to visualize exactly and in detail the occlusion site and access vessels for planning of the interventional procedure. Furthermore, the characterization and dynamic evaluation of leptomeningeal collateral circulation has been shown to be a crucial imaging information in regard to clinical outcome [7]. Therefore, in our opinion, a complete diagnostic cerebral angiography including the right and left common carotid artery and the dominant vertebral artery territories is essential prior to endovascular treatment approaches and should be performed in less than 10 minutes.

Technical developments of modern angiography systems, especially so-called flat panel detector (FPD) technology, have further improved diagnostic accuracy. FPD-mounted C-arm angiography systems have been widely introduced into neurointerventional suites. These detector systems permit the acquisition of high-quality 3-dimensional vascular imaging, so called 3D rotational angiography. Postprocessing of such a data set allows detailed 3-dimensional reconstruction of the intracranial vessel anatomy, which is especially helpful for the analysis, treatment planning, peri-interventional treatment monitoring, and follow-up imaging of complex intracranial vascular anatomy, such as in endovascular aneurysm treatment. Furthermore, FPD imaging allows CT-like cross-sectional

soft-tissue imaging of the brain parenchyma to be obtained. Applications include assessment of the extent of subarachnoid or intracerebral hemorrhage and the width of the ventricles as well as immediate control of coil and intra- and extracranial stent placement [8, 9]. FPD technology permits fast imaging without the need for time-consuming patient transfer to a CT facility and, therefore, has become a helpful tool for immediate "on the table" evaluation of treatment results and intra-procedural complications. Recently, the possibility of performing whole-brain parenchymal cerebral blood volume (CBV) measurements by means of intravenous contrast media injection has been added to the spectrum of FPD imaging [10, 11]. Current promising developments aim at further extending this technology to dynamic perfusion measurements such as cerebral blood flow (CBF) and further improving the quality of CT-like imaging of the brain parenchyma [12].

> Digital subtraction angiography (DSA), based on cerebral catheter angiography, is able to differentiate between occlusion and pseudo-occlusion of a brain-supplying vessel and to visualize exactly and in detail the occlusion site and access vessels for planning of the interventional procedure.

Intra-arterial pharmacological thrombolysis

Intravenous administration of thrombolytic drugs has been evaluated in several randomized stroke trials using recombinant tissue plasminogen activator (rtPA) demonstrating efficiency up to 3–4.5 hours after symptom onset [13, 14]. However, studies have shown a limited effect in patients with severe stroke and proximal vessel occlusion, such as the M1 segment or the ICA, with a high thrombus burden compared to more peripherally located occlusions [15–17]. In addition, due to the limited time window only a minority of patients admitted to stroke centers are eligible for intravenous stroke treatment. The advantage of intra-arterial application of thrombolytic drugs at the occlusion site is the delivery of a higher effective concentration of the thrombolytic agent directly to the thrombus. This increases the chance of clot dissolution, especially in occlusions with larger thrombus burden, resulting in higher recanalization rates. Furthermore, reduction of systemic exposure to the thrombolytic drug potentially reduces systemic side-effects and the risk of intracranial hemorrhage, expanding the time window for treatment. Technically, in intra-arterial thrombolysis a microcatheter is navigated over a microwire at the occlusion site and placed proximally to or directly into the thrombus. The landmark study for intra-arterial pharmacological thrombolysis is the Prolyse in Acute Cerebral Thrombembolism II (PROACT II) [18]. One hundred and eighty patients with angiographically confirmed M1 and M2 occlusions were randomized within 6 hours after symptom onset to be treated with 9 mg intra-arterial prourokinase and heparin or heparin only (control group). According to the study protocol prourokinase had to be administered into the proximal surface of the thrombus. Any mechanical manipulation of the thrombus, e.g. probing with the microwire, was prohibited. Favorable clinical outcome (modified Rankin Scale [mRS] ≤2) was achieved in 40% of the endovascularly treated patients and in 25% of the control group with a mortality rate of 25% and 27%, respectively. Recanalization rate defined as TIMI 2–3 was significantly higher in the prourokinase group (66%) than in the control group (18%). Intracranial hemorrhage with neurological deterioration within 24 hours was lower in the control group (2%) compared to the patients treated with prourokinase (10%). The PROACT study was able to demonstrate that despite the higher incidence of symptomatic intracranial hemorrhage intra-arterial application of prourokinase within 6 hours after symptom onset improves significantly clinical outcome without increasing mortality after 90 days in patients with M1 and M2 occlusions. However, despite the positive results of PROACT II, prourokinase has not been approved by the US Food and Drug Administration (FDA).

> **Intra-arterial application of thrombolytic drugs** at the occlusion site has the advantage of delivering a higher effective concentration of the thrombolytic agent directly to the thrombus while reducing the systemic exposure.

Mechanical treatment approaches

Although pharmacological intravenous and intra-arterial thrombolysis have been shown to be effective in some patients, the limited recanalization rate and time window for treatment with an increasing risk for intracranial hemorrhage over time leaves room for further improvement. Mechanical recanalization approaches aim at fast blood flow restoration by rapid direct thrombus removal, especially in the case of large thrombotic burden. Therefore, various endovascular mechanical treatment approaches have been advocated to overcome the limitations of pharmacological thrombolysis, i.e. to increase recanalization rate and accelerate time-to-recanalization. Furthermore, reduction or even waiving of thrombolytic drugs may reduce the risk of intracranial hemorrhage and may further enhance the time window of opportunity for recanalization and re-establishing of CBF. Endovascular mechanical treatment approaches can be divided into four major groups according to their mechanical mechanism of action:

1. Thrombus disruption
2. Thrombectomy
3. Stent recanalization
4. Retrievable stents (stent retriever).

Thrombus disruption

Different techniques for thrombus disruption and fragmentation have been reported. The most widely used is probing the thrombus with the microwire and/or advancing the microcatheter into or distally to the thrombus [19, 20]. This simple mechanical maneuver has been shown to be able to improve the rate of successful recanalization. Using this technique as an adjunct to intra-arterial thrombolysis successful recanalization of M1 occlusions has been reported in 79% [21] compared to 66% in the PROACT II trial [18], where mechanical clot disruption was not allowed. Another method of mechanical clot disruption is the use of percutaneous transluminal balloon angioplasty (PTA). The largest study compared 34 patients with M1 occlusions undergoing PTA as the first-line treatment to 36 patients treated with intra-arterial thrombolysis alone [22]. Sufficient recanalization was achieved in 91.2% in the PTA group as compared to 63.9% in the thrombolysis group with a favorable clinical outcome (mRS at 90 days of ≤2) in 73.5% versus 50%, respectively. However, 64.5% of patients required additional intra-arterial thrombolysis after PTA due to distal emboli occurring during the procedure. Therefore, due to the risk of procedural complications and distal vessel occlusion due to emboli associated with PTA, this technique has not become accepted as a first-line treatment. More elaborated thrombus disruption devices apply ultrasound or laser technology. The EKOS system (EKOS, Bothell, USA) consists of a 2.5F microcatheter

(MicroLysUS infusion catheter) with a 2.1-MHz piezoelectric sonography probe at its distal tip. Ultrasonic vibration applied at the thrombus is supposed to increase fluid penetration within the clot in order to ease and augment the effect of intra-arterial thrombolysis. Successful recanalization was reported in the initial clinical study with 14 patients in 57% with a favorable clinical outcome in 43% [23]. However, a 14% rate of intracranial hemorrhage was observed. The EKOS system has subsequently been investigated in the Interventional Management of Stroke (IMS) II [24] and IMS III trials [25] with successful recanalization rates of 73% and 71%, respectively. The EPAR system (EPAR, Endovasix, Belmont, USA) applies laser technology to emulsify the thrombus by application of microcavitation bubbles at the microcatheter tip. The initial clinical study [26] enrolled 34 patients but the device could only be used as intended in 18 patients (53%), with a successful recanalization rate of 61.1% in this subset. One severe adverse event due to a vessel rupture, a 5.9% rate of intracranial hemorrhage, and a mortality rate of 38.2% were reported.

> Disruption and fragmentation of the thrombus leads to a higher successful recanalization rate, but also a higher rate of intracranial hemorrhage.

Thrombectomy

All thrombectomy devices are delivered by endovascular access proximal to the occlusion site. Thrombectomy techniques can be divided according to where they apply force on the thrombus into two major approaches (Figure 19.1):

1. Proximal thrombectomy:

   Proximal devices apply force on the proximal aspect of the thrombus and include aspiration techniques using different aspiration catheters.

2. Distal thrombectomy:

   Distal devices are advanced proximally to the thrombus, but then are advanced by guide wire and microcatheter to pass the thrombus at the occlusion site and are unsheathed distally to it. These devices apply force at the distal aspect of the thrombus and include snare-like, basket-like, corkscrew-like, and brush-like devices.

Both approaches have been evaluated in several in-vivo animal studies. It has been demonstrated that proximal devices are faster to apply, with a low complication rate. Application of force on the proximal base of the thrombus results in thrombus elongation. On the other hand, distal devices were more successful in removing the thrombus. Application of force on the distal base of the thrombus results in thrombus

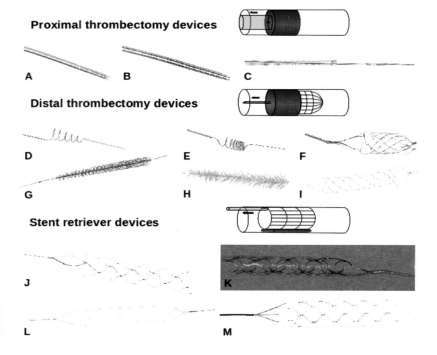

Figure 19.1. Mechanical thrombectomy devices. Overview of different mechanical thrombectomy devices and approaches. A: Vasco +35 Aspi (BALT, Montmorency, France). B: Distal Access Catheter (DAC; Concentric Medical, Mountain View, USA). C: Penumbra System (Penumbra Inc., Almeda, USA). D: Merci retriever X6 (Concentric Medical, Mountain View, USA). E: Merci retriever V (Concentric Medical, Mountain View, USA). F: Catch (BALT, Montmorency, France). G: pCR clot retriever (Phenox GmBH, Bochum, Germany). H: CRC clot retriever CAGE (Phenox GmBH, Bochum, Germany). I: BONnet (Phenox GmBH, Bochum, Germany). J: Solitaire FR (Ev3/Covidien, Irvine, USA). K: pREset (Phenox GmBH, Bochum, Germany). L: Capture LP short (Mindframe Inc., Irvine, USA). M: ReVive SE (Codman & Shurtleff Inc., Raynham, USA).

compression, which increases friction during retrieval and increases the risk of distal thromboembolic events [27–29]. Therefore, the use of proximal balloon occlusion and aspiration during retrieval of a distal device is recommended. Thrombectomy approaches have been advocated alone or in combination with adjuvant intravenous or intra-arterial thrombolysis.

Proximal thrombectomy

Manual suction thrombectomy is performed by advancing an aspiration catheter (usually 4.5–5.5F) to the proximal surface of the thrombus. Manual aspiration is then applied using a syringe. The aspiration catheter is then retrieved under constant negative pressure. Aspiration catheters have to be flexible enough to pass the tortuosity of the cranial vessels, such as the carotid siphon, and braided enough not to collapse during aspiration. Although this approach is widely used usually in the setting of a multimodal treatment approach in proximal vessel occlusion, such as the distal cervical ICA, the carotid terminus, or the basilar artery, only a few systematic studies have been published on this approach [21, 30–33]. Two recent studies reported recanalization rates of 81.9% and 71% and good clinical outcome in 45.5% and 54% of patients, respectively [34, 35] with larger catheters associated with a higher recanalization rate. These results suggest that manual aspiration used as part of a multimodality recanalization strategy is associated with favorable recanalization rates, clinical outcomes, and equivalent safety profiles compared with other mechanical revascularization methods. The drawback of this technique is the possible fragmentation of thrombotic material due to elongation of the thrombus during aspiration. Thrombotic fragments obstruct the aspiration catheter and prohibit further aspiration with the necessity for retrieval and repositioning of the system. A further development of the manual aspiration approach is targeted fragmentation and simultaneous continuous aspiration of thrombotic material.

The Penumbra System (Penumbra, Almeda, USA) is a modification of the manual proximal aspiration technique and consists of a dedicated reperfusion catheter connected to a pumping system applying continuous aspiration. A microwire with an olive-shaped tip, the separator, is used to clean the tip of the reperfusion catheter of clot fragments in order to avoid obstruction. The system was FDA approved for acute stroke treatment in 2007 and has been investigated in several trials. The Penumbra Pivotal Stroke Trial [36] prospectively recruited 125 stroke patients (mean National Institute of Health Stroke Scale [NIHSS] 18) within 8 hours of symptom onset. Recanalization of the target vessel was successful in 81.6% of patients. Nevertheless, good clinical outcome was achieved in only 25% of all patients and in 29% of patients with recanalization of the target vessel. Mortality was comparatively high (32.8%) and symptomatic intracranial hemorrhage occurred in 11.2%. The poor clinical outcome despite the relatively high recanalization rate in this trial prompted discussion of the impact of recanalization using mechanical thrombectomy. Subsequent single-center studies showed better clinical results using the Penumbra System. Kulcsar et al. reported successful recanalization in 93% of 27 patients with large-vessel occlusion (mean NIHSS 14) and good clinical outcome in 48% with a mortality rate of 11%[37]. Mean procedure time was 1.6 hours.

Distal thrombectomy

Compared to proximal thrombectomy approaches, distal thrombectomy is technically more challenging because the occlusion site has to be passed with a microcatheter in order to deliver the device distally to the thrombus. Proximal balloon occlusion using a balloon guide catheter placed in the cervical ICA and aspiration during device retrieval is recommended for most devices to avoid thromboembolic complications. Several distal thrombectomy devices have been introduced into clinical practice (e.g. Catch, BALT, Montmorency, France; Phenox pCR/CRC/Bonnet, Phenox GmbH, Bochum, Germany). Large clinical studies have been performed and published using the Merci device (Concentric Medical, Mountain View, USA), which was the first distal thrombectomy device that received FDA approval, in 2004.

The Merci retrieval system has been investigated in the MERCI trial (Mechanical Embolus Removal in Cerebral Ischemia) [38]. The trial included 151 patients with large-vessel occlusion of the anterior (90%) and posterior (10%) circulation ineligible for intra-arterial thrombolysis within 8 hours of symptom onset (mean NIHSS 20). Successful recanalization was achieved in 46% with good clinical outcome in 27.7% of patients. Mean procedure time was 2.1 hours and clinically significant procedural complications occurred in 7.1% with a rate of symptomatic intracranial hemorrhage of 7.8%. The subsequent Multi-MERCI trial [39] was an international single-arm trial including 164 patients (mean NIHSS 19), again within 8 hours of symptom onset. In contrast to the MERCI trial, intravenous rtPA, intra-arterial thrombolysis, or other mechanical treatment approaches were allowed in addition to the Merci device, and new modified versions of the Merci device were included. Successful recanalization was achieved in 57.3% using the Merci retriever alone and in 69.5% using additional recanalization modalities. Overall, favorable clinical outcome was achieved in 36%. Mean procedure time was 1.6 hours, with clinically significant procedural complications in 5.5% and symptomatic intracranial hemorrhage in 9.8%. The MERCI and Multi-MERCI trials promoted the introduction of the Merci device into wider clinical practice by providing clinical data from an early phase of the device introduction. Furthermore, both trials demonstrated a significant improvement in favorable clinical outcome in patients with recanalization compared to those without successful recanalization.

Proximal thrombectomy is faster to apply, distal thrombectomy more successful in removing the thrombus. Both techniques lead to a possible fragmentation of the thrombus.

Stent recanalization

The limitations of pharmacological thrombolysis and mechanical thrombectomy have led to a further pursuit of devices that can further improve recanalization rate. Placement of a permanent intracranial stent achieves immediate flow restoration and recanalization by compressing the thrombus against the vessel wall (Figure 19.2). Stenting allows fast and effective recanalization without the need of repetitive passing of the occlusion site and retrieval attempts compared to thrombectomy devices. However, this straightforward concept has some disadvantages in general and especially in the setting of acute stroke treatment. Thrombus compression may lead to permanent side branch or perforator occlusion. Moreover, permanent stent placement needs double platelet antiaggregation medication in order to prevent in-stent thrombosis

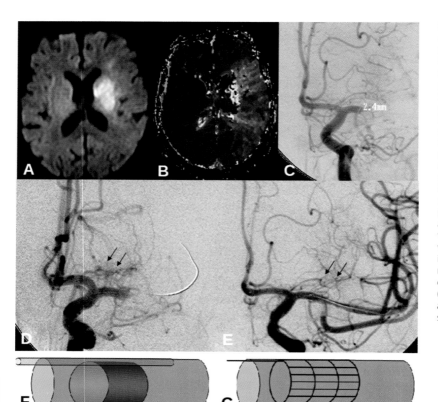

Figure 19.2. Stent recanalization. An 81-year-old patient presenting with aphasia and right hemiplegia (NIHSS 18). MR examination showing diffusion restriction in the left basal ganglia (A) and perfusion deficit (prolonged mean transit time; MTT) in the left middle cerebral artery territory (B). DSA demonstrating a left M1 occlusion (C). Passing of the occlusion site with the microwire and microcatheter in the cranial aspect of the occluding thrombus (D). Control angiogram after deployment of a permanent stent (Wingspan 3 × 15 mm) showing immediate and complete recanalization of the M1 segment. Note preservation of the lateral lenticulostriate arteries due to compression of the thrombus against the contralateral vessel wall (arrows in D and E). Schematic illustration of the principle of stent recanalization depicting passing of the occlusion site with the microcatheter (F) and compression of the thrombus against the contralateral vessel wall after stent deployment (G).

and re-occlusion. This preventive medication may increase the risk of symptomatic intracranial hemorrhage in the setting of acute stroke [40]. Furthermore, an in-stent restenosis rate of bare metal stents has been reported in up to 32% of patients in the treatment of intracranial arteriosclerotic stenosis after a follow-up period of 9 months [41].

The use of different stent systems has been reported in case reports and small case series. In general, self-expandable stents are preferentially used over balloon-mounted stents. Recanalization rates are reported to be between 79% and 92% with moderate clinical outcome in 33–50% [42, 43]. The Stent-Assisted Recanalization in Acute Ischemic Stroke (SARIS) trial is the first FDA-approved prospective trial investigating stenting in acute stroke treatment. Twenty patients (mean NIHSS 14) were included within 6 hours after symptom onset. Recanalization rate was 100% with adjuvant therapies such as angioplasty, intravenous rtPA, and intra-arterial thrombolysis applied in 63% of patients. Moderate clinical outcome was achieved in 60% of patients [44, 45]. Despite the high recanalization rate reported in these studies, the use of intracranial stenting in acute stroke treatment is debatable due to the risks associated with permanent stent deployment and the recent success of thrombectomy. However, stenting has a clear value in selective cases of rescue therapy, where other recanalization methods have failed. Furthermore, permanent stent deployment has its role in the acute phase of stroke treatment in the case of an underlying intracranial stenosis in order to achieve recanalization and to reduce the risk of re-occlusion due to insufficient flow across a stenosis.

> Stenting allows fast and effective recanalization, but has the disadvantage of the need of double platelet anti-aggregation medication in order to prevent in-stent thrombosis and re-occlusion. This may increase the risk of symptomatic intracranial hemorrhage in the setting of acute stroke. Furthermore, there is a risk of in-stent thrombosis or delayed stenosis.

Stent retriever

The most recently introduced mechanical treatment approaches are so-called "stent retrievers" or "stentrievers." Stent retrievers are self-expandable, re-sheathable, and re-constrainable stent-like devices. Wakhloo *et al.* demonstrated the technical feasibility of using a retrievable, closed cell, self-expanding stent

(Enterprise, Codman) for extraction of foreign bodies and clot in in-vitro and in animal testing by partially deploying and then retracting the device [46]. Kelly *et al.* first described the use of a partially unconstrained stent (Enterprise, Codman) to provide a temporary endovascular bypass to achieve recanalization of a M1 occlusion refractory to previous thrombolytic and mechanical treatment [47]. The original intention of the temporary bypass was to deploy the stent across the thrombus to facilitate intra-arterial thrombolysis with consecutive recovery of the stent into the microcatheter after clot dissolution without primary intention for thrombectomy. Henkes and coworkers [48] reported their first use of a fully deployable, self-expanding stent (Solitaire AB, ev3/Covidien) as a thrombectomy device for emergency treatment of a M1 occlusion after previously failed mechanical thrombectomy with a distal clot retriever. Mechanical thrombectomy using stent retrievers is an emerging treatment approach for acute ischemic stroke. The concept of stent retrievers combines the advantages of intracranial stent deployment with immediate flow restoration and a thrombectomy device with definitive clot removal from the occluded artery. The complete removal of the device avoids the major disadvantages associated with permanent stent implantation, such as the need for double antiplatelet medication, which potentially increases the risk of hemorrhagic complications [42, 49], and the risk of in-stent thrombosis or delayed stenosis [50].

The application of stent retrievers is comparable to that of intracranial stents. Initially, the occlusion site is passed with a microcatheter (0.0165–0.027 in) and the stent retriever is deployed by retrieving the microcatheter and un-sheathing the device covering the entire thrombus. The radial force of the stent retriever is able to immediately generate a channel by compressing the thrombus and to partially restore blood flow to the distal territory in most cases, creating a channel for a temporary bypass (Figures 19.3 and 19.4). Adjuvant intra-arterial thrombolysis can be applied and the temporary bypass effect can be used to facilitate clot dissolution by increasing the thrombus surface in contact with thrombolytic drugs. However, the device is typically left in place for an embedding time of 5–10 minutes allowing engagement of the thrombus within the stent struts [51–53]. During retrieval of the stent retriever into the guide catheter, proximal balloon occlusion and flow reversal by additional aspiration at the guide catheter

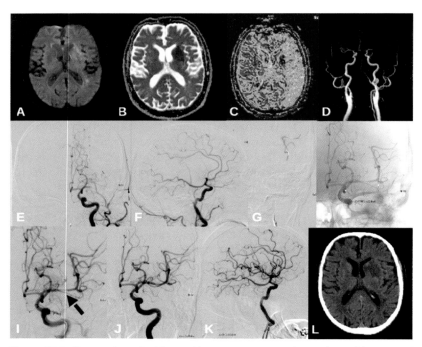

Figure 19.3. Stent retriever. An 85-year-old patient presenting 3 hours after sudden onset of aphasia and right hemiparesis (NIHSS 6). Emergency MRI revealing diffusion restriction in the basal ganglia, the head of the caudate nucleus, and the anterior limb of the internal capsule on the left with corresponding apparent diffusion coefficient (ADC) hypointensity (A, B). Perfusion imaging demonstrating impaired perfusion with prolonged MTT in the entire left middle cerebral artery territory (C). Contrast-enhanced MRA showing an occlusion of the left M1 segment (D). DSA confirming the left M1 occlusion in antero-posterior and lateral view. Distal angiogram after passing of the occlusion site with the microcatheter to confirm proper microcatheter localization distal to the occlusion (G). Mechanical thrombectomy was performed using a retrievable stent (Solitaire FR Revascularization Device 4 × 20 mm). The Solitaire FR was placed through the microcatheter and deployed by retracting the microcatheter through the occlusion site under fluoroscopic control (H). Once fully deployed a control angiogram was obtained to assess immediate recanalization effect, which showed immediate partial recanalization of the middle cerebral artery (arrow in I). Control angiogram after device retrieval demonstrated complete recanalization of the M1 segment corresponding to a TICI 3 grade (J and K). Control CT after 24 hours showed infarction restricted to the basal ganglia corresponding to the pre-existing DWI lesion on the pre-interventional MRI without further ischemic demarcation in the middle cerebral artery territory (L).

is again recommended. In-vivo experimental studies have illustrated incorporation of the thrombus within the stent struts. During mobilization and retrieval of the device, the thrombus–device complex remains in a straight position without obvious compression or elongation of the clot material [51, 53]. This might result in an increased retrieval force required to mobilize the thrombus and lower retrieval success rate [27, 28, 53]. Therefore, straight thrombus position during retrieval and firm clot engagement appear to be key features of stent retrievers compared to the mechanical principle of action of other thrombectomy devices and may explain their high success rates [51, 53]. However, since the optimal design of stent retrievers allowing maximal clot engagement remains unclear, variations of retriever designs have been developed. The different designs vary in terms of radial force ("lower" vs. "higher," zones with variable

radial force), stent design (open-end vs. closed-end, delivery profile), stent cell design (open-cell vs. closed-cell vs. hybrid), and material (Figure 19.1). Distinctive properties of currently available stent retrievers are summarized in Table 19.1.

The concept of stent retrievers combines the advantages of intracranial stent deployment with immediate flow restoration and a thrombectomy device with definitive clot removal from the occluded artery. The complete removal of the device avoids the major disadvantages associated with permanent stent implantation.

The first dedicated combined flow restoration and thrombectomy device for acute stroke treatment was the Solitaire FR (ev3/Covidien, Irvine, USA), receiving the CE mark in 2009 and FDA approval in 2012. The device is based on the Solitaire AB Neuro-vascular Remodeling Device, originally developed for stent-assisted treatment of wide-neck intracranial

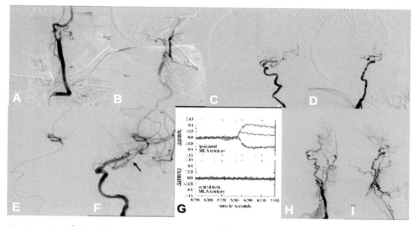

Figure 19.4. Stent retriever recanalization and NIRS measurements. A 66-year-old patient presenting with aphasia and right hemiparesis (NIHSS 8). DSA demonstrating left ICA pseudo-occlusion due to a high-grade ICA stenosis (A and B). Control DSA after PTA of the stenosis using proximal balloon protection showing reconstitution of flow in the ICA and concomitant left M1 occlusion (C and D). Passing of the occlusion site with the microcatheter and distal injection to confirm proper microcatheter localization (E). Deployment of a stent retriever (Solitaire FR 4 × 20 mm) using triple access technique with additional aspiration demonstrating immediate partial recanalization effect (arrow in F). Simultaneous near-infra-red spectroscopy measurements (NIRS; courtesy of Ch. Rummel, PhD, Bern) revealing immediate increase in oxyhemoglobin (red curve) and total hemoglobin (green curve) as well as decrease in deoxyhemoglobin (blue curve) in the ipsilateral MCA territory (upper row in G) corresponding to reconstitution of perfusion after recanalization. No change in oxygenation measurements are seen in the contralateral MCA territory (lower row in G). Final angiogram showing complete recanalization of the M1 segment and the ICA corresponding to a TICI 3 grade (H and I).

aneurysms. Within a short period of time, numerous studies have reported the in-vivo and clinical application of the Solitaire FR for stroke treatment [51, 52, 54, 55]. The first clinical case series published by Castano *et al.* [54] included 20 patients with M1 and carotid terminus occlusions and showed the ability for fast and efficient clot retrieval using the Solitaire AB with successful recanalization (TICI 3 or 2b) in 90% of patients and good clinical outcome (mRS ≤2) in 45% of patients. Subsequent single-center studies have demonstrated the potential to reduce the procedure time (42–55 minutes) and to increase recanalization rates to over 80–90% in large cerebral arteries, with favorable clinical outcome in a large percentage of patients (42–54%) [52, 54, 55], indicating the potential of this technique to be established as a major approach to endovascular stroke treatment. The largest retrospective study reported results from six large European stroke centers [56] treating 141 patients (median NIHSS 18) for large-vessel occlusion with the Solitaire FR as the first-choice mechanical thrombectomy device. In 52%, intravenous rtPA was administered prior to mechanical thrombectomy. Median recanalization time was 40 minutes, and successful recanalization was achieved in 85% of target vessels with favorable clinical outcome in 55%.

Symptomatic intracranial hemorrhage occurred in 6% with an overall mortality of 20.5%. Subgroup analysis demonstrated a significantly lower rate of collateral infarcts using proximal balloon occlusion (6%) than with procedures without proximal balloon occlusion (32%).

The SWIFT study (Solitaire FR with the Intention for Thrombectomy) [57] was a prospective, randomized, multicenter trial comparing the efficacy and safety of the Solitaire FR with the Merci device. The trial recruited 113 patients with ischemic stroke randomly assigned to undergo endovascular treatment with the Solitaire FR or the Merci device within 8 hours of symptom onset. The trial was halted a year sooner than anticipated on the advice of the safety monitoring committee due to a significantly better clinical outcome in the Solitaire FR patient group. Successful recanalization was achieved in 83.3% with the Solitaire FR compared with 48.1% with the Merci retriever, with good clinical outcome of 58.2% versus 33.3% respectively. Overall, 40% of patients had already been treated with intravenous rtPA, but failed to improve. Symptomatic intracranial hemorrhage occurred in 2% of the Solitaire FR group and in 11% of the Merci device group with mortality rates of 17% and 38% respectively.

Table 19.1. Overview of currently available stent retrievers

Device/company	Properties	Delivery system min ID (inch)	Sizes (mm)	Vessel diameter range (mm)
Solitaire FR *ev3/Covidien*	Honeycomb-like closed-cell design, longitudinal open-slit design	0.021 0.027	4 × 15/20 6 × 20/30	2–4 3–5.5
Trevo Pro 4 *Concentric Medical/ Stryker Neurovascular*	Active area with lower radial force, vertical strut orientation to enhance clot integration, wide cell area, guidewire-like tip	0.021	4 × 20	1.5–4
ReVive SE *Codman*	Decreased cell size from proximal to distal retrieval zone to enhance clot engagement, high radial force, closed distal end	0.021	4.5 × 22	1.5–5.5
Aperio/Aperio 1.9F *Acandis*	Hybrid open-closed cell design, reduced low profile design	0.027 0.0165	4.5 × 30/40	2–4
Capture/ Capture LP *Mindframe*	Closed-cell design, constant radial force to minimize cell deformation	0.027 0.0165	3 × 30 5 × 30	2–3 2.5–4.5
pREset *Phenox*	Helically shaped slit design, closed ring design with a proximal cell connector	0.021	4 × 20	2–4
Separator 3D *Penumbra*	Four intraluminal 3D chambers to support aspiration, minimal wall contact	0.025	4.5 × 26	≥3
CATCH+ *BALT*	longitudinal open-slit design	0.021	4 × 20	2–4

ID = inner diameter.

The TREVO 2 study (Thrombectomy REvascularization of large Vessel Occlusions in acute ischemic stroke) [58] was a randomized, multicenter trial comparing the Trevo Pro retriever (Concentric Medical/Stryker Neurovascular, USA) with the Merci device. The 178 patients were randomized (median NIHSS 18) within 8 hours of symptom onset. Successful recanalization was achieved in 89.7% in the Trevo group compared to 63.3% in the Merci group with good clinical outcome in 55% and 40%, respectively. Symptomatic intracranial hemorrhage occurred in 6.8% in the Trevo group and in 8.9% of the Merci group with mortality rates of 33% versus 24%, respectively.

The results of these trials support the assumption that there are distinctive mechanical mechanisms of action and therefore different success and efficacy rates depending on the mechanical approaches applied with superiority of stent retrievers over distal thrombectomy devices. This has to be taken into consideration in planning future studies investigating the efficacy of endovascular treatment strategies.

The recently published IMS III [25], Synthesis [59], and MR Rescue (Mechanical Retrieval and Recanalization of Stroke Clots Using Embolectomy) trials [60] were the first randomized controlled trials comparing endovascular stroke treatment to standard intravenous rtPA administration. All three trials reported negative results for endovascular stroke treatment.

The IMS III trial [25] was a randomized, open-label, clinical trial comparing a combined approach of intravenous thrombolysis followed by endovascular treatment with standard intravenous thrombolysis using rtPA within the 4.5-hour time window. Endovascular approaches approved were the Merci device, the Penumbra device, and the EKOS Micro-Sonic SV infusion system. Only in the final phase of the study a stent retriever device, the Solitaire FR, was cleared. The 656 subjects were randomized (434 endovascular therapy, 222 intravenous therapy). The IMS III trial has been suspended because of equipoise using mechanical approaches compared to intravenous thrombolysis. The prespecified primary outcome of a 10% difference in good clinical outcome (mRS ≤2) in favor of endovascular treatment was not achieved (40.8% endovascular, 38.7% intravenous treatment group). Mortality as well as symptomatic intracranial hemorrhage did not differ significantly (19.1% endovascular group vs. 21.6% intravenous treatment group and 6.2% vs. 5.9%, respectively). However, the study design has several flaws. First, during a relatively long inclusion period (2006–2012), diagnostic imaging modalities and endovascular techniques have significantly evolved. Especially the lack of multimodal diagnostic imaging including vessel imaging for demonstration of a major arterial occlusion and evaluation of the penumbra is a major weakness of the trial. Only 46% of patients underwent CTA, which was not used for inclusion resulting in patients undergoing therapy without major arterial occlusion. Second, the approved endovascular techniques were heterogeneous and some already outdated. Only 1.5% of patients were treated using latest-generation stent retrievers due to the late clearance for the study. As the SWIFT and TREVO 2 trials demonstrated, stent retrievers are superior to distal thrombectomy devices in terms of recanalization results and clinical outcome. In the light of these arguments the results of the IMS III study were already outdated at the time of its publication.

The Synthesis trial [59] was another randomized trial comparing standard intravenous rtPA treatment initiated within 4.5 hours after symptom onset to endovascular treatment within 6 hours after symptom onset. Randomization occurred within 4.5 hours after symptom onset, with 181 patients in each group. Patients undergoing endovascular treatment did not receive intravenous rtPA. Endovascular treatment included intra-arterial thrombolysis and guidewire thrombus fragmentation (66.1%) and endovascular devices (33.9%), including the Merci device and Penumbra device (8.5%) and stent retrievers (13.9%). The primary endpoint defined as a mRS of 0–1 was similar in both groups (30.4% endovascular, 34.8% intravenous treatment group). There was no

significant difference in the rate of intracranial hemorrhage (6% each) and mortality (14.4% endovascular, 9.9% intravenous treatment group). The criticisms of the IMS III trial apply to the Synthesis trial as well, i.e. lack of appropriate diagnostic imaging protocols and use of outdated devices in the majority of endovascular treatment cases. Furthermore, patients with a NIHSS score as low as 2 were included, who are known to have a high chance of good outcome even without treatment. Finally, the Synthesis trial in fact compares standard intravenous thrombolysis with endovascular treatment as sole therapy approach using obsolete devices.

The MR Rescue trial [60] was a randomized, multicenter trial enrolling patients with large anterior circulation vessel occlusion to undergo mechanical thrombectomy (Merci device or Penumbra device) or standard medical care within 8 hours of symptom onset. All patients underwent pretreatment diagnostic multimodal CT or MR imaging allowing stratification according to a favorable penumbral pattern (substantial salvageable tissue and small infarct core) and non-penumbral pattern (large core or small or absent penumbra). A total of 118 patients were enrolled, of whom 64 received endovascular treatment and 54 standard care. Fifty-eight percent of patients showed a favorable penumbral pattern. Successful recanalization was achieved in 67% of patients undergoing endovascular treatment. The patients were classified into four groups: endovascular therapy/penumbral pattern; standard care/penumbral pattern; endovascular therapy/non-penumbral pattern; and standard care/non-penumbral pattern. Clinical outcome measured as mean mRS did not significantly differ between the groups (3.9 vs. 3.9, p = 0.99). Endovascular therapy was not superior to standard care in patients with either favorable penumbral pattern (3.9 vs. 3.4, p = 0.23) or non-penumbral pattern (4.0 vs. 4.4, p = 0.32). The percentage of patients with good outcome and mortality was not significantly different between the groups (endovascular therapy/penumbral pattern: 21%/18%; standard care/penumbral pattern: 26%/21%; endovascular therapy/non-penumbral pattern: 17%/20%; and standard care/non-penumbral pattern: 10%/30%). Therefore, a favorable penumbral pattern was not able to identify patients who would benefit from endovascular therapy and mechanical thrombectomy was not superior to standard medical care. In contrast to the IMS III and Synthesis trials pretreatment diagnostic imaging

321

was more sophisticated, using multimodal imaging to evaluate major vessel occlusion and the penumbra. However, the assignment to a penumbral pattern using a dedicated software was not easy to handle and only 58% of patients could be processed in real time with a shift of pattern assignment in 8% after final core laboratory postprocessing. Furthermore, subgroups were rather small and therefore with limited statistical power. Finally, similar to the IMS III and Synthesis trials the latest generation of thrombectomy devices were not used.

The recently terminated STAR trial (Solitaire FR Thrombectomy for Acute Revascularization) [61] is the largest prospective multicenter trial on mechanical thrombectomy to date. The STAR trial was an international, multicenter, prospective, single-arm study evaluating the Solitaire FR in patients with anterior circulation strokes due to large-vessel occlusion within 8 hours of symptom onset. Strict selection criteria for participating sites were applied and 202 patients were enrolled (median NIHSS 17). All patients underwent pretreatment multimodal CT or MR imaging. ICA occlusions were found in 18% and middle cerebral artery occlusions in 82% of patients. Fifty-nine percent of patients underwent combined intravenous rtPA and mechanical thrombectomy and 41% mechanical thrombectomy only. Successful revascularization was achieved in 79.2% of patients. Device- or procedure-related events occurred in 7.4%. Favorable clinical outcome was achieved in 57.9% with a mortality rate of 6.9%. The rate of symptomatic intracranial hemorrhage was considerably low with 1.5%. Procedural time to final recanalization was the fastest reported so far with a median of 20 minutes indicating a learning curve in experienced centers. This study overall demonstrated improvement of clinical outcome compared to previous studies as well as low mortality and symptomatic intracranial hemorrhage rates. Crucial points of the study include the pretreatment multimodal imaging protocol, participation of only experienced, high-volume comprehensive stroke centers, and independently monitored data acquisition and core lab reviewing of recanalization results. On the other hand, the findings of the STAR trial are limited by the non-randomized, single-arm study design and the inclusion of only anterior circulation strokes. However, the data support further investigation of stent retrievers in randomized trials against best medical treatment alone.

Chapter summary

Successful recanalization with endovascular catheter-based treatment approaches (including intra-arterial thrombolysis using thrombolytic agents and various mechanical recanalization techniques) increases the chance of favorable outcome and reduces mortality.

Cerebral catheter angiography is based on the use of X-ray technology and intra-arterial application of iodinated contrast material. The established technical principle for image acquisition is digital subtraction angiography (**DSA**). DSA is able to differentiate between occlusion and pseudo-occlusion of a brain-supplying vessel and to visualize exactly and in detail the occlusion site and access vessels for planning of the interventional procedure.

Flat panel detector (**FPD**) technology permits the acquisition of high-quality 3-dimensional vascular imaging and furthermore allows CT-like cross-sectional soft-tissue imaging of the brain parenchyma to be obtained.

Intra-arterial application of thrombolytic drugs at the occlusion site has the advantage of delivering a higher effective concentration of the thrombolytic agent directly to the thrombus while reducing the systemic exposure. In the PROACT study, the intra-arterial application of prourokinase within 6 hours after symptom onset improved significantly clinical outcome without increasing mortality after 90 days, but intracranial hemorrhage with neurological deterioration was lower in the control group. Prourokinase has not been approved by the US Food and Drug Administration (FDA) yet.

Mechanical treatment approaches
Thrombus disruption
Disruption and fragmentation of the thrombus by probing the thrombus with a microwire, PTA (percutaneous balloon angioplasty) or devices applying ultrasound or laser technology leads to a higher successful recanalization rate, but also a higher rate of intracranial hemorrhage.

Thrombectomy
All thrombectomy devices are delivered by endovascular access proximal to the occlusion site. Proximal thrombectomy apply force on the proximal aspect of the thrombus and include aspiration techniques using different aspiration catheters. Distal devices are advanced proximally to the thrombus, but then are advanced by guide wire and microcatheter to

pass the thrombus at the occlusion site and are unsheathed distally to it. Proximal thrombectomy is faster to apply, distal thrombectomy more successful in removing the thrombus. Both techniques lead to a possible fragmentation of the thrombus. Devices such as the Penumbra System (for proximal thrombectomy) and the Merci device (for distal thrombectomy) have been approved by the FDA and investigated in clinical studies.

Stent recanalization

Stenting allows fast and effective recanalization without the need of repetitive passing of the occlusion site and retrieval attempts compared to thrombectomy devices, but has the disadvantage of the need of double platelet antiaggregation medication in order to prevent in-stent thrombosis and re-occlusion. This may increase the risk of symptomatic intracranial

hemorrhage in the setting of acute stroke. Furthermore, there is a risk of in-stent thrombosis or delayed stenosis.

Retrievable stents (stent retriever)

Mechanical thrombectomy using stent retrievers is an emerging treatment approach for acute ischemic stroke. The concept of stent retrievers combines the advantages of intracranial stent deployment with immediate flow restoration and a thrombectomy device with definitive clot removal from the occluded artery. The complete removal of the device avoids the major disadvantages associated with permanent stent implantation. Randomized, multicenter clinical trials investigated and compared different retriever devices or intravenous thrombolysis followed by endovascular treatment.

References

1. Rha JH, Saver JL. The impact of recanalization on ischemic stroke outcome: a meta-analysis. *Stroke* 2007; **38**(3):967–73.

2. Lindsberg PJ, Mattle HP. Therapy of basilar artery occlusion: a systematic analysis comparing intra-arterial and intravenous thrombolysis. *Stroke* 2006; **37**(3):922–8.

3. Willinsky RA, Taylor SM, TerBrugge K, *et al.* Neurologic complications of cerebral angiography: prospective analysis of 2,899 procedures and review of the literature. *Radiology* 2003; **227**(2):522–8.

4. Heiserman JE, Dean BL, Hodak JA, *et al.* Neurologic complications of cerebral angiography. *AJNR Am J Neuroradiol* 1994; **15**(8):1401–7; discussion 1408–11.

5. Cloft HJ, Joseph GJ, Dion JE. Risk of cerebral angiography in patients with subarachnoid hemorrhage, cerebral aneurysm, and arteriovenous malformation: a meta-analysis. *Stroke* 1999; **30**(2):317–20.

6. Dion JE, Gates PC, Fox AJ, Barnett HJ, Blom RJ. Clinical events

following neuroangiography: a prospective study. *Stroke* 1987; **18**(6):997–1004.

7. Jung SG, Slotboom J, El-Koussy M, *et al.* Factors that determine penumbral tissue loss in acute ischemic stroke. *Brain* 2013; **136**(pt 12):3554–60.

8. Doelken M, Struffert T, Richter G, *et al.* Flat-panel detector volumetric CT for visualization of subarachnoid hemorrhage and ventricles: preliminary results compared to conventional CT. *Neuroradiology* 2008; **50**(6):517–23.

9. White PM, Gilmour JN, Weir NW, Innes B, Sellar RJ. AngioCT in the management of neurointerventional patients: a prospective, consecutive series with associated dosimetry and resolution data. *Neuroradiology* 2008; **50**(4):321–30.

10. Struffert T, Deuerling-Zheng Y, Kloska S, *et al.* Flat detector CT in the evaluation of brain parenchyma, intracranial vasculature, and cerebral blood volume: a pilot study in patients with acute symptoms of cerebral ischemia. *AJNR Am J Neuroradiology* 2010; **31**(8):1462–9.

11. Mordasini P, El-Koussy M, Brekenfeld C, *et al.* Applicability of tableside flat panel detector CT parenchymal cerebral blood volume measurement in neurovascular interventions: preliminary clinical experience. *AJNR Am J Neuroradiol* 2012; **33**(1):154–8.

12. Royalty K, Manhart M, Pulfer K, *et al.* C-arm CT measurement of cerebral blood volume and cerebral blood flow using a novel high-speed acquisition and a single intravenous contrast injection. *AJNR Am J Neuroradiol* 2013; **34**(11):2131–8.

13. The National Institute of Neurologic Disorders and Stroke rt-PA Stroke Study Group. Tissue plasminogen activator for acute ischemic stroke. *N Engl J Med* 1995; **333**(24):1581–7.

14. Hacke W, Kaste M, Bluhmki E, *et al.* Thrombolysis with alteplase 3 to 4.5 hours after acute ischemic stroke. *N Engl J Med* 2008; **359**(13):1317–29.

15. Ingall TJ, O'Fallon WM, Asplund K, *et al.* Findings from the reanalysis of the NINDS tissue plasminogen activator for acute ischemic stroke treatment trial. *Stroke* 2004; **35**(10):2418–24.

16. Fischer U, Arnold M, Nedeltchev K, *et al.* NIHSS score and arteriographic findings in acute ischemic stroke. *Stroke* 2005; **36**(10):2121–5.

17. Riedel CH, Zimmermann P, Jensen-Kondering U, *et al.* The importance of size: successful recanalization by intravenous thrombolysis in acute anterior stroke depends on thrombus length. *Stroke* 2011; **42**(6):1775–7.

18. Furlan A, Higashida R, Wechsler L, *et al.* Intra-arterial prourokinase for acute ischemic stroke. The PROACT II study: a randomized controlled trial. Prolyse in Acute Cerebral Thromboembolism. *JAMA* 1999; **282**(21):2003–11.

19. Noser EA, Shaltoni HM, Hall CE, *et al.* Aggressive mechanical clot disruption: a safe adjunct to thrombolytic therapy in acute stroke? *Stroke* 2005; **36**(2):292–6.

20. Barnwell SL, Clark WM, Nguyen TT, *et al.* Safety and efficacy of delayed intraarterial urokinase therapy with mechanical clot disruption for thromboembolic stroke. *AJNR Am J Neuroradiol* 1994; **15**(10):1817–22.

21. Arnold M, Schroth G, Nedeltchev K, *et al.* Intra-arterial thrombolysis in 100 patients with acute stroke due to middle cerebral artery occlusion. *Stroke* 2002; **33**(7):1828–33.

22. Nakano S, Iseda T, Yoneyama T, Kawano H, Wakisaka S. Direct percutaneous transluminal angioplasty for acute middle cerebral artery trunk occlusion: an alternative option to intra-arterial thrombolysis. *Stroke* 2002; **33**(12):2872–6.

23. Mahon BR, Nesbit GM, Barnwell SL, *et al.* North American clinical experience with the EKOS MicroLysUS infusion catheter for the treatment of embolic stroke. *AJNR Am J Neuroradiol* 2003; **24**(3):534–8.

24. IMS II Trial Investigators. The Interventional Management of Stroke (IMS) II Study. *Stroke* 2007; **38**(7):2127–35.

25. Broderick JP, Palesch YY, Demchuk AM, *et al.* Endovascular therapy after intravenous t-PA versus t-PA alone for stroke. *N Engl J Med* 2013; **368**(10):893–903.

26. Berlis A, Lutsep H, Barnwell S, *et al.* Mechanical thrombolysis in acute ischemic stroke with endovascular photoacoustic recanalization. *Stroke* 2004; **35**(5):1112–16.

27. Gralla J, Schroth G, Remonda L, *et al.* Mechanical thrombectomy for acute ischemic stroke: thrombus-device interaction, efficiency, and complications in vivo. *Stroke* 2006; **37**(12):3019–24.

28. Brekenfeld C, Schroth G, El-Koussy M, *et al.* Mechanical thromboembolectomy for acute ischemic stroke: comparison of the catch thrombectomy device and the Merci Retriever in vivo. *Stroke* 2008; **39**(4):1213–19.

29. Mordasini P, Hiller M, Brekenfeld C, *et al.* In vivo evaluation of the Phenox CRC mechanical thrombectomy device in a swine model of acute vessel occlusion. *AJNR Am J Neuroradiol* 2010; **31**(5):972–8.

30. Chapot R, Houdart E, Rogopoulos A, *et al.* Thromboaspiration in the basilar artery: report of two cases. *AJNR Am J Neuroradiol* 2002; **23**(2):282–4.

31. Lutsep HL, Clark WM, Nesbit GM, Kuether TA, Barnwell SL. Intraarterial suction thrombectomy in acute stroke. *AJNR Am J Neuroradiol* 2002; **23**(5):783–6.

32. Nedeltchev K, Brekenfeld C, Remonda L, *et al.* Internal carotid artery stent implantation in 25 patients with acute stroke: preliminary results. *Radiology* 2005; **237**(3):1029–37.

33. Galimanis A, Jung S, Mono ML, *et al.* Endovascular therapy of 623 patients with anterior circulation stroke. *Stroke* 2012; **43**(4):1052–7.

34. Kang DH, Hwang YH, Kim YS, *et al.* Direct thrombus retrieval using the reperfusion catheter of the penumbra system: forced-suction thrombectomy in acute ischemic stroke. *AJNR Am J Neuroradiol* 2011; **32**(2):283–7.

35. Jankowitz B, Aghaebrahim A, Zirra A, *et al.* Manual aspiration thrombectomy: adjunctive endovascular recanalization technique in acute stroke interventions. *Stroke* 2012; **43**(5):1408–11.

36. Penumbra Pivotal Stroke Trial Investigators. The penumbra pivotal stroke trial: safety and effectiveness of a new generation of mechanical devices for clot removal in intracranial large vessel occlusive disease. *Stroke* 2009; **40**(8):2761–8.

37. Kulcsar Z, Bonvin C, Pereira VM, *et al.* Penumbra system: a novel mechanical thrombectomy device for large-vessel occlusions in acute stroke. *AJNR Am J Neuroradiol* 2010; **31**(4):628–33.

38. Smith WS, Sung G, Starkman S, *et al.* Safety and efficacy of mechanical embolectomy in acute ischemic stroke: results of the MERCI trial. *Stroke* 2005; **36**(7):1432–8.

39. Smith WS, Sung G, Saver J, *et al.* Mechanical thrombectomy for acute ischemic stroke: final results of the Multi MERCI trial. *Stroke* 2008; **39**(4):1205–12.

40. Diener HC, Bogousslavsky J, Brass LM, *et al.* Aspirin and clopidogrel compared with clopidogrel alone after recent ischemic stroke or transient ischemic attack in high-risk patients (MATCH): randomised, double-blind, placebo-controlled trial. *Lance* 2004; **364**(9431):331–7.

41. SSYLVIA Study Investigators. Stenting of Symptomatic Atherosclerotic Lesions in the Vertebral or Intracranial Arteries (SSYLVIA): study results. *Stroke* 2004; **35**(6):1388–92.

42. Levy EI, Mehta R, Gupta R, *et al.* Self-expanding stents for recanalization of acute cerebrovascular occlusions. *AJNR Am J Neuroradiol* 2007; **28**(5):816–22.

43. Brekenfeld C, Schroth G, Mattle HP, *et al.* Stent placement in acute cerebral artery occlusion: use of a self-expandable intracranial stent for acute stroke treatment. *Stroke* 2009; **40**(3):847–52.

44. Levy EI, Rahman M, Khalessi AA, *et al.* Midterm clinical and angiographic follow-up for the first Food and Drug Administration-approved prospective, Single-Arm Trial of Primary Stenting for Stroke: SARIS (Stent-Assisted Recanalization for Acute Ischemic Stroke). *Neurosurgery* 2011; **69**(4):915–920; discussion 920.

45. Levy EI, Siddiqui AH, Crumlish A, *et al.* First Food and Drug Administration-approved prospective trial of primary intracranial stenting for acute stroke: SARIS (stent-assisted recanalization in acute ischemic stroke). *Stroke* 2009; **40**(11):3552–6.

46. Wakhloo AK, Gounis MJ. Retrievable closed cell intracranial stent for foreign body and clot removal. *Neurosurgery* 2008; **62**(5 Suppl 2):ONS390–3; discussion ONS393–4.

47. Kelly ME, Furlan AJ, Fiorella D. Recanalization of an acute middle cerebral artery occlusion using a self-expanding, reconstrainable, intracranial microstent as a temporary endovascular bypass. *Stroke* 2008; **39**(6):1770–3.

48. Perez MA, Miloslavski E, Fischer S, Bazner H, Henkes H. Intracranial thrombectomy using the Solitaire stent: a historical vignette. *J Neurointerv Surg* 2012; **4**(6):e32.

49. Zaidat OO, Wolfe T, Hussain SI, *et al.* Interventional acute ischemic stroke therapy with intracranial self-expanding stent. *Stroke* 2008; **39**(8):2392–5.

50. Levy EI, Turk AS, Albuquerque FC, *et al.* Wingspan in-stent restenosis and thrombosis: incidence, clinical presentation, and management. *Neurosurgery* 2007; **61**(3):644–50; discussion 650–1.

51. Mordasini P, Frabetti N, Gralla J, *et al.* In vivo evaluation of the first dedicated combined flow-restoration and mechanical thrombectomy device in a swine model of acute vessel occlusion. *AJNR Am J Neuroradiol* 2011; **32**(2):294–300.

52. Brekenfeld C, Schroth G, Mordasini P, *et al.* Impact of retrievable stents on acute ischemic stroke treatment. *AJNR Am J Neuroradiol* 2011; **32**(7):1269–73.

53. Mordasini P, Brekenfeld C, Byrne JV, *et al.* Experimental evaluation of immediate recanalization effect and recanalization efficacy of a new thrombus retriever for acute stroke treatment in vivo. *AJNR Am J Neuroradiol* 2013; **34**(1):153–8.

54. Castano C, Dorado L, Guerrero C, *et al.* Mechanical thrombectomy with the Solitaire AB device in large artery occlusions of the anterior circulation: a pilot study. *Stroke* 2010; **41**(8):1836–40.

55. Costalat V, Machi P, Lobotesis K, *et al.* Rescue, combined, and stand-alone thrombectomy in the management of large vessel occlusion stroke using the solitaire device: a prospective 50-patient single-center study: timing, safety, and efficacy. *Stroke* 2011; **42**(7):1929–35.

56. Davalos A, Pereira VM, Chapot R, *et al.* Retrospective multicenter study of Solitaire FR for revascularization in the treatment of acute ischemic stroke. *Stroke* 2012; **43**(10):2699–705.

57. Saver JL, Jahan R, Levy EI, *et al.* Solitaire flow restoration device versus the Merci Retriever in patients with acute ischemic stroke (SWIFT): a randomised, parallel-group, non-inferiority trial. *Lancet* 2012; **380**(9849):1241–9.

58. Nogueira RG, Lutsep HL, Gupta R, *et al.* Trevo versus Merci retrievers for thrombectomy revascularisation of large vessel occlusions in acute ischemic stroke (TREVO 2): a randomised trial. *Lancet* 2012; **380**(9849):1231–40.

59. Ciccone A, Valvassori L, Nichelatti M, *et al.* Endovascular treatment for acute ischemic stroke. *N Engl J Med* 2013; **368**(10):904–13.

60. Kidwell CS, Jahan R, Gornbein J, *et al.* A trial of imaging selection and endovascular treatment for ischemic stroke. *N Engl J Med* 2013; **368**(10):914–23.

61. Pereira J, Gralla J, Davalos A, *et al.* Prospective Multi-Centre Single-Arm Study of Mechanical Thrombectomy using Solitaire FR in Acute Ischemic Stroke. *Stroke* 2013; **44**:2802–7.

Management of acute ischemic stroke and its late complications

Natan M. Bornstein and Eitan Auriel

General management of elevated blood pressure, blood glucose, and body temperature

Monitoring the blood pressure (BP), glucose levels, and temperature in acute stroke patients is an often neglected matter although it may have an important impact upon the patients' outcome. In the Tel Aviv stroke register, recorded between the years 2001 and 2003, 32% of acute stroke patients in the emergency room had glucose levels higher than 150 mg/dl, systolic BP higher than 140 mmHg was found in 77% of the patients, and 17% of patients had temperatures above 37 °C on admission. These numbers are representative of other centers as well. This chapter will summarize the current knowledge regarding the management of the above.

Hypertensive blood pressure values in acute ischemic stroke

Several observations have demonstrated spontaneous elevation of BP in the first 24–48 hours after stroke onset with a significant spontaneous decline after a few days [1–3]. Several mechanisms may be responsible for the increased BP, including stress, pain, urinary retention, and Cushing effect due to increased intracranial pressure and the activation of the sympathetic, renin–angiotensin, and adrenocorticotropic (ACTH)–cortisol pathways. Despite the increased prevalence of hypertension following stroke, optimal management has not been yet established. Several arguments speak for lowering the elevated BP: risks of hemorrhagic transformation, cerebral edema, recurrence of stroke, and hypertensive encephalopathy. On the other hand, it may be important to maintain the hypertensive state due to the damaged autoregulation in the ischemic brain and the risk of cerebral hypoperfusion exacerbated by the lowered systemic BP.

Blood pressure and outcome

Analysis of 17 398 patients in the International Stroke Trial [4] demonstrated a U-shaped relationship between baseline systolic BP and both early death and late death or dependency. Both high BP and low BP were independent prognostic factors for poor outcome. Early death increased by 17.9% for every 10 mmHg below 150 mmHg ($p < 0.0001$) and by 3.8% for every 10 mmHg above 150 mmHg ($p = 0.016$). A prospective study among 1121 patients admitted within 24 hours from stroke onset and followed up for 12 months demonstrated similar findings of the "U-shape" phenomenon [5]. Elevated pulse pressure (difference between the systolic and diastolic BP) during the acute phase of ischemic stroke was also found to be an independent predictor of poor early outcome at hospital discharge and 30-day mortality [6].

It should be taken into consideration that prolongation of the elevated BP may be caused by more severe stroke as compensation for the persistent vessel occlusion.

On the other hand, the GAIN study [7], done among 1455 patients with ischemic stroke, demonstrated that baseline mean arterial pressure was not associated with poor outcome. However, variables describing the course of BP over the first days have a marked and independent relationship with 1- and 3-month outcomes.

In a Cochrane systematic review of 32 studies involving 10 892 patients after ischemic and hemorrhagic stroke [8], death was found to be significantly associated with elevated mean arterial BP (odds ratio[OR] 1.61; 95% confidence interval[CI] 1.12–2.31) and high diastolic BP (OR 1.71; 95% CI 1.33–2.48).

> A U-shaped relationship between baseline systolic BP and both early and late death or dependency after ischemic stroke has been demonstrated in clinical trials.

Blood pressure and outcome in thrombolysed patients

Several observations, including the National Institute of Neurological Disorders and Stroke (NINDS)-rtPA trial [9, 10], found an association between high BP on admission, and its prolongation, with poor outcome and mortality. Although in one study no such association was found in alert patients, stroke patients with impaired consciousness showed higher mortality rates with increasing BP [11]. The Safe Implementation of Thrombolysis in Stroke (SITS) thrombolysis register prospectively recorded 11 080 stroke patients treated with intravenous thrombolysis. BP values were recorded at baseline, 2 hours, and 24 hours after thrombolysis [12]. High systolic BP was associated with poor outcome. Withholding antihypertensive therapy up to 7 days in patients with a history of hypertension was associated with worse outcome, whereas initiation of antihypertensive therapy in newly recognized moderate hypertension was associated with a favorable outcome.

The association between elevated BP and recanalization was evaluated in 149 patients after intra-arterial thrombolysis using angiography [13]. The study demonstrated that the course of elevated systolic BP, but not diastolic BP, after acute ischemic stroke was inversely associated with the degree of vessel recanalization. When recanalization failed, systolic BP remained elevated longer than when it succeeded.

Controlling blood pressure in the acute stroke phase

The theory that elevated systemic BP may compensate for the decreased cerebral blood flow in the ischemic region led to attempts to elevate BP as a treatment for acute ischemic stroke. The hemodynamic and metabolic impact of pharmacologically increased systemic BP on the ischemic core and penumbra was evaluated in rats. The mild induced hypertension was found to increase collateral flow and oxygenation and to improve cerebral metabolic rate of oxygen in the core and penumbra [14]. Several small studies in humans have addressed this question by investigating the responses to vasopressors, including phenylephrine and norepinephrine, in patients with acute stroke [15–17]. Despite a documented improvement in cerebral blood flow [18], the concept was abandoned because of the increased risk of hemorrhage and brain edema. In a systematic review of 12 relevant publications including 319 subjects, the small size of the trials and the inconclusive results limit conclusion as to the effects on outcomes, both benefits and harms. A randomized controlled trial is needed to determine the role of vasopressors in acute ischemic stroke [19].

> Elevated systemic blood pressure may compensate for the decrease of cerebral blood flow in the ischemic region, but raises the risks of hemorrhagic transformation, cerebral edema, recurrence of stroke, and hypertensive encephalopathy.

According to a systematic review of the literature [3] no conclusive evidence to support the lowering of BP in the acute phase of ischemic stroke was found and more research is needed to identify the effective strategies for BP management in that phase [3]. Despite the controversy over the management of BP in the acute phase, the benefit of BP reduction as a secondary prevention of stroke is well established and has been demonstrated in many studies. However, in most of these studies antihypertensive agents were administered several weeks after stroke onset. Only a few trials were performed in the acute stage. The ACCESS trial [20] was a prospective, double-blind, placebo-controlled, randomized study evaluating the angiotensin-receptor blocker candesartan vs. placebo for 342 hypertensive patients in the first week following stroke. Treatment was started with 4 mg candesartan or placebo on day 1 and dosage was increased to 8 or 16 mg candesartan or placebo on day 2, depending on the BP values. Treatment was aimed at a 10–15% BP reduction within 24 hours. Although no difference was found in stroke outcome at 3 months, a significantly lower recurrent cardiovascular event rate and lower mortality after 1 year were documented in the treatment group. The authors concluded that when there is need for or no contraindication against early antihypertensive therapy, candesartan is a safe therapeutic option.

In the UK's Controlling Hypertension and Hypotension Immediately Post-Stroke (CHHIPS) pilot trial [21], researchers randomized 179 patients who had suffered ischemic or hemorrhagic strokes within the previous 36 hours and who also had hypertension defined as systolic BP greater than 160 mmHg. Patients received doses of either the antihypertensive drugs lisinopril at a dosage of 5 mg or labetalol at a dosage of 50 mg or a placebo for 14 days. Three months after treatment began; the active treatment group had a significantly lower mortality compared to the placebo group. However, the recent SCAST study [22] showed no indication that BP-lowering treatment with candesartan is beneficial in patients with acute stroke and raised BP (>140 mmHg systolic). If anything, the evidence suggested a harmful effect.

Another important issue for consideration is whether patients who are already on antihypertensive treatment should continue or stop their pre-existing drugs. In the Continue or Stop Post-Stroke Antihypertensives Collaborative Study (COSSACS) [23], continuation of antihypertensive drugs did not reduce death or dependency at 2 weeks, cardiovascular event rate, or mortality at 6 months. However due to early termination, the study was underpowered.

It should be considered that stroke patients in these studies have been treated as a homogeneous group, without distinguishing between those who do and do not have hypoperfused brain tissue by perfusion imaging [24]. It stands to reason that the former might benefit from hypertension, whereas the latter would not, and might only suffer the side-effects of elevated BP.

Despite the somewhat confusing and unclear data the current European Stroke Organisation (ESO) 2008 Guidelines [25] recommend that BP up to 220 mmHg systolic or 120 mmHg diastolic may be tolerated in the acute phase without intervention unless there are cardiac complications. According to the American guidelines [26] it is generally agreed that patients with markedly elevated BP may have their BP lowered by not more than 15% during the first 24 hours after the onset of stroke. There is an indication to treat BP only if it is above 220 mmHg systolic or if the mean BP is higher than 120 mmHg. No data are available to guide selection of medication for the lowering of BP in the setting of acute ischemic stroke. The recommended medication and doses are based on general consensus. More studies are needed to identify the optimal strategy for BP management.

Several ongoing clinical trials such as the Efficacy of Nitric Oxide in Stroke (ENOS) trial may help answer the remaining questions.

> Guidelines recommend blood-pressure-lowering therapy above 220 mmHg systolic blood pressure (European Stroke Organisation (ESO) 2008 Guidelines and American Guidelines).

Hyperglycemia

It has been well established that elevated glucose levels play a major role in microvascular and macrovascular morbidity and in hematological abnormalities as well. Several processes were found to be associated with these conditions, including impaired vascular tone and flow, disruption to endothelial function, changes at the cellular level, intracellular acidosis, and increased aggregation and coagulability. Some animal studies [27, 28] have demonstrated the relations between acute ischemic stroke and hyperglycemia. In these models the administration of glucose to animals resulted in worsened brain ischemia. Those findings were attributed to the accumulation of lactate, decreased intracellular pH, increase in free radicals and excitatory amino acids, damage to the blood–brain barrier, formation of edema, and elevated risk of hemorrhagic transformation. Pretreatment with insulin was found to limit the ischemia.

As mentioned, 30–40% of acute stroke patients are found to have elevated glucose levels on admission, about half of them have known diabetes, while the others are newly diagnosed or suffer from stress-induced hyperglycemia [29].

In one systematic study it was shown that glucose pathology is seen in up to 80% of acute patients [30], many of them showing a high probability of previously unrecognized diabetes. Out of 238 consecutive acute stroke patients, 20.2% had previously known diabetes; 16.4% were classified as having newly diagnosed diabetes, 23.1% as having impaired glucose tolerance (IGT), and 0.8% as having impaired fasting glucose; and only 19.7% showed normal glucose levels.

Increased mortality was found in both diabetic and stress-induced hyperglycemia groups, independent of age, stroke type, and stroke size [31]. Stress hyperglycemia was associated with a 3-fold increase in risk of fatal 30-day outcome and 1.4-fold increase in risk of poor functional outcome in non-diabetic patients with acute ischemic stroke. Similar findings were also demonstrated in the NINDS rtPA stroke trial. Hyperglycemia on admission was correlated with decreased neurological improvement and the risk of hemorrhagic transformation in reperfused thrombolysed patients but not in non-reperfused rtPA-treated patients [32]. On the other hand, in the NINDS study, glucose level on admission was not associated with altered effectiveness of thrombolysis. All of these findings suggest that glucose level is an important risk factor for morbidity and mortality after stroke. However, it is not clear whether hyperglycemia itself affects stroke outcome or reflects, as a marker, the severity of the event due to the activation of stress hormones such as cortisol or norepinephrine. Diffusion–perfusion MRI analysis supports the first hypothesis. Hyperglycemia greater than 12.1 mmol/l in patients with perfusion–diffusion mismatch, shown on diffusion-weighted imaging–perfusion-weighted imaging (DWI/PWI) MRI, was associated with higher lactate production and with reduced salvage of mismatch tissue and increased conversion of tissue "at risk" to infarcted tissue compared with patients who arrived with the value of 5.2 mmol/l [33].

Among the factors found to contribute to the post-acute-stroke hyperglycemia [34] are the involvement of the insular cortex, which is known to play a role in sympathetic activation, involvement of the internal capsule, pre-existing diabetes, elevated systolic BP, and National Institute of Health Stroke Scale (NIHSS) higher than 14 points.

> Glucose level is an important risk factor for morbidity and mortality after stroke, but it is unclear whether hyperglycemia itself affects stroke outcomes or reflects the severity of the event as a marker.

Control of hyperglycemia

The previous data raise the question how, and especially to what extent, should post-acute-stroke hyperglycemia be treated. Intensive insulin therapy administered intravenous (i.v.) and aimed at maintaining blood glucose levels at 4.5–6.1 mmol/l in the surgical intensive care set-up was found to reduce mortality by more than 40% [35]. Similar results were documented among patients after myocardial infarction [36]. The question remains regarding the application in acute stroke patients. The UK Glucose Insulin in Stroke Trial (GIST-UK) addressed this question [37]. The study was conducted among 933 hyperglycemic acute stroke patients who received glucose-potassium-insulin (GKI) infusion versus placebo. In the treatment group significantly lowered glucose and BP values were documented; however, no clinical benefit was found among the treated patients. The time window for treating post-stroke hyperglycemia still remains uncertain. There are a variety of methods of insulin administration, including continuous i.v. infusion, repeated subcutaneous dosing, and i.v. infusion containing insulin and dextrose with potassium supplementation [38]. Ongoing trials address the role of i.v. insulin for hyperglycemic stroke patients. The Glucose Regulation in Acute Stroke Patients Trial (GRASP) is continuing recruitment. Patients with hyperglycemia (glucose >6.1 mmol/l) within 24 hours of symptom onset are randomized to tight glucose control (3.9–6.1 mmol/l), loose glucose control (6.1–11.1 mmol/l), or normal care. The insulin is delivered as a GKI infusion. The primary outcome of the GRASP trial is the rate of hypoglycemic events, and definitive information on clinical endpoints is not expected [39].

A randomized, multicenter, blinded pilot trial, Treatment of Hyperglycemia in Ischemic Stroke (THIS) [40], compared the use of aggressive treatment with continuous i.v. insulin, with no glucose or potassium in the insulin solution, with insulin administered subcutaneously in acute stroke patients. The aggressive-treatment group was associated with somewhat better clinical outcomes, which were not statistically significant. In the recently published INSULINFARCT study [41] 180 patients with acute ischemic stroke were randomized to receive either intensive insulin therapy or usual subcutaneous insulin for 24 hours. The former regimen was found to improve glucose control in the first 24 hours of stroke but was associated with larger infarct growths as measured by MRI. The 3-month functional outcome, death, and serious adverse events were similar in both groups.

According to the ESO 2008 recommendations [25], a blood glucose of 180 mg/dl (10 mmol/l) or higher is an indication for treatment with i.v. insulin. According to the American guidelines [26], even lower serum glucose levels, possibly between 140 and 180 mg/dl, should trigger administration of insulin. Many questions surrounding the role of glucose lowering therapy remain unanswered [38]. What level of blood glucose is best for intervention? What is the therapeutic time window? Will identification of

329

the penumbra with CT and MR imaging help in selecting appropriate patients? How long should the insulin infusion last? What level of monitoring is required? All these questions are still to be answered.

> Guidelines recommend i.v. insulin therapy for blood glucose levels equal to or greater than 180 mg/dl (10 mmol/l). In pre-thrombolysis patients, an even more aggressive approach may be advisable.

Hyperthermia

Several animal studies demonstrated the correlation of elevated temperature and poor outcome in ischemic stroke models [42,43]. Similar results were found in human observations. In the Copenhagen stroke study, stroke severity was correlated with hyperthermia higher than 37.5 °C, while a temperature lower than 36.5 °C was associated with a favorable outcome [44].

Other studies limited the correlation between stroke severity and hyperthermia to only the first 24 hours following stroke onset. In a prospective study temperature was recorded every 2 hours for 72 hours in 260 patients with a hemispheric ischemic stroke. Hyperthermia initiated only within the first 24 hours from stroke onset, but not afterward, was associated with larger infarct volume and worse outcome [45].

Therapeutic hypothermia

The above-mentioned animal studies and human observations raised the question regarding the role of hypothermia as a treatment for acute stroke. Hypothermia was introduced more than 50 years ago as a protective measure for the brain [46]. Mild induced hypothermia was found to improve neurological outcomes and reduce mortality following cardiac arrest due to ventricular fibrillation [47]; on the other hand, treatment with hypothermia aiming at 33 °C within the first 8 hours after brain injury was not found to be effective [48]. Other applications for which therapeutic hypothermia was suggested include acute encephalitis, neonatal hypoxia, and near drowning [45].

The use of antipyretics, such as acetaminophen, in high doses ranging between 3900 and 6000 mg daily [49, 50] caused only very mild reduction in body temperature, ranging from 0.2 to 0.4 °C respectively. The clinical benefit of this reduction is not well established. The use of external cooling aids [51], such as cooling blankets, cold infusions and cold washing, aiming at a body temperature of 33 °C for 48–72 hours in patients with severe middle cerebral artery (MCA) infarction, was not associated with severe side-effects and was found to help control elevated intracranial pressure values in cases of severe space-occupying edema. Similar results, of decreasing acute post-ischemic cerebral edema, were found in a small pilot study of endovascular-induced hypothermia [52]. The use of an endovascular cooling device which was inserted into the inferior vena cava was evaluated among patients with moderate to severe anterior circulation territory ischemic stroke in a randomized trial. Although no difference was found in the clinical outcome between the treatment group and the group randomized to standard medical management, the results suggest that this approach is feasible and that moderate hypothermia can be induced in patients with ischemic stroke quickly and effectively and is generally safe and well tolerated in most patients [53]. However, the current data do not support the use of induced hypothermia for treatment of patients with acute stroke. In conclusion, despite its therapeutic potential, hypothermia as a treatment for acute stroke has been investigated in only a few very small studies. Therapeutic hypothermia is feasible in acute stroke but owing to side-effects such as hypotension, cardiac arrhythmia, and pneumonia it is still thought of as experimental, and evidence of efficacy from clinical trials is needed [54]. According to the 2008 ESO recommendations [25], at a temperature of 37.5 °C or above reducing the body temperature should be advised. The American Heart and Stroke Association [26] recommend that antipyretic agents should be administered in post-stroke febrile patients but the effectiveness of treating either febrile or non-febrile patients with antipyretics is not proven.

> Hyperthermia within the first 24 hours from stroke onset was associated with larger infarct volume and worse outcome, but the current data do not support the use of induced hypothermia aiming at a body temperature of 33 °C for treatment of patients with acute stroke. The 2008 ESO Guidelines recommend reducing body temperature only if above 37.5 °C.

In summary, hypertension, hyperglycemia, and hyperthermia are common conditions following acute stroke. All three have a major and independent impact on the severity of outcome. Occasionally, the benefit of this impact is no less than that of more "heroic" strategies such as intravenous and intra-arterial thrombolysis. Despite the lack of consensus on the data and optimal management, one should carefully monitor these three "hyper-links" and treat them appropriately.

Summary

Optimal management of hypertension following stroke has not been yet established. A U-shaped relationship between baseline systolic BP and both early death and late death or dependency has been demonstrated in clinical trials: early death increased by 17.9% for every 10 mmHg below 150 mmHg and by 3.8% for every 10 mmHg above 150 mmHg. Stroke patients with impaired consciousness showed higher mortality rates with increasing BP. On the other hand, elevated systemic BP may compensate for the decrease in cerebral blood flow in the ischemic region. The benefit of BP reduction as a secondary prevention of stroke is well established, but only a few trials have been performed in the acute stage. However, these few trials demonstrate a beneficial effect of lowering BP. The current ESO 2008 Guidelines recommend that blood pressure up to 200 mmHg systolic or 120 mmHg diastolic may be tolerated in the acute phase. According to the American guidelines, lowering of markedly elevated BP should not exceed 15% during the first 24 hours after the onset of stroke

(Table 20.1). The latter applies for patients who do not receive thrombolysis,

Increased mortality was found in both diabetic and stress-induced hyperglycemia groups, independent of age, stroke type, and stroke size. Glucose level is an important risk factor for morbidity and mortality after stroke, but it is unclear whether hyperglycemia itself affects stroke outcomes or reflects the severity of the event as a marker. According to the ESO 2008 recommendations (Table 20.2) a blood glucose of 180 mg/dl (10 mmol/l) or higher is an indication for treatment with i.v. insulin. The American guidelines recommend treating hyperglycemia to achieve blood glucose levels in a range of 140–180 mg/dl (Table 20.1).

Hyperthermia within the first 24 hours from stroke onset was associated with larger infarct volume and worse outcome. Mild induced hypothermia was found to improve neurological outcome and reduce mortality following cardiac arrest due to ventricular fibrillation, but the current data (a few very small studies) do not support the use of induced hypothermia for treatment of patients with acute stroke. Because of side-effects such as hypotension, cardiac arrhythmia, and pneumonia, therapeutic hypothermia aiming at a body temperature of 33 °C is feasible in acute stroke, but is still thought of as experimental. The 2008 ESO recommendations are to reduce body temperature at temperatures of 37.5 °C or above.

Table 20.1. ESO 2008 and American Heart and Stroke Association recommendations in the acute stroke phase

	European Stroke Organisation (ESO) 2008 [25]	American Heart Association/American Stroke Association 2013 [26]
Blood pressure	Treat only if higher than 220/120 mmHg unless there are cardiac complications	In patients with markedly elevated blood pressure who do not receive fibrinolysis, a reasonable goal is to lower blood pressure by 15% during the first 24 hours after onset of stroke. The level of blood pressure that would mandate such treatment is not known, but consensus exists that medications should be withheld unless the systolic blood pressure is >220 mmHg or the diastolic blood pressure is >120 mmHg
Hyperglycemia	Treat with i.v. insulin if glucose levels are higher than 180 mg/dl	It is reasonable to treat hyperglycemia to achieve blood glucose levels in a range of 140 to 180 mg/dl and to closely monitor to prevent hypoglycemia in patients with acute ischemic stroke
Hyperthermia	Antipyretics should be administered if body temperature higher than 37.5 °C	Sources of hyperthermia (temperature >38 °C) should be identified and treated, and antipyretic medications should be administered to lower temperature in hyperthermic patients with stroke

Table 20.2. General stroke treatment recommendations according to current European Guidelines of the European Stroke Organisation [25].

Recommendations

- Intermittent monitoring of neurological status, pulse, blood pressure, temperature and oxygen saturation is recommended for 72 hours in patients with significant persisting neurological deficits **(Class IV, GCP)**
- It is recommended that oxygen should be administered if the oxygen saturation falls below 95% **(Class IV, GCP)**
- Regular monitoring of fluid balance and electrolytes is recommended in patients with severe stroke or swallowing problems **(Class IV, GCP)**
- Normal saline (0.9%) is recommended for fluid replacement during the first 24 hours after stroke **(Class IV, GCP)**
- Routine blood pressure lowering is not recommended following acute stroke **(Class IV, GCP)**
- Cautious blood pressure lowering is recommended in patients with extremely high blood pressures (>220/120 mmHg) on repeated measurements, with severe cardiac failure, aortic dissection, or hypertensive encephalopathy **(Class IV, GCP)**
- It is recommended that abrupt blood pressure lowering be avoided **(Class II, Level C)**
- It is recommended that low blood pressure secondary to hypovolemia or associated with neurological deterioration in acute stroke should be treated with volume expanders **(Class IV, GCP)**
- Monitoring serum glucose levels is recommended **(Class IV, GCP)**
- Treatment of serum glucose levels >180 mg/dl (>10 mmol/l) with insulin titration is recommended **(Class IV, GCP)**
- It is recommended that severe hypoglycemia (<50 mg/dl [<2.8 mmol/l]) should be treated with intravenous dextrose or infusion of 10–20% glucose **(Class IV, GCP points)**
- It is recommended that the presence of pyrexia (temperature >37.5 °C) should prompt a search for concurrent infection **(Class IV, GCP)**
- Treatment of pyrexia (temperature >37.5 °C) with paracetamol and fanning is recommended **(Class III, Level C)**
- Antibiotic prophylaxis is not recommended in immunocompetent patients **(Class II, Level B)**

Management of post-stroke complications

Stroke is a major cause of long-term physical, cognitive, emotional, and social disability. In addition to the neurological impairment appearing in the acute phase, there are infrequently late complications which are often neglected. These complications have a great impact on the quality of life, outcome, and chances of rehabilitation and may include post-stroke epilepsy, dementia, depression, and fatigue. Other complications, such as infections, are dealt with in Chapter 21. Table 20.3 gives an overview of the recommendations of the ESO for the prevention and management of complications [20].

Post-stroke seizures

Epilepsy is one of the most common serious neurological disorders and is associated with numerous social and psychological consequences. Stroke is the most commonly identified etiology of secondary epilepsy and accounts for 30% of newly diagnosed seizures in patients older than 60 years [55]. Although recognized as a major cause of epilepsy in the elderly, many questions still arise regarding the epidemiology, treatment, and outcome of post-stroke seizures.

The common definition of epilepsy includes at least two seizures with a time interval of at least 24 hours between the episodes. The current clinical classification of post-stroke seizures is made according to the period between the stroke and the first epileptic episode. A post-stroke seizure is defined as early if it occurs in the first 2 weeks after the stroke. A seizure occurring later is defined as late [56].

The estimated rate of early post-ischemic stroke seizures ranges from 2% to 33% and that of late seizures varies from 3% to 67% [57–65]. The wide range is due to the different methodologies, terminologies, and sizes of the populations in the different studies. The overall rate of post-stroke epilepsy, as previously defined as at least two episodes, is 3–4% and is higher in patients who have had a late seizure [65].

In an observational study among 1428 patients after stroke [65], 51 patients (3.6%) developed epilepsy. Post-stroke epilepsy was found to be more common among patients with hemorrhagic strokes, venous infarctions, and localization in the right hemisphere and MCA territory. The SASS (Seizures After

Table 20.3. Prevention and management of complications according to current European Guidelines of the European Stroke Organisation [25].

Recommendations

- It is recommended that infections after stroke should be treated with appropriate antibiotics **(Class IV, GCP)**
- Prophylactic administration of antibiotics is not recommended, and levofloxacin can be detrimental in acute stroke patients **(Class II, Level B)**
- Early rehydration and graded compression stockings are recommended to reduce the incidence of venous thromboembolism **(Class IV, GCP)**
- Early mobilization is recommended to prevent complications such as aspiration pneumonia, DVT, and pressure ulcers **(Class IV, GCP)**
- It is recommended that low-dose subcutaneous heparin or low molecular weight heparins should be considered for patients at high risk of DVT or pulmonary embolism **(Class I, Level A)**
- Administration of anticonvulsants is recommended to prevent recurrent post-stroke seizures **(Class I, Level A)**. Prophylactic administration of anticonvulsants to patients with recent stroke who have not had seizures is not recommended **(Class IV, GCP)**
- An assessment of risk of falls is recommended for every stroke patient **(Class IV, GCP)**
- Calcium/vitamin D supplements are recommended in stroke patients at risk of falls **(Class II, Level B)**
- Bisphosphonates (alendronate, etidronate, and risedronate) are recommended in women with previous fractures **(Class II, Level B)**
- In stroke patients with urinary incontinence, specialist assessment and management are recommended **(Class III, Level C)**
- Swallowing assessment is recommended but there are insufficient data to recommend a specific approach for treatment **(Class III, GCP)**
- Oral dietary supplements are only recommended for non-dysphagic stroke patients who are malnourished **(Class II, Level B)**
- Early commencement of nasogastric (NG) feeding (within 48 hours) is recommended in stroke patients with impaired swallowing **(Class II, Level B)**
- It is recommended that percutaneous enteral gastrostomy (PEG) feeding should not be considered in stroke patients in the first 2 weeks **(Class II, Level B)**

Stroke Study) was a prospective multicenter study held among 1897 patients after an ischemic or hemorrhagic stroke [56]. In that study 14% of the patients with ischemic stroke and 20% of patients with hemorrhagic stroke had seizures during the first year; a second episode, required to establish epilepsy, was found in 2.5% of the patients. Most of the patients with post-stroke epilepsy have simple partial seizures, while complex partial seizures are relatively rare. The risk of status epilepticus varies from 0.14% to 13%. It should be emphasized that it is not always clear whether the patient has had a seizure; seizures in the elderly are sometimes difficult to diagnose and may present as acute confusion, behavioral changes, or syncope of unknown origin [66].

> Post-stroke epilepsy is defined as at least two episodes of seizures. The overall rate is 3–4% of stroke patients.

Other predictors for post-stroke seizures found in various studies are cortical location, large infarct, evaluated clinically or radiologically, intracerebral hemorrhage, and cardiac emboli, most probably due to the tendency of the last to involve the cortex [61–64]. Post-stroke seizures are also more common among patients with pre-existing dementia evaluated using the validated IQCODE questionnaire (risk ratio of 4.66, CI 1.34–16.21). A recent cohort study found major stroke and sinus thrombosis as the two major predictors for post-stroke epilepsy [67]. In that study, conventional vascular risk factors were not associated with the occurrence of post-stroke seizures. Patients in high-risk populations should be advised to avoid factors increasing the risk of seizures, such as certain drugs [68]. In a retrospective study the presence of chronic obstructive pulmonary disease (COPD) was found to be an independent risk factor for the development of seizures in stroke patients [69].

The pathophysiology of early seizures is thought to be due to the increased excitatory activity mediated by the release of glutamate from the hypoxic tissue [70]. Late seizures are due to the development of tissue gliosis and neuronal damage in the infarct area [71]. An interesting question is whether post-stroke seizures worsen the outcome of patients after stroke. A cortical cerebral infarction disability was found to be greater in patients with seizures; on the other hand, in patients with cortical hemorrhage disability was found to be less [56].

The attending physician is required to deal with two important questions, the first being whether to start treatment after the first episode and the second being which antiepileptic drug to prefer. According to the common clinical approach, treatment should be initiated only after the second episode. Observational studies suggest that isolated early seizures after stroke do not require treatment [59, 60]. Beginning treatment after early-onset seizures has not been associated with reduction of recurrent seizures after discontinuing the medication [72].

At this stage there are no evidence-based studies to recommend one drug over the others. It is best to avoid the old drugs, especially phenytoin, because of their pharmacokinetic profile and interactions with anticoagulants and salicylates [73]. "New-generation" drugs (lamotrigine, gabapentin, and levetiracetam, etc.) in low doses would be a reasonable option because of their efficacy, improved safety profile, and fewer interactions with other drugs compared with first-generation drugs [74]. A single study has found gabapentin to be a safe and effective treatment; however, this recommendation should be taken with caution since the study had no control group [75]. In a prospective study comparing lamotrigine versus carbamazepine in 64 patients with post-stroke epilepsy, lamotrigine was found to be significantly better tolerated and with a trend to be also more efficacious (p = 0.06) [76].

> There is no evidence to prefer one antiepileptic drug over the others, but it is advised to avoid phenytoin because of interactions with anticoagulants and salicylates.

Post-stroke depression

Post-stroke depression is considered to be the most frequent and important neuropsychiatric consequence of stroke and has a major impact on functional recovery, cognition, and even survival.

The incidence of post-stroke depression ranges in various studies between 18% and 61%. Once again, the large variation in frequencies is due to methodological differences, including the point in time at which patients were assessed relative to the stroke onset and the different instruments and criteria for diagnosing depression that were used in the different studies.

A systematic review of collected data from 51 observational studies conducted between 1977 and 2002 found that the frequency of post-stroke depression is 33% (95% CI 29–36) and that

the depression resolves spontaneously within several months of onset in most of the patients [77]. The Italian multicenter observational study of post-stroke depression (DESTRO) assessed 1064 patients with ischemic or hemorrhagic stroke in the first 9 months after the event [78]. Patients with depression were followed for 2 years. post-stroke depression was detected in 36% of the patients, most of whom had minor depression with dysthymia, rather than major depression, and adaptation disorder. Although no correlation between post-stroke depression and mortality was found in the DESTRO study, an Australian study [79] found that among stroke patients in rehabilitation the depressed ones were eight times more likely to have died by 15-month follow-up than the non-depressed. In a recent Chinese multicentered prospective cohort study the diagnosis of post-stroke depression was associated with an increased risk of recurrent stroke at 1 year in a multivariate model (OR 1.49; 95% CI 1.03–2.15) [80].

The potential etiology for post-stroke depression [81] includes neuroanatomical mechanisms such as disruption of monoaminergic pathways and depletion of cortical biogenic amines, especially in the case of lesions in the left frontal and left basal ganglia territories [82], and psychological mechanisms such as the difficulty in adjusting to the new limitations and requirements of the disease. In a systematic review of 26 studies regarding the correlation of left hemispheric stroke and the risk of post-stroke depression no significant correlation was found [83]. Differences in the measurement of depression, study design, and presentations of results may also have contributed to the heterogeneity of the findings. Other risk factors for post-stroke depression include female gender, severe physical disability, previous depression, and history of psychiatric and emotional liability during the first days after stroke. Some studies have found aphasia as a risk factor, while others have not obtained similar results [84]. Dementia was also found to be an important predictor for the development of post-stroke depression [85].

> The frequency of post-stroke depression is 33% and it resolves spontaneously within several months of onset in most patients.

The treating physician should be aware of the diagnosis of depression in stroke survivors since it may be hindered by a number of conditions, including aphasia, agnosia, apraxia, and memory disturbances. The differential diagnosis of post-stroke depression includes anosognosia, apathy, fatigue, and disprosody [85]. Despite some encouraging data regarding the prophylactic use of antidepressants in post-stroke patients there is still insufficient randomized evidence to support this approach in routine post-stroke management [77]. A single recent double-blind placebo-controlled study evaluated the administration of escitalopram in a population of non-depressed patients following stroke [86]. Patients who received placebo were significantly more likely to develop depression than ones who received escitalopram after 12 months follow-up. Problem-solving therapy did not achieve significant results over placebo. A retrospective study held among 870 post-stroke patients showed that selective serotonin reuptake inhibitor (SSRI) treatment was associated with longer survival even though depression diagnosis was associated with greater risk of mortality [87].

According to the ESO 2008 recommendations [25] antidepressant drugs such as SSRIs and heterocyclics can improve mood after stroke, but there is less evidence that these agents can effect full remission of a major depressive episode or prevent depression. SSRIs are better tolerated than heterocyclics. There is no good evidence to recommend psychotherapy for treatment or prevention of post-stroke depression, although such therapy can elevate mood.

In spite of growing information, many questions still surround various aspects of post-stroke depression, including the development of standardized measure of depression, the optimal time after stroke onset to screen for post-stroke depression, the creation of predictors for post-stroke depression, and identifying the appropriate management.

> Antidepressant drugs can improve mood after stroke, but there is less evidence that these agents can be effective in a major depressive episode or prevention.

Post-stroke dementia

Stroke is an important risk factor for dementia and cognitive decline. According to the NINDS-AIREN criteria, in order to make the diagnosis of post-stroke dementia (PSD) the patient has to be demented, with either historical, clinical, or radiological evidence of cerebrovascular disease and the two disorders must be reasonably related [88]. On the other hand, according to the fourth edition (DSM-4) [89], vascular dementia is diagnosed by the development of multiple cognitive

deficits manifested by memory impairment and at least one of the following cognitive disturbances: aphasia, apraxia, agnosia, and disturbance in executive functioning with the presence of focal neurological signs and symptoms or laboratory evidence indicative of cerebrovascular disease that is judged to be etiologically related to the disturbance. The deficits should not occur exclusively during the course of an episode of delirium.

Despite the lack of accurate data due to poor definition of the disorder, the use of different tools and diagnostic difficulties in distinguishing between PSD and other types of dementia, PSD is considered to be the second most common type of dementia. Since several studies used different tools for the diagnosis of PSD and there were also differences in the methodologies and study populations, the incidence varies in the different studies from 8% to 30%. One study, done among a population of elderly demented patients, demonstrated that the frequency of dementia was found to depend upon the diagnostic criteria used [90]. For instance, using the NINDS-AIREN criteria only 14% of the patients were diagnosed with PSD, compared to 76% using the DSM-4 as a diagnostic tool. Interestingly there are also noticeable differences in the incidence rates between countries; an almost 3-fold difference in the age-standardized incidence ratios (SIR) of PSD rates between Germany and the Netherlands was demonstrated (1.23 and 0.42, respectively) [91], indicating that geographical variation is still present after taking into account the countries' differential age distributions. It is unclear whether these differences are due to genetic or environmental factors since, as in the previous trials mentioned, there were methodological differences between the studies.

Despite the conflicting data the overall estimated frequency of dementia in post-stroke patients is about 28% and the fact that stroke is a major risk factor for dementia is well established [92]. The mechanisms of PSD [93, 94] consist of large-vessel disease, including multi-infarcts or single infarcts in a strategic area such as the thalamus, hippocampus, basal forebrain, or the angular gyrus, or small-vessel disease such as lacunes or leukoaraiosis. Other mechanisms include hypoperfusion, hypoxic-ischemic disorders, and shared pathogenic pathways with degenerative dementia, especially Alzheimer type.

Risk factors for PSD include large and left-sided infarcts, bilateral infarcts, frontal lobe infarcts, large

MCA infarcts, and previous strokes. Diabetes, hyperlipidemia, and atrial fibrillation were also found as predictors for the development of PSD [93–95]. Silent brain infarcts demonstrated on CT, however, were not found to predict the development of PSD in one prospective study [96], while in another, higher grades of white matter findings on MRI were associated with impaired cognitive function [97]. Since it has also been shown in that study that the extent of white matter lesions is related to the BP level, even in normotensive patients, and since these lesions are correlated with the risk of PSD, it would be reasonable to assume that lowering BP would lower the risk of PSD. Abnormal EEG performed close to the ischemic stroke appears to be an indicator of subsequent PSD in a prospective study done among 199 patients, probably because it indicates cortical involvement [98].

The borders between dementia of the neurodegenerative type and vascular dementia are nowadays less visible and both types of dementia include many similar risk factors and clinical and pathological characteristics. It is suggested that cerebrovascular disease may play an important role in the presence and severity of Alzheimer's disease [99].

There is no evidence-based treatment for PSD. In a meta-analysis of randomized controlled trials cholinesterase inhibitors, which are administered for the treatment of degenerative-type dementia, were found to produce only small benefits in cognition of uncertain clinical significance in patients with mild to moderate vascular dementia. There are insufficient data to recommend the use of these agents in PSD [100].

> The frequency of dementia (PSD) in post-stroke patients is about 28%. There is no evidence-based treatment for PSD.

Post-stroke fatigue

Another common and disabling late sequel of stroke is general fatigue [101, 102]. It is important to distinguish between "normal" fatigue, which is a state of general tiredness that is a result of overexertion and can be ameliorated by rest, and "pathological" fatigue, which is a more chronic condition, not related to previous exertion and not ameliorated by rest. Many other central and peripheral neurological conditions, beside stroke, are known to be a cause of fatigue, including multiple sclerosis, amyotrophic lateral sclerosis, Parkinson's disease, post-polio syndrome, HIV, collagen diseases, and others [103–106]. It is

important to emphasize that post-stroke fatigue is not always a part of post-stroke depression and can occur in the absence of depressive features [100, 107]. It is estimated that about 70% of post-stroke patients experience "pathological" fatigue. However, the biological mechanisms of post-stroke fatigue are uncertain 108]. Fatigue was also rated by 40% of stroke patients as either their worst symptom or among their worst symptoms. Fatigue was found to be an independent predictor of functional disability and mortality [109, 110]]. Risk factors for post-stroke fatigue include older age and female sex, activities of daily living impairment, living alone or in an institution, anxiety, pre-stroke depression, leukoaraiosis, myocardial infarction, diabetes mellitus, pain, and sleeping disturbances [102, 110]. Some studies suggest the involvement of the brainstem, basal ganglia, and thalamus [102, 108].

The caring physician should be alert to identify possible predisposing factors and to diagnose "pathological" fatigue. The initial treatment should focus on optimizing the management of potential factors, exercise, sleep hygiene, stress reduction, and cognitive behavior therapy. The pharmacological therapy includes the stimulant agents amantadine and modafinil.

> It is estimated that about 70% of post-stroke patients experience fatigue and 40% of patients rate it among their worst symptoms. Pharmacological treatment includes the stimulating agents amantadine and modafinil.

Appropriate diagnosis and treatment of the late complications of stroke, which are often underdiagnosed and undertreated, are a crucial component in the management of stroke and should always be taken into consideration when dealing with stroke patients.

Chapter summary

> The overall rate of **post-stroke epilepsy**, defined as at least two episodes, is 3–4%. It is higher in patients who have a late seizure (early post-stroke seizures occur within the first 2 weeks after a stroke, late post-stroke seizures occur later). Predictors for post-stroke seizures are cortical location, large infarct, intracerebral hemorrhage and the presence of cardiac emboli, and pre-existing dementia. Treatment should be initiated only after the second episode. There is no evidence to recommend one drug over the others but it is advised to avoid phenytoin

because of interactions with anticoagulants and salicylates.

The frequency of **post-stroke depression** is 33% and it resolves spontaneously within several months of onset in most patients. Risk factors for post-stroke depression are female gender, severe physical disability, previous depression, and dementia. According to the ESO 2008 recommendations antidepressant drugs such as selective serotonin reuptake inhibitors (SSRIs) and heterocyclics can improve mood after stroke.

For the diagnosis of **post-stroke dementia** (PSD) the patient has to be demented, with either historical, clinical, or radiological evidence of cerebrovascular disease, and the two disorders must be reasonably related. PSD is the second most common type of dementia. The frequency of dementia in post-stroke patients is about 28%. Risk factors for PSD are large and left-sided infarcts, bilateral infarcts, frontal lobe infarcts, large MCA infarcts, previous strokes, diabetes, hyperlipidemia, and atrial fibrillation. There is no evidence-based treatment for PSD. Cholinesterase inhibitors were found to produce only small benefits in patients with mild to moderate vascular dementia.

Post-stroke fatigue is not related to previous exertion and is not ameliorated by rest and can occur in the absence of depressive features. It is estimated that about 70% of post-stroke patients experience fatigue and 40% of the patients rate it among their worst symptoms. The initial treatment should focus on the management of potential risk factors; pharmacological therapy includes the stimulant agents amantadine and modafinil.

References

1. Wallace JD, Levy LL. Blood pressure after stroke. *JAMA* 1981; **246**(19):2177–80.

2. Carlberg B, Asplund K, Hägg E. Factors influencing admission blood pressure levels in patients with acute stroke. *Stroke* 1991; **22**:527–30.

3. Urrutia VC, Wityk RJ. Blood pressure management in acute stroke. *Crit Care Clin* 2006; **22**(4):695–711.

4. Leonardi-Bee J, Bath PM, Phillips SJ, Sandercock PA; IST Collaborative Group. Blood pressure and clinical outcomes in the International Stroke Trial. *Stroke* 2002; **33**:1315–20.

5. Vemmos KN, Tsivgoulis G, Spengos K, *et al.* U-shaped relationship between mortality and admission blood pressure in patients with acute stroke. *J Intern Med* 2004; **255**:257–65.

6. Grabska K, Niewada M, Sarzyńska-Długosz I, Kamiński B, Członkowska A. Pulse pressure–independent predictor of poor early outcome and mortality following ischemic stroke. *Cerebrovasc Dis* 2009; **27**:187–92.

7. Aslanyan S, Fazekas F, Weir CJ, Horner S, Lees KR; GAIN International Steering Committee and Investigators. Effect of blood pressure during the acute period of ischemic stroke on stroke outcome: a tertiary analysis of the GAIN International Trial. *Stroke* 2003; **34**:2420–5.

8. Willmot M, Leonardi-Bee J, Bath PM. High blood pressure in acute stroke and subsequent outcome: a systematic review. *Hypertension* 2004; **43**(1):18–24.

9. Brott T, Lu M, Kothari R, *et al.* Hypertension and its treatment in the NINDS rt-PA Stroke Trial. *Stroke* 1998; **29**:1504–9.

10. Chamorro A, Vila N, Ascaso C, *et al.* Blood pressure and functional recovery in acute ischemic stroke. *Stroke* 1998; **29**:1850–3.

11. Carlberg B, Asplund K, Hägg E. The prognostic value of admission blood pressure in patients with acute stroke. *Stroke* 1993; **24**:1372–5.

12. Ahmed N, Wahlgren N, Brainin M, *et al.*; SITS Investigators. Relationship of blood pressure, antihypertensive therapy, and outcome in ischemic stroke treated with intravenous thrombolysis: retrospective analysis from Safe Implementation of Thrombolysis in Stroke-International Stroke Thrombolysis Register (SITS-ISTR). *Stroke* 2009;**40**:2442–9.

13. Mattle HP, Kappeler L, Arnold M, *et al.* Blood pressure and vessel recanalization in the first hours after ischemic stroke. *Stroke* 2005; **36**:264–8.

14. Shin HK, Nishimura M, Jones PB, *et al.* Mild induced hypertension improves blood flow and oxygen metabolism in transient focal cerebral ischemia. *Stroke* 2008; **39**:1548–55.

15. Rordorf G, Koroshetz WJ, Ezzeddine MA, Segal AZ, Buonanno FS. A pilot study of drug-induced hypertension for treatment of acute stroke. *Neurology* 2001; **56**:1210–13.

16. Marzan AS, Hungerbühler HJ, Studer A, Baumgartner RW, Georgiadis D. Feasibility and safety of norepinephrine-induced arterial hypertension in acute ischemic stroke. *Neurology* 2004; **62**:1193–5.

17. Hillis AE, Ulatowski JA, Barker PB, *et al.* A pilot randomized trial of induced blood pressure elevation: effects on function and

focal perfusion in acute and subacute stroke. *Cerebrovasc Dis* 2003; **16**:236–46.

18. Olsen TS, Larsen B, Herning M, Skriver EB, Lassen NA. Blood flow and vascular reactivity in collaterally perfused brain tissue. Evidence of an ischemic penumbra in patients with acute stroke. *Stroke* 1983; **14**:332–41.

19. Mistri AK, Robinson TG, Potter JF. Pressor therapy in acute ischemic stroke: systematic review. *Stroke* 2006; **37**(6):1565–71.

20. Schrader J, Lüders S, Kulschewski A, *et al.*; Acute Candesartan Cilexetil Therapy in Stroke Survivors Study Group. The ACCESS Study: evaluation of Acute Candesartan Cilexetil Therapy in Stroke Survivors. *Stroke* 2003; **34**:1699–703.

21. Potter JF, Robinson TG, Ford GA, *et al.* Controlling hypertension and hypotension immediately post-stroke (CHHIPS): a randomised, placebo-controlled, double-blind pilot trial. *Lancet Neurol* 2009; **8**:48–56.

22. Sandset EC, Bath PM, Boysen G, *et al.*; SCAST Study Group. The angiotensin-receptor blocker candesartan for treatment of acute stroke (SCAST): a randomised, placebo-controlled, double-blind trial. *Lancet* 2011;**377**:741–50

23. Robinson TG, Potter JF, Ford GA, *et al.*; COSSACS Investigators. Effects of antihypertensive treatment after acute stroke in the Continue or Stop Post-Stroke Antihypertensives Collaborative Study (COSSACS): a prospective, randomised, open, blinded-endpoint trial. *Lancet Neurol* 2010; **9**:767–75.

24. Copen WA, Schaefer PW, Wu O. MR perfusion imaging in acute ischemic stroke. *Neuroimaging Clin N Am* 2011; **21**:259–83.

25. The European Stroke Organisation (ESO) Executive Committee and the ESO Writing Committee. Guidelines for management of ischaemic stroke and transient ischaemic attack 2008. *Cerebrovasc Dis* 2008; **25**:457–507.

26. Jauch EC, Saver JL, Adams HP Jr, *et al.*; American Heart Association Stroke Council, Council on Cardiovascular Nursing, Council on Peripheral Vascular Disease, and Council on Clinical Cardiology. Guidelines for the early management of patients with acute ischemic stroke: a guideline for healthcare professionals from the American Heart Association/ American Stroke Association. *Stroke* 2013; **44**:870–947.

27. Vázquez-Cruz J, Martí-Vilalta JL, Ferrer I, Pérez-Gallofré A, Folch J. Progressing cerebral infarction in relation to plasma glucose in gerbils. *Stroke* 1990; **21**(11):1621–4.

28. Martín A, Rojas S, Chamorro A, *et al.* Why does acute hyperglycemia worsen the outcome of transient focal cerebral ischemia? Role of corticosteroids, inflammation, and protein O-glycosylation. *Stroke* 2006; **37**(5):1288–95. Epub 2006/05/06.

29. Kiers L, Davis SM, Larkins R, *et al.* Stroke topography and outcome in relation to hyperglycaemia and diabetes. *J Neurol Neurosurg Psychiatry* 1992; **55**:263–70.

30. Matz K, Keresztes K, Tatschl C, *et al.* Disorders of glucose metabolism in acute stroke patients: an underrecognized problem. *Diabetes Care* 2006; **29**:792–7.

31. Capes SE, Hunt D, Malmberg K, Pathak P, Gerstein HC. Stress hyperglycemia and prognosis of stroke in nondiabetic and diabetic patients: a systematic overview. *Stroke* 2001; **32**:2426–32.

32. Alvarez-Sabín J, Molina CA, Montaner J, *et al.* Effects of admission hyperglycemia on stroke outcome in reperfused tissue plasminogen activator-treated patients. *Stroke* 2003; **34**:1235–41.

33. Parsons MW, Barber PA, Desmond PM, *et al.* Acute hyperglycemia adversely affects stroke outcome: a magnetic resonance imaging and spectroscopy study. *Ann Neurol* 2002; **52**(1):20–8.

34. Allport LE, Butcher KS, Baird TA, *et al.* Insular cortical ischemia is independently associated with acute stress hyperglycemia. *Stroke* 2004; **35**:1886–91.

35. van den Berghe G, Wouters P, Weekers F, *et al.* Intensive insulin therapy in critically ill patients. *N Engl J Med* 2001; **345**(19):1359–67.

36. Malmberg K. Prospective randomized study of intensive insulin treatment on long term survival after acute myocardial infarction in patients with diabetes mellitus. DIGAMI (Diabetes Mellitus, Insulin Glucose Infusion in Acute Myocardial Infarction) Study Group. *BMJ* 1997; **314**:1512–15.

37. Gray CS, Hildreth AJ, Sandercock PA, *et al.*; GIST Trialists Collaboration. Glucose-potassium-insulin infusions in the management of post-stroke hyperglycaemia: the UK Glucose Insulin in Stroke Trial (GIST-UK). *Lancet Neurol* 2007; **6**:397–406.

38. McCormick MT, Muir KW, Gray C, Walters MR. Management of hyperglycemia in acute stroke: how, when, and for whom? *Stroke* 2008; **39**(7):2177–85.

39. Glucose Regulation in Acute Stroke Patients Trial (GRASP). *The Internet Stroke Center.* American Stroke Association. 2008.

40. Bruno A, Kent TA, Coull BM, *et al.* Treatment of hyperglycemia in ischemic stroke (THIS): a randomized pilot trial. *Stroke* 2008; **39**(2):384–9.

41. Rosso C, Corvol JC, Pires C, *et al.* Intensive versus subcutaneous insulin in patients with hyperacute stroke: results from the randomized INSULINFARCT trial. *Stroke* 2012; **43**:2343–9.

42. Memezawa H, Zhao Q, Smith ML, Siesjö BK. Hyperthermia nullifies the ameliorating effect of dizocilpine maleate (MK-801) in focal cerebral ischemia. *Brain Res* 1995; **670**(1):48–52.

43. Wass CT, Lanier WL, Hofer RE, Scheithauer BW, Andrews AG. Temperature changes of > or = 1 degree C alter functional neurologic outcome and histopathology in a canine model of complete cerebral ischemia. *Anesthesiology* 1995; **83**:325–35.

44. Reith J, Jørgensen HS, Pedersen PM, *et al.* Body temperature in acute stroke: relation to stroke severity, infarct size, mortality, and outcome. *Lancet* 1996; **347**:422–5.

45. Castillo J, Dávalos A, Marrugat J, Noya M. Timing for fever-related brain damage in acute ischemic stroke. *Stroke* 1998; **29** (12):2455–60.

46. Varon J, Acosta P. Therapeutic hypothermia: past, present, and future. *Chest* 2008; **133**:1267–74.

47. Hypothermia After Cardiac Arrest Study Group. Mild therapeutic hypothermia to improve the neurological outcome after cardiac arrest. *N Engl J Med* 2002; **346**:549–56.

48. Clifton GL, Miller ER, Choi SC, *et al.* Lack of effect of induction of hypothermia after acute brain injury. *N Engl J Med* 2001; **344**:556–63.

49. Kasner SE, Wein T, Piriyawat P, *et al.* Acetaminophen for altering body temperature in acute stroke: a randomized clinical trial. *Stroke* 2002; **33**:130–4.

50. Dippel DW, van Breda EJ, van Gemert HM, *et al.* Effect of paracetamol (acetaminophen) on body temperature in acute ischemic stroke: a double-blind, randomized phase II clinical trial. *Stroke* 2001; **32**:1607–12.

51. Schwab S, Schwarz S, Spranger M, *et al.* Moderate hypothermia in the treatment of patients with severe middle cerebral artery infarction. *Stroke* 1998; **29**:2461–6.

52. Guluma KZ, Oh H, Yu SW, *et al.* Effect of endovascular hypothermia on acute ischemic edema: morphometric analysis of the ICTuS trial. *Neurocrit Care* 2008; **8**(1):42–7.

53. Olsen TS, Weber UJ, Kammersgaard LP, *et al.* Therapeutic hypothermia for acute stroke. *Lancet Neurol* 2003; **2**:410–16.

54. De Georgia MA, Krieger DW, Abou-Chebl A, *et al.* Cooling for Acute Ischemic Brain Damage (COOL AID): a feasibility trial of endovascular cooling. *Neurology* 2004; **63**(2):312–17.

55. Forsgren L, Bucht G, Eriksson S, Bergmark L. Incidence and clinical characterization of unprovoked seizures in adults: a prospective population-based study. *Epilepsia* 1996; **37**:224–9.

56. Bladin CF, Alexandrov AV, Bellavance A, *et al.* Seizures after stroke: a prospective multicenter study. *Arch Neurol* 2000; **57**:1617–22.

57. Lesser RP, Luders H, Dinner DS, Morris HH. Epileptic seizures due to thrombotic and embolic cerebrovascular disease in older patients. *Epilepsia* 1985; **26**:622–30.

58. So EL, Annegers JF, Hauser WA, O'Brien PC, Whisnant JP. Population-based study of seizure disorders after cerebral infarction. *Neurology* 1996; **46**:350–5.

59. Kilpatrick CJ, Davis SM, Tress BM, *et al.* Epileptic seizures in acute stroke. *Arch Neurol* 1990; **47**:157–60.

60. Shinton RA, Gill JS, Melnick AK. The frequency, characteristics, and prognosis of epileptic seizures at the onset of stroke. *J Neurol Neurosurg Psychiatry* 1988; **51**:273–6.

61. Arboix A, Garcia-Eroles L, Massons JB, Oliveres M, Comes E. Predictive factors of early seizures after acute cerebrovascular disease. *Stroke* 1997; **28**:1590–4.

62. Reith J, Jørgensen HS, Nakayama H, Raaschou HO, Olsen TS. Seizures in acute stroke: the Copenhagen Stroke Study. *Stroke* 1997; **28**:1585–9.

63. Giroud M, Gras P, Fayolle H, *et al.* Early seizures after stroke: a study of 1,640 cases. *Epilepsia* 1994; **35**:959–64.

64. Olsen TS. Post-stroke epilepsy. *Curr Atheroscler Rep* 2001; **3** (4):340–4. Review.

65. Benbir G, Ince B, Bozluolcay M. The epidemiology of post-stroke epilepsy according to stroke sub-types. *Acta Neurol Scand* 2006; **114**:8–12.

66. Myint PK, Staufenberg EF, Sabanathan K. Post-stroke seizure and post-stroke epilepsy. *Postgrad Med J* 2006; **82**:568–72.

67. Conrad J, Pawlowski M, Dogan M, *et al.* Seizures after cerebrovascular events: risk factors and clinical features. *Seizure* 2013; **22**(4):275–82

68. Cordonnier C, Hénon H, Derambure P, Pasquier F, Leys D. Influence of pre-existing dementia on the risk of post-stroke epileptic seizures. *J Neurol Neurosurg Psychiatry* 2005; **76**:1649–53.

69. De Reuck J, Proot P, Van Maele G. Chronic obstructive pulmonary disease as a risk factor for stroke-related seizures. *Eur J Neurol* 2007; **14**:989–92.

70. Sun DA, Sombati S, DeLorenzo RJ. Glutamate injury-induced epileptogenesis in hippocampal

339

neurons: an in vitro model of stroke-induced "epilepsy". *Stroke* 2001; **32**:2344–50.

71. Stroemer RP, Kent TA, Hulsebosch CE. Neocortical neural sprouting, synaptogenesis, and behavioral recovery after neocortical infarction in rats. *Stroke* 1995; **26**:2135–44.

72. Gilad R, Lampl Y, Eschel Y, Sadeh M. Antiepileptic treatment in patients with early postischemic stroke seizures: a retrospective study. *Cerebrovas Dis* 2001; **12**:39–43.

73. Ryvlin P, Montavont A, Nighoghossian N. Optimizing therapy of seizures in stroke patients. *Neurology* 2006; **67**(12 Suppl 4):S3–9.

74. Gilad R. Management of seizures following a stroke: what are the options? *Drugs Aging* 2012; **29**:533–8.

75. Alvarez-Sabín J, Montaner J, Padró L, *et al*. Gabapentin in late-onset poststroke seizures. *Neurology* 2002; **59**(12):1991–3.

76. Gilad R, Sadeh M, Rapoport A, *et al*. Monotherapy of lamotrigine versus carbamazepine in patients with poststroke seizure. *Clin Neuropharmacol* 2007; **30**:189–95.

77. Hackett ML, Yapa C, Parag V, Anderson CS. Frequency of depression after stroke: a systematic review of observational studies. *Stroke* 2005; **36**:1330–4.

78. Paolucci S, Gandolfo C, Provinciali L, Torta R, Toso V; DESTRO Study Group. The Italian multicenter observational study on post-stroke depression (DESTRO). *J Neurol* 2006; **253**:556–62.

79. Morris PL, Robinson RG, Samuels J. Depression, introversion and mortality following stroke. *Aust N Z J Psychiatry* 1993; **27**:443–9.

80. Yuan HW, Wang CX, Zhang N, *et al*. Poststroke depression and risk of recurrent stroke at 1 year in a Chinese cohort study. *PLoS One* 2012; 7:e46906.

81. Gainotti G, Marra C. Determinants and consequences of post-stroke depression. *Curr Opin Neurol* 2002; **15**(1):85–9.

82. Narushima K, Kosier JT, Robinson RG. A reappraisal of poststroke depression, intra- and inter-hemispheric lesion location using meta-analysis. *J Neuropsychiatry Clin Neurosci* 2003; **15**:422–30.

83. Bhogal SK, Teasell R, Foley N, Speechley M. Lesion location and poststroke depression: systematic review of the methodological limitations in the literature. *Stroke* 2004; **35**:794–802.

84. Gaete JM, Bogousslavsky J. Post-stroke depression. *Expert Rev Neurother* 2008; **8**:75–92.

85. Brodaty H, Withball A, Sachdev PS. Rates of depression at 3 and 15 months poststroke and their relationship with cognitive decline: the Sydney Stroke Study. *Am J Geriatr Psychiatry* 2007; **15**:477–86.

86. Robinson RG, Jorge RE, Moser DJ, *et al*. Escitalopram and problem-solving therapy for prevention of poststroke depression: a randomized controlled trial. *JAMA* 2008; **299**:2391–400.

87. Ried LD, Jia H, Feng H, *et al*. Selective serotonin reuptake inhibitor treatment and depression are associated with poststroke mortality. *Ann Pharmacother* 2011; **45**:888–97.

88. Román GC, Tatemichi TK, Erkinjuntti T, *et al*. Vascular dementia: diagnostic criteria for research studies. Report of the NINDS-AIREN International Workshop. *Neurology* 1993; **43**(2):250–60.

89. American Psychiatric Association. *Diagnostic and Statistical Manual of Mental Disorders (DSM-4)*, 4th edn. Washington DC: American Psychiatric Association; 1994.

90. Wetterling T, Kanitz RD, Borgis KJ. Comparison of different diagnostic criteria for vascular dementia (ADDTC, DSM-IV, ICD-10, NINDS-AIREN). *Stroke* 1996; **27**:30–6.

91. Dubois MF, Hébert R. The incidence of vascular dementia in Canada: a comparison with Europe and East Asia. *Neuroepidemiology* 2001; **20**(3):179–87.

92. Hénon H, Durieu I, Guerouaou D, *et al*. Poststroke dementia: incidence and relationship to prestroke cognitive decline. *Neurology* 2001; **57**:1216–22.

93. Ince PG, Fernando MS. Neuropathology of vascular cognitive impairment and vascular dementia. *Int Psychogeriatr* 2003; **15** (Suppl1):71–5.

94. Jellinger KA. Pathology and pathophysiology of vascular cognitive impairment. A critical update. *Panminerva Med* 2004; **46**(4):217–21.

95. Skoog I. Status of risk factors for vascular dementia. *Neuroepidemiology* 1998; **17**(1):2–9.

96. Bornstein NM, Gur AY, Treves TA, *et al*. Do silent brain infarctions predict the development of dementia after first ischemic stroke? *Stroke* 1996; **27**:904–5.

97. Longstreth WT Jr, Manolio TA, Arnold A, *et al*. Clinical correlates of white matter findings on cranial magnetic resonance imaging of 3301 elderly people. The Cardiovascular Health Study. *Stroke* 1996; **27**:1274–82.

98. Gur AY, Neufeld MY, Treves TA, *et al*. EEG as predictor of

dementia following first ischemic stroke. *Acta Neurol Scand* 1994; **90**(4):263–5.

99. Snowdon DA, Greiner LH, Mortimer JA, *et al.* Brain infarction and the clinical expression of Alzheimer disease. The Nun Study. *JAMA* 1997; **277**:813–17.

100. Kavirajan H, Schneider LS. Efficacy and adverse effects of cholinesterase inhibitors and memantine in vascular dementia: a meta-analysis of randomised controlled trials. *Lancet Neurol* 2007; **6**:782–92.

101. Ingles JL, Eskes GA, Phillips SJ. Fatigue after stroke. *Arch Phys Med Rehabil* 1999; **80**(2):173–8.

102. Staub F, Bogousslavsky J. Fatigue after stroke: a major but neglected issue. *Cerebrovasc Dis* 2001; **12**:75–81.

103. Fisk JD, Pontefract A, Ritvo PG, Archibald CJ, Murray TJ. The impact of fatigue on patients with multiple sclerosis. *Can J Neurol Sci* 1994; **21**:9–14.

104. Rose L, Pugh LC, Lears K, Gordon DL. The fatigue experience: persons with HIV infection. *J Adv Nurs* 1998; **28**:295–304.

105. Riemsma RP, Rasker JJ, Taal E, *et al.* Fatigue in rheumatoid arthritis: the role of self-efficacy and problematic social support. *Br J Rheumatol* 1998; **37**:1042–6.

106. Zwarts MJ, Bleijenberg G, van Engelen BG. Clinical neurophysiology of fatigue. *Clin Neurophysiol* 2008; **119**:2–10.

107. van der Werf SP, van den Broek HL, Anten HW, Bleijenberg G. Experience of severe fatigue long after stroke and its relation to depressive symptoms and disease characteristics. *Eur Neurol* 2001; **45**:28–33.

108. Kutlubaev MA, Duncan FH, Mead GE. Biological correlates of post-stroke fatigue: a systematic review. *Acta Neurol Scand* 2012; **125**:219–27.

109. Glader EL, Stegmayr B, Asplund K. Poststroke fatigue: a 2-year follow-up study of stroke patients in Sweden. *Stroke* 2002; **33**:1327–33.

110. Naess H, Lunde L, Brogger J, Waje-Andreassen U. Fatigue among stroke patients on long-term follow-up. The Bergen Stroke Study. *J Neurol Sci* 2012; **312**:138–41.

Infections in stroke

Achim J. Kaasch and Harald Seifert

Introduction

Bacterial, viral, and parasitic infections are associated with stroke in several ways. First, at least 20% of strokes are preceded by a bacterial infection in the month prior to stroke. Second, many pathogens that affect the central nervous system are able to directly cause stroke. Third, patients who suffer a stroke are prone to develop infectious complications due to post-stroke immunodepression and impaired swallow and cough reflexes.

In this chapter, we will briefly summarize available evidence on how bacterial infections can trigger stroke. Then, specific infectious diseases that are a direct cause of stroke, such as endocarditis, vasculitis, and chronic meningitis, are reviewed. Furthermore, aspiration pneumonia is discussed, as an example of an early infectious complication that arises within the first week after stroke. Other infectious complications, such as ventilator-associated pneumonia or catheter-related infections, will not be covered since they are common infections in the hospital with no specific link to stroke.

Infections preceding stroke

Recent infection and stroke

Several studies have supplied evidence that acute infection in the week preceding stroke is an independent risk factor for cerebral infarction (odds ratio 3.4–14.5) [1–3]. Especially bacterial respiratory and urinary tract infections can trigger ischemic stroke [4]. Since a heterogeneous group of microbial pathogens is involved, the systemic inflammatory response is probably more important than microbial invasion per se. However, a detailed molecular understanding of events that lead to a higher susceptibility to

cerebral infarction is lacking. Numerous mechanisms have been discussed [5]. For example, inflammation has been implicated in atheroma instability and subsequent plaque rupture, alteration of the coagulation system, platelet aggregation, adhesion, and lysis. Furthermore, alteration of the lipid metabolism, spasms in vascular smooth muscle, antiphospholipid antibody formation, and impairment of endothelial function by endotoxin and bacterial toxins have been reported. Apart from these factors, dehydration, bed rest, and mechanical factors such as sneezing may play a role.

Aside from bacterial infection, common viral diseases such as seasonal flu may trigger stroke. Several observational studies suggest that influenza and pneumococcal vaccinations lower the risk of myocardial infarction and stroke in the elderly [6, 7]. However, conclusive evidence for a protective effect is still lacking.

Chronic infections and stroke

Atherosclerosis is a common disease and a major risk factor for stroke. Its etiology can largely be explained by the classic risk factors (age, gender, genetic predisposition, hypertension, diabetes, hypercholesterolemia, high-fat diet, smoking, low physical activity, etc.). Additionally, pathogens such as *Helicobacter pylori*, cytomegalovirus, herpes simplex virus, and *Chlamydia pneumoniae* have been proposed to be associated with atherosclerosis.

Most studies on the infectious etiology of atherosclerosis have been focused on *C. pneumoniae* (for review see Watson and Alp [8]). *C. pneumoniae* is an obligate intracellular bacterium and usually causes mild upper respiratory tract infection, and occasionally pneumonia. Exposure to this agent is common and by the age of 20 years 50% of individuals are seropositive.

Animal models support a role of *C. pneumoniae* in the initiation, maintenance, and rupture of atherosclerotic lesions, but clinical and epidemiological studies have not come to conclusive results. This shortcoming might be explained by the difficulty in attributing causality to a common pathogen and a multifactorial disease.

As with atherosclerosis, the contribution of chronic bacterial infections to the etiology of stroke is unclear. Some studies found an increased risk of stroke in patients with elevated antibody titers suggesting previous *C. pneumoniae* infection, *H. pylori* gastritis, and periodontal disease (caused by a great variety of bacteria). For these pathogens conflicting information has been published [9, 10] and randomized interventional trials, for example, aiming at the eradication of *C. pneumoniae* by macrolide therapy, failed to reduce the incidence of vascular events [11, 12]. In one study the "infectious burden," defined as previous infections with above-mentioned pathogens measured by serological studies, was associated with a higher risk for first stroke [13]. However, which bacteria should be included in a stroke-risk panel and how the microbial burden is measured remains an open question, as does, even more so, whether and when antimicrobial intervention may be appropriate.

Acute and chronic infections can raise the risk of cerebral infarction.

Infectious diseases that cause stroke

Multiple pathophysiological mechanisms can lead to stroke in bacterial, viral, and parasitic diseases. An overview of organisms implicated in infectious diseases that may lead to stroke and their associated pathophysiology is presented in Table 21.1. For example, (i) emboli from infected heart valves in bacterial or fungal endocarditis may obstruct cerebral arteries; (ii) direct microbial invasion and inflammation of the vessel wall can lead to wall destruction and obliteration of the lumen, as in obliterative vasculitis or necrotizing panarteritis; (iii) chronic inflammation of the meninges leads to stroke through several mechanisms; (iv) mycotic aneurysms can rupture and cause hemorrhagic stroke. In the following section we will review some of these diseases and associated pathogenic principles.

Table 21.1. Infectious causes of stroke and associated mechanisms

Embolism

Bacteria and fungi

Infective endocarditis	*Staphylococcus aureus*, *Streptococcus* spp., *Enterococcus* spp., *Aspergillus* spp., and others

Protozoa

Chagas disease	*Trypanosoma cruzi*

Meningitis

Bacteria

Acute meningitis	*Neisseria meningitidis*, *Haemophilus influenzae*, *Streptococcus pneumoniae*, and others
Chronic meningitis	*Mycobacterium tuberculosis*, *Borrelia burgdorferi*, *Treponema pallidum*

Fungi

Chronic meningitis	*Cryptococcus neoformans*, *Coccidioides immitis*

Helminths

Chronic meningitis	*Taenia solium* (cysticercosis)

Vasculitis

Virus

Vasculopathy	Varicella zoster virus, HIV

Mycotic aneurysm

Bacteria

	Staphylococcus aureus, *Salmonella enteritidis*, and others

Fungi

	Aspergillus spp., *Candida* spp.

Embolic stroke

Infective endocarditis

Infective endocarditis (IE) is an infection of the endocardium, a thin tissue layer that lines heart valves and mural myocardium (Figure 21.1). The incidence of IE is about 5–10 cases per 100 000 person-years and it is a serious disease with about 20% mortality. The main risk factors for endocarditis are an underlying structural heart disease (such as congenital heart defects or degenerative valvular lesions), injection drug use,

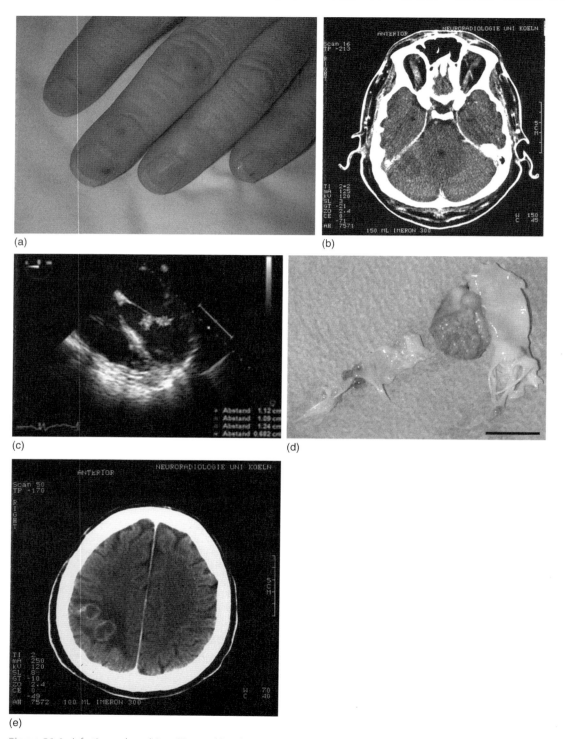

Figure 21.1. Infective endocarditis: a 53-year-old male presented with a 1-week history of malaise, fever (up to 41 °C), behavioral changes, and headache. On clinical examination mild meningeal signs, left-sided ataxia, and splinter hemorrhages (a) were noted. Computed tomography (CT) of the brain showed several ischemic lesions in both hemispheres and right cerebellum (b). *Staphylococcus aureus* was cultured from blood and cerebrospinal fluid. Transesophageal echocardiography revealed a large mitral valve vegetation (c) which was subsequently removed surgically (d, bar = 1 cm). A CT scan 3 weeks after initial symptoms showed abscess formation with contrast enhancement and marked edema (e). (Courtesy of K. Lackner, Department of Radiology, F. Dodos, Department of Cardiology, and J. Wippermann, Department of Cardiac Surgery, University Hospital of Cologne).

hemodialysis, and invasive intravascular procedures. Carriers of a prosthetic heart valve are especially at risk, with a 1–4% chance of developing IE within the first year following surgery[14].

IE is caused by bacteria or fungi that attach to and damage the endocardium or the prosthetic valve and grow into vegetations measuring up to several centimeters in size. If left untreated, destruction of the heart valve ultimately leads to heart failure and death. Complications, e.g. stroke, can arise when emboli break off from the vegetation and occlude blood vessels, leading to infarction of the dependant cerebral tissue.

Microbiology of IE

Many bacteria and fungi can cause IE, some of which are listed with their overall frequency of isolation in Table 21.2. Different clinical conditions favor certain microbes, e.g. right-sided endocarditis in injection drug users is commonly caused by *Staphylococcus aureus* (>80%). In patients with prosthetic heart valves, late IE (i.e. more than 2 months after surgery) is less often caused by *S. aureus* than by

coagulase-negative staphylococci (about 30% of all cases). Although fungal pathogens are rarely a cause of IE, *Candida* or *Aspergillus* spp. may occur in immune compromised patients.

Depending on the causative organisms different clinical courses can be observed. *S. aureus* and Enterobacteriaceae such as *Escherichia coli* or *Klebsiella pneumoniae* are associated with an acute course and high mortality. Patients with IE due to enterococci or viridans group streptococci usually report several weeks of symptoms before a clinical diagnosis is made.

Clinical presentation and diagnostic criteria in IE

Clinical signs and symptoms for IE are highly variable and often misleading. Fever, heart murmur, malaise, anorexia, weight loss, night sweats, and myalgia may or may not occur. The clinical course can be acute or subacute. Therefore IE is often recognized late, e.g. when complications have occurred.

To facilitate diagnosis of IE, diagnostic criteria have been developed. From the results of the clinical examination, blood cultures, and ultrasound imaging (preferably transesophageal echocardiography, TEE) a clinical score is derived that describes the likelihood of IE in a specific patient (e.g. Duke criteria, see Table 21.3).

Neurological complications of IE are common (about 20–40%) and are associated with a worse outcome [15]. They include stroke, intracranial or subarachnoidal hemorrhage, meningitis, seizures, encephalopathy, brain abscess, and mycotic aneurysm (frequencies in Table 21.4). Most neurological complications may go unnoticed. In a study by Snygg-Martin *et al.* cerebrovascular events were detected by MRI in 65% of patients with left-sided IE, but clinical symptoms were observed in only 35% of patients [16].

Pathogenesis of IE

IE is the result of a complex interaction between microorganism, matrix molecules, and platelets at the site of endocardial cell damage. The pathophysiological process can be divided into several stages: formation of non-bacterial thrombotic endocarditis (NBTE), bacterial colonization of the lesion, and growth into vegetations [17].

Endocardial damage is the starting point of IE pathogenesis. It is caused by congenital or acquired heart diseases that are associated with a turbulent blood flow. Then, fibrin and platelets are deposited

Table 21.2. Distribution of etiological agents in 2781 patients with definite endocarditis from 58 locations worldwide

Pathogen	Mean
Staphylococci	
Staphylococcus aureus	31%
Coagulase-negative staphylococci	11%
Streptococci	
Viridans group streptococci	17%
Streptococcus bovis	6%
Other streptococci	6%
Enterococcus species	10%
Gram-negative aerobic bacilli (e.g. HACEK group*)	2%
Fungi/yeast (e.g. *Candida* spp., *Aspergillus* spp.)	2%
Other bacteria	4%
Polymicrobial infections	1%
Culture negative	10%

HACEK: *Haemophilus aphrophilus, Aggregatibacter actinomycetemcomitans, Cardiobacterium hominis, Eikenella corrodens,* and *Kingella kingae.*
Source: Adapted from Murdoch *et al.* [18].

Table 21.3. Modified Duke criteria for the diagnosis of infective endocarditis. The diagnosis of IE is *definite* when (i) pathological/microbiological examination of vegetation shows active endocarditis, or (ii) two major criteria, or (iii) one major and three minor, or (iv) five minor criteria are met. IE is *possible* when (i) one major and one minor, or (ii) three minor criteria are met. It is *rejected* when (i) a firm alternative diagnosis explaining evidence of IE or (ii) resolution of IE syndrome with ≤4 days of antimicrobial treatment, or (iii) no pathological evidence of IE at surgery or autopsy with ≤4 days of antimicrobial treatment, or criteria for possible or (iv) definite IE are not met.

Major criteria

Blood culture positive for IE

Typical microorganism consistent with IE isolated from two separate blood cultures (viridans group streptococci, *Streptococcus bovis*, HACEK group, *Staphylococcus aureus; or* community-acquired enterococci, in the absence of a primary focus)

or Microorganism consistent with IE from persistently positive blood cultures (defined as at least two positive cultures of blood samples drawn >12 hours apart; *or* all of three or a majority of four or more separate cultures of blood, with first and last sample drawn at least 1 hour apart)

or Single positive blood culture for *Coxiella burnetti* or a high phase I IgG antibody titer (>1:800)

Evidence of endocardial involvement

Echocardiogram positive for IE[*] as follows: oscillating intracardiac mass on valve or supporting structures, in the path of regurgitant jets, or on implanted material in the absence of an alternative anatomical explanation; abscess; new partial dehiscence of prosthetic valve

or New valvular regurgitation (worsening or changing of pre-existing murmur not sufficient)

Minor criteria

Predisposition (predisposing heart condition or injection drug use)
Fever (temperature >38 °C)
Vascular phenomena

major arterial emboli, septic pulmonary infarcts, mycotic aneurysm, intracranial hemorrhage, conjunctival hemorrhage, and Janeway lesions

Immunological phenomena

glomerulonephritis, Osler nodes, Roth spots, and rheumatoid factor

Suggestive microbiological findings

positive blood culture not meeting major criterion[**] or serological evidence of active infection with organism consistent with IE

Notes: [*] Transesophageal echocardiography (TEE) recommended in patients with prosthetic valves, rated at least "possible IE" by clinical criteria, or complicated IE (paravalvular abscess). TTE as first test in other patients.
[**] Excludes single positive culture findings for coagulase-negative staphylococci and organisms that do not cause endocarditis.
Source: Adapted from Li *et al.* [53]

Table 21.4. Frequencies of neurological complications in infective endocarditis based on 1365 cases from seven studies

Complication	Frequency
Emboli	20–57%
Intra- or subarachnoidal hemorrhage	7–25%
Mycotic aneurysm	3–16%
Meningitis	6–39%
Abscess	2–16%
Encephalopathy	17–33%
Seizure	2–29%
Headache	9–25%

Source: Adapted from Cavassini *et al.* [54].

on traumatized endothelium, which results in NBTE. Microorganisms that have gained access to the bloodstream (bacteremia) and possess the necessary virulence factors may now colonize the lesion and lead to IE.

A frequent cause of bacteremia is damage of the skin or a mucosal surface. The skin and mucosal surfaces, such as oral cavity, nasopharynx, gastrointestinal tract, urethra, or vagina, are populated by a dense endogenous flora with many diverse bacterial species. Even a minor trauma such as tooth brushing or tooth extraction may lead to a temporary occurrence of bacteria in the bloodstream (transient bacteremia).

After having gained access to the bloodstream, IE-causing pathogens adhere to the NBTE. Adhesion to fibrin and platelets or to the surface of medical devices, such as artificial heart valves, is facilitated by microbial surface components recognizing adhesive matrix molecules (MSCRAMM), many of which have been identified in staphylococci, streptococci, and enterococci.

Following adhesion, bacteria stimulate the deposition of further fibrin and platelets and a secluded compartment is formed, which hides bacteria from the host immunological defense. The microorganisms proliferate and produce a thick mucilaginous polysaccharide matrix which is called biofilm. In a biofilm less than 10% of bacteria divide actively and responsiveness to antimicrobials is decreased. Since antimicrobials need to penetrate the biofilm to reach the bacterial targets, optimal antimicrobial treatment is crucial for a successful therapy of IE.

Pathogenic mechanisms leading to stroke in IE

Septic or sterile emboli that originate from vegetations and occlude cerebral arteries are a common cause of stroke in IE. Impairment of the cerebral blood flow can lead to a transient ischemic attack (TIA) or stroke. Depending on the localization and duration of reduced blood flow, focal clinical signs occur. When multiple emboli occlude several independent vessels, multifocal clinical signs may become apparent.

The source of emboli to the central nervous system is usually the left heart, from vegetations on the mitral or aortic valve. Emboli from the right heart are filtered by intrapulmonary arteries and cause pulmonary embolism. Therefore, tricuspid valve endocarditis, which is common among intravenous drug users, rarely leads to stroke. However, in rare cases paradoxical embolism has been reported.

Other complications of IE, such as brain abscesses and meningitis, may also lead to stroke. A brain abscess occurs when bacteria have seeded via the bloodstream to the brain parenchyma. Brain abscesses are a rare complication of IE and occur in less than 1% of patients with IE [15]. A brain abscess typically develops over 2–3 weeks. Initial imaging studies show a poorly demarcated lesion with localized edema. Over the weeks a clearly defined lesion develops, often accompanied by an extensive edema. The early stage is called cerebritis and is histologically defined by acute inflammation without tissue necrosis.

During abscess development tissue necrosis, liquefaction, and a fibrotic capsule become more prominent. A typical histological finding is a central necrotic area containing bacteria and debris and a hyperemic margin with bacteria and immune cells. In many cases antimicrobial therapy of a brain abscess alone is unsuccessful and has to be backed by surgical drainage.

Bacterial meningitis is caused by hematogenous seeding of microorganisms to the meninges. The inflammatory response can damage arterial vessel walls and cause mycotic aneurysms (see below). Ischemic stroke occurs through obstruction of inflamed vessels, hemorrhagic stroke through rupture of a mycotic aneurysm. The contribution of immune-mediated injury, e.g. by immune-complex deposition, is unknown.

Therapy of IE

Before the advent of antimicrobials, IE has inadvertently led to death. Despite major advances in antimicrobial and surgical therapy, in-hospital mortality is still 15–20% [18].

Antimicrobial therapy should be carefully selected according to the results of antimicrobial susceptibility testing of etiological organisms. Many scientific societies have issued guidelines that recommend specific drug treatment schemes for different organisms [19, 20]. The standard duration of antimicrobial therapy is at least 4–6 weeks and in some cases a combination therapy of two antimicrobials with different modes of action is advised.

To perform susceptibility testing, the offending organism needs to be isolated from blood or valve tissue. With the use of current technology, an initial culture of 40–60 ml of blood (corresponding to 2–3 pairs of blood culture bottles) is considered sufficient. Chances of a successful isolation increase when blood cultures are drawn at the beginning of a fever slope, and before antimicrobial drugs are administered. Blood cultures need to be repeated when IE is suspected and initial cultures did not yield a plausible organism.

In addition to antimicrobial drug treatment, surgical therapy needs to be considered. Indications for surgery are severe heart failure, uncontrolled infection (e.g. persistently positive blood cultures or a paravalvular abscess), and prevention of embolism [20].

Patients who have suffered a recent stroke are at risk of hemorrhagic transformation of a non-hemorrhagic infarct due to the anticoagulation necessary for the cardiopulmonary bypass. Whether heart valve replacement can be safely performed within the first 2 weeks after stroke is a matter of debate. In a recent multicenter study delay of surgery did not lead to a survival benefit [21]. However, each individual patient needs to be carefully evaluated by a multidisciplinary team.

347

Occlusion of cerebral arteries by septic or sterile emboli that originate from the vegetations is a common cause for stroke in infective endocarditis (IE). IE is often diagnosed late and should be treated with a carefully selected antimicrobial therapy for at least 4–6 weeks. Additionally, surgical therapy needs to be considered.

Embolic stroke due to Chagas disease

Chagas disease is an infection with the protozoan parasite *Trypanosoma cruzi*, which is most prevalent in South and Central America. The parasite is transmitted by the feces of an insect vector (*Triatoma* and other assassin bug species). Additionally, transmission occurs by vertical transmission from mother to child, contaminated foods, blood products, and organ transplant. Once inside the host, the parasite multiplies within various host cells and is distributed via the bloodstream. After an often asymptomatic acute infection, the parasite can persist in various tissues, including adipose tissue. Chronic infection can persist for years or decades and may be asymptomatic. In 10–30% of patients parasitic invasion of the heart muscle leads to cardiomyopathy, probably through chronic inflammation [22].

Embolic stroke may be the first sign of cardiac Chagas disease. Conditions that predispose to cardiac emboli in Chagas disease are cardiac arrhythmias, congestive heart failure, apical aneurysms, and mural thrombus formation. By the time stroke occurs, the damage to the heart is irreversible. Thus effort needs to be directed towards prevention of *Trypanosoma* infection by vector control and improvement of basic housing conditions, as well as early diagnosis and treatment.

Meningitis as a cause of stroke

Meningitis denotes the inflammation of the leptomeninges, which consist of the pia mater and arachnoid mater. These layers ensheath the spinal cord and brain and confine the subarachnoidal space, which contains cerebrospinal fluid (CSF). Infection of the meninges by bacteria or fungi leads to an inflammatory response which causes the typical clinical symptoms, headache and nuchal rigidity. Depending on the time course, meningitis can be classified as acute or chronic.

Acute bacterial meningitis is prevalent worldwide and accounts for an estimated 1.2 million cases with 185 000 deaths per year. Patients present with fever,

Table 21.5. Acute bacterial meningitis: age groups and most common causative organisms.

Age group	Main pathogens
Neonates (≤1 month)	Enterobacteriaceae, *Streptococcus agalactiae* (group B streptococcus), coagulase-negative staphylococci (in preterm infants)
Children (1 month to 15 years)	*Neisseria meningitidis*, *Streptococcus pneumoniae*, *Haemophilus influenzae*[*]
Adults (>15 years)	*Streptococcus pneumoniae*, *Neisseria meningitidis*

Note: [*] *Haemophilus influenzae* meningitis has become rare with the introduction of vaccination in almost all regions of the world.

nuchal rigidity, and lethargy or confusion. Other less frequent symptoms are photophobia, seizures, petechial bleeding, and arthritis. The disease occurs in all age groups, but the causative organisms vary depending on age (Table 21.5). If left untreated, the disease is fatal.

Diagnosis is based on clinical symptoms, CSF analysis, and microbiological testing. Empiric antimicrobial treatment needs to be initiated as early as possible with antimicrobials that reach adequate bactericidal concentrations in the CSF. The choice of antimicrobial agent needs to be reconsidered when the causative organism is identified and susceptibility testing results become available.

Common complications of acute bacterial meningitis include elevated intracranial pressure, seizures, and hyponatremia. A recent study described cerebral infarction in about 25% of meningitis cases [23].

The underlying molecular mechanisms of stroke in meningitis are not well explored. Most likely, the spreading inflammation involves intracranial vessels and leads to thrombosis and subsequent ischemia or hemorrhage [24].

Chronic meningitis lasts for more than 4 weeks, has a subacute onset, and is often accompanied by fever, headache, and vomiting. There are many infectious and non-infectious causes of chronic meningitis and despite advances in diagnostic techniques, such as PCR, about 30% of cases are idiopathic. In the following sections we will discuss several organisms that cause chronic meningitis with a high incidence of stroke.

Tuberculous meningitis

Tuberculous meningitis is caused by *Mycobacterium tuberculosis*, a hardy slow-growing bacterium whose only natural reservoir is the human. It is taken up by inhalation, phagocytosed by alveolar macrophages, and transported to the lung tissue, where an exudative inflammation is initiated. During the first couple of weeks, mycobacteria are undetected by the cellular immune system and spread to the draining hilar lymph nodes. There they slowly proliferate and the host immune system finally mounts a T-cell response. Depending on the capacity of the host immune system the infection can be cleared or mycobacteria survive within granulomata.

Granulomata are caseous foci with a fibrotic capsule that enwraps viable mycobacteria. They are formed by the host immune system to keep the bacteria contained and prevent further spread of infection. However, they allow the pathogen to persist within its host for decades, until the conditions for growth become more favorable, e.g. when the host immune system is impaired.

The concurrent presence of a granuloma at the site of initial infection and of swollen hilar lymph nodes is a typical feature of early tuberculosis, called "primary complex." Lymphogenous and hematogenous spread may occur to various distant organs, e.g. the meninges, where further granulomata are formed.

When reactivation of the disease occurs, the center of a granuloma liquefies, mycobacteria proliferate, and the granuloma ruptures. Bacteria are released into the surrounding tissue, which leads, in the case of a meningeal granuloma, to tuberculous meningitis.

In tuberculous meningitis, the meningeal inflammation produces a basilar, gelatinous inflammatory exudate in the subarachnoid space. The walls of small and medium-sized arteries that traverse the exudate are invaded by inflammatory cells. Furthermore, disturbance of CSF circulation leads to an increased intracranial pressure.

Ischemic stroke is a relatively frequent complication of tuberculous meningitis and occurs in up to 60% of cases within 12 months [25]. Most cerebral infarcts occur in the anterior circulation. Strangulation and spasm of blood vessels by an intense inflammatory exudate, periarteritis or necrotizing panarteritis, and stretching of blood vessels by increased intracranial pressure are pathogenic mechanisms. Compression of the M1 or M2 segment of the middle cerebral artery by the exudate causes large artery infarctions, whereas multiple infarcts are most likely due to secondary thrombosis.

When tuberculous meningitis is suspected in a patient, the diagnosis needs to be confirmed by microbiological techniques, i.e. direct microscopic examination, culture, or PCR-based techniques, before a long-lasting drug therapy is initiated.

Cryptococcal meningitis

The fungus *Cryptococcus neoformans* is a soil pathogen with a high potential to invade the central nervous system. The infection is often fatal despite antimycotic therapy. Especially immunocompromised individuals with a defect in cellular immunity (e.g. acquired immunodeficiency syndrome [AIDS] patients) are at risk of developing cryptococcal disease. The frequency of ischemic complications is unknown, but stroke is associated with a worse outcome [26, 27].

Coccidioidomycosis

Coccidioides immitis is a fungal pathogen restricted to the deserts of south-western USA, Central, and South America. Inhalation of contaminated soil normally leads to asymptomatic infection or mild pulmonary symptoms. Fewer than 2% of patients develop disseminated disease within weeks to months after exposure. Most common extrapulmonary sites of infection are skin and subcutaneous soft tissue, the meninges, and the skeleton.

Patients with basilar, coccidioidal meningitis have a 30–40% risk of developing cerebral infarcts and they often develop communicating hydrocephalus [28, 29]. Standard antifungal treatment is a lifelong course of oral fluconazole. However, there is a significant risk of relapse.

Neurosyphilis and neuroborreliosis

Other bacterial infections that have been implicated in stroke are the spirochetes *Treponema pallidum* and *Borrelia burgdorferi*. Meningovascular syphilis, caused by *T. pallidum*, is now a rare complication, since syphilis is most often recognized and treated at an earlier stage.

Stroke in syphilis develops as a result of inflammatory infiltration of medium to large arteries. Most often the middle cerebral artery and to a lesser extent basilar arteries are involved [30]. Typically, the onset of stroke is subacute. A diagnosis is based on serological testing of CSF. Additionally, syphilis can cause stroke by other mechanisms, e.g. compression of the left carotid artery by a large aneurysm of the thoracic aorta has been reported [31].

Chronic meningitis in neuroborreliosis, an infection with *B. burgdorferi*, rarely causes stroke [32].

Neurocysticercosis

Neurocysticercosis is the most common parasitic central nervous system infection. The pork tapeworm *Taenia solium* is prevalent worldwide, especially in developing countries. In humans, the definite host, *Taenia solium* lives as a tapeworm in the small intestine and sheds eggs with the feces. The cystic larval form (termed cysticercus) is usually found in the pig. However, when humans ingest shed tapeworm eggs invasive larvae develop in the intestines, penetrate the mucosa, enter the bloodstream, migrate to the tissues, and mature into cysticerci.

Cysticerci have a predilection for neural tissue and often settle in the brain, subarachnoid space, and ventricle. Symptoms depend on localization and size of the larvae and include seizures, headache, visual problems, confusion, and hydrocephalus. About 50% of patients develop arteritis with associated lacunar infarcts and corresponding lacunar syndromes [33]. Erosion of large vessels can occasionally lead to a large artery stroke, preferentially in the territory of the middle cerebral artery.

The diagnosis in non-endemic areas can be difficult and is generally made by a combination of clinical, radiographic, and serological criteria. Cysticerci normally die within 5–7 years after arrival in the brain, a process which can be accelerated by antiparasitic drug treatment. In many cases of symptomatic disease, drug treatment is not sufficient and neurosurgical procedures are required.

> Chronic meningitis, caused by, for example, tuberculosis, neurosyphilis, or neuroborreliosis, can lead to stroke when the spreading inflammation involves intracranial vessels and leads to thrombosis.

Infectious diseases causing vasculitis

Varicella zoster virus vasculopathy

Varicella zoster virus (VZV) can lead to stroke due to viral infection of the cerebral artery walls (for review see Nagel *et al.* [34]). Two different types of infection can be differentiated depending on the immune status of the patient. Immunocompromised individuals, e.g. organ transplant or AIDS patients, show a diffuse inflammation of cerebral blood vessels of all sizes. Immunocompetent patients may develop herpes zoster-associated cerebral angiitis, a granulomatous angiitis that usually affects larger arteries. In both cases, histopathological features include multinucleated giant cells, Cowdry A inclusion bodies, and VZV particles.

Diagnosis of VZV vasculopathy can be difficult, and is based on patient history, imaging studies, and analysis of the CSF. It should be suspected in patients with ischemic lesions in MRI or CT, combined with a positive VZV PCR or serological detection of VZV IgG. Patient history often reveals a typical herpetiform rash. The rash can precede the manifestation of stroke by up to several months. When cerebral angiography is performed, unifocal or multifocal vascular lesions with corresponding lesions in CT or MRI imaging studies can be found.

Randomized clinical trials for standard treatment are lacking. Based on expert opinion, current treatment includes intravenous acyclovir in combination with steroids. A vaccination for VZV is available and has significantly diminished VZV-related morbidity and mortality in children.

HIV-associated vasculopathy and vasculitis

Several cohort studies around the world have shown that stroke in patients with AIDS is more frequent than in an age-adjusted HIV-negative population. However, a firm causal relationship between HIV infection and stroke has yet to be proven (for review see Singer *et al.* [35]). A cohort study on young patients with stroke in South Africa suggests that the mechanisms leading to stroke in HIV-positive patients are largely similar to those in HIV-negative controls [36]. In this study, frequent causes were opportunistic infections (tuberculosis, neurosyphilis, varicella zoster vasculopathy, cryptococcal meningitis), coagulopathy, and cardioembolism. In 10–20% of the cases, HIV-associated vasculitis was suspected as a cause of stroke.

Several molecular mechanisms may promote ischemic stroke in patients with HIV: induction of autoantibodies (e.g. anticardiolipin, antiphospholipid, and anti-prothrombin antibodies), vasculitis, aneurysmal arteriopathy, and accelerated atherosclerosis [35]. In the early stages of HIV infection an intracranial vasculopathy of small arteries can be found [37].

Histological features are thickening of the vessel wall, perivascular space dilatation, rarefaction, pigment deposition, and occasional perivascular inflammatory cell infiltrates. This condition is associated with asymptomatic microinfarcts and may predispose to ischemic stroke. In later stages of AIDS, HIV-associated vasculitis can be found, a poorly characterized entity that involves large or medium-sized intra- or extracranial arteries. It results in fusiform aneurysms, stenosis, or thrombosis and can lead to ischemic or hemorrhagic stroke. Whether HIV-associated vasculitis is directly caused by HIV infection or is due to an undetected opportunistic infection is still under debate [38].

The use of combination antiretroviral therapy also increases the risk of stroke and heart disease [35]. Adverse effects that may predispose to stroke are dyslipidemia and glucose intolerance.

> Vasculitis from infectious diseases, e.g. varicella zoster virus and HIV, can result in ischemic stroke.

Mycotic aneurysms as cause of stroke

Mycotic aneurysms are caused by bacteria or fungi and account for a minority (about 3%) of all intracranial aneurysms. They develop in a significant fraction of patients with IE (3–16%), due to microemboli that congest the vasa vasorum of the cerebral arteries. In these patients, rupture of a mycotic aneurysm without adequate antimicrobial therapy is frequent (57%) but the risk after a full course of antimicrobial treatment is very low; however, it is a potentially devastating event [39].

Different mechanisms have been implicated in aneurysm formation; (1) septic microemboli to the vasa vasorum; (2) hematogenous seeding of bacteria to atherosclerotic vessels; (3) extension from a contiguous infected focus; and (4) direct contamination through trauma of the arterial wall. Infection of the vessel wall leads to necrosis, local hemorrhage, and abscess formation. The muscularis and elastica layers are destroyed, but the intima often remains intact. Bacterial aneurysms are usually small, saccular, and localized at multiple sites, whereas fungal aneurysms are long, large, and fusiform.

The causative organisms of intracerebral aneurysms are the same as for IE, mainly viridans group streptococci, *S. aureus*, enterococci, and other *Streptococcus* spp. Enterobacteriaceae, in particular non-typhi *Salmonella* spp., play an important role in

extracranial aneurysms but rarely cause intracranial aneurysms.

Among the fungi, *Aspergillus* spp. are a well-described cause of true fungal mycotic aneurysms. An important virulence factor of *Aspergillus* spp. is the enzyme elastase, which degrades elastic fibers of the vessel wall [40].

Central nervous system aspergillosis usually occurs in immunocompromised patients and manifests as a triad: mycotic aneurysm, stroke, and granuloma formation. The mortality associated with intracranial aspergillosis is high and patients with mycotic aneurysms who survived have not been reported. Aside from aneurysm rupture, *Aspergillus* spp. can lead to stroke by thrombotic occlusion due to vascular extension of hyphae.

> In patients with infective endocarditis and in immunocompromised patients, rupture of mycotic aneurysms can be the cause of stroke.

Infectious diseases with similarities to stroke: toxoplasmosis and malaria encephalitis

Cerebral toxoplasmosis, an infection with the protozoan parasite *Toxoplasma gondii*, mainly occurs as an opportunistic infection in immunocompromised individuals, especially in AIDS patients. The parasite is transmitted by undercooked meat or cat feces and taken up by the oral route.

During often asymptomatic initial infection, the parasite disseminates into various tissues and forms dormant tissue cysts, especially in the brain and muscle tissue. Reactivation of dormant parasites during an impaired immune response leads to lesions with a necrotic central area, hyperemic border, and sometimes a thin fibrotic capsule. A feature that distinguishes these lesions from an abscess is a hypertrophic arteritis with or without thrombotic arterial occlusion that causes discrete infarcts. Thus cerebral toxoplasmosis results in a slowly expanding ischemic lesion [41].

Clinical signs depend on the localization of the lesions and, in contrast to acute ischemic stroke, onset is often subacute. MR and CT imaging studies often show multiple ring enhancing lesions that can occur anywhere in the brain or spinal cord, but are most often localized in the basal ganglia. Definite diagnosis requires histological demonstration of the organism

351

or PCR-based methods. To prevent the occurrence of toxoplasmosis in immunocompromised patients, antimicrobial prophylaxis (e.g. with trimethoprim-sulfamethoxazole) is initiated depending on CD4$^+$ T-cell counts.

The pathogenesis of cerebral malaria shares some similarity with stroke (for review see Idro et al. [42]). The causative organism of falciparum malaria is the protozoan parasite *Plasmodium falciparum*, which is transmitted by mosquitoes (*Anopheles* spp.). Common clinical manifestations of cerebral malaria are seizures, respiratory distress, and impaired consciousness.

During infection *P. falciparum* invades red blood cells and alters their surface properties. As a result, erythrocytes stick to the endothelium of the cerebral blood vessels and reduce the microvascular flow. Additionally, the membrane of infected erythrocytes becomes less deformable and thus travelling through narrow capillaries is more difficult.

As in stroke, the reduced blood flow impairs the delivery of substrates, which causes hypoxia, reduction of the blood–brain barrier, and ultimately brain swelling. At autopsy petechial hemorrhages are regularly observed, but infarction, necrosis, and large hemorrhages are rare.

> In the course of malaria and toxoplasmosis, ischemic lesions mimicking stroke can occur.

Infectious diseases as complication of stroke

Early-onset infectious complications

Infectious complications after acute stroke are common. In a recent meta-analysis of 87 studies that included 137 817 patients with stroke, 30% of patients developed infections. The most prominent infections were pneumonia (10%) and urinary tract infections (10%) [43]. In this meta-analysis infections increased the risk of death and particularly pneumonia was significantly associated with death (odds ratio 3.6).

Diagnostic workup of infections post-stroke

When clinical signs or laboratory testing results (e.g. fever or hypothermia, leukocytosis, elevated C-reactive protein [CRP] serum levels) point towards an infection, diagnostic specimens should be obtained for microbiological testing. A diagnostic workup is guided by the clinical signs and symptoms and should include blood cultures, urine culture, and a chest X-ray. If pneumonia is suspected, sputum or tracheal aspirate should be sampled. Microbiological specimens should be obtained before antimicrobial therapy is initiated.

Aspiration pneumonia

Pneumonia in stroke patients is most often caused by dysphagia and secondary aspiration. In up to 70% of stroke patients the cough and swallow reflexes are impaired and oropharyngeal or gastric content may gain access to the lungs, where bacteria originating from oropharyngeal or gastric secretions can initiate an infectious process [44]. However, aspiration is not sufficient to initiate infection, since aspiration of nasopharyngeal secretions regularly occurs in healthy individuals during sleep, at an estimated volume of 0.01–0.2 ml [45]. Major risk factors for aspiration pneumonia are older age, stroke, altered mental state, poor oral hygiene, and gastroesophageal reflux disease (for review see Shigemitsu and Afshar [46]).

Patients that are at increased risk of developing pneumonia within 7 days after stroke can be identified by the PANTHERIS score, which is based on age, Glasgow Coma Scale, white blood cell count, and systolic arterial blood pressure [47].

The high frequency of pneumonia in stroke patients has led to the concept of post-stroke immunosuppression. Although this concept is largely based on experimental stroke models, data suggest that release of catecholamines and steroids by sympathetic activation after stroke increases susceptibility to infection [48]. Downregulation of the immune system during a life-threatening condition seems paradoxical but it may serve to prevent damage to the brain by immune cells [49].

To reduce the risk of aspiration pneumonia, post-stroke patients need to be observed for potential aspiration of fluids or semi-solids and the diet should be adapted accordingly [50]. Other measures (positioning, oral hygiene, tube feeding) have been proposed for the prevention of aspiration pneumonia. However, controlled clinical trials in stroke patients are lacking.

Antimicrobial therapy to prevent aspiration pneumonia has been shown to be effective in a mouse model [51], and four randomized clinical trials have been carried out to assess its usefulness in patients with stroke. A meta-analysis demonstrated that preventive antimicrobial therapy reduced the risk of infection but did not reduce mortality [52]. Larger, multicenter studies are needed to assess the usefulness of preventive antimicrobial therapy.

Therapy of aspiration pneumonia is largely based on appropriate antimicrobial treatment. Empiric regimens should cover *S. pneumoniae*, *S. aureus*, *Haemophilus influenzae*, and Gram-negative enteric bacilli and anaerobic bacteria and should follow local treatment guidelines. To guide further treatment, proper specimens for microbiological analysis, preferably bronchoalveolar lavage fluid and blood cultures, should be obtained.

Urinary tract infections

Urinary tract infections (UTI) are common infections post-stroke, since many patients have indwelling catheters in place, which convey a significant risk of infection. Intermittent catheterization has not been shown to reduce the risk of infection. Asymptomatic occurrence of bacteria in the urine (bacteriuria) needs to be distinguished from a true infection. Signs of UTI include mild irritative symptoms, such as frequency and urgency, dysuria, fever, and severe systemic manifestations, such as bacteremia and sepsis.

Microbiological examination of a urine specimen confirms the diagnosis, identifies the causative organism, and provides susceptibility testing results. Since antimicrobial treatment is initiated only in symptomatic infections, routine culture is not recommended.

Initial treatment is strongly dependent on local resistance patterns and should follow local guidelines. Urine cultures should be obtained prior to the start of antimicrobial therapy.

> Infectious complications after acute stroke are common, mostly pneumonia and urinary tract infections.

Chapter summary

> Acute infection in the week preceding stroke is an independent risk factor for cerebral infarction; the "infectious burden concept" states that the aggregate burden of microbial antigens determines stroke risk rather than the occurrence of a single pathogen.
>
> **Embolic stroke** can be caused by infective endocarditis (IE). The main risk factors for endocarditis are an underlying structural heart disease (especially prosthetic valves), injection drug use, hemodialysis, and invasive intravascular procedures. Clinical signs and symptoms of IE are highly variable and often misleading, therefore IE is often diagnosed late.
>
> Occlusion of cerebral arteries by septic or sterile emboli that originate from vegetations, usually in the left heart, is a common cause of stroke in IE. To recover the causative organism, at least two blood cultures need to be drawn (40–60 ml). Antimicrobial therapy should be carefully selected according to the results of antimicrobial susceptibility testing and be given for at least 4–6 weeks. In addition, surgical therapy needs to be considered. Embolic stroke may also be the first sign of cardiac Chagas disease.
>
> **Meningitis** can lead to stroke. Most likely the spreading inflammation involves intracranial vessels and leads to thrombosis and subsequent ischemia or hemorrhage. Organisms that cause chronic meningitis with a high incidence of stroke are:
> - Tuberculosis. Ischemic stroke is a relatively frequent complication of tuberculous meningitis and occurs in about 30% of cases.
> - Coccidioidomycosis. Patients with basilar, coccidioidal meningitis have a 40% risk of developing cerebral infarcts and they often develop communicating hydrocephalus.
> - Neurosyphilis and neuroborreliosis.
> - Neurocysticercosis.
>
> **Vasculitis** from infectious diseases, e.g. varicella zoster virus and HIV, can result in ischemic stroke.
>
> **Mycotic aneurysms** account for about 3% of all intracranial aneurysms. Rupture of a mycotic aneurysm without adequate antimicrobial therapy is frequent.
>
> **Cerebral toxoplasmosis** results in a slowly expanding ischemic lesion because it leads to a hypertrophic arteritis with or without thrombotic arterial occlusion that causes discrete infarcts. In **cerebral malaria** the infected erythrocytes stick to the endothelium of the cerebral blood vessels and reduce the microvascular flow.
>
> **Infectious complications** after acute stroke are common, mostly pneumonia and urinary tract infections. Pneumonia in stroke patients is most often caused by dysphagia and secondary aspiration. To prevent aspiration pneumonia, post-stroke patients need to be screened for potential aspiration of fluids or semi-solids and the diet should be adapted accordingly.

References

1. Grau AJ, Buggle F, Heindl S, *et al.* Recent infection as a risk factor for cerebrovascular ischemia. *Stroke* 1995; **26**:373–9.

2. Paganini-Hill A, Lozano E, Fischberg G, *et al.* Infection and risk of ischemic stroke: differences among stroke subtypes. *Stroke* 2003; **34**:452–7.

3. Smeeth L, Thomas SL, Hall AJ, *et al.* Risk of myocardial infarction and stroke after acute infection or vaccination. *N Engl J Med* 2004; **351**:2611–18.

4. Lichy C, Grau AJ. Investigating the association between influenza vaccination and reduced stroke risk. *Expert Rev Vaccines* 2006; **5**:535–40.

5. Grau AJ, Urbanek C, Palm F. Common infections and the risk of stroke. *Nat Rev Neurol* 2010; **6**:681–94.

6. Vila-Corcoles A, Ochoa-Gondar O, Rodriguez-Blanco T, *et al.* Clinical effectiveness of pneumococcal vaccination against acute myocardial infarction and stroke in people over 60 years: the capamis study, one-year follow-up. *BMC Pub Health* 2012; **12**:222.

7. Hung IF, Leung AY, Chu DW, *et al.* Prevention of acute myocardial infarction and stroke among elderly persons by dual pneumococcal and influenza vaccination: a prospective cohort study. *Clin Infect Dis* 2010; **51**:1007–16.

8. Watson C, Alp NJ. Role of *Chlamydia pneumoniae* in atherosclerosis. *Clin Sci (Lond)* 2008; **114**:509–31.

9. Elkind MS, Cole JW. Do common infections cause stroke? *Semin Neurol* 2006; **26**:88–99.

10. Grau AJ, Marquardt L, Lichy C. The effect of infections and vaccinations on stroke risk. *Expert Rev Neurother* 2006; **6**:175–83.

11. Grayston JT, Kronmal RA, Jackson LA, *et al.* Azithromycin for the secondary prevention of coronary events. *N Engl J Med* 2005; **352**:1637–45.

12. O'Connor CM, Dunne MW, Pfeffer MA, *et al.* Azithromycin for the secondary prevention of coronary heart disease events: the wizard study: a randomized controlled trial. *JAMA* 2003; **290**:1459–66.

13. Elkind MS, Ramakrishnan P, Moon YP, *et al.* Infectious burden and risk of stroke: the northern Manhattan study. *Arch Neurol* 2010; **67**:33–8.

14. Bayer AS. Infective endocarditis. *Clin Infect Dis* 1993; **17**:313–20.

15. Garcia-Cabrera E, Fernandez-Hidalgo N, Almirante B, *et al.* Neurological complications of infective endocarditis: risk factors, outcome, and impact of cardiac surgery: a multicenter observational study. *Circulation* 2013; **127**:2272–84.

16. Snygg-Martin U, Gustafsson L, Rosengren L, *et al.* Cerebrovascular complications in patients with left-sided infective endocarditis are common: a prospective study using magnetic resonance imaging and neurochemical brain damage markers. *Clin Infect Dis* 2008; **47**:23–30.

17. Garrison PK, Freedman LR. Experimental endocarditis I. Staphylococcal endocarditis in rabbits resulting from placement of a polyethylene catheter in the right side of the heart. *Yale J Biol Med* 1970; **42**:394–410.

18. Murdoch DR, Corey GR, Hoen B, *et al.* Clinical presentation, etiology, and outcome of infective endocarditis in the 21st century: the international collaboration on endocarditis-prospective cohort study. *Arch Intern Med* 2009; **169**:463–73.

19. Baddour LM, Wilson WR, Bayer AS, *et al.* Infective endocarditis: diagnosis, antimicrobial therapy, and management of complications: a statement for healthcare professionals from the Committee on Rheumatic Fever, Endocarditis, and Kawasaki Disease, Council on Cardiovascular Disease in the Young, and the Councils on Clinical Cardiology, Stroke, and Cardiovascular Surgery and Anesthesia, American Heart Association: endorsed by the Infectious Diseases Society of America. *Circulation* 2005; **111**: e394–434.

20. Habib G, Hoen B, Tornos P, *et al.* Guidelines on the prevention, diagnosis, and treatment of infective endocarditis (new version 2009): the Task Force on the Prevention, Diagnosis, and Treatment of Infective Endocarditis of the European Society of Cardiology (ESC). Endorsed by the European Society of Clinical Microbiology and Infectious Diseases (ESCMID) and the International Society of Chemotherapy (ISC) for Infection and Cancer. *Eur Heart J* 2009; **30**:2369–413.

21. Barsic B, Dickerman S, Krajinovic V, *et al.* Influence of the timing of cardiac surgery on the outcome of patients with infective endocarditis and stroke. *Clin Infect Dis* 2013; **56**:209–17.

22. Carod-Artal FJ. Chagas cardiomyopathy and ischemic stroke. *Expert Rev Cardiovasc Ther* 2006; **4**:119–30.

23. Schut ES, Lucas MJ, Brouwer MC, *et al.* Cerebral infarction in adults with bacterial meningitis. *Neurocrit Care* 2012; **16**:421–7.

24. Takeoka M, Takahashi T. Infectious and inflammatory disorders of the circulatory system and stroke in childhood. *Curr Opin Neurol* 2002; **15**:159–64.

25. Brancusi F, Farrar J, Heemskerk D. Tuberculous meningitis in adults: a review of a decade of developments focusing on prognostic factors for outcome. *Future Microbiol* 2012; **7**:1101–16.

26. Ecevit IZ, Clancy CJ, Schmalfuss IM, Nguyen MH. The poor prognosis of central nervous system cryptococcosis among nonimmunosuppressed patients: a call for better disease recognition and evaluation of adjuncts to antifungal therapy. *Clin Infect Dis* 2006; **42**:1443–7.

27. Leite AG, Vidal JE, Bonasser Filho F, Nogueira RS, Oliveira AC. Cerebral infarction related to cryptococcal meningitis in an HIV-infected patient: case report and literature review. *Braz J Infect Dis* 2004; **8**:175–9.

28. Williams PL, Johnson R, Pappagianis D, *et al.* Vasculitic and encephalitic complications associated with coccidioides immitis infection of the central nervous system in humans: report of 10 cases and review. *Clin Infect Dis* 1992; **14**:673–82.

29. Mathisen G, Shelub A, Truong J, Wigen C. Coccidioidal meningitis: clinical presentation and management in the fluconazole era. *Medicine* 2010; **89**:251–84.

30. Flint AC, Liberato BB, Anziska Y, Schantz-Dunn J, Wright CB. Meningovascular syphilis as a cause of basilar artery stenosis. *Neurology* 2005; **64**:391–2.

31. Nakane H, Okada Y, Ibayashi S, Sadoshima S, Fujishima M. Brain infarction caused by syphilitic aortic aneurysm. A case report. *Angiology* 1996; **47**:911–17.

32. Scheid R, Hund-Georgiadis M, von Cramon DY. Intracerebral haemorrhage as a manifestation of Lyme neuroborreliosis? *Eur J Neurol* 2003; **10**:99–101.

33. Marquez JM, Arauz A. Cerebrovascular complications of neurocysticercosis. *Neurologist* 2012; **18**:17–22.

34. Nagel MA, Mahalingam R, Cohrs RJ, Gilden D. Virus vasculopathy and stroke: an under-recognized cause and treatment target. *Infect Disord Drug Targets* 2010; **10**:105–11.

35. Singer EJ, Valdes-Sueiras M, Commins DL, Yong W, Carlson M. HIV stroke risk: evidence and implications. *Ther Adv Chronic Dis* 2013; **4**:61–70.

36. Tipping B, de Villiers L, Wainwright H, Candy S, Bryer A. Stroke in patients with human immunodeficiency virus infection. *J Neurol Neurosurg Psychiatry* 2007; **78**:1320–4.

37. Connor MD, Lammie GA, Bell JE, *et al.* Cerebral infarction in adult AIDS patients: observations from the Edinburgh HIV Autopsy Cohort. *Stroke* 2000; **31**:2117–26.

38. Ortiz G, Koch S, Romano JG, Forteza AM, Rabinstein AA. Mechanisms of ischemic stroke in HIV-infected patients. *Neurology* 2007; **68**:1257–61.

39. Salgado AV, Furlan AJ, Keys TF. Mycotic aneurysm, subarachnoid hemorrhage, and indications for cerebral angiography in infective endocarditis. *Stroke* 1987; **18**:1057–60.

40. Ho CL, Deruytter MJ. CNS aspergillosis with mycotic aneurysm, cerebral granuloma and infarction. *Acta Neurochir (Wien)* 2004; **146**:851–6.

41. Huang TE, Chou SM. Occlusive hypertrophic arteritis as the cause of discrete necrosis in CNS toxoplasmosis in the acquired immunodeficiency syndrome. *Hum Pathol* 1988; **19**:1210–14.

42. Idro R, Jenkins NE, Newton CR. Pathogenesis, clinical features, and neurological outcome of cerebral malaria. *Lancet Neurol* 2005; **4**:827–40.

43. Westendorp WF, Nederkoorn PJ, Vermeij JD, Dijkgraaf MG, van de Beek D. Post-stroke infection: a systematic review and meta-analysis. *BMC Neurol* 2011; **11**:110.

44. Martino R, Foley N, Bhogal S, *et al.* Dysphagia after stroke: incidence, diagnosis, and pulmonary complications. *Stroke* 2005; **36**:2756–63.

45. Gleeson K, Eggli DF, Maxwell SL. Quantitative aspiration during sleep in normal subjects. *Chest* 1997; **111**:1266–72.

46. Shigemitsu H, Afshar K. Aspiration pneumonias: under-diagnosed and under-treated. *Curr Opin Pulm Med* 2007; **13**:192–8.

47. Harms H, Grittner U, Droge H, Meisel A. Predicting post-stroke pneumonia: the pantheris score. *Acta Neurol Scand* 2013; **128**:178–84.

48. Kamel H, Iadecola C. Brain-immune interactions and ischemic stroke: clinical implications. *Arch Neurol* 2012; **69**:576–81.

49. Dirnagl U, Klehmet J, Braun JS, *et al.* Stroke-induced immunodepression: experimental evidence and clinical relevance. *Stroke* 2007; **38**:770–3.

50. European Stroke Organisation (ESO) Executive Committee; ESO Writing Committee. Guidelines for management of ischaemic stroke and transient ischaemic attack 2008. *Cerebrovasc Dis* 2008; **25**:457–507.

51. Meisel C, Prass K, Braun J, *et al.* Preventive antibacterial treatment improves the general medical and neurological outcome in a mouse model of stroke. *Stroke* 2004; **35**:2–6.

52. Westendorp WF, Vermeij JD, Vermeij F, *et al.* Antibiotic therapy for preventing infections in patients with acute stroke. *Cochrane Database Syst Rev* 2012; **1**:CD008530.

53. Li JS, Sexton DJ, Mick N, *et al.* Proposed modifications to the duke criteria for the diagnosis of infective endocarditis. *Clin Infect Dis* 2000; **30**:633–8.

54. Cavassini M, Meuli R, Francioli P. Complications of infective endocarditis. In: Scheld WM, Whitley RJ, Marra CM, eds. *Infections of the Central Nervous System*. Philadelphia: Lippincott Williams and Wilkins; 2004:537–68.

355

Secondary prevention

Hans-Christoph Diener, Sharan K. Mann, and Gregory W. Albers

Introduction

Secondary prevention aims at preventing a stroke after a transient ischemic attack (TIA) or a recurrent stroke after a first stroke. About 80–85% of patients survive a first ischemic stroke [1, 2]. Of those between 8% and 15% suffer a recurrent stroke in the first year. Risk of stroke recurrence is highest in the first few weeks and declines over time [3–5]. The risk of recurrence depends on concomitant vascular diseases (coronary heart disease [CHD], peripheral artery disease [PAD]) and vascular risk factors and can be estimated by risk models [6, 7]. Stroke risk after a TIA is highest in the first 3 days [8]. Therefore, immediate evaluation of patients with stroke or TIA, identification of the pathophysiology, and initiation of pathophysiology-based treatment is of major importance [9]. In the following sections, we will deal with the treatment of risk factors, antithrombotic therapy, and surgery or stenting of significant stenosis of extra- or intracranial arteries. Each paragraph will be introduced by recommendations, followed by the scientific justification.

Treatment of risk factors

Hypertension

- Antihypertensive therapy reduces the risk of stroke. The combination of an angiotensin-converting enzyme (ACE) inhibitor (perindopril) with a diuretic (indapamide) is significantly more effective than placebo, and an angiotensin-receptor blocker (ARB, eprosartan) is more effective than a calcium-channel blocker (nitrendipine). Ramipril reduces vascular events in patients with vascular risk factors.

- Early initiation of antihypertensive therapy with telmisartan in addition to standard antihypertensive therapy is not more effective than placebo.

- Most likely all antihypertensive drugs are effective in secondary stroke prevention. Beta-blockers, such as atenolol, show the lowest efficacy. More important than the choice of a class of antihypertensives is to achieve the systolic and diastolic blood pressure targets (<140/90 mmHg in non-diabetics and <130/80 mmHg in diabetics). In many cases this requires combination therapy. Concomitant diseases (kidney failure, congestive heart failure) have to be considered.

- Lifestyle modification will lower blood pressure and should be recommended in addition to drug treatment.

There are very few studies investigating the efficacy of classes of antihypertensive drugs in secondary stroke prevention. One has to remember that two concepts exist in this field. Placebo-controlled trials may try to achieve a maximum lowering of blood pressure in patients with high blood pressure. Vascular protective studies such as the Heart Outcomes Prevention Evaluation (HOPE) study [10] include patients with vascular risk factors even with normal blood pressure under the assumption that end organs such as the brain will be protected. A meta-analysis comprised seven studies of 15 527 patients with TIA, or ischemic or hemorrhagic stroke, who were followed for 2–5 years. Treatment with antihypertensives reduced the risk of stroke by 24%, non-fatal stroke by 21%, risk of myocardial infarction (MI) by 21%, and the risk of all vascular events by 21% [11]. For the endpoint stroke the combination of an ACE inhibitor with a diuretic was more effective (45% risk reduction) than a diuretic as monotherapy (32%), monotherapy with an ACE inhibitor (7%), or a beta-blocker (7%).

ACE inhibitors and ARBs were thought to have pleiotropic and protective vascular effects beyond lowering high blood pressure. Therefore the HOPE study compared ramipril with placebo. In the subgroup of patients with TIA or stroke as the qualifying event, ramipril resulted in a relative reduction of the combined endpoint of stroke, MI or vascular death by 24% and an absolute risk reduction (ARR) of 6.3% in 5 years [12].

The Perindopril Protection Against Recurrent Stroke Study (PROGRESS) was the first large-scale trial specifically performed in patients after stroke. Patients (n = 6105) were treated with perindopril as monotherapy or in combination with indapamide or placebo. Across the 4-year observation time blood pressure was lowered on average by 9/4 mmHg. The ARR for recurrent stroke was 4% and the relative risk reduction (RRR) was 28%. Monotherapy with the ACE inhibitor was not superior to placebo, but also did not achieve the same level of blood pressure lowering as the combination therapy. The RRR for combination therapy was 43% [13].

Acute Candesartan Cilexetil Therapy in Stroke Survivors (ACCESS) was a small phase II safety study in stroke patients with high blood pressure (>200/110 mmHg) in the early phase after an acute stroke. Patients were randomized to receive either the ARB candesartan or placebo in the first 7 days after stroke and continued with candesartan [14]. In the 12-month observation period the rate of vascular events was significantly lower in the candesartan group (9.8% vs. 18.7%, RRR = 52%).

The Morbidity and Mortality After Stroke, Eprosartan Compared with Nitrendipin for Secondary Prevention (MOSES) study included 1352 patients with hypertension who had suffered a stroke in the previous 24 months. Patients were treated either with eprosartan (600 mg) or with nitrendipine (10 mg) on top of additional antihypertensive therapy when appropriate. For an identical drop in blood pressure, eprosartan was superior to nitrendipine in preventing recurrent vascular events (21% RRR). Optimal systolic blood pressure in the MOSES trial was 120–140 mmHg.

The Prevention Regimen For Effectively avoiding Secondary Stroke (PRoFESS) study randomized 20 332 patients with a recent ischemic stroke to receive telmisartan at 80 mg/day or placebo in addition to other therapies, for a median duration of 2.4 years. Mean blood pressure over the trial period was lower in the telmisartan group by 3.8/2.0 mmHg. Recurrent strokes occurred in 8.7% in the telmisartan group compared to 9.2% in the placebo group, which was not significant. Therefore initiation of telmisartan early after a stroke, and continuation for a median of 2.4 years, did not significantly lower the rate of recurrent strokes, other major vascular events, or new diabetes [15].

The Secondary Prevention in Small Subcortical Strokes Trial (SPS3) randomized 3020 patients with recent, MRI-confirmed symptomatic lacunar strokes into two blood pressure target groups: 130–140 mmHg or <130 mmHg. Patients were followed for a mean of 3.7 years. The primary outcome was reduction in all stroke, both ischemic and hemorrhagic. After 1 year, the mean blood pressure was 138 mmHg in the higher target group and 127 mmHg in the lower target group. There was no significant difference in the rate of recurrent stroke between the two groups but the rate of intracerebral hemorrhage was significantly reduced in the lower target group [16].

> Antihypertensive therapy reduces the risk of stroke. Most likely all antihypertensive drugs are effective in secondary stroke prevention.
>
> In patients with lacunar stroke, there is no additional benefit with a lower systolic blood pressure target of <130 mmHg compared to the conventional target of <140 mmHg.

High cholesterol

- Patients with TIA or ischemic stroke and CHD should be treated with a statin irrespective of the initial low-density lipoprotein (LDL) cholesterol level. The target range of LDL is 70–100 mg/dl. Patients with atherosclerotic ischemic stroke or TIA without CHD and LDL cholesterol levels between 100 and 190 mg/dl will benefit from a treatment with 80 mg atorvastatin. Statin therapy reduces the rate of recurrent stroke and vascular events.
- Lowering high LDL is more important than the use of a particular statin. Therefore lowering LDL cholesterol <100 mg/dl or ≥50% of the initial LDL cholesterol level is recommended.

The association of cholesterol levels and the risk of recurrent stroke is not as strong as the association with the risk of MI. Statins will, however, lower the risk of stroke in patients with CHD [17]. The RRR calculated from a meta-analysis is 21% [18]. NCEP ATP III (National Cholesterol Education Program Adult Treatment Panel III) guidelines recommend treating stroke patients with CHD with a statin. The LDL cholesterol level should be <100 mg/dl and <70 mg/dl in high-risk patients [19].

Patients with stroke without CHD were investigated in a subgroup of the Heart Protection Study (HPS) and the trial. Within the HPS patient population of 20 536 high-risk patients, 3280 patients had TIA or stroke, 1820 of them without concomitant CHD. The RRR achieved by simvastatin given for 5 years for vascular events was 20% and the ARR 5.1% [20]. In the overall population the RRR for stroke was 25%, whereas there was no significant reduction in the stroke rate in the subgroup of patients with TIA or stroke as the qualifying event [21]. Stroke Prevention by Aggressive Reduction in Cholesterol Levels (SPARCL) was performed in 4731 patients with TIA or stroke without CHD and LDL cholesterol levels between 100 and 190 mg/dl. Patients received either 80 mg atorvastatin or placebo. After an average of 4.9 years the primary endpoint (stroke) was reduced by 16% relative and 2.2% absolute [22]. The discrepancy with the HPS trial might be explained by the fact that HPS recruited patients on average 4.3 years after the initial vascular event whereas this time interval was only 6 months in SPARCL. The RRR for the combined endpoint of stroke, MI, and vascular death was 20% and the ARR 3.5%. The rate of ischemic stroke was reduced (218 vs. 274) whereas hemorrhagic strokes were more frequent with atorvastatin (55 vs. 33).

Therapy with a statin should be initiated early after an ischemic stroke or TIA. The sudden discontinuation of a statin in patients with a stroke or acute coronary syndrome might be associated with higher morbidity and mortality [23, 24]. Therefore, patients on a statin should continue treatment following an acute ischemic event.

> Patients with TIA or ischemic stroke and coronary heart disease (CHD) should be treated with a statin irrespective of the initial LDL cholesterol level.

Diabetes mellitus

Randomized controlled studies were unable to show an effect of glitazones on vascular events in stroke patients with diabetes mellitus [25]. Aggressive lowering of blood glucose does not reduce the risk of stroke and might even increase mortality [26, 27]. Therefore, treatment of diabetes mellitus should not be restricted to drug treatment but should also include diet, weight loss, and regular exercise.

Supplementation of vitamins

- Treatment of increased plasma levels of homocysteine with vitamin B6, vitamin B12, and folic acid is not effective in secondary stroke prevention.

The VISP study was unable to show a benefit of the treatment of high homocysteine in stroke patients with B-vitamins and folic acid [28]. The HOPE-2 study also failed to demonstrate benefit [29]; the study included 5522 patients aged >55 years who had a vascular event or diabetes mellitus and were treated for 5 years with either placebo or a combination of 2.5 mg folic acid, 50 mg vitamin B6, and 1 mg vitamin B12. This resulted in a significant reduction in homocysteine levels but not in a reduction of vascular events.

Hormone replacement therapy after menopause

- Hormone replacement after menopause is not effective in the secondary prevention of stroke and may even increase the risk of fatal strokes.

A randomized, placebo-controlled study in women receiving hormone replacement therapy after menopause who suffered a stroke found an increase in stroke mortality and a poorer prognosis in non-fatal strokes [30]. Therefore, in general, hormone replacement should be avoided following a stroke.

Antiplatelet therapy

- Patients with TIA or ischemic stroke should receive antiplatelet drugs. The choices are acetylsalicylic acid (ASA 50–150 mg), the combination of ASA (2 × 25 mg) and extended-release dipyridamole (ER-DP 2 × 200 mg) or clopidogrel (75 mg).
- ASA is recommended in patients with a low risk of recurrence (<4%/year). Patients with a higher risk of recurrent stroke should be treated with ASA + ER-DP or clopidogrel. ASA + ER-DP and clopidogrel appear to be equally effective. ASA + ER-DP has more side-effects.

- Doses of ASA >150 mg/day result in an increased risk of bleeding complications.
- The combination of clopidogrel plus ASA is not more effective than either ASA or clopidogrel monotherapy, and carries a higher bleeding risk.
- The efficacy of antiplatelet therapy beyond 4 years after the initial event has not been studied in randomized trials. Theoretically, treatment should continue beyond that period.
- In the case of a recurrent ischemic event the pathophysiology of the ischemic event should be evaluated. When there is an indication for antiplatelet therapy the recurrence risk should be evaluated and the antiplatelet therapy adapted to the new risk. There is no evidence that changing antiplatelet therapy from ASA plus ER-DP to clopidogrel or vice versa provides greater protection.
- Patients with a history of TIA or ischemic stroke and an acute coronary syndrome should receive the combination of clopidogrel and ASA for at least 3 months. The same is true for patients with a coronary stent. This therapy is also typically extrapolated to patients with carotid stents.
- In patients with lacunar stroke, there is no significant benefit of dual antiplatelet therapy with clopidogrel and aspirin over aspirin alone. Moreover, the combination can increase the risk of hemorrhagic side-effects.
- A short-term course of dual antiplatelet therapy may be considered after an acute stroke or TIA.

Antiplatelet drugs are effective in secondary stroke prevention after TIA or ischemic stroke. This has been shown in many placebo-controlled trials and in several meta-analyses [31–33]. The RRR for non-fatal stroke achieved by antiplatelet therapy in patients with TIA or stroke is 23% (reduced from 10.8% to 8.3% in 3 years) [32]. The combined endpoint of stroke, MI, and vascular death is reduced by 17% (from 21.4% to 17% in 29 months).

A meta-analysis of 11 randomized and placebo-controlled trials investigating ASA monotherapy in secondary stroke prevention found a RRR of 13% (95% confidence interval [CI] 6–19) for the combined endpoint of stroke, MI, and vascular death [34]. There is no relationship between the dose of ASA and its efficacy in secondary stroke prevention [32, 34, 35]. Therefore, the recommended dose of ASA is 75–150 mg/day. Gastrointestinal adverse events and bleeding complications are, however, dose-dependent and bleeding rates increase significantly beyond a daily ASA dose of 150 mg [36, 37].

Clopidogrel monotherapy (75 mg/day) was compared to ASA (325 mg/day) in almost 20 000 patients with stroke, MI, or PAD. The combined endpoint of stroke, MI, and vascular death showed a RRR of 8.7% in favor of clopidogrel. The ARR was 0.51% [38]. The highest benefit of clopidogrel was seen in patients with PAD. The risk of gastrointestinal bleeds (1.99% versus 2.66%) and gastrointestinal side-effects (15% versus 17.6%) were smaller with clopidogrel than with ASA.

The MATCH study compared the combination of clopidogrel 75 mg and ASA 75 mg with clopidogrel monotherapy in high-risk patients with TIA or ischemic stroke [39] and failed to show the superiority of combination antiplatelet therapy for the combined endpoint of stroke, MI, vascular death, and hospitalization due to a vascular event. The combination resulted in a significant increase in bleeding complications, and therefore is not recommended.

The CHARISMA trial (Clopidogrel for High Atherothrombotic Risk and Ischemic Stabilization, Management, and Avoidance) was a combined primary and secondary prevention study in 15 603 patients and compared the combination of clopidogrel and ASA with ASA monotherapy [40]. Similarly to MATCH, the study failed to show a benefit of combination therapy and displayed a higher bleeding rate with the combination. Symptomatic patients, however, showed a trend towards a benefit for combination antiplatelet therapy [41].

The combination of low-dose ASA and ER-DP was investigated in the second European Stroke Prevention Study (ESPS2) with 6602 patients with TIA or stroke [42]. Patients were randomized to ASA (25 mg bid), ER-DP (200 mg bid), the combination of ASA and ER-DP, or placebo. For the primary endpoint of stroke, the combination was superior to ASA monotherapy (RRR 23%, ARR 3%) and placebo (RRR 37%, ARR 5.8%). ASA monotherapy lowered the risk of stroke by 18% (ARR 2.9%) and DP monotherapy by 16% (ARR 2.6%) compared to placebo. Major bleeding complications were seen more frequently with ASA and the ASA + ER-DP combination, whereas DP monotherapy had a similar bleeding rate to placebo. Cardiac events occurred at similar frequency in the groups treated with DP compared to ASA [43]. The industry-independent ESPRIT study [44] randomized 2739 patients with presumed atherothrombotic TIA or

Table 22.1. Strategies for prevention of recurrent stroke after an initial TIA or ischemic stroke

Intervention	Relative RR	Absolute RR/year	NNT/year	Comments
Antihypertensive therapy	24%	0.46%	217	Proven for perindopril + indapamide and eprosartan
Statins	16%	0.4%	250	Proven for atorvastatin and simvastatin
ASA 50–150 mg after TIA or ischemic stroke	18–22%	1.3%	77	ASA doses >150 mg = higher bleeding risk
ASA 50 mg + dipyridamole 400 mg versus ASA	23%	1.0–1.5%	33–100	Combination also superior to placebo
Clopidogrel versus ASA	8%	0.5%	200	Based on a subgroup analysis from CAPRIE
Surgery of a high-degree carotid stenosis*	65%	3.1%	32	Efficacy declines with time interval from event
Oral anticoagulation in cardiac source of embolism (AF) INR 2.0–3.0	68%	8%	12	Only one placebo-controlled study available (EAFT)
ASA in AF	19%	2.5%	40	In patients with contraindications for warfarin

Notes: * Outcome stroke and death.
NNT = number needed to treat; RR = risk reduction; AF = atrial fibrillation; INR = international normalized ratio.

minor stroke to ASA (30–325 mg) or the combination of ASA with DP and followed them for a mean period of 3.5 years. The primary endpoint was the combination of vascular death, stroke, MI, and major bleeding complications. The event rate for the primary endpoint was 16% with ASA monotherapy and 13% with ASA + DP, resulting in a RRR of 20% (ARR 1%). In the combination arm 34% of patients terminated the trial prematurely, mostly because of adverse events such as headache (13% in the ASA arm of the study). A meta-analysis of all stroke prevention trials testing ASA monotherapy versus ASA + DP showed a RRR of 18% (95% CI 9–26) in favor of the combination for the combined vascular endpoint [44].

A head-to-head comparison of clopidogrel and ASA + ER-DP was performed in the PRoFESS study [45]. The study randomized 20 332 patients with ischemic stroke and followed them for a mean period of 2.4 years. There was no difference in efficacy across all endpoints and no subgroup of patients. ASA + ER-DP resulted in more intracranial bleeds and a higher drop-out rate due to headache compared with clopidogrel (5.9% vs. 0.9%).

Table 22.1 gives an overview of ARR and RRR for different approaches in secondary stroke prevention.

The calculation of the Essen risk score is shown in Table 22.2 [8, 46, 47].

Glycoprotein (GP)-IIb/IIIa receptor antagonists are effective in the acute coronary syndrome [48]. Oral GP-IIb/IIIa-antagonists are not superior to ASA and carry a higher bleeding risk as shown in the BRAVO trial [36].

The use of dual antiplatelet therapy in patients with lacunar stroke was investigated in the SPS3 trial, which randomized 3020 patients with recent, MRI-confirmed symptomatic lacunar strokes into two antiplatelet groups: aspirin 325 mg daily and clopidogrel 75 mg daily versus aspirin 325 mg daily and placebo. Patients were followed for a mean of 3.4 years. The primary outcome was reduction in all stroke, both ischemic and hemorrhagic. The risk of recurrent ischemic stroke was not significantly different between the two groups. The risk of major hemorrhage was significantly higher in the dual antiplatelet therapy group, 2.1% per year, compared with 1.1% per year risk in the aspirin-only group. Hence, there was no significant benefit of dual antiplatelet therapy in this patient population and in fact, there is evidence that this combination leads to increased adverse events [49].

Table 22.2. Essen risk score for the calculation of the risk of a recurrent stroke after an initial ischemic stroke of atherothrombotic origin. A score of ≥3 points indicates a recurrence risk of ≥4%/year

Risk factor	Points
Age <65 years	0
Age 65–75 years	1
Age >75 years	2
Hypertension	1
Diabetes mellitus	1
Myocardial infarction	1
Other cardiovascular events	1
Peripheral arterial disease	1
Smoking	1
Additional TIA or ischemic stroke	1

The question of whether a short-term use of aggressive, dual antiplatelet therapy in patients with acute minor stroke or TIA prevents recurrent stroke has been addressed in one large randomized clinical trial. The Clopidogrel in High-risk patients with Acute Non-disabling Cerebrovascular Events (CHANCE) trial randomized over 5000 Chinese patients with acute TIA or minor stroke to receive either clopidogrel initiated with a loading dose of 300 mg followed by 75 mg/day for the first 21 days or placebo. Both groups received aspirin 75 mg/day for a 3-month period. Patients were randomized within 24 hours after TIA or stroke. The primary efficacy endpoint was any recurrent stroke (ischemic or hemorrhagic) at 3 months. The results of the trial were recently presented at the International Stroke Conference in February, 2013. The dual antiplatelet group had a significantly lower rate of any recurrent stroke (hazard ratio 0.68). The recurrent ischemic stroke rate was also significantly lower in the dual antiplatelet group compared to aspirin alone (7.9% versus 11.4%, ARR 3.5%). The brain hemorrhage rates were surprisingly low with both groups having a rate of only 0.3% [50, 51].

A similar North American trial called the Platelet Oriented Inhibition in New TIA and ischemic stroke (POINT) trial is currently underway. The POINT trial has a shorter randomization window compared with CHANCE (12 hours vs. 24 hours) and a higher loading dose of clopidogrel (600 mg vs. 300 mg) [52].

Patients with TIA or ischemic stroke should receive an antiplatelet agent. Short-term use of aggressive, dual antiplatelet therapy may be considered in patients with acute minor stroke or TIA.

Anticoagulation in cerebral ischemia due to cardiac embolism

- Patients with a high-risk cardiac source of embolism, in particular atrial fibrillation (AF), should typically be treated with oral anticoagulation. Options for patients with AF include dose-adjusted warfarin (INR 2.0 to 3.0), dabigatran, rivaroxaban, and apixaban.
- Patients with contraindications or unwilling to use oral anticoagulation should receive ASA 81–325 mg/day.
- Patients with mechanical heart valves should be anticoagulated with an INR between 2.0 and 3.5, depending upon the valve.
- Patients with biological heart valves are anticoagulated for 3 months.
- In patients with TIA or minor stroke, oral anticoagulation can be initiated immediately after the exclusion of cerebral hemorrhage.
- The combination of ASA plus clopidogrel is inferior to oral anticoagulation with warfarin and carries a similar bleeding risk.
- There is no evidence that the use of anticoagulation in patients with low left ventricular ejection fraction is superior to antiplatelet therapy.

The evidence that oral anticoagulation prevents recurrent strokes in patients with AF results from the European Atrial Fibrillation Trial [53]. This randomized placebo-controlled trial showed a 68% RRR for a recurrent stroke for patients treated with warfarin compared to only 19% for patients receiving 300 mg ASA. Numbers needed to treat (NNT) are 12/year [53]. Therefore, oral anticoagulation in patients with AF is by far the most effective treatment for secondary stroke prevention. A Cochrane analysis concluded that oral anticoagulation is more effective than ASA for the prevention of vascular events (odds ratio [OR] 0.67; 95% CI 0.50–0.91) or recurrent stroke (OR 0.49; 95% CI 0.33–0.72) [54]. The risk of major bleeding complications is significantly increased but not the risk of intracranial bleeds. Patients with intermittent AF have a similar stroke risk to patients with permanent AF [55, 56]. The optimal INR range for oral anticoagulation is between 2.0 and 3.0 [57]. INR values >3.0 lead to an increased risk of major bleeding complications in particular in the elderly [58].

The ACTIVE study compared the combination of ASA and clopidogrel versus oral anticoagulation with warfarin in patients with AF [59]: the study was terminated prematurely due to a significant reduction of stroke and systemic embolism in favor of warfarin. The rate of major bleeding complications was not different between the two regimens.

More recently, several newer oral anticoagulants have become available as an alternative to dose-adjusted warfarin in non-valvular AF. Currently, three agents have been approved for use by the United States Food and Drug Administration (FDA): dabigatran, rivaroxaban, and apixaban. These three agents have all been studied in large clinical trials.

Dabigatran is a direct thrombin inhibitor, which was compared with warfarin in the RE-LY trial. In RE-LY, 18 113 patients were randomly assigned to receive dabigatran 150 mg twice a day, dabigatran 110 mg twice a day, or dose-adjusted warfarin. Patients were followed for a mean of 2.0 years. The primary outcome was hemorrhagic stroke, ischemic stroke, or systemic embolism. The 150 mg dabigatran group had a significantly lower rate of the primary outcome compared with the warfarin group (1.11% per year for dabigatran versus 1.69% per year for warfarin, $p \leq 0.001$ for superiority) and had a similar rate of major bleeding (3.11% per year for dabigatran versus 3.36% per year in the warfarin group, $p = 0.31$). The 110 mg dabigatran group had a similar rate of the primary outcome compared with warfarin (1.53% per year for dabigatran versus 1.69% per year for warfarin, $p < 0.001$ for noninferiority) but had a lower risk of hemorrhagic stroke (2.71% per year for dabigatran versus 3.36% per year for warfarin) [60].

Rivaroxaban, a factor X inhibitor, was compared with warfarin in the ROCKET AF trial. In the trial, 14 264 patients with non-valvular AF and at increased risk for stroke were randomized to receive either rivaroxaban 20 mg daily or dose-adjusted warfarin. The primary endpoint was hemorrhagic stroke, ischemic stroke, or systemic embolism. The median follow-up was 1.9 years. In the intention-to-treat analysis, the rate of the primary endpoint was 2.1% per year for the rivaroxaban group compared with 2.4% per year in the warfarin group ($p < 0.001$ for noninferiority). The rate of major and non-major

clinically relevant bleeding was not significantly different between the two groups (14.9% per year for rivaroxaban versus 14.5% per year for warfarin, $p = 0.44$) [61].

The ARISTOTLE trial compared another factor X inhibitor, apixaban, with warfarin. The trial randomized 18 201 patients with AF and at least one additional stroke risk factor to either apixaban 5 mg twice a day or dose-adjusted warfarin. The primary outcome was a combination of hemorrhagic stroke, ischemic stroke, or systemic embolism. The median follow-up was 1.8 years. The rate of the primary outcome was 1.27% per year in the apixaban group versus 1.60% per year in the warfarin group ($p \ll 0.001$ for noninferiority and $p = 0.01$ for superiority). The rate of major bleeding was lower in the apixaban group compared to the warfarin group: 2.13% per year for apixaban and 3.09% per year for warfarin ($p < 0.001$) [62].

The AVERROES trial evaluated apixaban 5 mg twice daily versus aspirin 81–324 mg daily in patients with AF and increased risk of stroke that were felt to be unsuitable for vitamin K antagonist therapy. Patients were followed for a mean of 1.1 years for the primary outcome of stroke (hemorrhagic or ischemic) or systemic embolism. The study was terminated early as recommended by the data safety monitoring board because of a clear benefit in favor of apixaban [63].

The Warfarin versus Aspirin in Reduced Cardiac Ejection Fraction (WARCEF) trial was designed to determine whether anticoagulation was superior to antiplatelet therapy in patients with heart failure and low left ventricular ejection fraction. The trial randomized 2305 patients to either dose-adjusted warfarin with a target INR range of 2.0–3.5 or aspirin 325 mg daily. The mean follow-up was 3.5 years and the primary outcome a composite endpoint of ischemic stroke, intracerebral hemorrhage, or death from any cause. The rate of the primary outcome was not significantly different between the two groups: 7.47 events per 100 patient-years in the warfarin group and 7.93 in the aspirin group ($p = 0.40$). The warfarin group had a lower rate of ischemic stroke compared to aspirin: 0.72 events per 100 patient-years for warfarin versus 1.36 per 100 patient-years for aspirin ($p = 0.005$). However, as expected, the rate of major hemorrhage was higher in the warfarin group: 1.78 events per 100 patient-years for warfarin as opposed to 0.87 for aspirin ($p < 0.001$) [64].

At present there are no prospectively collected data as to when it is safe to initiate oral anticoagulation after a TIA or ischemic stroke. Patients with acute ischemic events were excluded from the trials with the novel anticoagulants. The recommendation is to start anticoagulation in patients with TIA on day 1, in patients with mild strokes on day 3, and in patients with moderate strokes on day 6. In patients with severe stroke anticoagulation can be initiated after 2 weeks provided that a repeat CT does not show major hemorrhagic transformation.

> Patients with a cardiac source of embolism, in particular atrial fibrillation (AF), should be treated with oral anticoagulation. Options include dose-adjusted warfarin (INR 2.0–3.0), dabigatran, rivaroxaban, and apixaban.

Patent foramen ovale closure

Autopsy and imaging studies have shown that patent foramen ovale (PFO) occurs in about 25% of the normal population but PFOs can be detected in up to 44% of younger stroke patients [65, 66]. Recently, there have been three clinical, randomized trials of PFO closure versus medical management alone.

The first trial to be published was the Closure or Medical Therapy for Cryptogenic Stroke with Patent Foramen Ovale (CLOSURE) trial, which randomized 909 patients between the ages of 18 and 60 with cryptogenic stroke or TIA in the previous 6 months to PFO closure versus medical management alone. The primary endpoint was a composite of stroke or transient ischemic attack during 2 years of follow-up, death from any cause during the first 30 days, or death from neurological causes between 31 days and 2 years. There was no significant difference between the two groups; 5.5% of the surgical group had a primary endpoint event vs. 6.8% of the medical group (p = 0.37) [67].

The Closure of Patent Foramen Ovale versus Medical Therapy after Cryptogenic Stroke (RESPECT) trial randomized 980 patients of ages 18 to 60 with ischemic stroke or TIA in the prior 6 months to PFO closure versus medical management alone. The primary results of the trial were analyzed after 25 primary endpoints occurred. The primary endpoint was defined as a composite of stroke or TIA during 2 years of follow-up, death from any cause during the first 30 days, and death from neurological causes between 31 days and 2 years. In the intention-to-treat (ITT) analysis, 9 events occurred in the closure group versus 16 in the medical group. There was no significant difference between the two groups in the ITT analysis (hazard ratio with closure = 0.49; 95% CI 0.22–1.11, p = 0.08). There was a significant difference between the two groups favoring the closure in the per protocol analysis (hazard ratio = 0.37; 95% CI 0.14–0.96, p = 0.03) [68].

Finally, the Percutaneous Closure of Patent Foramen Ovale in Cryptogenic Embolism trial (PC-Trial) randomized 414 patients age 18 to 60 with ischemic stroke, TIA, or a peripheral thromboembolic event and a PFO to either PFO closure or medical management alone. The primary endpoint was a composite of death, non-fatal stroke, TIA, or peripheral embolism. The primary endpoint was not significantly different in the two groups with 3.4% of closure patients and 5.2% of medical patients experiencing a primary endpoint after a mean follow-up of 4 years [69].

In summary, none of the three clinical trials demonstrated that PFO closure was significantly better than medical management in patients with cryptogenic stroke or TIA and the rate of recurrent stroke was low in all three studies. Therefore, in general, PFO patients should be managed medically. However, as trends favoring closure were noted in all three studies, PFO closure may be considered for highly selected patients such as individuals with recurrent cryptogenic stroke despite medical management [67–69].

> Patent foramen ovale (PFO) closure should not be recommended as first-line treatment in patients with cryptogenic stroke. PFO closure may be considered for patients with recurrent cryptogenic stroke despite medical management.

Anticoagulation in cerebral ischemia of non-cardiac origin

- Oral anticoagulation is not superior to ASA and is not recommended.
- The benefit of anticoagulation for patients with dissection of the vertebral or carotid arteries versus antiplatelet drugs has not been studied in head-to-head trials.
- Patients with cryptogenic stroke and coagulation disorders, e.g. protein C or S deficiency or factor V (Leiden) mutation, may benefit from oral anticoagulation. The optimal treatment duration and specific coagulation disorders that warrant anticoagulation are not clear.

The Stroke Prevention in Reversible Ischemia Trial (SPIRIT) studied oral anticoagulation with an INR between 3.0 and 4.5 versus ASA 30 mg in patients with TIA or minor stroke without a cardiac source of embolism [70]. The study was terminated due to a significantly increased bleeding risk with anticoagulation. The risk of bleeding was increased by a factor of 1.43 (95% CI 0.96–2.13) for an increase of the INR by 0.5. The Warfarin Aspirin Recurrent Stroke Study (WARSS) had a similar rate of ischemic events and bleeding complications comparing warfarin (INR 1.4–2.8) and ASA in stroke patients without a cardiac source of embolism [71]. This result was replicated in the European/Australasian Stroke Prevention in Reversible Ischemia Trial (ESPRIT) study [72]. ESPRIT found a lower rate of ischemic events with anticoagulation counterbalanced by an increased risk of intracranial bleeds.

A Cochrane analysis of five trials, with 4076 patients, was unable to show that anticoagulants are more or less efficacious in the prevention of vascular events than antiplatelet therapy (medium-intensity anticoagulation relative risk [RR] 0.96, 95% CI 0.38–2.42; high-intensity anticoagulation RR 1.02, 95% CI 0.49–2.13). The relative risk of major bleeding complications for low-intensity anticoagulation was 1.27 (95% CI 0.79–2.03) and for medium-intensity anticoagulation 1.19 (95% CI 0.59–2.41). High-intensity oral anticoagulants with INR 3.0–4.5 resulted in a higher risk of major bleeding complications (RR 9.0; 95% CI 3.9–21) [73].

The Antiphospholipid Antibodies and Stroke Study (APASS) found no difference in stroke, MI, or vascular death in patients with antiphospholipid antibodies (aPL) treated with warfarin (INR 1.4–2.8) compared to 325 mg ASA [74]. There was in addition no difference in event rates between patients positive or negative for aPL. The evidence for anticoagulation in patients with protein C, protein S, or antithrombin deficiency is derived from patients with deep vein thrombosis and not from patients with stroke.

The possible benefit of oral anticoagulation, compared with antiplatelet drugs, for the long-term treatment of dissections has never been studied in a randomized trial. An observational study from Canada in 116 patients with angiographically proven dissection of the vertebral or carotid arteries found a rate of TIA, stroke, or death in the first year of 15%. The event rate in patients with anticoagulation

was 8.3% and in patients receiving ASA 12.4%; the difference was not statistically significant [75]. A Cochrane review of 26 observational studies in 327 patients found no difference between anticoagulation and antiplatelet drugs for the endpoints death and severe disability [76]. A more recent review came to a similar conclusion [77].

Carotid endarterectomy and stenting with balloon angioplasty

- Symptomatic patients with significant stenosis of the internal carotid artery (ICA) should undergo carotid endarterectomy. The benefit of surgery increases with the degree of stenosis between 70% and 95%. The benefit of surgery is highest in the first 2–4 weeks after the initial TIA or minor stroke.
- The benefit of surgery is lower in patients with a stenosis between 50% and 70%, in high-degree stenosis (pseudo-occlusion), in women, and in cases when surgery is performed 12 weeks or later after the initial event.
- The benefit of surgery is no longer present when the complication rate exceeds 6%.
- Patients should receive ASA prior to, during, and after endarterectomy. Clopidogrel should be replaced by ASA 5 days before surgery.
- At present carotid stenting has a slightly higher short-term complication rate and similar medium-term outcomes. The use of protection systems does not decrease the complication rate. The restenosis rate is higher after stenting. Whether this translates into higher long-term event rates is not yet known. The complication rate of carotid stenting is age dependent and increases beyond the age of 65–68 years.
- The combination of clopidogrel (75 mg) plus ASA (75–100 mg) is recommended in patients after carotid stenting for 1–3 months based on extrapolation from studies of coronary stents.

Two large randomized trials (NASCET and ESC) found a clear benefit of carotid surgery compared to medical treatment in patients with high-degree stenosis of the ICA [78–84]. Taken together the trials found an ARR of 13.5% over 5 years for the combined endpoint of stroke and death in favor of carotid endarterectomy [84]. The risk reduction is even higher in stenosis >90%. In patients with 50–69%

ICA stenosis the 5-year ARR for the endpoint ipsilateral stroke is 4.6%. This benefit is mainly seen in males. Patients with <50% ICA stenosis do not benefit from carotid endarterectomy. The short-term complication rates (stroke and death) were 6.2% for stenosis >70% and 8.4% for 50–69% stenosis. ASA should be given prior to, during, and after carotid surgery [85].

Several studies randomized patients with significant ICA stenosis to carotid endarterectomy or balloon angioplasty with stenting. Surgeons and interventional neuroradiologists had to pass a quality control. SPACE randomized 1200 symptomatic patients with a >50% stenosis (NASCET criteria) or >70% (ESC criteria) within 6 months after TIA or minor stroke to carotid endarterectomy or stenting [86]. The primary endpoint, ipsilateral stroke or death within 30 days, was 6.84% in patients undergoing stenting and 6.34% in patients who were operated on. A post-hoc subgroup analysis identified age <68 years as a factor in a lower complication rate in patients treated with stenting. The complication rate of surgery was not age dependent [87]. The use of a protection system did not influence the complication rate. The EVA3S study was terminated prematurely after 527 patients were randomized due to a significant difference in the 30-day complication rate favoring carotid surgery (9.6% vs. 3.9%; OR 2.5; 95% CI 1.25–4.93) [88]. Taken together the results of the two studies show a lower complication rate for endarterectomy [89]. The reported medium-term outcomes were comparable and the restenosis rate was higher after carotid stenting.

The CREST trial compared stenting versus endarterectomy for the treatment of carotid artery stenosis (CAS). Patients who were either symptomatic or asymptomatic were included in the study. Patients were considered symptomatic if they experienced a TIA, amaurosis fugax, or minor non-disabling stroke in the territory of the study carotid artery within 180 days prior to randomization. Symptomatic patients were required to have stenosis of 50% or more on angiography, 70% or more on ultrasonography, or 70% or more on computed tomographic angiography or magnetic resonance angiography to be included in the study. Asymptomatic patients were eligible to participate if the degree of carotid stenosis was 60% or more on angiography, 70% or more on ultrasonography, or 80% or more on computed tomographic angiography or magnetic resonance

angiography. The primary endpoint was a composite of either (1) stroke, myocardial infarction, or death from any cause during the periprocedural period or (2) any ipsilateral stroke within 4 years after randomization. The study followed 2502 patients for a median follow-up period of 2.5 years. The estimated 4-year rate of the primary endpoint was not significantly different between the two groups (7.2% for stenting and 6.8% for endarterectomy, p = 0.51). However, there was a difference in the periprocedural risk of stroke and myocardial infarction between the two groups. The rate of periprocedural stroke was higher in the stenting group (4.1% for stenting versus 2.3% for endarterectomy, p = 0.01) whereas the risk of periprocedural myocardial infarction was higher in the endarterectomy group (1.1% for stenting versus 2.3% for endarterectomy, p = 0.03). The rate of ischemic stroke after the periprocedural period was similar between the groups (2.0% and 2.4%, respectively; p = 0.85). Lastly, there was a significant relationship between age and treatment efficacy (p = 0.02): patients <70 tended to do better with stenting whereas those >70 did better with endarterectomy [90].

> Symptomatic patients with significant stenosis of the internal carotid artery (ICA) should undergo carotid endarterectomy. Carotid artery stenting is a reasonable alternative to endarterectomy in patients who are deemed to be unsuitable or at high risk for endarterectomy.

Intracranial stenosis

- Symptomatic patients with intracranial stenosis or occlusions should be treated with antiplatelet therapy.
- In patients with recurrent events, angioplasty can be considered.

The WASID-II study recruited 569 patients with intracranial stenosis and randomized them to either oral anticoagulation (INR 2.0–3.0) or ASA (1300 mg/day). The study was terminated prematurely due to a higher rate of bleeding complications with warfarin [91]. Therefore ASA is recommended in these patients. Whether the high dose of ASA is needed is not known. Lower doses are better tolerated and appear to have equal efficacy in other ischemic stroke etiologies. Predictors for a recurrent ischemic event were the degree of stenosis, stenosis in the vertebrobasilar system, and female sex [92]. In patients with recurrent ischemic events stenting might be considered [93, 94], although not based on the results of randomized trials.

The Stenting versus Aggressive Medical Therapy for Intracranial Arterial Stenosis (SAMMPRIS) trial randomized patients with recent TIA or stroke due to high-grade intracranial stenosis (70–99%) to aggressive medical management alone or aggressive medical management plus stenting. The primary endpoint was either (1) stroke or death within 30 days after enrollment or after a revascularization procedure, or (2) stroke in the territory of the qualifying artery beyond 30 days. Enrollment was stopped early after 451 patients were randomized because the 30-day rate of stroke or death was 14.7% in the stenting arm and only 5.8% in the medical-management group (p = 0.002). One year rates of the primary endpoint were 20.0% in the stenting group and 12.2% in the medical-management group. Given the significantly higher stroke rates in the stenting arm, patients with TIA or stroke due to intracranial stenosis should typically be managed with medical therapy alone. If recurrent stroke or TIA events occur in the distribution of the stenotic intracranial vessel despite optimal medical management, then angioplasty (preferably without stenting) may be considered. However, there are no randomized clinical trials comparing medical management alone with medical management and angioplasty without stenting in patients with intracranial stenosis [95].

Chapter summary

- **Antihypertensive therapy** reduces the risk of stroke. Most likely all antihypertensive drugs are effective in secondary stroke prevention. More important than the choice of a class of antihypertensives is to achieve the systolic and diastolic blood pressure targets (<140/90 mmHg in non-diabetics and <130/80 mmHg in diabetics). In many cases this requires combination therapy and lifestyle modification.
- **Statin** therapy reduces the rate of recurrent stroke and vascular events. The target range of LDL is 70–100 mg/dl.
- Aggressive lowering of **blood glucose** does not reduce the risk of stroke and might even increase mortality.

- Treatment of increased plasma levels of **homocysteine** with vitamin B6, vitamin B12, and folic acid is not effective in secondary stroke prevention.
- **Hormone replacement** after menopause is not effective in the secondary prevention of stroke and may even increase the risk of fatal strokes.
- Patients with **TIA or ischemic stroke** should receive antiplatelet drugs. The choices are acetylsalicylic acid (ASA 50–150 mg), the combination of ASA (2 × 25 mg) and extended-release dipyridamole (ER-DP 2 × 200 mg) or clopidogrel (75 mg). Short-term use of aggressive, dual antiplatelet therapy may be considered in patients with acute minor stroke or TIA.
- Patients with a **cardiac source of embolism**, in particular atrial fibrillation (AF), should be treated with oral anticoagulation. Options for patients with AF include dose-adjusted warfarin (INR 2.0–3.0), dabigatran, rivaroxaban, and apixaban. Patients with contraindications or unwilling to use oral anticoagulation should receive ASA 100–300 mg/day.
- In cerebral ischemia of **non-cardiac** origin oral anticoagulation is not superior to ASA and is not recommended.
- Patent foramen ovale (PFO) closure should not be recommended as first-line treatment in patients with cryptogenic stroke. PFO closure may be considered for patients with recurrent cryptogenic stroke despite medical management.
- Symptomatic patients with significant **stenosis** of the **internal carotid artery** (ICA) (degree of stenosis between 70% and 95%) should undergo carotid endarterectomy. Carotid artery stenting is a reasonable alternative to endarterectomy in patients who are deemed to be unsuitable or at high risk for endarterectomy. Patients should receive ASA prior to, during, and after endarterectomy or the combination of clopidogrel (75 mg) plus ASA (75–100 mg) after carotid stenting for 1–3 months.
- Symptomatic patients with **intracranial stenosis** or occlusions should be treated with optimal medical management, which includes antiplatelet therapy and high-dose statins (if deemed appropriate). In patients with recurrent events, angioplasty can be considered.

References

1. Grau AJ, Weimar C, Buggle F, *et al*. Risk factors, outcome, and treatment in subtypes of ischemic stroke: the German stroke data bank. *Stroke* 2001; **32**:2559–66.

2. Wolf PA, Cobb JL, D'Agostino RB. Epidemiology of stroke. In Barnett HJM, Mohr JP, Stein BM, Yatsu FM, eds. *Stroke: Pathophysiology, Diagnosis and Management*. New York: Churchill Livingstone; 1992: 3–27.

3. Hill MD, Yiannakoulias N, Jeerakathil T, *et al*. The high risk of stroke immediately after transient ischemic attack: a population-based study. *Neurology* 2004; **62**:2015–20.

4. Lovett J, Coull A, Rothwell P. Early risk of recurrence by subtype of ischemic stroke in population-based incidence studies. *Neurology* 2004; **62**:569–73.

5. Weimar C, Roth MP, Zillessen G, *et al*. Complications following acute ischemic stroke. *Eur Neurol* 2002; **48**:133–40.

6. Coutts SB, Eliasziw M, Hill MD, *et al*. An improved scoring system for identifying patients at high early risk of stroke and functional impairment after an acute transient ischemic attack or minor stroke. *Int J Stroke* 2008; **3**(1):3–10.

7. Weimar C, Goertler M, Rother J, *et al*. Systemic Risk Score Evaluation in Ischemic Stroke Patients (SCALA): a prospective cross sectional study in 85 German stroke units. *J Neurol* 2007; **254**(11):1562–8.

8. Giles MF, Rothwell PM. Risk of stroke early after transient ischemic attack: a systematic review and meta-analysis. *Lancet Neurol* 2007; **6**(12):1063–72.

9. Rothwell PM, Giles MF, Chandratheva A, *et al*. Effect of urgent treatment of transient ischemic attack and minor stroke on early recurrent stroke (EXPRESS study): a prospective population-based sequential comparison. *Lancet* 2007; **370**(9596):1432–42.

10. Yusuf S, Teo KK, Pogue J, *et al*. Telmisartan, ramipril, or both in patients at high risk for vascular events. *N Engl J Med* 2008; **358**(15):1547–59.

11. Rashid P, Leonardi-Bee J, Bath P. Blood pressure reduction and secondary prevention of stroke and other vascular events. A systematic review. *Stroke* 2003; **34**:2741–8.

12. Flather MD, Yusuf S, Kober L, *et al*. Long-term ACE-inhibitor therapy in patients with heart failure or left-ventricular dysfunction: a systematic overview of data from individual patients. *Lancet* 2000; **355**:1575–81.

13. Progress Collaborative Group. Randomised trial of a perindopril-based blood-pressure lowering regimen among 6105 individuals with previous stroke or transient ischemic attack. *Lancet* 2001; **358**:1033–41.

14. Schrader J, Lüders S, Kulschewski A, *et al*.; The ACCESS Study: evaluation of acute candesartan cilexetil therapy in stroke survivors. *Stroke* 2003; **34**:1699–703.

15. Yusuf S, Diener HC, Sacco RL, *et al*. Randomized trial of telmisartan therapy to prevent recurrent strokes and major vascular events among 20,332 individuals with recent stroke. *N Engl J Med* 2008; **359**:1225–37.

16. The SPS3 Study Group. Blood-pressure targets in patients with recent lacunar stroke: the SPS3 randomised trial. *Lancet* 2013; **382**(9891): 507–15. Erratum in *Lancet* 2013; **382**(9891): 506.

17. Paciaroni M, Hennerici M, Agnelli G, Bogousslavsky J. Statins and stroke prevention. *Cerebrovasc Dis* 2007; **24**(2–3): 170–82.

18. Amarenco P, Labreuche J, Lavallee P, Touboul PJ. Statins in stroke prevention and carotid atherosclerosis: systematic review and up-to-date meta-analysis. *Stroke* 2004; **35**(12):2902–9.

19. Grundy SM, Cleeman JI, Merz CN, *et al*. Implications of recent clinical trials for the National Cholesterol Education Program Adult Treatment Panel III Guidelines. *J Am Coll Cardiol* 2004; **44**(3):720–32.

20. Heart Protection Study Collaborative Group. MRC/BHF Heart Protection Study of cholesterol lowering with simvastatin in 20,536 high-risk individuals: a randomised placebo-controlled trial. *Lancet* 2002; **360**:7–22.

21. Collins R, Armitage J, Parish S, Sleight P, Peto R; Heart Protection Study Collaborative Group. Effects of cholesterol-lowering with simvastatin on stroke and other major vascular events in 20536 people with cerebrovascular disease or other high-risk conditions. *Lancet* 2004; **363**:757–67.

22. The Stroke Prevention by Aggressive Reduction in Cholesterol Levels (SPARCL) Investigators. High-dose atorvastatin after stroke or transient ischemic attack. *N Engl J Med* 2006; **355**:549–59.

23. Endres M, Laufs U. Discontinuation of statin treatment in stroke patients. *Stroke* 2006; **37**(10):2640–3.

24. Blanco M, Nombela F, Castellanos M, *et al*. Statin treatment withdrawal in ischemic stroke: a controlled randomized study. *Neurology* 2007; **69**(9):904–10.

25. Wilcox R, Bousser MG, Betteridge DJ, *et al*. Effects of pioglitazone in patients with type 2 diabetes with or without previous stroke: results from PROactive (PROspective

pioglitAzone Clinical Trial In macroVascular Events 04). *Stroke* 2007; **38**(3):865–73.

26. Gerstein HC, Miller ME, Byington RP, *et al*. Effects of intensive glucose lowering in type 2 diabetes. *N Engl J Med* 2008; **358**(24):2545–59.

27. Patel A, MacMahon S, Chalmers J, *et al*. Intensive blood glucose control and vascular outcomes in patients with type 2 diabetes. *N Engl J Med* 2008; **358**(24): 2560–72.

28. Toole JF, Malinow MR, Chambless LE, *et al*. Lowering homocysteine in patients with ischemic stroke to prevent recurrent stroke, myocardial infarction, and death: the Vitamin Intervention for Stroke Prevention (VISP) randomized controlled trial. *JAMA* 2004; **291**(5):565–75.

29. Lonn E, Yusu FS, Arnold MJ, *et al*.; Heart Outcomes Prevention Evaluation (HOPE) 2 Investigators. Homocysteine lowering with folic acid and B vitamins in vascular disease. *N Engl J Med* 2006; **354**:1567–77.

30. Viscoli CM, Brass LM, Kernan WN, *et al*. A clinical trial of estrogen-replacement therapy after ischemic stroke. *N Engl J Med* 2001; **345**:1243–9.

31. Antiplatelet Trialists' Collaboration. Collaborative overview of randomised trials of antiplatelet therapy – I: prevention of death, myocardial infarction, and stroke by prolonged antiplatelet therapy in various categories of patients. *BMJ* 1994; **308**:81–106.

32. Antithrombotic Trialists' Collaboration. Collaborative meta-analysis of randomised trials of antiplatelet therapy for prevention of death, myocardial infarction, and stroke in high risk patients. *BMJ* 2002; **524**: 71–86.

33. Born G, Patrono C. Antiplatelet drugs. *Br J Pharmacol* 2006; **147**(Suppl 1):S241–51.

34. Algra A, van Gijn J. Cumulative meta-analysis of aspirin efficacy after cerebral ischemia of arterial origin. *J Neurol Neurosurg Psychiatry* 1999; **65**:255.

35. Patrono C, Garcia Rodriguez LA, Landolfi R, Baigent C. Low-dose aspirin for the prevention of atherothrombosis. *N Engl J Med* 2005; **353**(22):2373–83.

36. Topol E, Easton D, Harrington R, *et al*. Randomized, double-blind, placebo-controlled, international trial of the oral IIb/IIIa antagonist lotrafiban in coronary and cerebrovascular disease. *Circulation* 2003; **108**:16–23.

37. Yusuf S, Zhao F, Mehta SR, *et al*. Effects of clopidogrel in addition to aspirin in patients with acute coronary syndromes without ST-segment elevation. *N Engl J Med* 2001; **345**:494–502.

38. CAPRIE Steering Committee. A randomised, blinded, trial of clopidogrel versus aspirin in patients at risk of ischemic events (CAPRIE) CAPRIE steering committee. *Lancet* 1996; **348**:1329–39.

39. Diener H, Bogousslavsky J, Brass L, *et al*. Acetylsalicylic acid on a background of clopidogrel in high-risk patients randomised after recent ischemic stroke or transient ischemic attack: the MATCH trial results. *Lancet* 2004; **364**:331–4.

40. Bhatt DL, Fox KA, Hacke W, *et al*. Clopidogrel and aspirin versus aspirin alone for the prevention of atherothrombotic events. *N Engl J Med* 2006; **354**(16): 1706–17.

41. Bhatt DL, Flather MD, Hacke W, *et al*. Patients with prior myocardial infarction, stroke, or symptomatic peripheral arterial disease in the CHARISMA trial. *J Am Coll Cardiol* 2007; **49**(19): 1982–8.

42. Diener HC, Cuhna L, Forbes C, *et al*.; European Stroke Prevention Study 2. Dipyridamole and acetylsalicylic acid in the secondary prevention of stroke. *J Neurol Sci* 1996; **143**:1–13.

43. Diener HC, Darius H, Bertrand-Hardy JM, Humphreys M. Cardiac safety in the European Stroke Prevention Study 2 (ESPS2). *Int J Clin Pract* 2001; **55**:162–3.

44. The ESPRIT Study Group. Aspirin plus dipyridamole versus aspirin alone after cerebral ischemia of arterial origin (ESPRIT): randomised controlled trial. *Lancet* 2006; **367**:1665–73.

45. Diener HC, Sacco R, Yusuf S; Steering Committee; PRoFESS Study Group. Rationale, design and baseline data of a randomized, double-blind, controlled trial comparing two antithrombotic regimens and telmisartan vs. placebo in patients with strokes: the Prevention Regimen for Effectively Avoiding Second Strokes (PRoFESS) trial. *Cerebrovasc Dis* 2007; **23**:368–80.

46. Diener HC, Ringleb PA, Savi P. Clopidogrel for secondary prevention of stroke. *Expert Opin Pharmacother* 2005; **6**:755–64.

47. Diener HC. Modified-release dipyridamole combined with aspirin for secondary stroke prevention. *Aging Health* 2005; **1**:19–26.

48. Topol EJ, Byzova TV, Plow EF. Platelet GPIIb-IIIa blockers. *Lancet* 1999; **353**:227–31.

49. The SPS3 Study Group. Effects of clopidogrel added to aspirin in patients with recent lacunar stroke. *N Engl J Med* 2012; **367**:817–25.

50. Wang Y, Johnston SC; CHANCE Investigators. Rationale and design of a randomized, double-blind trial comparing the effects of a 3-month clopidogrel-aspirin regimen versus aspirin alone for the treatment of high-risk patients

with acute nondisabling cerebrovascular event. *Am Heart J.* 2010; **160**(3):380–6.

51. Wang Y, Johnston SC; CHANCE Investigators. Clopidogrel and aspirin versus aspirin alone for the treatment of high-risk patients with acute non-disabling cerebrovascular event (CHANCE): a randomized, double-blind, placebo-controlled multicenter trial. Presented at: The International Stroke Conference; 2013; February 6–8; Honolulu, Hawaii.

52. University of California, San Francisco. Platelet-Oriented Inhibition in New TIA and Minor Ischemic Stroke (POINT) Trial. In: ClinicalTrials.gov [Internet]. Bethesda (MD): National Library of Medicine (US). 2000-[cited 2013 Jun 22]. Available from: http://clinicaltrials.gov/ct2/show/NCT00991029 NLM Identifier: NCT00991029.

53. EAFT Group. Secondary prevention in non-rheumatic atrial fibrillation after transient ischemic attack or minor stroke. *Lancet* 1993; **342**:1255–62.

54. Saxena R, Koudstaal PJ. Anticoagulants for preventing stroke in patients with nonrheumatic atrial fibrillation and a history of stroke or transient ischemic attack. *Stroke* 2004; **35**:1782–3.

55. Hart R, Pearce L, Miller V, *et al.* Cardioembolic vs. noncardioembolic strokes in atrial fibrillation: frequency and effect of antithrombotic agents in the stroke prevention in atrial fibrillation studies. *Cerebrovasc Dis* 2000; **10**:39–43.

56. Nieuwlaat R, Capucci A, Camm AJ, *et al.* Atrial fibrillation management: a prospective survey in ESC member countries: the Euro Heart Survey on Atrial Fibrillation. *Eur Heart J* 2005; **26**(22):2422–34.

57. Fuster V, Ryden LE, Cannom DS, *et al.* ACC/AHA/ESC 2006 guidelines for the management of patients with atrial fibrillation: full text: a report of the American College of Cardiology/American Heart Association Task Force on practice guidelines and the European Society of Cardiology Committee for Practice Guidelines (Writing Committee to Revise the 2001 guidelines for the management of patients with atrial fibrillation) developed in collaboration with the European Heart Rhythm Association and the Heart Rhythm Society. *Europace* 2006; **8**(9):651–745.

58. Hylek EM, Evans-Molina C, Shea C, Henault LE, Regan S. Major hemorrhage and tolerability of warfarin in the first year of therapy among elderly patients with atrial fibrillation. *Circulation* 2007; **115**(21):2689–96.

59. ACTIVE Writing Group on behalf of the ACTIVE Investigators, Connolly S, Pogue J, *et al.* Clopidogrel plus aspirin versus oral anticoagulation for atrial fibrillation in the Atrial fibrillation Clopidogrel Trial with Irbesartan for prevention of Vascular Events (ACTIVE W): a randomised controlled trial. *Lancet* 2006; **367**:1903–12.

60. Connolly SJ, Ezekowitz MD, Yusuf S, *et al.* Dabigatran versus warfarin in patients with atrial fibrillation. *N Engl J Med* 2009; **361**:1139–51.

61. Patel MR, Mahaffey KW, Garg J, *et al.* Rivaroxaban versus warfarin in nonvalvular atrial fibrillation. *N Engl J Med* 2011; **365**:883–91.

62. Granger CB, Alexander JH, McMurray JJV, *et al.* Apixaban versus warfarin in patients with atrial fibrillation. *N Engl J Med* 2011; **365**:981–92.

63. Connolly SJ, Eikelboom J, Joyner C, *et al.* Apixaban in patients with atrial fibrillation. *N Engl J Med* 2011; **364**:806–17.

64. Homma S, Thompson JLP, Pullicino PM, *et al.* Warfarin and aspirin in patients with heart failure and sinus rhythm. *N Engl J Med* 2012; **366**:1859–69.

65. Hagen PT, Scholz DG, Edwards WD. Incidence and size of patent foramen ovale during the first 10 decades of life: an autopsy study of 965 normal hearts. *Mayo Clin Proc* 1984; **59**:17–20.

66. Handke M, Harloff A, Olschewski M, Hetzel A, Geibel A. Patent foramen ovale and cryptogenic stroke in older patients. *N Engl J Med* 2007; **357**:2262–8.

67. Furlan AJ, Reisman M, Massaro J, *et al.* Closure or medical therapy for cryptogenic stroke with patent foramen ovale. *N Engl J Med* 2012; **366**:991–9.

68. Carroll JD, Saver JL, Thaler DE, *et al.* Closure of patent foramen ovale versus medical therapy after cryptogenic stroke. *N Engl J Med* 2013; **368**:1092–100.

69. Meier B, Kalesan B, Mattle HP, *et al.* Percutaneous closure of patent foramen ovale in cryptogenic embolism. *N Engl J Med* 2013; **368**:1083–91.

70. The Stroke Prevention in Reversible Ischemia Trial (SPIRIT) Study Group. A randomized trial of anticoagulants versus aspirin after cerebral ischemia of presumed arterial origin. *Ann Neurol* 1997; **42**:857–65.

71. Mohr JP, Thompson JL, Lazar RM, *et al.* A comparison of warfarin and aspirin for the prevention of recurrent ischemic stroke. *N Engl J Med* 2001; **345**:1444–51.

72. The ESPRIT Study Group. Medium intensity oral anticoagulants versus aspirin after cerebral ischemia of arterial origin (ESPRIT): a randomised

controlled trial. *Lancet Neurol* 2007; **6**(2):115–24.

73. Algra A, De Schryver E, van Gijn J, Kappelle L, Koudstaal P. Oral anticoagulants versus antiplatelet therapy for preventing further vascular events after transient ischemic attack or minor stroke of presumed arterial origin. *Cochrane Database Syst Rev* 2006; 3:CD001342.

74. Levine SR, Brey RL, Tilley BC, *et al.* Antiphospholipid antibodies and subsequent thrombo-occlusive events in patients with ischemic stroke. *JAMA* 2004; **291**(5):576–84.

75. Beletsky V, Nadareishvili Z, Lynch J, *et al.* Cervical arterial dissection. Time for a therapeutic trial? *Stroke* 2003; **34**:2856–60.

76. Lyrer P, Engelter S. Antithrombotic drugs for carotid artery dissection. *Stroke* 2004; **35**(2):613–14.

77. Engelter ST, Brandt T, Debette S, *et al.* Antiplatelets versus anticoagulation in cervical artery dissection. *Stroke* 2007; **38**(9): 2605–11.

78. Barnett HJ, Taylor DW, Eliasziw M, *et al.* Benefit of carotid endarterectomy in patients with symptomatic moderate or severe stenosis. *N Engl J Med* 1998; **339**:1415–25.

79. European Carotid Surgery Trialists' Collaborative Group. Randomised trial of endarterectomy for recently symptomatic carotid stenosis: final results of the MRC European Carotid Surgery Trial (ECST). *Lancet* 1998; **351**:1379–87.

80. European Carotid Surgery Trialists' Collaborative Group. MRC European carotid surgery trial: interim results for symptomatic patients with severe carotid stenosis and with mild carotid stenosis. *Lancet* 1991; **337**:1235–43.

81. Ferguson GG, Eliasziw M, Barr HWK, *et al.* The North American symptomatic carotid endarterectomy trial: surgical result in 1415 patients. *Stroke* 1999; **30**:1751–8.

82. Rothwell PM, Warlow CP, on behalf of the European Carotid Surgery Trialists' Collaborative Group. Prediction of benefit from carotid endarterectomy in individual patients: a risk-modelling study. *Lancet* 1999; **353**:2105–10.

83. Rothwell PM, Eliasziw M, Gutnikov SA, *et al.* Analysis of pooled data from the randomized controlled trials of endarterectomy for symptomatic carotid stenosis. *Lancet* 2003; **361**:107–16.

84. Rothwell P, Eliasziw M, Gutnikov S, *et al.* Endarterectomy for symptomatic carotid stenosis in relation to clinical subgroups and timing of surgery. *Lancet* 2004; **363**:915–24.

85. Chaturvedi S, Bruno A, Feasby T, *et al.* Carotid endarterectomy – an evidence-based review: report of the Therapeutics and Technology Assessment Subcommittee of the American Academy of Neurology. *Neurology* 2005; **65**(6):794–801.

86. Ringleb PA, Allenberg J, Bruckmann H, *et al.* 30 day results from the SPACE trial of stent-protected angioplasty versus carotid endarterectomy in symptomatic patients: a randomised non-inferiority trial. *Lancet* 2006; **368**(9543):1239–47.

87. Stingele R, Berger J, Alfke K, *et al.* Clinical and angiographic risk factors for stroke and death within 30 days after carotid endarterectomy and stent-protected angioplasty: a subanalysis of the SPACE study. *Lancet Neurol* 2008; **7**(3):216–22.

88. Mas JL, Chatellier G, Beyssen B, *et al.*; EVA-3S Investigators. Endarterectomy versus stenting in patients with symptomatic severe carotid stenosis. *N Engl J Med* 2006; **355**:1660–71.

89. Kern R, Ringleb PA, Hacke W, Mas JL, Hennerici MG. Stenting for carotid artery stenosis. *Nat Clin Pract Neurol* 2007; **3**(4): 212–20.

90. Brott TG, Hobson RW, Howard G, *et al.* Stenting versus endarterectomy for treatment of carotid-artery stenosis. *N Engl J Med* 2010; **363**:11–23.

91. Chimowitz MI, Lynn MJ, Howlett-Smith H, *et al.* Comparison of warfarin and aspirin for symptomatic intracranial arterial stenosis. *N Engl J Med* 2005; **352**(13): 1305–16.

92. Kasner SE, Chimowitz MI, Lynn MJ, *et al.* Predictors of ischemic stroke in the territory of a symptomatic intracranial arterial stenosis. *Circulation* 2006; **113**(4): 555–63.

93. Zaidat OO, Klucznik R, Alexander MJ, *et al.* The NIH registry on use of the Wingspan stent for symptomatic 70–99% intracranial arterial stenosis. *Neurology* 2008; **70**(17):1518–24.

94. Jiang WJ, Xu XT, Du B, *et al.* Comparison of elective stenting of severe vs. moderate intracranial atherosclerotic stenosis. *Neurology* 2007; **68**(6):420–6.

95. Chimowitz MI, Lynn MJ, Derdeyn CP, *et al.* Stenting versus aggressive medical therapy for intracranial arterial stenosis. *N Engl J Med* 2011; **365**:993–1003.

Introduction and overview

Stroke is the most common cause of long-term disability in adults. Although progress in the acute treatment of stroke (e.g. thrombolysis, the concept of stroke units, dysphagia management) as well as improvements of the organization of stroke services has occurred over recent years, neurorehabilitation (mainly organized inpatient multidisciplinary rehabilitation) remains one of the cornerstones of stroke treatment. The overall benefit of stroke units results not only from thrombolysis – only a small proportion of all stroke patients (overall about 10–15%) are treated with this regimen – but more generally from the multidisciplinary stroke unit management, including treatment optimization, minimization of complications, and elements of early neurorehabilitation [1–3].

After the acute treatment, stroke patients with relevant neurological deficits should in general be treated by a specialized neurorehabilitation clinic or unit. The best timing for transferring a patient after initial treatment (e.g. on a stroke unit) to a specialized neurorehabilitation ward or clinic is dependent on several factors, but early initiation of rehabilitation is mandatory for outcome optimization (whereas ultra-early high-intensity training in the first hours to few days might be problematic).

Neurorehabilitation of stroke nowadays is considered as a multidisciplinary and multimodal concept to improve physiological functioning, activity, and participation by creating therapeutic "learning situations," inducing several means of recovery including restitution, functional remodeling, compensation, and reconditioning [2]. A key point in successfully diminishing negative long-term effects after stroke and achieving recovery is the *work of a specialized multidisciplinary neurorehabilitation team* (physicians, nursing staff, therapists, others) with structured organization and processes and the stroke patient taking part in a multimodal, intense treatment program which is well adapted in detail to the individual goals of rehabilitation and deficits.

There is growing evidence indicating a better outcome of neurorehabilitation in stroke with early initiation of treatment; high intensity, specifically aimed, and active therapies; and the coordinated work and multimodality of a specialized team [4]. In this context, interdisciplinary goal-setting and regular assessments of the patient are important. The WHO's ICF (The International Classification of Functioning, Disability and Health; 2001) is now widely accepted as a useful tool in goal-setting in clinical practice. It also adds a social perspective with emphasis on participation. Furthermore, several additional potential enhancers of neural plasticity, e.g., peripheral and brain stimulation techniques, pharmacological augmentation, and use of robotics, are under evaluation. Clinical research makes use of clinical evaluation/assessments, neurophysiological techniques, as well as imaging modalities such as positron emission tomography (PET), functional magnetic resonance imaging (fMRI) and the more recently introduced diffusion tensor imaging (DTI).

Neuroplasticity in stroke recovery
Mechanisms of neuroplasticity

For many decades of the last century it was believed that, "once development is complete, the sources of growth and regeneration of axons and dendrites are irretrievably lost. In the adult brain the nerve paths are fixed and immutable: everything can die, nothing can be regenerated" [5], but afterwards – from a clinical point of view – there have been limited but important reports on observations that therapeutic exercises influence the course of spontaneous recovery of a brain affection [6]. It has been a long way, however, until a paradigm shift has taken place to what we now know, first by measurement of the effects of rehabilitation, that the central nervous system of the adult human being has an astounding potential for recovery and adaptability, which can be selectively promoted [7].

The extent of recovery in stroke is dependent on many factors, the initial size and location of the cerebral lesion and the degree of success of recanalization therapies being predominant factors. With a varying individual relevance, the recovery curve flattens in the course of time from the initial incidence.

Such recovery of the central nervous system over the course of time after onset of stroke is possible due to mechanisms described as neural plasticity or neuroplasticity, which can be observed and investigated by different approaches, e.g., from a clinical to a neurobiological and neuropathological point of view. Hebb first described neuroplasticity with regard to the function of synapses [8], and later this principle was also linked to the functioning of neurons in the wider context of neuronal networks. The term "neural plasticity" might refer to transiently achieved functional changes in the context of learning and recovery, as well as structural changes (overviewed by Møller [9]) describing the basis for neural plasticity as plastic changes in the nervous system which are supposed to occur in four main ways, including functional changes in synaptic efficacy, modifying protein synthesis and proteinase activity in nerve cells, creation of new anatomical connections or by altering synapses morphologically, and by specific apoptosis. However, the role of neurogenesis in human adult stroke recovery still remains somewhat unclear.

Several (overlapping and interacting) mechanisms of neuronal plasticity can be identified [9–13], which include:

- *Vicariation* (vice = instead of) describes the hypothesis that the functions of damaged areas can be taken over by different regions of the brain. In clinical practice this ability may vary widely and may be insufficient for a large group of patients with remaining difficulties after brain damage. With functional imaging, however, it

could be demonstrated that vicariation takes place in cortical representation areas (see below). Another clinical example is the change in lateralization of speech in some younger patients.

- *Plasticity of areas of cortical representation* was described in animal models in connection with the variable size of cortical representation "loco typico" of motor fields [14, 15]. Later such enlargement of cortical representations was also demonstrated in humans. By using transcranial magnetic stimulation (TMS) mapping in stroke patients, the area of cortical representation of the abductor minimi muscle (ADM) transiently increased even after a single training session. These findings suggest a very variable cortical representation [16]. Using positron emission tomography (PET) and functional magnetic resonance imaging (fMRI) different patterns of activation have been described (for a summary refer to Ward [13]). In an illustrative longitudinal study [17], a small group of stroke patients with comparable circumscribed M1 lesions (similar to experimental lesions in animal models) affecting the motor control of the contralateral hand were assessed over several months. In the first follow-up, ipsi- and contralateral activation patterns were noted. After several months, activation was again ipsilesional and closer to the former representation and more dorsal for the function of finger-extension as compared to controls, reflecting functional reorganization in the motor cortex adjacent to the lesion.

To summarize TMS and functional imaging studies using fMRI and PET after focal ischemic brain lesions resulting in motor deficits with damage to the corticospinal tract, it is suggested that interruption of projections from the primary motor cortex (M1) leads to increased recruitment of secondary motor areas such as the dorsolateral premotor cortex and supplementary motor areas[18]:

1. For the phase of early *compensation* in longitudinal fMRI studies an initial upregulation in primary and secondary motor regions (ipsi- and/or contralateral) but also activity of other nonprimary structures of the sensorimotor network could be observed, followed by

2. More precise activation patterns with more focused and efficient brain activity in a later phase reflecting *recovery* and accordingly *reorganization*, and which are – in case of success – reminiscent of

normal mostly ipsilateral activation patterns. A precondition to accomplish this more successful course is the preservation of a sufficient amount of specialized cortical and subcortical brain tissue and especially the pyramid tract [15, 18–21].

For better understanding of these mechanisms a main strategy for recovery in such patients seems to be the goal of achieving the best results by recruitment and adaptation of surviving secondary motor areas in both hemispheres [18]: in addition to a static point-by-point view of the somatotopic organization of the motor homunculus recent studies also demonstrate the representation of movements within the primary sensorimotor cortex, and, on the other hand, secondary motor areas have direct projections to brainstem and spinal cord motor neurons, although they are less numerous than those from M1. These connections such as the cortico-rubro-spinal tract may have an important compensatory function in patients with pyramid lesions [22].

However, a persistent activation of many different areas may also indicate a less successful or failed reorganization in chronic stroke patients: the higher the involvement of the ipsilesional motor network, the better the recovery. In this respect *interaction between lesional and contralesional hemispheres* is supposed to play an important role (see below) [21, 23, 24].

Basic underlying mechanisms of these findings include both different functional use of existing networks and synapses, but also structural changes. In the early course of ischemic stroke, pathophysiological mechanisms in the perilesional region are initiated, which include upregulation of plasticity-related proteins, brain-derived neurotrophic factor, synapsin I, and certain neurotransmitters. These modifications probably lead to morphological changes, e.g. synaptic plasticity and sprouting as discussed below, especially in the early weeks after stroke [19, 25–27].

- *Sprouting of neurons* after damage of the neuron itself is well known in the peripheral nervous system, where axons may regrow after Wallerian degeneration. In the central nervous system of the adult, however, this mechanism is reduced (but not excluded) for several reasons, including the lack of Schwann cells (functioning as a leading structure for sprouting in the peripheral nervous system), barriers of gliosis produced by glia cells, incomplete remyelinization by oligodendrocytes, production of inhibitory factors by these cells, and low production of growth factor e.g. growth associated protein 43 (GAP-43) in the adult central nervous system, which is available in the peripheral nerve system over the entire lifespan [10]. However, in animal models sprouting of neurons after lesions and also after interventions to reduce production of inhibitory factors has already been shown to lead to a better outcome. Sprouting of dendrites is much more common than the limited sprouting of axons.

- *Collateral sprouting* can lead to a change of function in a damaged neuron by receiving new synaptic input from dendrites of non-lesioned sprouting neurons.

- *Synaptic plasticity* refers to the altered synaptic function when cells are communicating, leading to plastic changes, stated as "cells that fire together, wire together" by Hebb [8]. Changes in synaptic activity can be measured by alterations in the number of N-methyl-D-aspartate (NMDA receptors) and are morphologically seen as "spines" between two neurons.

- *Diaschisis* is a term used by von Monakow [28] to describe the phenomenon that a focal lesion may also lead to changes in brain functioning of areas located far away. An example demonstrated by several recent neuroimaging studies is an enhanced contralesional cerebellar activity after cortical infarction.

- Furthermore an *enriched environment* must also be mentioned in terms of neuroplasticity [18], as has been demonstrated in animal models: rats with an ischemic lesion due to middle cerebral artery occlusion showed much better recovery when held in an enriched environment with free access to physical activity and social interactions [29].

Neuroplasticity is the dynamic potential of the brain to reorganize itself during ontogeny, learning, or following damage. In clinical neurorehabilitation this potential is utilized by creating a stimulating learning atmosphere and using stimulation techniques.

Inducing and promoting neuroplasticity

One key principle of neurorehabilitation is the repetitive creation of specific learning situations to promote mechanisms of neural plasticity in stroke recovery. There are many parallels between postlesional neuroplasticity (relearning) and human learning as part of personal development, education, or training leading to changes of behavior and abilities or knowledge, e.g., by repetitive interactions with the social environment. In clinical neurorehabilitation, the main effect of the multidisciplinary teamwork and applied therapies is to create repetitive specified learning conditions and a stimulating learning atmosphere in a defined way, hereby considering interdisciplinary treatment goals that are adapted to the patient's individual needs and deficits. This is achieved by therapeutic sessions and methods (see below) as well as in everyday life on the neurorehabilitation ward in interactions with physicians, nursing team, therapists, and others, in which the patient is guided to the highest meaningful degree of mental and physical activity [3]. A valuable didactical principle to force the individual to learn is the use of *constraint-induced therapies (CIT)*, which, however, cannot be used in the treatment of the majority of stroke patients (see below). In addition, other *stimulation techniques* and *enhancement by use of medications* are under evaluation.

Supporting neuroplasticity by peripheral and brain stimulation techniques

Although not yet recommended and approved for clinical routine, several trials have been undertaken and are currently ongoing to evaluate non-invasive cortical stimulation techniques with the purpose of enhancing neuroplasticity and recovery, using clinical outcome measures or fMRI. Stimulation techniques can address e.g. motor, language, or neglect (see below) rehabilitation. The main techniques are repetitive transcranial magnetic stimulation (rTMS) and transcranial direct current stimulation (TDCS), which can be used for both cortical enhancement and inhibition, depending on the setup parameters. Furthermore, epidural electrical stimulation (EES) is an invasive approach using a grid of electrodes implanted neurosurgically. Therefore, its practical use in stroke patients is limited.

Beside therapeutically modifying cortical activity in certain cortex regions (e.g. motor or language-related areas), which might be altered by damage or indirectly due to mechanisms of neuroplasticity, another important theory behind influencing cortical activity is the hypothesis of contralesional hemisphere overexcitability, leading to a "vicious circle" of inhibition even of undamaged functions and hindering recovery. It is supposed that metabolic changes or neuronal reorganization around the ischemic lesion lead to alterations of transcallosal excitability, which is followed by motor cortical disinhibition in the unaffected hemisphere, even increasing the inhibition of ipsilesional motor cortex (see Figure 23.1) [21, 23, 24]. "Corrective"

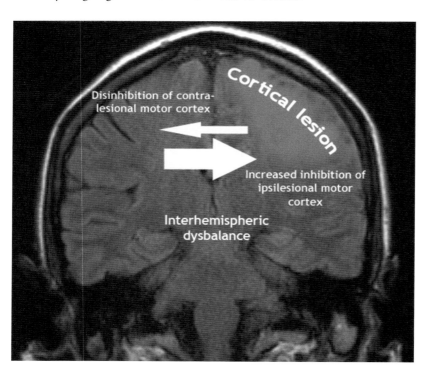

Figure 23.1. Non-invasive brain stimulation in stroke refers partly to the "contralesional hemisphere overexcitability hypothesis" – repetitive transcranial magnetic stimulation (rTMS) or transcranial direct current stimulation (TDCS) can be used for both cortical enhancement and inhibition, depending on the setup parameters used:

- Unaffected hemisphere – *Decrease excitability*:
  - cathodal TDCS
  - inhibitory low-frequency rTMS (including theta burst protocols)
- Affected hemisphere – *Increase excitability*:
  - anodal TDCS
  - excitatory rTMS > 5Hz

cortical activity modification can be achieved non-invasively in conscious humans using rTMS and TDCS.

In rTMS, an electric current is induced in the underlying cortex by a magnetic field, which then activates the axons of cortical neurons. Low-frequency rTMS around 1 Hz results in decreased cortical excitability (which persists after the application of rTMS) and is therefore used on the contralesional hemisphere for downregulation. Higher frequencies of more than 5 Hz increase cortical excitability and can be applied to stimulate the cortex on the ipsilesional hemisphere. Special patterns of inhibitory rTMS (theta bursts) have also been established and are reported to have longer-lasting modulatory capacity [30–33].

In TDCS, two electrodes (one active and one reference) are placed on the skin, delivering weak polarizing electrical current leading to different effects in the cortex, depending on the polarity: anodal TDCS has an excitatory effect, cathodal TDCS induces inhibition via presumed hyperpolarization. Usually 10–20 minutes of TDCS at 1–2 mA is regarded as safe and painless.

With the application of these newer treatment methods in stroke patients, recent findings suggest a 10% functional improvement in single sessions, and about 20% or more in multiple sessions has been reported. Long-term effects are widely unknown. As far as is known now, cortical stimulation appears to be a safe and promising intervention for stroke patients; however, more trials are needed to assess the long-term benefit and to optimize protocols [34]. Main potential side-effects (although rare overall) include seizure induction, possible syncope, transient headache or local pain, transient hearing changes, transient cognitive or neuropsychological changes, and others. Although there has been progress in standardization, however, many questions remain to be solved, including patient selection, optimal stimulation parameters, and localization, as well as the combination with other types of interventions. The heterogeneity of trials might contribute to a recent cautious interpretation of a meta-analysis concerning motor rehabilitation [30] despite promising single trials [11, 31–39].

Furthermore, peripheral techniques indirectly influencing cortical activity are under evaluation.

Increasing input from the paretic hand using somatosensory stimulation may also improve motor function [40, 41], but only limited data are available now. Motor training of the paretic hand itself increases somatosensory input as well as CIT (Figure 23.1).

Supporting neuroplasticity by pharmacological interventions

Pharmacological interventions can address several brain neurotransmitter systems that have been identified to be related to motor learning, e.g. glutamate, acetylcholine, 5-hydroxy tryptophan, norepinephrine, and dopamine. Drugs have been studied in animal models, healthy volunteers, and stroke patients in single or multiple dosages, with and without additional therapeutic tasks. No single medication evaluated for its beneficial effect of modulating plasticity has reached class I evidence so far. Several studies using this approach have been conducted for motor learning as well as aphasia therapy, but the results of some studies are contradictory. In detail levodopa, D-amphetamine, methylphenidate, donepezil, reboxetine, and fluoxetine are found to be beneficial in trials evaluating motor and/or aphasia recovery after stroke, but in one study D-amphetamine was found to have no effect [42–48]. In a recent study including 118 patients in a multicenter setting, fluoxetine was found to be beneficial (initiated 5–10 days after onset of stroke) in addition to standard inpatient rehabilitation in terms of promoting motor recovery and independence, demonstrated by significantly better scores using Fugl–Meyer and Rankin scales than in the placebo group [49]. The noradrenergic enhancement of reboxetine was found to be beneficial in reduction of cortical hyperactivity, especially in the ipsilesional ventral premotor cortex and supplementary motor area, as well as in improvements of pathological hypoconnectivity of ipsilesional supplementary motor area with the primary M1 [48], leading to functional improvements. For further description of models of functional network interactions and changes in neural networks after stroke, refer to Grefkes and Fink [50].

In a single-center observational study with various drugs, pharmacological augmentation was regarded as relatively safe [51].

Negative effects on outcome were noted for benzodiazepines, haloperidol, prazosin, and clonidine [52], leading to the advice to rather avoid these drugs during rehabilitation.

It is fair to conclude that larger controlled trials are needed, and findings need to be replicated as well as

375

patient selection criteria reapproved before pharmacological augmentation can be generally recommended. Meanwhile stroke patients presenting a reduced ability to take part in therapies due to diminished alertness and drive should be carefully evaluated for depression first. If treatment with stimulating antidepressants is not successful or not possible, the use of levodopa or a central stimulating agent may be an alternative treatment option, considering regulative issues of "off-label" use (see Table 23.1).

However, the most often used medications in neurorehabilitation of stroke patients are those addressing secondary prevention to diminish the risk of stroke recurrence.

> Non-invasive cortical stimulation techniques (repetitive transcranial magnetic stimulation and transcranial direct current stimulation) are used in rehabilitation to enhance neuroplasticity and recovery. In preliminary studies, some medications such as levodopa were found to be beneficial for motor recovery. Benzodiazepines, haloperidol, prazosin, and clonidine should rather be avoided.

Structured multidisciplinary neurorehabilitation

Importance of multidisciplinary teamwork for stroke recovery

In addition to thrombolysis, the multidisciplinary management in a stroke unit or by a stroke team has been shown to improve outcome significantly by reducing death rates and dependency (number needed to treat [NNT] 7 for thrombolysis versus NNT 9 for stroke unit treatment) [1]. The positive effect of stroke units is achieved by structural organization and interdisciplinary management, but also by early use of elements of neurorehabilitation[53, 54].

According to a large meta-analysis (n = 1437), the benefit of post-acute treatment in organized inpatient multidisciplinary rehabilitation (as compared with treatment on a general ward and other nonspecific rehabilitation clinics) is associated with reduced odds for death, institutionalization, and dependency. According to differences in place of stay with respect to independence after post-stroke rehabilitation, of 100 patients treated by organized multidisciplinary neurorehabilitation (as compared with general medical treatment), an extra 5 returned home in an independent state [55]. Therefore the beneficial elements of acute and post-acute stroke treatment should be combined.

The amount of rehabilitation treatment in the acute phase may vary widely, as a multicenter study examining physical activity within the first 14 days of acute stroke unit care has shown: in the daytime patients spent more than 50% of the time resting in bed, 28% sitting out of bed, and only 13% engaged in activities with the potential to prevent complications and improve recovery of mobility. Furthermore, patients were alone for 60% of their time [56]. The best timing for transferring a patient after initial treatment to a specialized neurorehabilitation ward or clinic is still under discussion, and concerns regarding optimal timing and intensity might also contribute to the problem (see below).

After acute stroke treatment medically stable patients with relevant neurological deficits should be treated in a specialized neurorehabilitation clinic or unit in an in- or outpatient setting to take advantage of the impact of the work of a specialized multidisciplinary team with structured organization and processes: the patient takes part in a multimodal, intensive treatment program which must be adapted to the individual goals of rehabilitation with regular interdisciplinary re-evaluation.

A short and useful definition for an *organized inpatient multidisciplinary rehabilitation* includes [55]:

- interdisciplinary goal-setting;
- input from a multidisciplinary team of medical, nursing, and therapy staff with an expertise in stroke and rehabilitation whose work is coordinated through regular weekly meetings under medical leadership;
- involvement of patients and family in the rehabilitation process;
- program of staff training.

This approach should be centered on the individual patient and family/caregivers, interacting closely with a multidisciplinary team consisting of physicians, nurses, physical and occupational therapists, kinesiotherapists, speech and language pathologists (SLPs), psychologists, recreational therapists, and social workers [4]. The required equipment in a neurorehabilitation department must be defined in detail to ensure structural quality. A continuous improvement process with description of medical and organizational processes using a quality-management system, as well as a positive error culture, e.g. using a critical incidence reporting system (CIRS), is also important for rehabilitation centers.

Table 23.1. Selected medications used in the course of neurorehabilitation

Indication	Substance	Remarks
Post-stroke depression	Venlafaxine	75–300(+) mg/day
	Citalopram	20–40 mg/day; also useful in pathological crying
	Mirtazapine	With sleep disorders; 15–45 mg/day (at bedtime); combination with venlafaxine and other possible
	Trazodone	With agitation; 50–200 mg/day (main dosage at bedtime); can also be used in the elderly
Diminished drive	Levodopa/benserazide	Evaluate 100/25–200/50 mg/day (studies for motor recovery undertaken with pulsed use in combination with physical therapies)
	Methylphenidate	Start with 10 mg/day, restricted substance, inpatient evaluation
Agitation, psychosis	Quetiapine	25–300(+) mg/day; in elderly patients start first application with 12.5–25 mg
Agitation, sleep disorder	Pipamperone	20–80(+) mg/day (at bedtime) for sleep disorder of the elderly
Post-stroke epilepsy	Levetiracetam	1000–3000 mg/day; 2000(+) mg/day in monotherapy
	Valproate	800–1800(+) mg/day; sometimes also used in central pain syndrome
	Carbamazepine	600–1200(+) mg/day; sometimes also used in central pain syndrome and paroxysmal symptoms
	Phenytoin and *other antiepileptic drugs*	250–300(+) mg/day
	Clonazepam, lorazepam *and other benzodiazepines*	i.v. application in status epilepticus; other indications include anxiety, sleep disorder, depression (temporarily) negative effect on cognition and learning; adverse drug reaction with agitation in the elderly
Pain/shoulder-arm pain	Ibuprofen *and other NSAIDs*	Combine with positioning and physical therapies
Shoulder-hand syndrome	Prednisone	Start trial with 50–70 mg/day
Central pain syndrome	Amitriptyline	Especially useful in constant burning pain; consider very slow initiation, e.g. 10 mg/day (50–75 mg/day) only second line in depression
	Pregabalin	Slow elevation diminishes side-effects; 75–300(600) mg/day
	Gabapentin	Slow elevation diminishes side-effects; 900–3600 mg/day
	Tramadol	Combination with pregabaline or gabapentine; 50–150(+) mg/day
	Oxycodone	In severe central pain syndrome; add-on; 5–50(+) mg/day
Bladder dysfunction	Oxybutynin	Detrusor spasticity; 5 –15(20) mg/day
	Darifenacin	1 × 7.5 mg (15 mg)/day
	Solifenacin	1 × 5 mg (10 mg)/day
	Tolterodine	1 × 4 mg (2 mg)/day

Table 23.1. (cont.)

Indication	Substance	Remarks
Bladder dysfunction (cont.)	Trospium chloride	2 × 20 mg/day
	Desmopressin	In severe nocturia; 20 µg/day given intranasally at bedtime
Reflux, gastritis, ulcers (prevention)	Omeprazole, pantoprazole *and other proton pump inhibitors*	Consider administration twice daily in critically ill patients
Spasticity	Botulinum toxin A	Period of >3 months between intramuscular injections to diminish risk of antibodies
	Baclofen	30–75(+) mg/day orally; intrathecal application in severe (spinal) spasticity
	Tizanidine	4–24 mg/day (orally baclofen and tizanidine have very limited effects in cerebral spasticity)

Notes: Please note that (1) substances mentioned are examples of their group; (2) several of the indications are "off-label"; please verify with your national regulation standards; (3) there are not enough data for all of the mentioned substances to provide evidence-based recommendations (expert opinion or observational studies); (4) medications for secondary prevention, dementia, cardiovascular diseases, and infections are not included.
NSAIDs = non-steroidal anti-inflammatory drugs.

At the onset of the rehabilitation process a multidisciplinary assessment of deficits and resources is mandatory, including clinical neurological examination, assessment of functional performance, activities of daily living (ADL), social and personal background, and coping strategies. To achieve recovery of physical and psychological functions and to reintegrate the patient into his/her social environment, therapies and other interventions must be adapted to the individual abilities and disabilities. In the course of rehabilitation the patients' progress and abilities are critically discussed and reevaluated in the multidisciplinary team in at least weekly sessions with an adaptation and reconsideration of treatment strategies and goals (see below), if necessary (Figure 23.2) [57].

> Treatment in an organized inpatient multidisciplinary setting improves the outcome after stroke significantly. The positive effect of stroke units is gained by structural organization and interdisciplinary management, but also by the early use of elements of neurorehabilitation.

Initiation and intensity of therapies

Clinical studies indicate that an early start and high intensity of therapies are decisive for a favorable long-term outcome. On the basis of pathophysiological data, the first 3 weeks after stroke are considered as a particularly promising period: in animal models active training leads to better functional recovery and sprouting, whereas inactivity results in additional loss of ability [14, 25, 26]. However, some experimental studies in rats show that very early (starting within 24 hours) and intense forced activity could lead to an enlargement of lesion areas. The occurrence of these negative consequences is explained by cytotoxic effects of glutamate, metabolic collapse of the penumbra region, inhibition of upregulation of signal proteins, focal hyperthermia, and other factors [58–60]. Other recent animal studies, however, support the early initiation of appropriate activation. Early motor activation starting at day 5 after focal ischemia had a superior outcome (functional measures and more dendritic sprouting) than a late beginning (at days 14 and 30) [25]. Furthermore, in primates reorganization of cortical representation areas was found to be more effective after early activation (within 7 days) [14, 61]. Finally, in contrast to the above-mentioned studies, a better functional result without signs of enlargement of lesion areas was achieved by early motor training in rats beginning 24 hours after maturation of ischemic lesions [62].

Clinical data are consistent with these findings. In humans, however, other factors should be taken into account: immobilization increases the rate of complications after acute stroke, including thrombosis, infections, and ulcers. Early mobilization in the first days and structured training at an early stage on a

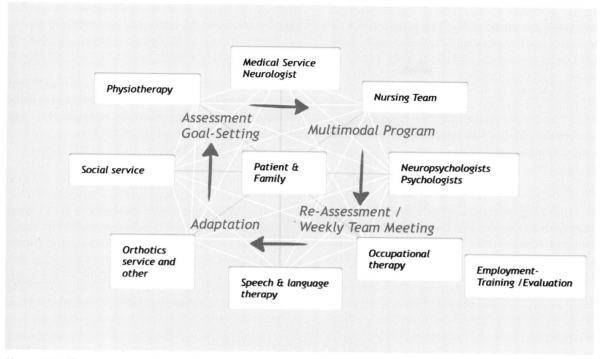

Figure 23.2. The patient-centered model of multidisciplinary specialized neurorehabilitation includes assessment, individual goal-setting, multimodal therapies, and reevaluation. The work of the multidisciplinary team of medical, nursing, and therapy staff with expertise in stroke rehabilitation is coordinated through regular weekly meetings with involvement of patients and family in the rehabilitation process.

stroke unit enhances the rate of discharges to the home with a lower degree of disabilities [63] as compared to later activation on a medical ward. Better long-term outcome is reported in stroke patients with early start of an organized inpatient multidisciplinary rehabilitation within 7 days in a multicenter study (n = 1760) with reduction of disability and better quality-of-life measures [64]. In another large study (n = 969) specifically examining the impact of the timing of the initiation of neurorehabilitation and functional recovery, a highly significant correlation of early treatment start and functional outcome was detected [65].

Not only early initiation of treatment but also the *intensity of rehabilitative therapies* is of significant importance, as shown in a meta-analysis [66], with higher mobility, autonomy, and improved executive functions when different therapeutic modalities are performed with increased intensity. Therapy intensity is also related to shorter lengths of stay and to improvements in patients' functional independence.

A higher intensity of therapies can also be achieved by the additional use of *rehabilitation robotics* in the multidisciplinary approach, as established for arm functioning and walking.

To summarize:

- immobilization after stroke is counterproductive (and should be reserved for specific rare situations, e.g. in the case of instable brain perfusion due to arterial stenosis) and
- an appropriate amount of activity should take place very early after the onset of stroke
- with the initiation of specific and intense individually adapted neurorehabilitation of the medically stable patient, ideally within the first days after stroke
- including in the course of treatment a high proportion of multimodal active therapies.

Early mobilization (within the first days) and structured training at an early stage improves the outcome after stroke.

Goal-setting and assessment in stroke rehabilitation

Structured assessment of deficits and resources in stroke, directly linked to the model of illness, can

379

provide the basis for definition of treatment goals: most widely accepted is the "The International Classification of Functioning, Disability and Health" (ICF) proposed by the WHO in 2001 providing a catalog of stroke-specific core-sets (2003). In determining treatment goals the medical model is extended by adding a social perspective and defining "participation" as an important objective. Treatment goals measure the physical and psychological status, examining the impact of deficits on social aspects such as everyday life, social communication, or ability to work. Even if some somatic functions cannot be regained directly, higher social goals can be reached by establishing compensatory strategies. Interdisciplinary goal-setting is crucial for determining the exact treatment schedule, for estimating the duration of neurorehabilitation, and for evaluating rehabilitative potential (Figure 23.3).

Assessment in stroke is crucial to demonstrate the course of recovery and benefit of neurorehabilitation

and also to deliver instruments for research purposes. Some assessment measures add *evaluation of quality of life* to *activity* as an outcome parameter. Activity can be assessed by *activity scales* and *scales of activities of daily living*.

Activity scales evaluate abilities and have their value in detailed measurement of aspects of specific therapies or in motor function research [49]. The most commonly used *activity scales* are:

• The Rivermead Mobility Index (RMI) [67]: a clinically relevant measure of disability which concentrates on body mobility. The RMI contains a series of 14 questions and one direct observation, and covers a range of activities from turning over in bed to running. Its validity as a measure of mobility after head injury and stroke was tested by concurrent measurement of mobility using gait speed and endurance, and by standing balance. The RMI forms a scale and can be used in hospital or at home. A modified version

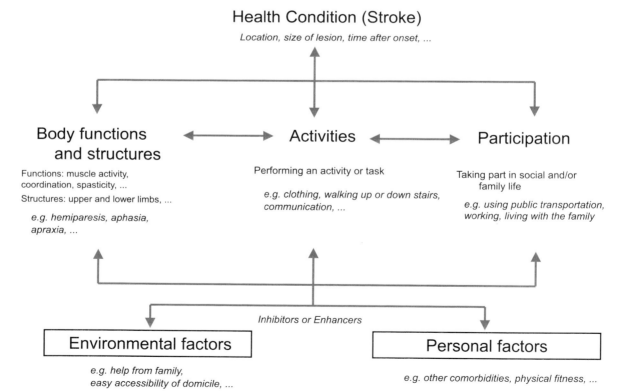

Figure 23.3. The ICF (The International Classification of Functioning, Disability and Health; WHO 2001) transforms the former WHO concept of "disability" into activity and stresses the interrelation of the several components: activity, body functions, body structures, participation, including two context factors: environmental and personal factors. (Figure adapted and examples added from "International Classification of Functioning, Disability and Health", World Health Organization, 2001.)

has been developed [68] in which the number of test items was reduced from 15 to 8 items in order to measure mobility-related items that physical therapists consider essential for demonstrating treatment effects in patients following stroke, with the aim of better sensitivity.

- The Motor Assessment Scale (MAS) [69] is a brief assessment of eight areas of motor function and one item related to muscle tone. Each item is scored on a scale from 0 to 6. It is aimed at the functional capacities of stroke patients, and the items are: supine to side lying, supine to sitting over the edge of a bed, balanced sitting, sitting to standing, walking, upper-arm function, hand movements, and advanced hand activities. Modified Motor Assessment Scale (MMAS): also included is a single item, general tonus, intended to provide an estimate of muscle tone on the affected side, which attracts criticism as being difficult to rate. In a special version [70] item descriptions were modified and the general tonus item was deleted.

- The Get-Up and Go Test [71] requires patients to stand up from a chair, walk a short distance, turn around, return, and sit down again. Balance function is scored on a five-point scale. In the development the same patients undergo laboratory tests for gait and balance, showing good correlation with laboratory tests. The Get-Up and Go Test is regarded as a satisfactory clinical measure of balance in elderly people.

- The Action Research Arm Test (ARAT) [72] is an evaluative measure to assess specific changes in limb function among individuals who have sustained cortical damage resulting in hemiplegia. The ARAT consists of 19 items grouped into four subscales: grasp, grip, pinch, and gross movement. It assesses the ability to handle objects differing in size, weight, and shape and therefore can be considered to be an arm-specific measure of activity limitation.

- The Nine Hole Peg Test (NHPT) [73] is composed of a square board with nine pegs and the patient is instructed to take pegs from a container, one by one, and place them into the holes on the board, as quickly as possible. It is aimed at measuring fine manual dexterity. The NHPT is easy to perform and estimates parts of the upper limb function.

Of the numerous scales to assess ADL the Barthel Index (BI) and the Functional Independence Measure (FIM), which includes additional items assessing the function of cognition, are most commonly used.

The BI [74] measures the extent to which somebody can function independently and has mobility in ADL; i.e. feeding, bathing, grooming, dressing, bowel control, bladder control, toilet use, transfers (bed to chair and back), mobility (on level surfaces), and stair climbing, resulting in a cumulative score between 0 and 100 and also indicating the need for assistance in care. The BI is a widely used measure of functional disability but there are numerous extensions and modifications, e.g. the modified 10-item version by Collin et al. [75], the extended BI (EBI) by Prosiegel et al. [76], and the Early Rehabilitation Barthel Index (ERI) proposed by Schönle [77].

The Functional Independence Measure (FIM) [78] was developed based on the BI and measures overall performance on ADL. It determines the need for assistance by another person (burden of care) and includes a cognitive domain score.

For assessing the ability of a person to live independently within a community an *instrumental activities of daily living* (IADL) is necessary, which includes several important and more complex functions that go beyond the items of basic self-care. It is debatable, however, which of the items, such as performing light housework, preparing a meal, taking medications, shopping for groceries or clothes, using the telephone and managing money, and many others, should be included.

For an overview on the scales used for *instrumental activities of daily living* and *measurements of quality of life* refer to Graham [79].

Stroke-specific instruments include the *Stroke Impact Scale* (SIS) [80], which is a self-report (patient and caregiver) health status measure to assess multidimensional stroke outcomes: in addition to functional status such as strength and hand function, ADL and other dimensions of health-related quality of life, such as communication, memory, and thinking, and social role function, are also considered. The SIS can show persisting difficulties in the physical domain of stroke patients who had been considered independent using ADL measures.

> Interdisciplinary goal-setting is crucial for determining the exact treatment schedule, for estimating duration as well as intensity of neurorehabilitation, and for evaluating rehabilitative potential. Assessment is obligatory using validated scales.

Methods and subtopics

Concepts of physiotherapy

The predominant common concepts of physiotherapy, the Bobath, Brunnstrom, proprioceptive neuromuscular facilitation (PNF), and Vojta methods, have in common that they claim to have a neurophysiological basis, in which facilitation and inhibition play a basic role. From an evidence-based point of view there is no doubt about the benefits of physiotherapy (see above) but there have not been sufficient data available to identify one of these special concepts as superior. The Bobath method is the leading approach in many central European countries, whereas in northern America and Scandinavia the Brunnstrom method is more common.

The Bobath concept was developed from the 1940s on by the physical therapist Berta Bobath and the physician Dr. Karel Bobath, who also supplied the neurophysiological background to their concept. Basically the Bobath concept involves "24 h management" in which first of all the patient's basal and everyday needs are targets of the therapeutic and nursing management. The concept of neuronal reorganization aims at preventing the development of pathological movements by recognizing variations of "normal central postural control mechanism" regulations. The evaluation according to Bobath includes assessments of tonus, reciprocal inhibition, and movement patterns. The treatment itself uses several stimuli, including positioning, tactile control, single movement elements, and others. As knowledge of neurophysiology has changed, it is no surprise that some of the former explanations may sound outdated from a modern point of view. But several modern principles of plasticity and learning can be identified in the concept, e.g. repetition, task specificity, goal orientation, avoidance of "learned non-use," and forced-use therapy. In addition the concept has developed, and changes in several aspects of its practical implementation have occurred.

The Brunnstrom approach is based on a concept developed by the Swedish physical therapist Signe Brunnstrom. It also uses facilitation techniques but, in contrast to the Bobath concept, in spastic hemiparesis synergetic patterns are regarded as early adaptations which are eventually transitioned by therapy into voluntary activation of movements.

The Bobath concept includes assessments of tonus, reciprocal inhibition, and movement patterns. The treatment itself uses several stimuli, including positioning, tactile control, single movement elements, and others. In comparative studies, no advantage has been found for one technique over the other, including the Bobath, Brunnstrom, and other techniques.

Motor rehabilitation

Motor impairment is the most common deficit in stroke, often resulting in reduced independence and mobility. Beside the concepts of physical, occupational, and other therapies (see below) the following methods are aimed especially at motor recovery.

Treadmill training

Walking is an important objective in stroke rehabilitation, conventional gait training programs on the floor being routine practice. With the aim of enhancing the efficacy of gait training and also of easing the burden on the therapists, three groups of treadmill training concepts have been developed and evaluated:

- body-weight supported treadmill training (BWSTT): partial body-weight support can be used to gain better stepping kinematics in stroke patients unable to walk;
- treadmill training without body-weight support;
- gait training devices or gait machines, such as the Lokomat or Gait Trainer GTI, in addition to BWSTT, can provide a "gait pattern" even for seriously paretic limbs.

In rehabilitation practice these methods are used in addition to conventional modalities, leaving no doubt about the benefit in terms of easing the burden on the therapists and overall being regarded as useful for certain patients. In addition, measurement of gait indicators such as velocity and distance can be easily monitored. Several studies investigated the efficacy on different outcome parameters of gait [81–85]. Most of the studies can be criticized for low treatment contrast since control groups also received intense conventional training, and in addition different outcome parameters and intensities make a comparison of the results harder. However a meta-analysis concludes that there is weak evidence for the overall effectiveness in improvement of gait endurance [86]. The authors recommend that currently BWSTT should be reserved for patients whose physical condition is too weak to tolerate intense training.

Gait training devices in stroke rehabilitation are currently being investigated regarding the potential benefit for walking training as well as for certain subgroups of stroke patients. It has been assumed that there might be an additional benefit for patients with neglect or pusher syndrome. In a recent study, patients took part either in conventional training or in robotic-assisted gait training, and the participants of the conventional group had better benefits, e.g., in improving their walking speed. The authors conclude that, for subacute stroke participants with moderate to severe gait impairments, the diversity of conventional gait training interventions appears to be more effective than robotic-assisted gait training for facilitating returns to walking ability [87]. However, benefits were found when integrating treadmill training with structured speed dependence as a complementary tool in gait rehabilitation of stroke patients including physiotherapy, resulting in better gait speed and cadence after a 2-week training program for hemiparetic outpatients. These findings were recently reproduced [88]: at the end of a 6-week trial including 67 patients in the first 3 months after subacute stroke, the subgroup that received locomotor therapy with the use of robotic-assisted gait training combined with regular physiotherapy showed promising effects on functional and motor outcomes as compared with regular physiotherapy alone, as expressed by a greater functional ambulatory capacity score and in their neurological status according to the National Institutes of Health Stroke Scale (NIHSS). However, for the primary outcome point (ability to walk independently) there were non-significant differences between the groups.

It is therefore concluded that patients who receive robot-assisted training in combination with physiotherapy after stroke are more likely to achieve better motor function than patients trained without these devices, or only with these devices [89]. Further data need to be collected.

Gait training with rhythmical acoustical pacing

Auditory stimulation is useful combined with treadmill training [70], resulting in gait symmetry improved with acoustic pacing. Non-blinded studies illustrate the positive effect of conventional gait training with rhythmic cueing by a metronome or embedded in music, resulting in better stride length and walking speed [90, 91].

Constraint-induced therapy (CIT)

The principles of CIT and constraint-induced movement therapy (CIMT) were described by Taub *et al.* in 1993 [92]; however, their relevance to practical neurorehabilitation and experimental neuroscience came later: at that time Taub argued that, after stroke, patients try unsuccessfully to use the affected side. Discouragement due to initial failure leads to "learned non-use." Later, three principles for this kind of therapy were formulated, consisting of constraining the unaffected limb, forcing use of the affected limb, and intensive practice. Using this method motor rehabilitation of the upper limb is possible, if a selective function for the paretic wrist and fingers is present before initiation of treatment with CIMT. Therefore its use as a general treatment method in stroke is limited. A placebo-controlled study applying CIMT over a 2-week period in patients with stroke onset at 3–9 months before therapies showed highly significantly greater improvements than in the control group in motor and functional improvement [93], still detectable at 2-year follow-up [94]. In a recent review including further studies, it was stated that the performed trials according to CIMT delivered a large effect size and showed robust effects on arm function, but not on hand function (Figure 23.4) [95].

Robotics for upper limb rehabilitation with/without elements of virtual reality

It has been stated that an estimated 30–60% of adult patients after stroke do not achieve satisfactory motor recovery of the upper limb despite intensive rehabilitation [96, 97]. Therefore, robotics for upper limb rehabilitation and elements of virtual reality (VR) have been combined in several technical devices and used for therapy and studies. In a recent meta-analysis of robot-assisted therapy of upper limb recovery after stroke, only a subsequent sensitivity analysis showed a significant improvement in upper limb motor function. No significant improvements were found in ADL function [98]. It has been concluded that larger samples; adequately controlled study design and follow-up; greater homogeneity in selection criteria; and parameters measuring severity of stroke, motor impairment, and recovery are necessary [96]. For an overview of different available robotics refer to Pignolo [99]. Comparable to gait machines, some devices provide training programs even for severely paretic limbs. In general the use of such robotics must

383

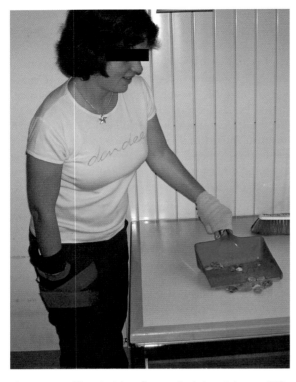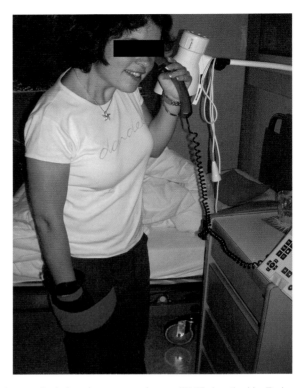

Figure 23.4. The principles of constraint-induced therapy (CIT) and constraint-induced movement therapy (CIMT) described by Taub are: constraining the unaffected limb, enforced use of the affected limb, and repetitive practice. The illustration shows a patient training the affected left arm in everyday life situations and therapeutic exercises.

be part of a multimodal rehabilitation program, while in most places upper limb rehabilitation is a special target of occupational therapy [100].

VR is a relatively recent approach that (in combination with robotics or interfaces) may enable simulated practice of functional tasks at a higher dosage than traditional therapies and therefore enhance the effect of repetitive task training as described above. VR uses computer technology to create environments that appear similar to real-world objects and situations, and furthermore VR technology has potentially the capability of creating an interactive, motivating environment in which practice intensity and feedback can be manipulated to create individualized treatments to retrain movement [96, 101]. Beside the development of robotics and VR devices for rehabilitation purposes, there has been rising interest in the use of available "off-the-shelf" gaming consoles, as models with sensors are available that enable participants to interact with games while performing wrist, arm, and hand movements [102], but more data need to be collected. As there is a

demand for cost-effective therapies and augmentation of therapies, also having in mind the worldwide burden of stroke in countries with lesser capacities to spend money on medical devices, further studies are regarded as valuable.

Repetitive training, aerobic exercises, and specific muscle strength training

According to learning theories and knowledge derived from studies of neuronal plasticity, a high repetition of tasks in rehabilitation in order to achieve better functional outcome is mandatory. A review of repetitive task training after stroke revealed modest improvement in lower limb function only, not in upper limb function [103, 104].

Stroke patients suffer not only from neurological deficits but also to varying extents from physical deconditioning and sometimes also from cardiac comorbidity [86]. Several studies address the possible benefit of general strengthening and aerobic exercises. In a retrospective analysis whole-body intensive rehabilitation was found to be feasible and effective in chronic stroke survivors [105]. In an observational study aerobic capacity and walking capacity were found to be decreased in hemiplegic stroke patients but were directly correlated with each other [106]. Adding physical fitness programs, e.g. by water-based exercise for cardiovascular fitness in stroke patients [107] or task-related circuit training [108], was found to be useful, leading to better outcome not only in physical fitness but also in various secondary measures such as walking speed and endurance, muscle strength, maximal workload, and others.

One concern in *specific muscle strength training* is increasing abnormal tone, leading to worsening of functional recovery. However, current opinions based on acquired data have changed; e.g. an observational study showed that targeted strength training significantly increased muscle power in patients with muscle weakness of central origin without any negative effects on spasticity [109]. Instead it was beneficial for functional outcome, showing that strength is related statistically to functional and walking performance.

Mirror therapy

Mirror therapy, mental practice, and enhanced feedback methods are regarded as promising strategies, especially in the management of the severely paretic limb. In mirror therapy a mirror is placed at 90° close to the midline of the patient, positioning the affected limb behind the mirror. Using this arrangement the patient is instructed to watch the non-affected limb in the mirror with both eyes and perform exercises. Hereby he or she is getting the visual impression that the limb in the mirror – attributed as the affected limb – is now fully functioning. The role of mirror therapy in motor rehabilitation is not clear yet, but recently, after methodologically weak publications, a promising randomized controlled trial (n = 40) has been published for upper limb rehabilitation of sub-acute stroke patients with severe motor affection without aphasia or apraxia [110]: approximately 1 hour of mirror therapy daily in addition to a conventional rehabilitation program was more beneficial in terms of motor recovery and hand-related functioning than a similar treatment without mirroring. The beneficial effect on hand functioning started post-treatment and continued during the 6-month follow-up evaluation rated by Functional Independence Measure subscales. Several underlying mechanisms have been discussed, e.g. substitution of mirror illusions of a normal movement of the affected hand for decreased proprioceptive information, thereby helping to activate the premotor cortex and promoting rehabilitation by enhancing connections between visual input and premotor areas [111]. Contralateral activation of visual fields was also shown using fMRI [112], with the result that healthy subjects view their hand as their opposite hand by mirroring, activating the visual cortex opposite to the seen hand. Mirror therapy could be an additional option for the rehabilitation of severely paretic limbs, but more data need to be collected.

Mental practice

Several studies examined the additional use of mental practice with motor imagery in stroke patients, especially in the management of the upper limb. While some studies reported promising results with improvements of motor functions (e.g. [113, 114]), there have also been reports of no benefit. Although the results of several publications suggest that mental practice can be a promising addition in motor rehabilitation of the severely affected limb, the role of mental practice for clinical routine remains unclear at the moment, and well-designed studies with sufficient numbers of patients are needed.

> Treadmill training, repetitive training, mirror therapy and constraint-induced therapy are newly investigated training principles and can be used especially for enhancing motor recovery.

Rehabilitation of speech disorders

Aphasia with its affection of different modalities, including speech, comprehension, reading, and writing, is a common consequence of stroke, mainly of the left hemisphere. Because of its enormous impact on patients' lives rehabilitative therapy is mandatory and uses principles such as forced-use for treatment concepts [115]. Even more than in other therapeutic modalities, the importance of a high treatment intensity has been demonstrated: a meta-analysis shows that studies which demonstrated a significant treatment effect of speech therapy on average provided 8.8 hours of therapy per week for about 11 weeks. In contrast, the negative studies only provided an average of 2 hours per week for about 23 weeks [116]. Furthermore, the total number of hours of aphasia therapy applied was directly linked to outcome, as measured by the Token Test, for example.

Rehabilitation of aphasia needs to be intense and newer studies correct the former uncertainty regarding the effectiveness of aphasia therapy. In the acute stage intense daily therapies are recommended. While spontaneous recovery can also be expected to some extent within the first year, only a minimal effect size is reported after 1 year post-onset [115]. Therefore, there is a need for therapy in chronic aphasia and an appeal for episodic concentration of therapies has been made, as positive effects were found after intensive (3 hours/day) short-term (10 consecutive days) intervention using communication language games in a group-therapy setting [91, 117]. For transfer of results from the therapeutic situation into the patients' environments there is also an indication for lower-frequency therapies of long duration.

The effect of aphasia therapy was also demonstrated using functional imaging such as PET. From functional imaging it is known that clinical aphasia syndromes in practice are not strictly linked to anatomical regions and furthermore, with these methods, the courses of recovery and less successful progress can be revealed [118, 119], showing that successful regeneration from post-stroke aphasia depends more on the integration of available language-related brain regions than on recruiting new brain regions. Using PET and rTMS interference, restoration (for the right-handed patient) of the left hemisphere network seems to be more effective. On the other hand, in some cases, right hemisphere areas are integrated successfully. This is especially relevant for severe aphasia, where the right hemisphere recruitment may play a larger role in supporting recovery, when there is a greater damage to left hemisphere language areas [120]. As summarized by Heiss and Thiel [121], responses due to tasks and therapies in the right superior temporal gyrus, especially in Wernicke's patients, and in the inferior frontal gyrus are seen, but more successful restoration of language is usually achieved only if left temporal areas are preserved and can be reintegrated into the functional network. Furthermore, the existence of a dual-pathway network for language and recovery with different functions for repetition and comprehension has been described, showing that the "classic" connection between the motor and sensory speech centers, the arcuate fascicle, is active during language repetition, even of pseudowords, whereas the function of language comprehension is linked to the integrity of the ventral pathway through the extreme capsule, providing

therefore a different anatomical course (implicating a potentially different location of damage) of these routes [122 ,123].

Several studies examined the additional benefit from brain stimulation techniques using TDCS [124] and rTMS [125, 126] as well as medication [45] on recovery from aphasia with positive results. However, it is premature to deduce a recommendation for clinical routine, as for aphasic patients there is currently not enough evidence that these task-specific improvements are persistent or have sufficient impact on real-life communication abilities [127]. In addition, for severe aphasia the use of intensive melodic intonation therapy is under evaluation.

Dysarthria is an impairment of speech intelligibility, which in about half of cases is due to lacunar syndrome [128]. Extracerebellar infarcts causing dysarthria were located in all patients along the course of the pyramidal tract. At follow-up evaluation of 38 patients, 40% were judged to have normal speech, 23 patients had mild residual dysarthria, and only seven suffered from ongoing severe speech disturbances, underlining the rather good prognosis under standard rehabilitation.

> Rehabilitation of aphasia needs to be intense and newer studies support the efficacy of speech therapy, if applied at sufficient frequency.

Dysphagia

Dysphagia is a potentially life-threatening complication of many neurological disorders, and stroke is the most common cause of neurogenic swallowing disorder.

The main dangers are:

- incidence of bolus, leading to acute blockage of airways;
- pneumonia due to aspiration;
- dysphagia can also lead to malnutrition and/or dehydration.

On the other hand, swallowing and food intake are important for the quality of life and autonomy of patients and will for many patients be considered an important goal of rehabilitation, according to the ICF (The International Classification of Functioning, Disability and Health; WHO 2001).

Dysphagia occurs in the acute state of stroke in more than 50% of patients, probably leading to aspiration in more than about 20% of them. In a meta-analysis of more than 15 studies using techniques such as fiberoptic endoscopic examination of swallowing (FEES) a wide range of dysphagia rates from 30% to 78% [129, 130] was identified. The rate of pneumonia in stroke is at least twice as high in dysphagic patients: in a meta-analysis nine trials were identified with a rate of pneumonia in patients identified as dysphagic ranging from 7% to 68%, with the highest number reflecting patients with proven aspiration [131]. In a study focusing on cause-specific mortality after first cerebral infarction of more than 440 patients in the first month after stroke, mortality resulted predominantly from neurological complications. Afterwards mortality remained high because of respiratory and cardiovascular factors, but mainly because of pneumonia [132]. It is therefore encouraging that the detection of dysphagia was found to be highly associated with the prevention of pneumonia, when appropriate treatment by the clinician was initiated, using, for example, variations in food consistency and fluid viscosity or implementation of swallowing techniques [133, 134]. The rate of detection, however, varies depending on the examination method and is highest for instrumental testing, which surpasses clinical testing protocols [130].

Neurogenic swallowing disorders are common in the course of stroke due to widespread involvement of different brain areas in swallowing, including cortical (mainly sensory and motor cortex, premotor cortex) and brainstem areas, e.g. nuclei of caudal cranial nerves and "central pattern generators" within the medulla oblongata.

Evaluation of swallowing functions includes *clinical evaluation*, consisting of:

- *clinical neurological examination* with emphasis on bulbar symptoms, dysarthria, disturbed sensation and reflexes of the oropharynx;
- noting the most important *warning signs*: (a) voice sounds wet or "gurgly," (b) bubbling sound during respiration, (c) drooling, (d) history of recurrent respiratory infections, (e) coughing, especially while/after eating or drinking;
- performing *clinical bedside tests*: various protocols exist, most of them using clear and clean water portions in ascending volume, with monitoring of warning signs (which can be combined with oximetry). A more structured, elaborated, and easy-to-use bedside test, the Gugging Swallowing Screen (GUSS) [134], allows a graded rating with separate evaluations for nonfluid and fluid

nutrition, starting with nonfluids, and assesses the severity of aspiration risk and recommends a special diet accordingly.

Particularly if technical evaluation is not performed, offering food should begin with food of simple consistencies.

If a stroke patient *presents with warning signs and/ or has failed a bedside test* at least three main targets should be considered:

- *avoiding aspiration*: mandatorily discontinue oral food/fluid intake until a detailed treatment plan is set up;
- *nutrition*: choose an alternative pathway, e.g. nasogastric tube (up to 4 weeks) or in many cases percutaneous endoscopic gastrostomy;
- *quality of life, regaining autonomy*: continuing diagnosis and description of the swallowing problems *previous* to individual therapy, which in most cases will include technical evaluation (adapted from Prosiegel *et al.* [135]).

The rate of detection of dysphagia is higher with *technical evaluation*, which furthermore allows determination of the degree of swallowing disorder and checking of, for example, the appropriateness of compensatory maneuvers and adaptation of food/fluid consistency. The methods predominantly used are:

- *Fiberoptic endoscopic examination of swallowing (FEES)* [136]: the value of laryngoscopy has become appreciated for its direct view of the larynx, functional structures, and mucosa, and its value in guiding treatment. Therefore FEES has become a standard procedure. At the onset of the swallow the pharyngeal air space is obliterated by tissue contacting other tissue and the bolus passing through, resulting in a so-called "swallow whiteout" without direct vision. However, when the swallow is over, its success or failure can be judged by the residue of colored test food and fluids [137]. FEES has only limited ability to assess the upper esophageal sphincter (UES) and its dysfunctioning.
- *Videofluoroscopic swallowing study (VFSS)*: the stroke patient must be able to sit in front of a fluoroscope. First, anatomical structures and landmarks are identified at rest without contrast. Then radiopaque material (usually barium) mixed with liquid and food of varying consistencies is administered [138].

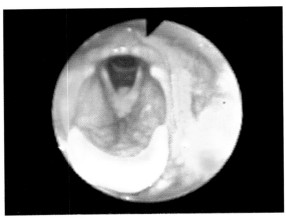

Figure 23.5. Fiberoptic Endoscopic Examination of Swallowing (FEES): Findings from an 18-year-old female (cerebral venous sinus thrombosis) with tracheostomy showing severe dysphagia with penetration, residuals, and postdeglutitive "silent" aspiration (patient shows no coughing at any time); rating score 8 on Rosenbek penetration-aspiration scale. Later withdrawal from the tracheostomy after structured laryngopharyngeal sensory-training (using a fenestrated and perforated cannula with a one-way speech valve) was successful.

The main *pathological findings* of the technical examinations include:

- leaking/pooling: fluids/food reach the pharynx in an uncontrolled way;
- penetration: fluids/food are reaching the aditus laryngis prematurely, above the vocal cords;
- retention: fluids/food remain in the hypopharynx after swallowing, e.g. in the sinus piriformis (carrying the risk of later aspiration);
- aspiration, including silent aspiration: fluids/food pass the vocal cords. It is especially dangerous if coughing or other cleaning procedures are not promptly initiated. To rate the findings of such examinations the Rosenbek penetration–aspiration scale is established (Figure 23.5) [139].

After defining the individual problems of swallowing dysfunction, an adequate treatment schedule can be set up, including several *therapeutic compensatory interventions*, for example:

- modify bolus volume, consistency, viscosity;
- change method of food/liquid delivery;
- modify sequence of delivery;
- change rate of food/liquid delivery;
- alter behavior (e.g. dry/clearing swallows, postural changes);

and *rehabilitative* techniques which include:

- swallow maneuvers (supraglottic swallow, effortful swallow);
- exercises (to increase strength of muscle groups); sensory stimulation techniques (thermal-tactile stimulation and others) [137].

In addition peripheral and central stimulation techniques for the treatment of dysphagia are under evaluation, but it is premature to conduct routine clinical use.

> Dysphagia is a common and dangerous problem after stroke and can be detected by clinical assessment and technical evaluation (fiberoptic endoscopy or videofluoroscopy). It must be treated by modification of the ingested substances and rehabilitative techniques.

Tracheostomy

Patients admitted with tracheostomy also need intense dysphagia management. Endoscopic evaluation of the cannula should be performed, looking for the correct distal position (to avoid lesions of the trachea by chronic pressure) and, if a model with fenestration is used, checking the fenestration (which is often closed by material or granuloma, or the fenestration of the cannula might not be suitable anatomically for the individual patient). Basically when withdrawal from the cannula is formulated as a goal because a patient with tracheostomy improves as regards dysphagia, level of consciousness, and/or pulmonary function, one should try to increase the duration of episodes with aeration of the larynx and pharynx in order to diminish sensory loss of the mucosa and to increase swallowing function. This can be achieved by using a cannula with fenestration and one-way speech valve and/or deblockage of the cannula. Respiration and swallowing function must be controlled carefully. If long-term tracheostomy is needed, percutaneous tracheotomy should be avoided because of the high rate of long-term complications, with high rates of bleeding, granulomas, pain, and other problems such as the often difficult exchange by caregivers [140, 141].

Treatment of spasticity

The treatment of spasticity requires mainly physiotherapy, nursing care, occupational therapy, and in many cases orthotic management. Whereas spasticity as a consequence of a stroke might in many cases also have a certain beneficial compensatory aspect, it can also lead to increased disability, loss of function, pain, and hindered care, and also carries the risk of secondary complications. If physical treatment reaches a limit, in generalized symptoms of spasticity one might want to consider the option of oral agents and intrathecal baclofen, but orally given medication such as baclofen in cortical or subcortical stroke has a disappointing effect to side-effect ratio in most cases. In focal or sometimes multifocal spasticity, *botulinum toxin* as a part of a longer-term strategy is an often successful treatment option in many cases, requiring patient assessment and definition of the goals of treatment [142]. Botulinum toxin (which exists in seven different serotypes, proteins A–G) acts on cholinergic neuromuscular junctions to block transmitter release. Type A was the first botulinum toxin for medical use. Applied into the muscles by injection, a positive effect can be expected after between several days and 1 week, lasting for 3–6 months. Often one or two treatment sessions with botulinum toxin are helpful to regain therapeutic benefit from intense physical therapies. In general, botulinum toxin is considered a safe therapeutic agent [143]; however, there have been safety warnings regarding the adherence to the maximum dosage per session and time interval between injections because of case reports about exacerbation of pre-existing swallowing disorders and neurological deterioration in higher-dosage applications.

Practically, the use of electromyography for application helps to improve the cost-effectiveness and the use of lower dosages. As several products of botulinum toxin A and B with different rates of effectiveness per unit are available, documentation of the product used is indispensable.

If multimodal treatment of spasticity (maybe also considering serial casting) fails, surgical therapy in some cases may finally be a therapeutic option.

In the event of an increase in spasticity in the course of treatment, symptomatic factors such as infections, bladder dysfunctioning, fractures, thrombosis, and many others should be considered.

> Spasticity can be treated with physiotherapy, nursing care, and occupational therapy. If physical treatment comes to a limit, in focal spasticity the use of botulinum toxin, or in severe cases surgical therapy are treatment options, whereas the use of oral agents in cerebral infarction is often limited due to side-effects.

Neuropsychological syndromes and cognitive recovery after stroke

Besides defined neuropsychological syndromes, cognitive impairment after a stroke is very common and may persist in the post-acute and also the chronic phase. Individual assessment includes evaluation of several aspects of attention, intelligence, memory, executive functions, and personality prior to devising an individual treatment schedule, which can be neuropsychologically specific but should also be interdisciplinary, as the impairment usually has an impact on several aspects of the rehabilitation progress and the ability to cope with the ADL. Depending on treatment goals, a more practical evaluation including out-of-hospital observations can also be useful. For detailed guidelines on cognitive rehabilitation refer to Cappa *et al.* [144].

> Restoration or preservation of cognition is an important and increasingly recognized field in stroke rehabilitation. Impairment of attention, memory, and other domains has to be considered when setting up treatment goals.

Spatial neglect

Spatial neglect is a common syndrome following stroke, most frequently of the right hemisphere, predominantly but not exclusively of the parietal lobe. It is a complex deficit in attention and awareness which can affect extrapersonal space and/or personal perception. Elements of spatial neglect may also be seen with infarctions of the left hemisphere; however, symptoms are clinically less consistent than in right hemispheric neglect [145].

The therapeutic process is often prolonged. In multidisciplinary neurorehabilitation, perception via the affected side is enforced as much as possible, and additional alertness training as well as visual, proprioceptive, and vestibular stimulation techniques are used [146, 147]. In addition to focal disturbances, in this condition an interhemispheric imbalance is supposed to be of predominant clinical relevance. Therefore, several studies have been published to evaluate the benefit of cortical stimulation techniques in neglect therapy, addressing the contralesional hemisphere overexcitability as a central pathophysiological mechanism in hemispatial neglect. For a review on technical considerations and recent data refer to Muri *et al.* [31]. The authors conclude that there are promising results especially for rTMS theta-burst stimulation, stressing its future role as an add-on therapy in the rehabilitation of neglect patients, despite overall methodological heterogeneity of available studies and still limitations of collected data.

> Spatial neglect is a frequent syndrome of right hemispheric stroke and needs active and prolonged attention in the rehabilitation process.

Other neuropsychological syndromes

Hemianopia has a large impact on daily activities which appears in problems in reading, orientation, and safety in traffic. Basic rehabilitative management includes stimulation from the hemianopic side (e.g. positioning of the bed, talking). While spontaneous recovery might occur at least up to several months, treatment options such as visual field training are controversial. Using compensatory visual field training compared with a control group no formal change of visual defect was reported by Nelles *et al.* [148], although the training improved detection of and reaction to visual stimuli. Other groups recently reported an improvement of the visual field of up to 5° for ischemic lesions and up to 10° benefit for stroke after a hemorrhage, using reaction perimetry treatment [149].

Space perception disorders can lead to spatial disorientation (affecting a person's topographical orientation), well known in right-hemisphere infarction. A misperception of the body's orientation in the coronal plane is seen in stroke patients with a "pusher syndrome." They experience their body as oriented upright when it is in fact tilted to one side, and therefore use the unaffected arm or leg to actively push away from the unparalyzed side and typically try to resist any attempt to passively correct their body posture. The syndrome is a distinctive clinical disorder after unilateral left or right brain lesions in the posterior thalamus or in the insula and postcentral gyrus [150]. The recovery under physical therapy, by trying to enhance sensorimotor input from the contralateral side, is often prolonged.

Apraxia is a syndrome of left-hemisphere infarction. It often severely hinders ADL independence (apart from contributing to speech disorders as speech apraxia) and treatment of apraxia should definitely be part of the overall neurorehabilitation program [144]. Although the literature on recovery and treatment is limited, apraxia has been shown to be improved by occupational therapy. For a review of apraxia treatment and also on other aspects of occupational therapy refer to Steultjens *et al.* [100].

Further reading in the topic of behavioral and cognitive aspects of stroke is provided by Godefroy [151].

> Hemianopia, visual perception deficits, and apraxia are frequent and disabling. They deserve active screening and should be considered in goal-setting.

Rehabilitation of brainstem syndromes

The locked-in syndrome (LiS) typically originates from a ventro-pontine lesion, resulting in a complete quadriplegia and anarthria without coma (in stroke caused by basilar artery occlusion or brainstem hemorrhage). In most cases communication remains possible (by simple or elaborate speech coding), using spared vertical eye movements or blinking. For the clinician it is important to know this syndrome and to make an early diagnosis. The levels of cognitive function in cases of pure brainstem lesions are normal in many cases, while additional brain injuries are most likely responsible for associated cognitive deficits in LiS [152]. Patients should receive early and intensive multidisciplinary rehabilitation with the goal of establishing communication, with evaluation of the use of patient–computer interfaces such as infrared eye-movement detectors and others. In the first treatment episode the prognosis is undetermined, as a small proportion of patients to some extent develop motor recovery [153]. According to the authors, in spite of severe disability most of these patients do not want to die.

> The locked-in syndrome – quadriplegia and anarthria without coma – is usually caused by severe pontine infarction often due to basilar artery occlusion or brainstem hemorrhage and represents a challenge to rehabilitation teams.

As in other brainstem syndromes, *pathological crying* can also occur in LiS (selective serotonin reuptake inhibitor [SSRI] medication should be evaluated; see Table 23.1).

Brainstem lesions should be carefully evaluated for dysphagia. Individual assessment is necessary in severe brainstem syndromes with vegetative state or minimally conscious state.

Other common problems in clinical practice

Bladder dysfunction: urine incontinence occurs frequently in the acute state of stroke and after 1 year 20% of survivors suffer from it. The patient should be investigated for residual urine by ultrasound or intermittent catheterization, and infection should be ruled out. Disorders of storage can be treated by bladder retraining and pelvic floor exercises. In storage problems provoked by detrusor spasticity, which can occur with or without urethral sphincter dysfunction, treatment with anticholinergic drugs such as oxybutynin, darifenacin, solifenacin, tolterodine, or trospium chloride should be evaluated (see Table 23.1).

Pain in the post-stroke episode may be due to different causes, e.g. associated with spasticity (see above) or related to a central post-stroke syndrome. Mostly affections of the brainstem, thalamic structures, or spinal stroke contribute to this problem. This specific pain can be episodic but more often is constant. Treatment options include physiotherapy, and medication (see Table 23.1) such as antidepressants, anticonvulsants, and opioid analgesics. Because of the chronic course, psychological support to improve coping may be necessary.

Hemiplegic shoulder (arm) pain has multiple causes. The shoulder joint in hemiplegia is sensitive to traumatization of various structures and inferior subluxation can lead to injuries, including tendons, capsule, or peripheral nerves and plexus. It is important to keep the shoulder correctly positioned to prevent subluxation. Hemiplegic shoulder pain in stroke may be due to adhesive capsulitis (50%), shoulder subluxation (44%), rotator cuff tears (22%), and shoulder-hand syndrome (16%) [154]. The etiology of shoulder-hand syndrome with pain of the shoulder or arm and edema of the hand and arm is controversial; many authors consider it a form of reflex sympathetic dystrophy/complex regional pain syndrome, probably initiated by mechanisms mentioned above. Management includes positioning, orthotic management, physical therapy including steps for reduction of edema, and analgesics. In more severe cases intermediate dosage treatment with oral prednisone is effective [155].

Depression: post-stroke depression occurs in at least one-third of patients in the first year after onset, although estimates differ widely between studies due to varying definitions, populations, exclusion criteria, and the timing of assessments [156]. Post-stroke depression often hinders the course of rehabilitation and influences recovery and outcome following stroke. It is often underdiagnosed because of overlapping symptoms with the stroke itself. It sometimes manifests itself in subtle signs, such as refusal to participate in treatments. Antidepressive treatment with SSRI and related substances (see Table 23.1) is the first treatment choice; in addition studies suggest adaptations of cognitive-behavioral therapy techniques and brief supportive therapy to be beneficial [4]. In a Cochrane review, however, there was no evidence for improvements of post-stroke depression by medication. The authors indicate that the heterogeneity of the studies and problematic patient selection, with exclusion of certain neurological deficits such as aphasia, might have led to the result [156].

Driving after stroke: in a study investigating relative crash risk associated with medical conditions (n = 4448) the diagnosis "previous stroke" was only a nearly significant risk [157]. There is no doubt that driving ability in the post-stroke period needs assessment, and a study by Fisk *et al.* shows that patients are in danger of making inappropriate decisions about their driving capabilities without professional advice and/or evaluation [158]. As a first step there are certain medical and neurological conditions where clinical judgment will confirm stroke patients as being incapable of driving, e.g. persistent complete hemianopia, neglect, recent seizures, and relevant cognitive impairment, whereas pure motor deficits can often be solved by car adaptation.

The extent of further evaluation ranges from screening tests, specific neuropsychological assessments, and simulator tests to full road tests. If a post-stroke patient is evaluated as not capable of driving, a reassessment in the further course of rehabilitation with appropriate therapies can be a goal. It has also been shown that simulator-based driving training improved driving ability, especially for well-educated and less disabled stroke patients [159].

Partnership and sexual functioning: partnership is in many cases affected by the post-stroke condition, owing to altered physical and psychological conditions with their implications for everyday life and communication. Couple psychotherapy can be initiated and also improvements to assistance in the various fields can indirectly help relieve the often serious problems. Summarized in a review by Rees *et al.* [160], observational studies suggest that the frequency and range of sexual disorders after stroke are high and a noticeable decline in sexuality occurs in both genders after stroke; furthermore, partner dissatisfaction is high. In addition to the direct consequences of stroke, psychosocial issues and depression are likely to contribute to the problem. Pre-existing vascular disorders may also cause erectile difficulties as well as antihypertensive agents and other drugs. As the problems are often complex, treatment suggestions have to

391

be comprehensive. Erectile dysfunctioning can be treated with phosphodiesterase type 5 inhibitors or intracavernosal prostaglandin E1 injections.

Hypersexuality rarely occurs, and is treatable with behavioral therapy, SSRI, and antiandrogens.

Social problems after stroke can severely affect various aspects of patients' lives, such as unemployment, invalidity, financial problems, problems with health insurance, difficulties with housing, family issues, social contacts, and other factors. Social counseling is therefore mandatory in the course of stroke rehabilitation, which includes, for example, information about social security systems, social services, self-help and stroke groups.

Chapter summary

Neuroplasticity is the dynamic potential of the brain to reorganize itself during ontogeny and learning, or following damage. The central nervous system of the adult human being has an astounding potential for regeneration and adaptability, which can be selectively supported and used for rehabilitation.

Several mechanisms of neuronal plasticity can be identified:

- *Vicariation* describes the hypothesis that functions of damaged areas can be taken over by different regions of the brain.
- *Plasticity of areas of cortical representation*: damage to the brain leads to an increased recruitment of secondary areas of representation as early compensation, followed by a later phase of reorganization.
- *Sprouting of neurons* as in the peripheral nervous system. In the central nervous system of the adult, however, this mechanism is reduced, but not absent.
- *Diaschisis* describes the phenomenon that a focal lesion may also lead to changes in brain functioning of areas located far away.

Neuroplasticity can be supported by:

- Early elements of neurorehabilitation in the stroke unit setting and later the work of a multidisciplinary specialized team in a neurorehabilitation clinic. In this setting input from a team of medical, nursing, and therapy staff; optimal timing and early initiation (i.e. within 7 days) of intensive rehabilitation; and the definition of treatment goals following physical

and psychological status evaluation are beneficial.

- Special training, such as treadmill training, constraint-induced therapy (CIT: the unaffected limb is constrained to enforce the use of the affected limb under intensive practice), repetitive training, or mirror therapy.
- Peripheral and brain stimulation techniques: repetitive transcranial magnetic stimulation (rTMS) leads to decreased or increased cortical excitability, depending on the frequency. It can be used for downregulation of the contralesional or stimulation of the ipsilesional hemisphere. With transcranial direct current stimulation (TDCS), a weak polarizing electrical current is delivered to the cortex.
- Pharmacological interventions: in preliminary studies, some medications such as levodopa and others were found to be beneficial for motor recovery, while others, e.g. benzodiazepines, had a negative effect on outcome.

Speech disorders need intense training because of their enormous impact on the patient's life. Newer studies with therapies taking place daily for several hours correct the former uncertainty regarding the effectiveness of aphasia therapy. Brain stimulation techniques and medication might add additional benefit.

Dysphagia occurs in the acute state of stroke in more than 50% of patients, probably leading to aspiration in more than about 20% of them. To detect dysphagia, clinical evaluation can be combined with technical tests such as fiberoptic endoscopic examination of swallowing (FEES) and videofluoroscopic swallowing studies (VFSS). After defining the individual problems in swallowing dysfunction, adequate therapeutic compensatory interventions, for example modification of bolus volume and viscosity, and rehabilitative techniques, such as exercise or sensory stimulation, can be set up. Patients admitted with tracheostomy often also need intense dysphagia management.

Spasticity can be treated with physiotherapy, nursing care, and occupational therapy. If physical treatment reaches a limit, oral agents, intrathecal baclofen, and especially botulinum toxin are treatment options.

For the treatment of **spatial neglect**, perception via the affected side is enforced as much as possible and additional alertness training as well as visual and proprioceptive stimulation techniques are used. Only a few pilot studies have been published to evaluate the benefit of cortical stimulation techniques (e.g. inhibitory low-frequency rTMS).

References

1. Warlow C, Sudlow C, Dennis M, Wardlaw J, Sandercock P. Stroke. *Lancet* 2003; **362**:1211–24.

2. Beer S, Clarke S, Diserens K, *et al.* Neurorehabilitation nach Hirnschlag. *Schweiz Med Forum* 2007; **7**:294–7.

3. Albert SJ, Kesselring J. Neurorehabilitation of stroke. *J Neurol* 2012; **259**:817–32.

4. Duncan PW, Zorowitz R, Bates B, *et al.* Management of Adult Stroke Rehabilitation Care: a clinical practice guideline. *Stroke* 2005; **36**: e100–43.

5. Cajal R. *Degeneration and Regeneration of The Nervous System.* London: Oxford University Press; 1928.

6. Foerster O. Übungstherapie. In: Bumke O, Foerster O, eds. *Handbuch der Neurologie*, Vol. **8**, *Allgemeine Neurologie.* 1936; 316–414.

7. Kesselring J. Neurorehabilitation: a bridge between basic science and clinical practice. *Eur J Neurol* 2001; **8**:221–5.

8. Hebb DO. *The Organization of Behavior: A Neuropsychological Approach.* New York: Wiley; 1949.

9. Møller A. Basis for neural plasticity. In: Møller AR, *Neural Plasticity and Disorders of the Nervous System.* Cambridge: Cambridge University Press; 2006: 7–32.

10. Nelles G. Neuronale Plastizität. In: Nelles G, *ed. Neurologische Rehabilitation.* Stuttgart: Thieme; 2004: 1–13.

11. Duffau H. Brain plasticity: from pathophysiological mechanisms to therapeutic applications. *J Clin Neurosci* 2006; **13**:885–97.

12. Nudo RJ. Mechanisms for recovery of motor function following cortical damage. *Curr Opin Neurobiol* 2006; **16**:638–44.

13. Ward NS. Future perspectives in functional neuroimaging in stroke recovery. *Eura Medicophys* 2007; **43**:285–94.

14. Nudo RJ, Milliken GW. Reorganization of movement representations in primary motor cortex following focal ischemic infarcts in adult squirrel monkeys. *J Neurophysiol* 1996; **75**:2144–9.

15. Nudo RJ, Milliken GW, Jenkins WM, Merzenich MM. Use-dependent alterations of movement representations in primary motor cortex of adult squirrel monkeys. *J Neurosci* 1996; **16**:785–807.

16. Liepert J, Graef S, Uhde I, Leidner O, Weiller C. Training-induced changes of motor cortex representations in stroke patients. *Acta Neurol Scand* 2000; **101**:321–6.

17. Jaillard A, Martin CD, Garambois K, Lebas JF, Hommel M. Vicarious function within the human primary motor cortex? A longitudinal fMRI stroke study. *Brain* 2005; **128**:1122–38.

18. Ward NS, Cohen LG. Mechanisms underlying recovery of motor function after stroke. *Arch Neurol* 2004; **61**:1844–8.

19. Ward NS, Brown MM, Thompson AJ, Frackowiak RS. Neural correlates of motor recovery after stroke: a longitudinal fMRI study. *Brain* 2003; **126**:2476–96.

20. Ward NS, Brown MM, Thompson AJ, Frackowiak RS. Neural correlates of outcome after stroke: a cross-sectional fMRI study. *Brain* 2003; **126**:1430–48.

21. Calautti C, Baron JC. Functional neuroimaging studies of motor recovery after stroke in adults: a review. *Stroke* 2003; **34**:1553–66.

22. Ruber T, Schlaug G, Lindenberg R. Compensatory role of the cortico-rubro-spinal tract in motor recovery after stroke. *Neurology* 2012; **79**:515–22.

23. Di Lazzaro V, Oliviero A, Profice P, *et al.* Direct demonstration of interhemispheric inhibition of the human motor cortex produced by transcranial magnetic stimulation. *Exp Brain Res* 1999; **124**:520–4.

24. Shimizu T, Hosaki A, Hino T, *et al.* Motor cortical disinhibition in the unaffected hemisphere after unilateral cortical stroke. *Brain* 2002;**125**:1896–907.

25. Biernaskie J, Chernenko G, Corbett D. Efficacy of rehabilitative experience declines with time after focal ischemic brain injury. *J Neurosci* 2004; **24**:1245–54.

26. Wall PD, Egger MD. Formation of new connections in adult rat brains after partial deafferentation. *Nature* 1971; **232**:542–5.

27. Witte OW. Lesion-induced plasticity as a potential mechanism for recovery and rehabilitative training. *Curr Opin Neurol* 1998;**11**:655–62.

28. Von Monakow C. *Die Lokalisation in Grosshirn und der Abbau der Funktion durch kortikale Herde.* Wiesbaden: Bergmann; 1914.

29. Johansson BB, Ohlsson AL. Environment, social interaction, and physical activity as determinants of functional outcome after cerebral infarction in the rat. *Exp Neurol* 1996; **139**:322–7.

30. Hao Z, Wang D, Zeng Y, Liu M. Repetitive transcranial magnetic stimulation for improving function after stroke. *Cochrane Database Syst Rev* 2013; **5**: CD008862.

31. Muri RM, Cazzoli D, Nef T, *et al.* Non-invasive brain stimulation in neglect rehabilitation: an update. *Front Hum Neurosci* 2013; 7:248.

32. Nyffeler T, Cazzoli D, Hess CW, Muri RM. One session of repeated parietal theta burst stimulation trains induces long-lasting improvement of visual neglect. *Stroke* 2009; **40**:2791–6.

33. Schlaug G, Marchina S, Wan CY. The use of non-invasive brain stimulation techniques to facilitate

recovery from post-stroke aphasia. *Neuropsychol Rev* 2011; **21**:288–301.

34. Harris-Love ML, Cohen LG. Noninvasive cortical stimulation in neurorehabilitation: a review. *Arch Phys Med Rehabil* 2006; **87**: S84–93.

35. Schlaug G, Renga V, Nair D. Transcranial direct current stimulation in stroke recovery. *Arch Neurol* 2008; **65**:1571–6.

36. Talelli P, Cheeran BJ, Teo JT, Rothwell JC. Pattern-specific role of the current orientation used to deliver Theta Burst Stimulation. *Clin Neurophysiol* 2007; **118**:1815–23.

37. Talelli P, Greenwood RJ, Rothwell JC. Exploring Theta Burst Stimulation as an intervention to improve motor recovery in chronic stroke. *Clin Neurophysiol* 2007; **118**:333–42.

38. Talelli P, Rothwell J. Does brain stimulation after stroke have a future? *Curr Opin Neurol* 2006; **19**:543–50.

39. Ward NS. Neural plasticity and recovery of function. *Prog Brain Res* 2005; **150**:527–35.

40. Alon G, Levitt AF, McCarthy PA. Functional electrical stimulation (FES) may modify the poor prognosis of stroke survivors with severe motor loss of the upper extremity: a preliminary study. *Am J Phys Med Rehabil* 2008; **87**:627–36.

41. Alon G, Levitt AF, McCarthy PA. Functional electrical stimulation enhancement of upper extremity functional recovery during stroke rehabilitation: a pilot study. *Neurorehabil Neural Repair* 2007; **21**:207–15.

42. Berthier ML, Green C, Higueras C, *et al.* A randomized, placebo-controlled study of donepezil in poststroke aphasia. *Neurology* 2006; **67**:1687–9.

43. Berthier ML, Green C, Lara JP, *et al.* Memantine and constraint-

induced aphasia therapy in chronic poststroke aphasia. *Ann Neurol* 2009; **65**:577–85.

44. Grade C, Redford B, Chrostowski J, Toussaint L, Blackwell B. Methylphenidate in early poststroke recovery: a double-blind, placebo-controlled study. *Arch Phys Med Rehabil* 1998; **79**:1047–50.

45. Kessler J, Thiel A, Karbe H, Heiss WD. Piracetam improves activated blood flow and facilitates rehabilitation of poststroke aphasic patients. *Stroke* 2000; **31**:2112–16.

46. Rosser N, Heuschmann P, Wersching H, *et al.* Levodopa improves procedural motor learning in chronic stroke patients. *Arch Phys Med Rehabil* 2008; **89**:1633–41.

47. Scheidtmann K, Fries W, Muller F, Koenig E. Effect of levodopa in combination with physiotherapy on functional motor recovery after stroke: a prospective, randomised, double-blind study. *Lancet* 2001; **358**:787–90.

48. Wang LE, Fink GR, Diekhoff S, *et al.* Noradrenergic enhancement improves motor network connectivity in stroke patients. *Ann Neurol* 2011; **69**:375–88.

49. Chollet F, Tardy J, Albucher JF, *et al.* Fluoxetine for motor recovery after acute ischaemic stroke (FLAME): a randomised placebo-controlled trial. *Lancet Neurol* 2011; **10**:123–30.

50. Grefkes C, Fink GR. Reorganization of cerebral networks after stroke: new insights from neuroimaging with connectivity approaches. *Brain* 2011; **134**:1264–76.

51. Engelter ST. Safety in pharmacological enhancement of stroke rehabilitation. *Eur J Phys Rehabil Med* 2013; **49**:261–7.

52. Ziemann U, Meintzschel F, Korchounov A, Ilic TV. Pharmacological modulation of

plasticity in the human motor cortex. *Neurorehabil Neural Repair* 2006; **20**:243–51.

53. Bernhardt J, Thuy MN, Collier JM, Legg LA. Very early versus delayed mobilisation after stroke. *Cochrane Database Syst Rev* 2009; 1:CD006187.

54. Stroke Unit Trialists Collaboration. How do stroke units improve patient outcomes? A collaborative systematic review of the randomized trials. *Stroke* 1997; **28**:2139–44.

55. Langhorne P, Duncan P. Does the organization of postacute stroke care really matter? *Stroke* 2001; **32**:268–74.

56. Bernhardt J, Dewey H, Thrift A, Donnan G. Inactive and alone: physical activity within the first 14 days of acute stroke unit care. *Stroke* 2004; **35**:1005–9.

57. Kesselring J. Neuroscience and clinical practice: a personal postscript. *Brain Res Brain Res Rev* 2001; **36**:285–6.

58. DeBow SB, McKenna JE, Kolb B, Colbourne F. Immediate constraint-induced movement therapy causes local hyperthermia that exacerbates cerebral cortical injury in rats. *Can J Physiol Pharmacol* 2004; **82**:231–7.

59. Humm JL, Kozlowski DA, James DC, Gotts JE, Schallert T. Use-dependent exacerbation of brain damage occurs during an early post-lesion vulnerable period. *Brain Res* 1998; **783**:286–92.

60. Kozlowski DA, James DC, Schallert T. Use-dependent exaggeration of neuronal injury after unilateral sensorimotor cortex lesions. *J Neurosci* 1996; **16**:4776–86.

61. Barbay S, Plautz EJ, Friel KM, *et al.* Behavioral and neurophysiological effects of delayed training following a small ischemic infarct in primary motor cortex of squirrel monkeys. *Exp Brain Res* 2006; **169**:106–16.

62. Marin R, Williams A, Hale S, *et al.* The effect of voluntary exercise exposure on histological and neurobehavioral outcomes after ischemic brain injury in the rat. *Physiol Behav* 2003; **80**:167–75.

63. Indredavik B, Bakke F, Slordahl SA, Rokseth R, Haheim LL. Treatment in a combined acute and rehabilitation stroke unit: which aspects are most important? *Stroke* 1999; **30**:917–23.

64. Musicco M, Emberti L, Nappi G, Caltagirone C. Early and long-term outcome of rehabilitation in stroke patients: the role of patient characteristics, time of initiation, and duration of interventions. *Arch Phys Med Rehabil* 2003; **84**:551–8.

65. Maulden SA, Gassaway J, Horn SD, Smout RJ, DeJong G. Timing of initiation of rehabilitation after stroke. *Arch Phys Med Rehabil* 2005; **86**:S34–40.

66. Jette DU, Warren RL, Wirtalla C. The relation between therapy intensity and outcomes of rehabilitation in skilled nursing facilities. *Arch Phys Med Rehabil* 2005; **86**:373–9.

67. Collen FM, Wade DT, Robb GF, Bradshaw CM. The Rivermead Mobility Index: a further development of the Rivermead Motor Assessment. *Int Disabil Stud* 1991; **13**:50–4.

68. Lennon S, Johnson L. The modified Rivermead mobility index: validity and reliability. *Disabil Rehabil* 2000; **22**:833–9.

69. Carr JH, Shepherd RB, Nordholm L, Lynne D. Investigation of a new motor assessment scale for stroke patients. *Phys Ther* 1985; **65**:175–80.

70. Loewen SC, Anderson BA. Reliability of the Modified Motor Assessment Scale and the Barthel Index. *Phys Ther* 1988; **68**: 1077–81.

71. Mathias S, Nayak US, Isaacs B. Balance in elderly patients: the "get-up and go" test. *Arch Phys Med Rehabil* 1986; **67**:387–9.

72. Lyle RC. A performance test for assessment of upper limb function in physical rehabilitation treatment and research. *Int J Rehabil Res* 1981; **4**:483–92.

73. Mathiowetz V, Kashman N, Volland G, *et al.* Grip and pinch strength: normative data for adults. *Arch Phys Med Rehabil* 1985; **66**:69–74.

74. Mahoney FI, Barthel DW. Functional Evaluation: The Barthel Index. *Md State Med J* 1965; **14**:61–5.

75. Collin C, Wade DT, Davies S, Horne V. The Barthel ADL Index: a reliability study. *Int Disabil Stud* 1988; **10**:61–3.

76. Prosiegel M, Böttger S, Schenk T, *et al.* Del Erweiterte Barthel-Index (EBI) – eine neue Skala zur Erfassung von Fähigkeitsstörungen bei neurologisachen patienten. *Neurol Rehabil* 1996; **2**:7–13.

77. Schönle PW. Der Frühreha-Barthelindex (FRB) – eine Frührehabilitationsorientiere Erwieterung des Barthelindex. *Rehabilitation (Stuttg)* 1995; **34**:69–73.

78. McDowell I, Newell C. *Measuring Health: A Guide to Rating Scales and Questionnaires.* New York: Oxford University Press; 1996.

79. Graham A. Measurement in stroke: activity and quality of life. In: Barnes M, Dobkin B, Bougousslavsky J, eds. *Recovery After Stroke.* Cambridge: Cambridge University Press; 2005: 135–60.

80. Duncan PW, Wallace D, Lai SM, *et al.* The stroke impact scale version 2.0. Evaluation of reliability, validity, and sensitivity to change. *Stroke* 1999; **30**:2131–40.

81. da Cunha IT Jr, Lim PA, Qureshy H, *et al.* Gait outcomes after acute stroke rehabilitation with supported treadmill ambulation training: a randomized controlled pilot study. *Arch Phys Med Rehabil* 2002; **83**:1258–65.

82. Kosak MC, Reding MJ. Comparison of partial body weight-supported treadmill gait training versus aggressive bracing assisted walking post stroke. *Neurorehabil Neural Repair* 2000; **14**:13–19.

83. Nilsson L, Carlsson J, Danielsson A, *et al.* Walking training of patients with hemiparesis at an early stage after stroke: a comparison of walking training on a treadmill with body weight support and walking training on the ground. *Clin Rehabil* 2001; **15**:515–27.

84. Sullivan KJ, Knowlton BJ, Dobkin BH. Step training with body weight support: effect of treadmill speed and practice paradigms on poststroke locomotor recovery. *Arch Phys Med Rehabil* 2002; **83**:683–91.

85. Visintin M, Barbeau H, Korner-Bitensky N, Mayo NE. A new approach to retrain gait in stroke patients through body weight support and treadmill stimulation. *Stroke* 1998; **29**:1122–8.

86. Wood-Dauphinee S, Kwakkel G. The impact of rehabilitation on stroke outcomes: what is the evidence. In: Barnes M, Dobkin B, Bougousslavsky J, eds. *Recovery After Stroke.* Cambridge: Cambridge University Press; 2005: 162–88.

87. Hidler J, Nichols D, Pelliccio M, *et al.* Multicenter randomized clinical trial evaluating the effectiveness of the Lokomat in subacute stroke. *Neurorehabil Neural Repair* 2009; **23**:5–13.

88. Schwartz I, Sajin A, Fisher I, *et al.* The effectiveness of locomotor therapy using robotic-assisted gait training in subacute stroke patients: a randomized controlled trial. *PM R* 2009; **1**:516–23.

89. Waldner A, Tomelleri C, Hesse S. Transfer of scientific concepts to clinical practice: recent

395

robot-assisted training studies. *Funct Neurol* 2009; **24**:173–7.

90. Mandel AR, Nymark JR, Balmer SJ, Grinnell DM, O'Riain MD. Electromyographic versus rhythmic positional biofeedback in computerized gait retraining with stroke patients. *Arch Phys Med Rehabil* 1990; **71**:649–54.

91. Thaut MH, McIntosh GC, Rice RR. Rhythmic facilitation of gait training in hemiparetic stroke rehabilitation. *J Neurol Sci* 1997; **151**:207–12.

92. Taub E, Miller NE, Novack TA, *et al.* Technique to improve chronic motor deficit after stroke. *Arch Phys Med Rehabil* 1993; **74**:347–54.

93. Wolf SL, Winstein CJ, Miller JP, *et al.* Effect of constraint-induced movement therapy on upper extremity function 3 to 9 months after stroke: the EXCITE randomized clinical trial. *JAMA* 2006; **296**:2095–104.

94. Wolf SL, Winstein CJ, Miller JP, *et al.* Retention of upper limb function in stroke survivors who have received constraint-induced movement therapy: the EXCITE randomised trial. *Lancet Neurol* 2008; **7**:33–40.

95. Langhorne P, Coupar F, Pollock A. Motor recovery after stroke: a systematic review. *Lancet Neurol* 2009; **8**:741–54.

96. Lucca LF. Virtual reality and motor rehabilitation of the upper limb after stroke: a generation of progress? *J Rehabil Med* 2009; **41**:1003–100.

97. Lucca LF, Castelli E, Sannita WG. An estimated 30–60% of adult patients after stroke do not achieve satisfactory motor recovery of the upper limb despite intensive rehabilitation. *J Rehabil Med* 2009; **41**:953.

98. Kwakkel G, Kollen BJ, Krebs HI. Effects of robot-assisted therapy on upper limb recovery after stroke: a systematic review.

Neurorehabil Neural Repair 2008; **22**:111–21.

99. Pignolo L. Robotics in neuro-rehabilitation. *J Rehabil Med* 2009; **41**:955–60.

100. Steultjens EM, Dekker J, Bouter LM, Leemrijse CJ, van den Ende CH. Evidence of the efficacy of occupational therapy in different conditions: an overview of systematic reviews. *Clin Rehabil* 2005; **19**:247–54.

101. Merians AS, Jack D, Boian R, *et al.* Virtual reality-augmented rehabilitation for patients following stroke. *Phys Ther* 2002; **82**:898–915.

102. Saposnik G, Teasell R, Mamdani M, *et al.* Effectiveness of virtual reality using Wii gaming technology in stroke rehabilitation: a pilot randomized clinical trial and proof of principle. *Stroke* 2010; **41**:1477–84.

103. French B, Thomas L, Leathley M, *et al.* Does repetitive task training improve functional activity after stroke? A Cochrane systematic review and meta-analysis. *J Rehabil Med* 2010; **42**:9–14.

104. French B, Thomas LH, Leathley MJ, *et al.* Repetitive task training for improving functional ability after stroke. *Cochrane Database Syst Rev* 2007; **4**:CD006073.

105. Wing K, Lynskey JV, Bosch PR. Whole-body intensive rehabilitation is feasible and effective in chronic stroke survivors: a retrospective data analysis. *Top Stroke Rehabil* 2008; **15**:247–55.

106. Courbon A, Calmels P, Roche F, *et al.* Relationship between maximal exercise capacity and walking capacity in adult hemiplegic stroke patients. *Am J Phys Med Rehabil* 2006; **85**:436–42.

107. Chu KS, Eng JJ, Dawson AS, *et al.* Water-based exercise for cardiovascular fitness in people

with chronic stroke: a randomized controlled trial. *Arch Phys Med Rehabil* 2004; **85**:870–4.

108. Dean CM, Richards CL, Malouin F. Task-related circuit training improves performance of locomotor tasks in chronic stroke: a randomized, controlled pilot trial. *Arch Phys Med Rehabil* 2000; **81**:409–17.

109. Badics E, Wittmann A, Rupp M, Stabauer B, Zifko UA. Systematic muscle building exercises in the rehabilitation of stroke patients. *NeuroRehabilitation* 2002; **17**:211–14.

110. Yavuzer G, Selles R, Sezer N, *et al.* Mirror therapy improves hand function in subacute stroke: a randomized controlled trial. *Arch Phys Med Rehabil* 2008; **89**:393–8.

111. Altschuler EL, Wisdom SB, Stone L, *et al.* Rehabilitation of hemiparesis after stroke with a mirror. *Lancet* 1999; **353**:2035–6.

112. Dohle C, Kleiser R, Seitz RJ, Freund HJ. Body scheme gates visual processing. *J Neurophysiol* 2004; **91**:2376–9.

113. Liu KP, Chan CC, Wong RS, *et al.* A randomized controlled trial of mental imagery augment generalization of learning in acute poststroke patients. *Stroke* 2009; **40**:2222–5.

114. Letswaart M, Johnston M, Dijkerman HC, *et al.* Mental practice with motor imagery in stroke recovery: randomized controlled trial of efficacy. *Brain* 2011; **134**(Pt 5):1373–86.

115. Barthel G, Meinzer M, Djundja D, Rockstroh B. Intensive language therapy in chronic aphasia: Which aspects contribute most? *Aphasiology* 2008; **22**:408–21.

116. Bhogal SK, Teasell R, Speechley M. Intensity of aphasia therapy, impact on recovery. *Stroke* 2003; **34**:987–93.

117. Meinzer M, Djundja D, Barthel G, Elbert T, Rockstroh B. Long-term stability of improved language

functions in chronic aphasia after constraint-induced aphasia therapy. *Stroke* 2005; **36**:1462–6.

118. Heiss WD, Thiel A, Kessler J, Herholz K. Disturbance and recovery of language function: correlates in PET activation studies. *Neuroimage* 2003; **20** (Suppl 1):S42–9.

119. Winhuisen L, Thiel A, Schumacher B, *et al.* The right inferior frontal gyrus and poststroke aphasia: a follow-up investigation. *Stroke* 2007; **38**:1286–92.

120. Naeser MA, Martin PI, Ho M, *et al.* Transcranial magnetic stimulation and aphasia rehabilitation. *Arch Phys Med Rehabil* 2012; **93**:S26–34.

121. Heiss WD, Thiel A. A proposed regional hierarchy in recovery of post-stroke aphasia. *Brain Lang* 2006; **98**:118–23.

122. Saur D, Kreher BW, Schnell S, *et al.* Ventral and dorsal pathways for language. *Proc Natl Acad Sci U S A* 2008; **105**:18 035–40.

123. Weiller C, Bormann T, Saur D, Musso M, Rijntjes M. How the ventral pathway got lost: and what its recovery might mean. *Brain Lang* 2011; **118**:29–39.

124. Monti A, Cogiamanian F, Marceglia S, *et al.* Improved naming after transcranial direct current stimulation in aphasia. *J Neurol Neurosurg Psychiatry* 2008; **79**:451–3.

125. Thiel A, Hartmann A, Rubi-Fessen I, *et al.* Effects of noninvasive brain stimulation on language networks and recovery in early poststroke aphasia. *Stroke* 2013; **44**:2240–6.

126. Kindler J, Schumacher R, Cazzoli D, *et al.* Theta burst stimulation over the right Broca's homologue induces improvement of naming in aphasic patients. *Stroke* 2012; **43**:2175–9.

127. Cappa SF. Current to the brain improves word-finding difficulties in aphasic patients. *J Neurol Neurosurg Psychiatry* 2008; **79**:364.

128. Urban PP, Wicht S, Vukurevic G, *et al.* Dysarthria in acute ischemic stroke: lesion topography, clinicoradiologic correlation, and etiology. *Neurology* 2001; **56**:1021–7.

129. Mann G, Hankey GJ, Cameron D. Swallowing disorders following acute stroke: prevalence and diagnostic accuracy. *Cerebrovasc Dis* 2000; **10**:380–6.

130. Martino R, Foley N, Bhogal S, *et al.* Dysphagia after stroke: incidence, diagnosis, and pulmonary complications. *Stroke* 2005; **36**:2756–63.

131. Smithard DG, O'Neill PA, Parks C, Morris J. Complications and outcome after acute stroke. Does dysphagia matter? *Stroke* 1996; **27**:1200–4.

132. Vernino S, Brown RD Jr, Sejvar JJ, *et al.* Cause-specific mortality after first cerebral infarction: a population-based study. *Stroke* 2003; **34**:1828–32.

133. Hinchey JA, Shephard T, Furie K, *et al.* Formal dysphagia screening protocols prevent pneumonia. *Stroke* 2005; **36**:1972–6.

134. Trapl M, Enderle P, Nowotny M, *et al.* Dysphagia bedside screening for acute-stroke patients: the Gugging Swallowing Screen. *Stroke* 2007; **38**:2948–52.

135. Prosiegel M, Aigner F, Diesener P, *et al.* Qualitätskriterien und Standards für die Diagnostik und Therapie von Patienten mit neurologischen Schluckstörungen. Neurogene Dysphagien – Leitlinien der DGNKN. *Neurol Rehabil* 2003; **9**(3–4):157–81.

136. Langmore SE, Schatz K, Olsen N. Fiberoptic endoscopic examination of swallowing safety: a new procedure. *Dysphagia* 1988; **2**:216–19.

137. Langmore SE. Endoscopic evaluation of oral and pharyngeal phases of swallowing. *GI Motility online* (2006), doi:101038/gimo28, naturecom 2006.

138. Gramigna GD. How to perform video-fluoroscopic swallowing studies. *GI Motility online* (2006), doi:101038/gimo95, naturecom 2006.

139. Rosenbek JC, Robbins JA, Roecker EB, Coyle JL, Wood JL. A penetration-aspiration scale. *Dysphagia* 1996; **11**:93–8.

140. Prosiegel M, Höling R, Heintze M, *et al.* Rehabilitation neurogener Dysphagien. In: Diener HC, *ed. Leitlinien für Diagnostik und Therapie in der Neurologie.* Stuttgart: Thieme; 2005:746–56.

141. Hess DR. Tracheostomy tubes and related appliances. *Respir Care* 2005; **50**:497–510.

142. Ward AB. Spasticity treatment with botulinum toxins. *J Neural Transm* 2008; **115**:607–16.

143. Rosales RL, Chua-Yap AS. Evidence-based systematic review on the efficacy and safety of botulinum toxin-A therapy in post-stroke spasticity. *J Neural Transm* 2008; **115**:617–23.

144. Cappa SF, Benke T, Clarke S, *et al.* EFNS guidelines on cognitive rehabilitation: report of an EFNS task force. *Eur J Neurol* 2005; **12**:665–80.

145. Beis JM, Keller C, Morin N, *et al.* Right spatial neglect after left hemisphere stroke: qualitative and quantitative study. *Neurology* 2004; **63**:1600–5.

146. Karnath HO, Christ K, Hartje W. Decrease of contralateral neglect by neck muscle vibration and spatial orientation of trunk midline. *Brain* 1993; **116**(Pt 2):383–96.

147. Thimm M, Fink GR, Kust J, Karbe H, Sturm W. Impact of alertness training on spatial neglect: a behavioural and fMRI study. *Neuropsychologia* 2006; **44**:1230–46.

148. Nelles G, Esser J, Eckstein A, *et al.* Compensatory visual field training for patients with hemianopia after stroke. *Neurosci Lett* 2001; **306**:189–92.

149. Schmielau F, Wong EK Jr. Recovery of visual fields in brain-lesioned patients by reaction perimetry treatment. *J Neuroeng Rehabil* 2007; **4**:31.

150. Karnath HO. Pusher syndrome–a frequent but little-known disturbance of body orientation perception. *J Neurol* 2007; **254**:415–24.

151. Godefroy OE. *The Behavioral and Cognitive Neurology of Stroke.* Cambridge: Cambridge University Press; 2013: 1–442.

152. Schnakers C, Majerus S, Goldman S, *et al.* Cognitive function in the locked-in syndrome. *J Neurol* 2008; **255**:323–30.

153. Smith E, Delargy M. Locked-in syndrome. *BMJ* 2005; **330**:406–9.

154. Lo SF, Chen SY, Lin HC, *et al.* Arthrographic and clinical findings in patients with hemiplegic shoulder pain. *Arch Phys Med Rehabil* 2003; **84**:1786–91.

155. Braus DF, Krauss JK, Strobel J. The shoulder-hand syndrome after stroke: a prospective clinical trial. *Ann Neurol* 1994; **36**:728–33.

156. Hackett ML, Anderson CS, House A, Halteh C. Interventions for preventing depression after stroke. *Cochrane Database Syst Rev* 2008; 3:CD003689.

157. Sagberg F. Driver health and crash involvement: a case-control study. *Accid Anal Prev* 2006; **38**:28–34.

158. Fisk GD, Owsley C, Pulley LV. Driving after stroke: driving exposure, advice, and evaluations. *Arch Phys Med Rehabil* 1997; **78**:1338–45.

159. Akinwuntan AE, De Weerdt W, Feys H, *et al.* Effect of simulator training on driving after stroke: a randomized controlled trial. *Neurology* 2005; **65**:843–50.

160. Rees PM, Fowler CJ, Maas CP. Sexual function in men and women with neurological disorders. *Lancet* 2007; **369**:512–25.

Index

ACA. *See* anterior cerebral artery (ACA)
ACCESS trial, 327, 357
ACE (angiotensin-converting enzyme) inhibitors, 128, 356–7
acetylsalicylic acid (ASA)
  acute stroke, 299–300
  AF management, 131, 361–3
  carotid endarterectomy, 364
  CVT management, 230
  patient criteria, 93
  secondary prevention, 358–63
  warfarin compared, 366
achromatopsia, 244
acidotoxicity, 18
acquired thrombophilias, 275
Action Research Arm Test (ARAT), 381
ACTIVE study, 362
activities of daily living (ADLs) assessment. *See also* Rankin Scale (modified)
  imaging in, 64
  scales, 381–2
activities scales, motor function, 380–1
acute coronary syndrome, prevention, 360
acute febrile neutrophilic dermatosis, 276
acute multifocal placoid pigment epitheliopathy, 273
acute reversible cerebral angiopathies, 274
acute strokes
  CT imaging, 45–9
  emboli monitoring, 90–4
  therapies, 294, 306–7
  thrombolysis in, 294–9
  ultrasound
    fast-track, 89–91, 99
    prognostic, 95–6
adenosine triphosphate (ATP), 16
aerobic exercises, 384–5
AF. *See* atrial fibrillation (AF)
age
  and AF, 130
  blood pressure and, 127–9
  stroke risk, 109, 128
aggression, in stroke, 247

agitation, 175–6
  management, 230
agnosia, 169, 243–4
agraphia, 237–9
AICA (anterior inferior cerebellar artery), 160–1
AIDS infection, vasculopathy, 350–1
akinesia, 176–7
Alberta Stroke Program Early CT Score (ASPECTS), 45–6, 65–6
alcohol consumption risks, 109–10, 122–3
  ICH and, 192
  SAH and, 207
alexia, 237–9
alien-hand syndrome, 157–8
alpha-galactosidase deficiency, 181–2
alteplase. *See* recombinant tissue plasminogen activator (rtPA)
Alteplase Thrombolysis for Acute Noninterventional Therapy in Ischemic Stroke Trials (ATLANTIS), 294–5
Alzheimer's disease (AD)
  and ICH, 193
  post-stroke dementia and, 260–1
  vascular risk factors, 133
amantadine, 336
amaurosis fugax, 158
American Academy of Neurology, on ultrasound accuracy, 88
American guidelines
  on BP in acute ischemic stroke, 328
  on hyperglycemia, 329
American Heart and Stroke Association
  on hyperthermia, 330
  on ischemic stroke complications, 332
amnesia
  boundary-zone infarcts, 169
  thalamic ischemia, 164
  uncommon stroke syndromes, 174–5
amnesic stroke syndromes, 241
amniotic emboli, 276
amyloid proteins, 3, 193
anastomotic steal phenomena, 12
aneurysms
  and SAH, 206–8

  false, 193
  monitoring and management, 211
  occlusion techniques, 212
  unruptured in young people, 275
anger, in stroke, 247
angiography. *See also* computed tomography angiography (CTA); digital subtraction angiography (DSA); magnetic resonance angiography (MRA)
  ACA vasospasm, 214
  cerebral, 210
angiopathies
  acute reversible, 274
  bleeding-prone, 193–4
  post-partum, 274, 296
angiotensin-converting enzyme (ACE) inhibitors, 128, 356–7
angiotensin-receptor blockers (ARBs), 128, 356–7
anhedonia, 250
animal studies, 9–10
  clinical application, 23–7
anomia, 237
anosognosia, 156
anterior cerebral artery (ACA), 155
  aneurysm, 214
  infarction, 157–8
    contralateral akinesia, 176
    PSD prediction, 260
  microembolus, 90, 103
  vasospasm, 214
anterior choroidal artery (AChA), 155, 158
anterior circulation syndromes, 155–8, 169–70
anterior communicating artery (ACoA), 157
anterior inferior cerebellar artery (AICA), 160–1
antibiotic treatment, septic CVT, 232
anticoagulant therapy
  acute stroke, 300–1
  antagonization in ICH, 200–1
  atrial fibrillation, 130–2
  cerebral ischemia, 361–4
  CVT, 224, 228–9
    long-term, 229–30
  CVT recurrence, 232

anticoagulant therapy (cont.)
    ICH and, 189–92
    in pregnancy, 233
    post-stroke, young people, 279
Anticoagulation and Risk Factors in
    Atrial Fibrillation (ATRIA)
    study, 112
antidepressants, post-stroke, 335, 391
antiepileptic drugs (AEDs), 230–1,
    333–4
antihypertensive drugs, 128
    secondary prevention, 356–7
Antihypertensive Treatment of Acute
    Cerebral Hemorrhage
    (ATACH) study, 305
antimicrobial therapy, in IE, 347
Antiphospholipid Antibodies and
    Stroke Study (APASS), 364
antiphospholipid syndrome, 275
antiplatelet agents. See also
    acetylsalicylic acid (ASA)
    after stent recanalization, 316–17
    anticoagulation compared, 363–4
    in acute stroke, 300
    in AF, 131–2
    thrombolysis and, 298
antiplatelet therapy
    in secondary prevention, 358–61
    intracranial stenosis, 365–6
antithrombotic therapy, patient
    criteria, 93
anxiety disorders, post-stroke, 249
aortic arch
    atherosclerosis, 35–6
    dissection, 184
aortic valve, endocarditis, 146
apathy, 242–3, 251
aphasia, 78, 236–9
    AChA infarct, 158
    adynamic, 164
    Broca, 156
    classification, 237–8
    functional imaging, 73–5
    in PSD prediction, 260
    language evaluation, 237
    MCA infarct, 156–8
    rehabilitation, 385–6
    rTMS effects, 76
    thalamic, 158, 164
    Wernicke's, 157
apical ballooning, 148–9
apixaban, 132, 361–2
apoptosis, 8–9, 21–2
apperceptive visual object agnosia,
    243–4
apraxia, rehabilitation, 390
ARBs (angiotensin-receptor blockers),
    128, 356–7
ARISTOTLE trial, 362

arterial dissection
    anticoagulation, 363–4
    uncommon presentations, 182–4
arterial occlusion, clot evaluation,
    48–9
arterial spin labeling (ASL), 53–8
arteriopathies, hereditary, 1
arteriovenous malformation (AVM),
    188, 190
artery-to-artery embolism, 36
ASA (atrial septal aneurysm), 38, 148
aseptic CVT, 223, 225
Aspergillus spp., 345, 351
aspiration catheter thrombectomy,
    315
aspiration pneumonia, post-stroke,
    352–3
aspiration, in dysphagia, 386–8
aspirin. See acetylsalicylic acid (ASA)
assessments, stroke rehabilitation,
    378–82
astasia, thalamic, 164
astrocytes
    glutamate-induced glycolysis, 13
    in focal brain ischemia, 11–12
    in ischemic cell death, 7–9
astroglial scar formation, 8
ataxic hemiparesis, 165
atenolol, 356
atheromatous plaques, 1
atherosclerosis, 1–2, 27, 34–5,
        See also large-vessel
        atherosclerosis
    infectious etiology, 342–3
    ischemia mechanism, 36
    large artery, 33–6, 43
atherosclerotic occlusions, of ICA, 158
atherosclerotic plaques, 1–2
atorvastatin, 358
atrial fibrillation (AF)
    alcohol consumption, 123
    anticoagulant therapy, 130–2,
        361–3
    and ICH, 189–91
    embolism and, 178, 268
    in cardioembolic stroke, 37–8, 361–3
    in young people, 268
    management guidelines, 131
    prevalence, 141
    role in stroke, 140–3
    vascular risk factors, for PSD, 258–9
atrial natriuretic peptide (ANP), 142
atrial septal aneurysm (ASA), 38, 148
atrioventricular valve, 150
attention, cortical networks, 240
auditory hallucinations, 248
auditory stimulation, in gait training,
    383
aura, migrainous, 47, 184–5, 277

autoregulation, cerebral blood flow,
    10–11
AVERROES trial, 362
azetazolamide, 231

BA. See basilar artery (BA)
Babinski-Nageotte syndrome, 160
Babinski's sign, 156
baclofen, 389
bacterial infections. See also septic CVT
    in IE, 343–5
    meningitis, 347–9
    mycotic aneurisms and, 351
    pre-stroke, 342
    vasculopathies, 180–1
balance, Get-up and Go Test, 381
Balint's syndrome, 166
balloon angioplasty stenting, 364–5
Barthel Index (BI), 64, 381
basal forebrain strokes, 241
basal ganglia, ICH in, 188, 196–8
basilar artery (BA), 158 See also distal
        basilar artery
    intra-arterial thrombolysis, 298
    occlusion, 39–40, 89–90, 173–5
    premonitory stroke signs, 161
    stenosis, 89–90, 171–2
    stroke syndromes, 161–3
behavioral changes, 157
    MCA infarcts, 157–8
    thalamic ischemia, 164
behavioral neurology, 236, 251–2,
        See also delirium; depression
    anger and aggressiveness, 247
    anxiety disorders, 249
    emotional disturbances, 248–9
    executive deficits, 242–3
    language disorders, 236–9
    mania, 250
    memory disturbances, 240–2
    personality changes, 250–1
    psychotic disorders, 247–8
    PTSD, 250
    spatial neglect, 239–40
    visual agnosia, 243–5
benign oligemia, 13
beta-blockers
    comparative trials, 128
    secondary prevention, 356
beta thalassemia, 275
bioprosthesis. See prosthetic heart
        valves
bladder dysfunction,
        neurorehabilitation, 390–1
bleeding-prone angiopathy, 193–4
blind sight, 173–6
blindness, 173–4
blood flow. See cerebral blood flow
        (CBF)

blood glucose, 302–3,
See also hyperglycemia;
hypoglycemia
blood pressure. See also hypertension
age and stroke mortality, 128
changes in acute stroke, 326–7
lifestyle and, 110
outcome and, 301–2
Blood Pressure Lowering Treatment
Triallists' (BPLTT)
Collaboration, 128
blood vessels, CVD origins in, 1–3
Bobath concept, 382
body mass index (BMI), 109–10, 123
body temperature, 303,
See also hyperthermia;
hypothermia
borderzone infarcts, 3–4, 166–7
low flow as cause, 169–70
borreliosis, 349–50
botulinum toxin, in spasticity, 389
bradycardia, 143–4
stroke management, 143
brain abscesses, 347
brain activity, cortico-spinal damage
and, 74
brain blood supply, assessment,
67–8
brain edema, 20–1
brainstem compression, 160
etiology, 198–9
induced hypothermia, 330
malignant stroke, 156
management, 289, 303–4
pressure management, 231–2
brain microbleeds. See cerebral
microbleeds (CMBs)
brain perfusion imaging, diagnostic,
94–5
brain stimulation, for neuroplasticity,
374–5
brainstem lesions, 159
brainstem syndromes, 162, 390
BRAVO trial, 360
breath-holding index (BHI), 97
Broca aphasia, 156
Brunnstrom approach, 382
Buerger disease, 273

CADASIL. See cerebral autosomal
dominant arteriopathy with
subcortical infarcts and
leukoencephalopathy
(CADASIL)
calcium antagonists, 128
calcium-channel blockers, 213, 356
calcium toxicity, in ischemic
damage, 19
calcium, dietary, 125

cancer, non-bacterial thrombotic
endocarditis and, 177
candesartan, 327–8, 357
Candida spp., 345
Capgras syndrome, 247
capsular warning syndrome, 166, 173
carbamazepine, 334
carbon dioxide (CO_2), reactivity,
11, 97
cardiac arrhythmias, 140–4, 150
cardiac diseases, 140–51
bradycardia in, 143
in cardioembolic stroke, 36–9
stroke risk, 150–1
tachycardia in, 144
cardiac event monitoring, 140–2
cardioembolic strokes, 36–9, 43
anticoagulant therapy, 361–3
embolism sources and risks, 37
features, 39–43
cardioembolism, in young people,
268–70
cardiomyopathy
dilated, 38
peripartum, 270
carotid arteries. See also common
carotid artery (CCA); external
carotid artery (ECA); internal
carotid artery (ICA)
intimal medial thickness, 86, 98
stroke syndromes, 155–8
carotid bifurcation disease, 33–4, 83
carotid endarterectomy, 364–5
carotid occlusion, 86–9, 94
carotid stenosis, 35–6
sonography, 82–9, 98–9
CAST (Chinese Acute Stroke Trial),
299–300
catheter angiography. See digital
subtraction angiography
(DSA)
caudate hemorrhage, 5
causality criteria, ischemic stroke
studies, 114
Causative Classification System (CCS),
ischemic strokes, 34
cavernous sinus, thrombosis, 224
CCA (common carotid artery),
83, 86
cell therapy, regeneration, 22
cellular pathology, ischemic strokes,
6–9
central nervous system, primary
vasculitis, 274
cerebellar arteries
anterior inferior, 160–1
posterior inferior, 89, 160
cerebellar hemorrhages, 6, 189
cerebellar infarction, 304

cerebral amyloid angiopathy (CAA),
193
cerebral aneurysms. See aneurysms
cerebral angiography. See angiography
cerebral arteries. See also anterior
cerebral artery (ACA); middle
cerebral artery (MCA);
posterior cerebral artery (PCA)
cerebral autosomal dominant
arteriopathy with subcortical
infarcts and
leukoencephalopathy
(CADASIL), 181
family history, 267
in young people, 271–2
post-stroke dementia, 260–1
white matter hyperintensities, 182
cerebral blood flow (CBF), 12, 46,
See also regional cerebral blood
flow (rCBF)
assessment, 77
Doppler ultrasonography, 82–3
hyperviscosity, 169–73
in thrombolysis, 95–6
mapping, 70–2
outcome prediction, 24
PCT data, 46–7
PET imaging, 23–4
reduction etiology, 33–4, 36
regulation, 10–11
vasopressors to increase, 327
velocities, 89
cerebral blood volume (CBV), 23
cerebral computed tomography
(CCT). See computed
tomography (CT)
cerebral edema. See brain edema
cerebral function, impairment, 102
cerebral ischemia. See also delayed
cerebral ischemia (DCI)
cardiac embolism, 361–3
mechanism, 36
non-cardiac origin, 363–4
cerebral metabolic rate for glucose
(CMRGlc), 12, 23, 70–1
assessment, 77
post-stroke aphasia, 73–5
cerebral metabolic rate for oxygen
($CMRO_2$), 12, 71–2
damage prediction, 24
PET images, 23–4
cerebral microbleeds (CMBs), 193–4
imaging, 54
PSD risk, 260
cerebral perfusion, assessment, 67–8
cerebral thrombosis, ultrasound
accuracy, 88
cerebral venous system, anatomy,
222

cerebral venous thrombosis (CVT), 6, 222, 233–4, *See also* septic CVT
  aseptic, 223, 225
  diagnostic workup, 225–8
  elderly patients, 233
  etiology, 223–8
  future study needs, 233
  imaging, 225–7
    CT scan, 225–6
    DSA, 244
    MRI, 226
  mortality rates, 232
  pregnancy and puerperium, 232–3
  prognosis, 232–3
  recurrence, 232
  risk factors, 223–8
  therapy, 228–32
  thrombophilia screening, 227–8
cerebrospinal fluid (CSF)
  in CVT, 228
  in SAH, 210
  in VZV, 350
  removal in edema, 231
cerebrovascular diseases (CVDs), 1–6
cerebrovascular reactivity (CVR), 97
cervical arteries
  atherosclerosis, 34
  cervical fibromuscular dysplasia, 272
cervical artery dissection (CAD), 182–4
  chiropractic manipulation, 183
  in young people, 268, 271
cervical fibromuscular dysplasia, 272
cesarean section, gas emboli, 276
Chagas disease, 348
CHD. *See* coronary heart disease (CHD)
chicken pox, VZV vasculopathy, 179–80, 350
childbirth. *See* puerperium
children. *See also* young people/children
  strokes, 266
    epidemiology, 266
    outcome, 279
Chinese Acute Stroke Trial (CAST), 299–301
Chinese CHANCE trial, 361
chiropractic manipulation, 183
Chlamydia pneumoniae, pre-stroke, 342–3
chocolate consumption, 126
cholesterol levels
  control in secondary prevention, 357–8
  ICH and, 192
  lifestyle risk factor, 109–10
  statin therapy, 129–30
choriocarcinoma, 276

choroidal arteries
  anterior, 155, 158
  posterior, 155
chronic infections, pre-stroke, 342–3
chronic meningitis, 348
cigarette smoking, 121–2, 207
circle of Willis, variant, 155
citicoline, 262
classic lacunar syndrome, 41
clinical management, use of experimental concepts, 23–7
clinical presentations, uncommon, 173–7
clinical trials, revascularization, 56
clopidogrel, 93, 300
  carotid endarterectomy, 364
  secondary prevention, 358–61
Clopidogrel and Aspirin for Reduction of Emboli in Symptomatic Carotid Stenosis Study (CARESS), 93
Clopidogrel for High Atherothrombotic Risk and Ischemic Stabilization, Management, and Avoidance (CHARISMA) trial, 359
Clopidogrel in High-risk patients with Acute Non-disabling Cerebrovascular Events (CHANCE) trial, 361
Closure or Medical Therapy for Cryptogenic Stroke with Patent Foramen Ovale trials, 363
clot. *See* thrombus
CMRGlc. *See* cerebral metabolic rate for glucose (CMRGlc)
$CMRO_2$. *See* cerebral metabolic rate for oxygen ($CMRO_2$)
coagulation disorders, anticoagulation therapy, 363
coagulopathy, in ICH, 304
coagulotherapy, in ICH, 305
coccidiomycosis, meningitis, 349
Cochrane review, antihypertensive drugs, 128
coffee intake, 126
cognitive disturbance, 157, *See also* dementia (post-stroke)
  MCA infarct, 156
  rehabilitation, 389–90
  thalamic ischemia, 164
  vascular risk factors, 132–3
coils, endovascular, 212
Collet Sicard syndrome, 190
Collier sign, 161
color agnosia, 244
coma, 175, 197
common carotid artery (CCA), 83, 86
communicating arteries

anterior, 157
posterior, 155
compression stockings, 305
computed tomography (CT), 77
  assessment for thrombolysis, 57–8
  CVT cord sign, 225–6
  in ICH, 45–9, 194–7
  in SAH, 209–10
  ischemic stroke detection, 46–7
  MRI compared, 58
  multimodal imaging, 54–8
  structural imaging, 64–6
computed tomography angiography (CTA)
  acute stroke, 45, 48–9
  assessment for thrombolysis, 57
  brain blood supply assessment, 68
confrontation naming, 237
congenital thrombophilia, 275
connective tissue disorders
  inflammatory vasculopathies, 177–9
  intracranial aneurysms and, 206–7
  saccular aneurysms, 207
consciousness impaired. *See also* delirium
  coma, 175, 197
  in CVT, 224
  in SAH, 208
constraint-induced therapy (CIT), 383, 388
continuous positive airways pressure (CPAP), 132–3
contralesional hemispheric overexcitability, 374–5
contrast agents. *See also* microbubbles; ultrasound contrast agents (UCAs)
  arterial spin labeling, 53–8
  brain perfusion imaging, 94–5
  nephrotoxicity, 49
  precautions, 45
Control of Hypertension and Hypotension Immediately Post-Stroke (CHHIPS) pilot trial, 328
cord sign, CT scan, 225–6
core infarcts, 4
coronary heart disease (CHD)
  alcohol consumption, 122–3
  hypertension reduction, 132
  stroke and, 144–50
  stroke prevention, 357–8
cortical representation, plasticity in, 372–3
cortical stimulation, for neuroplasticity, 374–5
cortical watershed infarcts (CWS), 166
corticospinal damage, brain activity and, 72

corticospinal tract, imaging, 66
CPAP (continuous positive airways pressure), 132–3
cranial arteritis, 179
cranial nerve palsy
    focal brainstem ischemia, 176
    ICA dissection, 183, 190
craniotomy, decompressive, 303–4
CREST trial, 365
criblures, 3
crying, pathological, 248–9, 390
cryptococcal meningitis, 349
cryptogenic strokes, 33, 43
    ASA and, 148
    PFO and, 147, 363
CT. See computed tomography (CT)
CTA. See computed tomography angiography (CTA)
Cushing's triad, 160
CVDs. See cerebrovascular diseases (CVDs)
CVT. See cerebral venous thrombosis (CVT)
cystic infarct, transformation to, 8
cysticercosis, 350
cytomegalovirus, pre-stroke, 342–3
cytotoxic edema, ischemic, 20–1

dabigatran, 132, 361–2
dairy products, consumption, 125
DASH (Dietary Approaches to Stop Hypertension) trial, 125–6
dCMP (dilated cardiomyopathy), 38
death rates, from stroke, 102–3
decompressive surgery, 289, 304
decompressive surgery in malignant middle cerebral artery infarcts (DECIMAL) study, 304
deep perforating artery system, 156
Déjerine syndrome, 160
delayed cerebral ischemia (DCI)
    detection, 209
    in SAH, 213–14
delirium, 175–6, 245–7
    clinical features, 245
    pathogenesis, 246–7
    pathophysiology, 246
    precipitating factors, 246
delta sign, CT scan, 225
delusional misidentification syndromes, 248
delusions, 247–8, 250
dementia (post-stroke), 262–3, 335–6
    causes, 260–1
    definitions, 255
    determinants, 258–60
    diagnostic criteria, 335
    epidemiology, 256
    incidence and impact, 255–6

literature search, 256
mechanisms, 335
mortality rates, 262
outcomes, 261–2
prevalence, 257–8
risk factors, 335–6
risk rates, 258
treatment, 262
depolarization, peri-infarct spreading depression, 17–18
depression (post-stroke), 249–50, 334–5, 391
    antidepressants, 335, 391
    etiology/risk factors, 334
    incidence, 334
    management, 334–5
    outcome, 334
    predictive factors, 250
diabetes mellitus (DM)
    control in secondary prevention, 358
    hypertension, 128–9
    risk factors for PSD, 258–9
diaschisis, 73–5, 373
diet
    dairy products, 125
    fruit and vegetables, 124–5
    lifestyle, 109–10, 124–6
Dietary Approaches to Stop Hypertension (DASH) trial, 125–6
diffusion tensor imaging (DTI), 66–7
diffusion tensor tractography (DTT), 67
diffusion-weighted imaging (DWI), 16, 40, 49, 77
    advantages, 50
    criteria for thrombolysis, 58
    lacunar infarcts, 42
    mismatch concept, 51–3
    penumbra and irreversible damage, 26–7
    structural imaging, 66
    techical aspects, 51
digital subtraction angiography (DSA), 311–12
    ACA aneurysm, 214
    in CVT, 227, 244
    neurological complications, 311–12
    SAH aneurysm, 210, 214
dilated cardiomyopathy (dCMP), 38, 148
dipyridamole, 300
dipyridamole extended release (ER-DP), 358–60
direct oral anticoagulants (DOACs). See anticoagulant therapy
disability-adjusted life years (DALYs), 102–3

diseases and pathological conditions, stroke risk, 133–4,
    See also individual disease
disinhibition. See uninhibited behavior
distal basilar artery, occlusion, 161
distal thrombectomy, 314–16
diuretics
    in brain edema, 231, 303, 307
    in secondary prevention, 356
DM. See diabetes mellitus (DM)
door-to-needle times, 286–8
    outcomes, 296–7
        clinical trials, 294–6
Doppler ultrasonography, 98–9,
    See also transcranial color Doppler (TCD) sonography
    carotid stenosis, 82–5
dorsolateral medullary stroke, 160
driving ability, 391
drop attacks, 171–2
drug abuse
    hemorrhage risk, 192
    SAH risk factor, 207
drug-induced QT prolongation, 144
DSA. See digital subtraction angiography (DSA)
DTT. See diffusion tensor tractography (DTT)
Duke criteria, in IE, 345–6
dysarthria, outcome, 386
dysarthria clumsy hand syndrome, 165
dysgraphia, 237–9
dyslexia, 237–9
dyslipidemia
    DM and, 129
    statin therapy, 129–30
dysphagia
    rehabilitation, 386–8
    swallowing evaluation, 387–8
    warning signs, 387

Eales disease, 273
eclampsia, 275
edema. See brain edema
EKOS thrombus disruption system, 313–14
electrocardiography (ECG), diagnostic workup, 289
electrolyte disturbances, in SAH, 214
electronic health records (EHRs), 112–14
embolic occlusions, of ICA, 158
embolic strokes, infectious causes, 343–50
embolism
    AF as cause, 178
    cardiogenic from MI, 145
    in young people, 268–70

embolism (cont.)
  large-vessel disease, 33–4
  mechanical removal, 299
  monitoring, acute stroke, 90–4
  paradoxical, 38, 147
  sources and risks, cardioembolic
      stroke, 37
emergency medical services (EMS),
      prehospital care, 285
emotional expression control
      disorders, 248–9
encephalopathy, inflammatory
      vasculopathies, 177–9
endocarditis. See also infective
      endocarditis (IE)
  and stroke, 38, 177
  aortic valve, 146
  non-bacterial thrombotic, 177, 345–7
endomyocardial fibrosis, 150
endoplasmic reticulum (ER), 20
endovascular coiling, aneurysm
      occlusion, 212
endovascular-induced hypothermia,
      330
endovascular treatment, for DCI,
      213–14
energy metabolism, brain tissue,
      12–13
environmental stimulation, in
      neuroplasticity, 373–4
EPAR thrombus disruption system,
      313–14
epileptic seizures, 332–4,
      See also antiepileptic drugs
      (AEDs)
  differential diagnosis, 143–4
  in CVT, 224–5, 230–1
  in SAH, 212
  management, 230–1, 333–4
  pathophysiology, 333
  predictors, 332–3
  Seizures After Stroke Study (SASS),
      333
  thrombolysis and, 298
  young people/children, 278
episodic memory deficits, 174–5
eprosartan, 356–7
erectile dysfunction, 391–2
ESC trial, 365
escitalopram, 335
ESO. See European Stroke
      Organisation (ESO)
ESPRIT study, 360, 364
Essen risk score, 360–1
estrogen replacement therapy, 126–7
ethnicity
  in ICH, 188
  mortality data, 103–5
  stroke risk, 109

stroke type, 34–5, 102
  strokes in young people, 266
European Atrial Fibrillation Trial,
      361–2
European Cooperative Acute Stroke
      Study (ECASS), 294–5
European Federation of Neurological
      Societies, guidelines, 86–7
European Stroke Initiative (ICH), on
      BP, 304
European Stroke Organisation (ESO)
  diagnostic procedures, 289–90
  emergency stroke care, 285–7, 289
  on BP, 328
  on complications, 291, 332–3
  on hyperglycemia, 329
  on hyperthermia, 330
  on intracranial pressure, 289, 291
  on stroke management, 289
  stroke unit facilities, 288–9
  treatment guidelines, 290–1, 332
European Stroke Prevention Study
      (ESPS2), 359
excitotoxicity, ischemic damage, 18–19
executive deficits, 242–3
external carotid artery (ECA), 83
external ventricular drainage (EVD),
      213
extracranial atherosclerosis, 34–6
extracranial carotid stenosis, 35
extracranial hemorrhages,
      anticoagulants and, 131
extracranial stenosis, ultrasonography,
      82–3
eye disorders. See also visual
      disturbance
  secondary vasculitis, 273
eye movements. See also nystagmus
  BA stroke, 161
  gaze paresis, 159, 161
  ICH presentation, 197
  posterior circulation infarcts, 159

Fabry disease, 181–2, 275–6
face recognition difficulties
      (prosopagnosia), 244–5
facial palsy, AICA syndrome, 160–1
factor Xa inhibitors, 132
family history
  stroke risk, 109
  young people/children, 267–8
fast-track neurovascular ultrasound,
      89–91, 99
fat emboli, 276
fat, dietary, 126
fatigue (post-stroke), 336
fever
  in acute stroke, 303
  in SAH, 211

Fiberoptic Endoscopic Examination of
      Swallowing (FEES), 387–8
fibrous cap, atherosclerotic lesion, 2
filament occlusion, of the MCA, 9–10
fish consumption, 125
flat-panel detector (FPD) technology,
      312
fluid attenuated inversion recovery
      (FLAIR), 49–51, 53
  criteria for thrombolysis, 58
flumazenil (FMZ), 24–6
fluoxetine, 375
focal brain ischemia, 11–12, 169, 185–6
  injury pathways, 18
  viability thresholds, 14
focal brainstem ischemia, cranial
      nerve palsy, 176
focal dysfunction, 102
focal neurological signs, in CVT, 224
focal paresis, 177–8
focal seizures, differential diagnosis,
      170
forebrain strokes, amnesia and, 241
Framingham Stroke Profile (FSP),
      112–13
Framingham study, 3, 9
free radicals, 19, 301
Fregoli syndrome, 248
frontal lobe lesions
  evaluation of function, 243
  executive deficits, 176–7, 242–3
fruit consumption, 124–5
functional imaging, 69–70, 72–3,
      See also functional magnetic
      resonance imaging (fMRI);
      positron emission tomography
      (PET)
Functional Independence Measure
      (FIM), 64, 381
functional magnetic resonance
      imaging (fMRI), 69–72, 77
  motor and sensory deficits, 72–3
  plasticity mapping, 372–3
functional outcome prediction.
      See also outcomes
  imaging in, 64–78
fungal infections
  in meningitis, 349
  infective endocarditis, 343–5
  mycotic aneurysms, 351

gait training, 382–3
gamma-aminobutyric acid (GABA),
      24–6
gas emboli, 276
gaze paresis, 159, 161
gender
  atherosclerosis in young people, 268
  in Fabry disease, 275–6

lifestyle risk factors, 110
mortality rates and, 103
physical activity benefit, 124
stroke epidemiology, 105–7
genetic factors
in stroke, 181–4
spontaneous ICH, 191–2
Get-up and Go Test, 381
ghost cells, ischemic cell death, 8
giant cell arteritis, 179
Glasgow Coma Scale (GCS), in SAH, 209
glucose metabolism, 12–13
post-stroke aphasia, 73–5
Glucose Regulation in Acute Stroke Patients Trial (GRASP), 329
glutamate neurotransmitter, 18–19
glutamate-induced glycolysis, 13
glycerol, for brain edema, 231, 303, 307
glycoprotein-IIb/IIIa-receptor antagonists, 360
goal-setting, stroke rehabilitation, 379–82
gradient echo (GRE), MRI imaging, 194–7
granulomata, in TB meningitis, 349
Gugging Swallowing Screen (GUSS), 387

hallucinations, 247–8, 250
hand function
jerky dystonic movements, 165
recovery, 73–4
thalamic hand, 164
headaches, 159, See also migraine
ICH presentation, 197
in CVT, 224–5
management, 230
thunderclap in SAH, 207–8
Health Professionals Follow-up Study, 119, 124–5
hearing loss, 160–1
heart valves. See also mitral valve; prosthetic heart valves
aortic, 146
atrioventricular valve, 150
valvular heart disease, 145–6, 268
Helicobacter pylori infection, 342–3
hematological diseases, 275
hematological diseases, hyperviscosity in, 172–3
hematoma expansion, 197
in ICH, 195–8
hemianopia, 169, 390
hemichorea-hemiballismus, 165, 177
hemi-medullary stroke, 160
hemiparesis
AChA infarcts, 158

ataxic, 165
BA stroke syndromes, 161
MCA infarcts, 156–7
pure motor, 165, 173
hemiplegia, fluctuating, 166
hemiplegic shoulder pain, 391
hemodynamic treatment, for DCI, 213–14
hemodynamics, in stroke, 10–12
hemoglobin, magnetic properties, 71–2
hemoglobinopathies, and stroke, 275
hemorrhagic infarctions, 4–5
hemorrhagic strokes
alcohol consumption, 122–3
imaging, 49–54
statins and, 129–30
hemorrhagic transformations, 39
heparin. See also low molecular weight heparin (LMWH)
in acute stroke, 228–9, 305
studies on, 300–1
hereditary disorders
arteriopathies, 1
causes of stroke, 181–4
spontaneous ICH, 191–2
Hereditary Endotheliopathy with Retinopathy and Stroke (HERNS) syndrome, 276
herpes simplex virus, 342–3
hiccup, 160
high-density lipoprotein (HDL), 130
hippocampus
amnesic strokes, 241
lesions in, 8–9
newly generated neurons, 22
history taking, young people/children, 267
HIV infection, 277, 350–1
Holter monitoring, 141, 143
homocystinurea, 276, 358
homonymous hemianopia, 156–7
HOPE study, 356–7
hormone replacement therapy, 126–7, 358
Horner's sign, 160
Horner's syndrome, 159–61
Horton's disease. See giant cell arteritis
hospital, Stroke Alarm protocol, 286
hyaline, in small-vessel disease, 3
hydrocephalus, 213, 305
hyperglycemia
in SAH, 211
management, 302–3, 328–30
stroke complication, 331
hyperkinetic movement disorders, 176–7
hypertension
in cerebral hemorrhages, 5–6, 192–3

management
hemorrhagic stroke, 199–200, 211, 304–5
ischemic stroke, 326–8
medically induced in ischemic stroke, 327
recurrence risk, 356–7
reduction, 127–9
stroke risk, 132
SAH risk factor, 207
stroke complication, 301–2, 331–6
stroke risk, 127–9
thrombolysis and, 298
Hypertension in the Very Elderly Trial (HYVET), 129
hyperthermia, stroke complication, 330–1
hyperventilation, therapeutic, 305
hyperviscosity, low flow and, 172–3
hypoglycemia, management, 302–3
hypokinesia, 176–7
hyponatremia, 214
hypothermia, induced, 303, 330

ICA. See internal carotid artery (ICA)
ICH. See intracerebral hemorrhage (ICH)
IE. See infective endocarditis (IE)
imaging. See also individual imaging modalities
functional outcome assessment, 77–8
patient criteria for thrombolysis, 57–8
venous system in parodoxical embolism, 155
young people/children, 267
implantable loop recorder, 141–2
IMT (intimal-medial thickness), 86, 98
indapamide, 356–7
infarcts
core imaging, 16
expansion, 16–22
growth, 17
types, 27, 260
infectious CVT. See septic CVT
infectious diseases
post-stroke complication, 352–3
pre-stroke, 342–51, 353
secondary vasculitis, 273–4
similar to stroke, 351–2
infective endocarditis (IE), 145–6
and stroke, 177, 343–8
diagnosis, 345–6
emboli in young people, 268
etiology, 345
imaging, 343, 374

infective endocarditis (IE) (cont.)
  microbiology, 345
  mortality rates, 347
  mycotic aneurysms, 351
  neurological complications, 346
  pathogenesis, 345–7
  symptoms and diagnosis, 345
  therapy, 347–8
inferolateral arteries, 164
inflammation response, in stroke, 20
inflammatory diseases, atherosclerosis
    in, 1–2
inflammatory vasculopathies, 177–9,
    274
influenza, pre-stroke, 342
injury pathways, 1–2, 13–14, 18
inner cerebral veins, thrombosis, 224
instrumental activities of daily living
    (IADL), 381
insulin therapy, in acute stroke,
    329–30
INSULINFARCT study, 329
Intensive Blood Pressure Reduction in
    Acute Cerebral Haemorrhage
    Trial (INTERACT), 304–5
interatrioseptal aneurysm (IASA),
    269–70
internal carotid artery (ICA)
  carotid endarterectomy, 364–5
  dissection, 183, 190, 272
  hypoplasia, 184
  IMT measurement, 86
  infarcts, 167
  occlusion, 158
    limb-shaking TIA, 171
    moyamoya disease, 274
  stenosis, 83–5
internal watershed infarcts (IWS), 166
International Classification of
    Functioning, Disability and
    Health (ICF), 379–80, 384, 386
International Stroke Trial (IST),
    295–6, 301
INTERSTROKE study, 119
interventional intravascular therapies,
    311, 322–3
  digital subtraction angiography,
    311–12
  mechanical approaches, 313–22
  thrombolytic intra-arterial therapy,
    312–13
intimal-medial thickness (IMT), 86, 98
intra-arterial thrombolysis, 298,
    312–13
intracardiac myxoma, 270
intracerebral hemorrhage (ICH), 5–6,
    188, 201–2
  anticoagulants and, 131, 200–1
  classification, 188–91

clinical features, 197, 224–5
complications, 197–9
etiology, 189
imaging, 54, 58, 194–7
  CT, 45–6, 49
  hematoma expansion, 198
  MRI staging, 194–5
  prognosis assessment, 195–7
  spot signs, 196–8
  in CVT, 224
management, 199–201, 304–5
morbidity in, 191
mortality rates, 197–9
pathophysiology, 192–4
prognostic factors, 191
risk factors, 191–2
site distribution, 189
thrombolysis, 48, 57–8
thrombus disruption systems,
    313–14
intracranial disease, ultrasound
    diagnosis, 86–9
intracranial dissections, 272
intracranial hemorrhage (ICH). See
    intracerebral hemorrhage (ICH)
intracranial pressure. See also brain
    edema
  emergency management, 289
  ESO Guidelines, 291
  in acute stroke, 303–4
  management in CVT, 231–2
  therapeutic hyperventilation, 305
intracranial stenosis
  flow velocities, 89
  management, 365–6
  ultrasound accuracy, 87–8
  ultrasound grading, 89
intracranial vessel occlusion, 67–8
intravascular therapies, recanalization,
    322–3
intravenous thrombolysis, 294–9, 306,
    See also recombinant tissue
    plasminogen activator (rtPA)
  administration, 298
  cerebral blood flow data, 48
  patient criteria, 45–6
intraventricular hemorrhage (IVH),
    198
irreversible damage
  penumbra detection, 23–4
  prediction, 24–5
  surrogate markers, 26–7
ischemia, viability thresholds, 13–14
ischemic cardioembolic strokes, 39–43
ischemic cell death, 27
ischemic injury
  mechanisms of infarct expansion,
    16–22
  pre- and postconditioning, 22

ischemic ophthalmopathy, 170
ischemic penumbra, 12–16
ischemic strokes, 3–4, See also young
    people/children
  alcohol consumption, 122–3
  blood pressure control, 326–8
  Causative Classification System
    (CCS), 34
  causes, 33, 42–3
  cellular pathology, 6–9
  cerebral blood flow data, 46–7
  classification, 33–4
  complications, 326, 332–7
    guidelines, 332
    late, 332–6
  hyperglycemia control, 328–30
  hyperthermia control, 330–1
  imaging
    CT data, 46–7
    MRI and MRA, 49–54
    ultrasound, 82–99
  low cerebral flow, 169–72
  major causes, 34
  obesity and, 123
  physical activity and, 124
  recurrence prevention, 360
  smoking and, 121–2
  statins and, 129–30

jerky dystonic unsteady hand, 165

Kawasaki syndrome, 276
Köhlmeier–Degos disease, 273

lactic acidosis, 182, 276
lacunar infarcts, 4, 43
  common sequelae, 42
  DWI, 42
  in post-stroke dementia, 260
  in young people, 271
  risk factors, 41
  silent, 41
  small-vessel disease, 40–2
lacunar state (status lacunaris), 3
lacunar stroke syndromes, 41–2,
    165–7
  AChA infarcts, 158
  in CADASIL, 181
lacunar strokes
  cognitive impairment, 262
  secondary prevention, 357, 360
LAIT (lesions amenable to
    intervention), 90
lamotrigine, 334
language disorders, 236–9,
    See also aphasia
language, functional organization, 238
large-vessel atherosclerosis, 33–6, 43,
    268

large-vessel infarcts, outcome, 260
large-vessel occlusion, outcome, 72
laser thrombus disruption, 313–14
laughter, pathological, 161, 248–9
LDL. *See* low-density lipoprotein (LDL)
left atrial appendage (LAA), 141–2
left atrial myxoma, 271
left hemispheric strokes, 73–5
    activation patterns, 75
    aphasia, 73–5, 236
    in PSD, 260
left ventricular hypertrabeculation/
       non-compaction (LVHT),
       149–50
left ventricular mural thrombi, 38
lenticulostriate arteries, 156–7
    capsular warning syndrome, 166,
       173
    infarcts, 157
leptomeningeal artery system, 156–7
lesions amenable to interventional
       treatment (LAIT), 90
leukoaraiosis, 260, 262
levetiracetam, 230–1
levodopa, 375–6
lifestyle
    healthy, 119
    stroke mortality data, 105
    stroke prevention, 119–27, 133
    stroke risk, 109–11, 113–14, 119–27
limb-shaking TIA, 158, 170–1
lipid-lowering drugs, 86
lipohyalinoic arteries, 192–3
lipohyalinosis, 271
LMWH. *See* low molecular weight
       heparin (LMWH)
lobar (white matter) hemorrhages, 5,
       188–9
locked-in syndrome (LiS), 161, 390
low molecular weight heparin
       (LMWH)
    in acute stroke, 228–9, 305
    in pregnancy, 233
    in SAH, 211
low-density lipoprotein (LDL), 129
    in inflammation, 1–2
    statin therapy, 130
    target range, 357
LVHT (left ventricular
       hypertrabeculation/non-
       compaction), 149–50

magnesium, dietary, 125
magnetic resonance angiography
       (MRA), 58
    CBF assessment, 77
    in SAH, 210
    ischemic and hemorrhagic strokes,
       49–54

patient criteria for thrombolysis,
       58
magnetic resonance imaging (MRI),
       16
    carotid stenosis, 35
    contraindications, 49
    CT compared, 58
    evaluation, 54
    hand function recovery, 74
    ICH assessment, 194–7
    in CVT, 226–7
    in SAH, 209–10
    ischemic and hemorrhagic strokes,
       49–54
    lacunar infarcts, 41
    MCA stenosis, 40
    multimodal, 52, 54–8, 77
    old microbleeds, 193–4
    patient criteria for thrombolysis, 58
    structural imaging, 66–7
    volumetric studies, 25
magnetic resonance venography
       (MRV), 226–7
malaria, differentiation from stroke,
       352
malignant atrophic papulosis, 273
malignant MCA stroke, 156
man-in-the-barrel presentation, 166
mania, post-stroke, 250
mannitol, for brain edema, 231, 303,
       307
manual dexterity tests, 381
MATCH study, 359
MCA. *See* middle cerebral artery
       (MCA)
Mechanical Embolectomy Removal in
       Cerebral Ischemia (MERCI),
       299
mechanical thrombectomy, 313–22
mechanical valve prosthesis, 146
medial medullary stroke, 160
medial temporal lobe atrophy
       (MTLA), 259
medications
    ICH and, 192
    in neurorehabilitation, 377–8
Mediterranean-style diet, 126
MELAS (mitochondrial
       encephalopathy lactic acidosis
       and stroke), 182, 276
membrane potential, 13–14
memory disturbances, 240–2,
       See also amnesia
memory, systems, 241
meningeal signs, in SAH, 208
meningitis
    bacterial, 180–1, 347–8
    stroke in, 348–50
    tuberculous, 180, 349

meningovascular syphilis, 180
mental practice, motor imagery, 385
MERCI thrombectomy device,
       315–16, 319–20
mercury, in fish consumption, 125
MES. *See* microembolic signs (MES)
metabolic disorders, young people,
       275–6
metabolic regulation, CBF, 10–11
microbleeds. *See* cerebral microbleeds
       (CMBs)
microbubbles, contrast agents, 94–7,
       99
microcirculation, disturbances, 11–12
microembolic signs (MES), on TCD,
       90–4, 99, 103
middle cerebral artery (MCA), 155
    aneurysms, 208
    intra-arterial thrombolysis, 298
    left hemisphere stroke, 236
    leptomeningeal branches, 157
    stenosis, 40, 89
middle cerebral artery (MCA)
       infarctions, 39, 156–7, 166–7
    brain edema, 303–4
    complete, 156–7
    induced hypothermia, 303, 330
    real-time visualization, 94–5
middle cerebral artery (MCA)
       occlusions, 89
    animal studies, 9–10
    biochemical imaging, 16
    neuronal plasticity, 7, 15
    prognosis, 95–6, 156
    spreading depressions, 17
    ultrasound, 90–1, 95–6
migraine, 181, 184–5
migraine with aura (MA), 47, 184–5,
       277
minimally invasive surgery, in ICH,
       199
mirror therapy, 385
mismatch concept, 51–3
mitochondria, 7–9, 20
mitochondrial encephalopathy lactic
       acidosis and stroke (MELAS),
       182
mitral valve
    endocarditis, 145–6
    prolapse, 39, 270
    repair, 146
mobility assessment tests, 380–1
mobilization, 378–9
modafinil, 336
modified Rankin Scale (mRS), 64–5,
       297
molecular injury cascades, 18
molecular mechanisms, ischemic
       damage, 18–20

Monitoring of Trends and Determinants in Cardiovasular Disease (MONICA) Stroke Study, 105–8
monocular transient retinal ischemia, 170
mood disorders. *See also* depression
    anxiety (post-stroke), 249
    apathy, 242–3
    emotional expression control disorders, 248–9
    mania (post-stroke), 250
mortality rates, 103–8, 262
    gender and, 103
    in ICH, 191, 197–9
    international, 103–5
    MONICA study, 105–8
Moschcowitz syndrome, 275
MOSES trial, 357
Motor Assessment Scale (MAS), 381
motor deficits. *See also* focal paresis; hemiparesis
    BA stroke syndromes, 161
    frontal lobe lesions, 176–7
    imaging, 72–3, 77
        DTI outcome prediction, 67
    in CVT, 224
    MCA infarcts, 157–8
    PCA infarcts, 163
    rehabilitation, 382–5
    thalamic ischemia, 164–5
moyamoya disease, 170, 172, 184, 273
    young person, 274
MRI. *See* magnetic resonance imaging (MRI)
multidisciplinary team. *See* stroke units
multimodal imaging, 50, 52, 54–8
    acute stroke, 55–6
    revascularization trials, 56–7
multiple infarcts, in PSD, 260
Mycobacterium tuberculosis infection, 180, 349
mycotic aneurysms, 177
    and stroke, 351
myocardial infarction (MI)
    embolism from, 145
    hyperglycemia control, 329
    in cardioembolic stroke, 38
    risk for PSD, 258–9
myocardial ischemia, detection, 144
myocardium, left ventricular non-compaction, 149–50
myxoma, 270–1

naming impairment (anomia), 237
NASCET trial, 84–5, 365
National Institute of Health Stroke Scale (NIHSS), 64–6, 288

National Institute of Neurological Disorders and Stroke (NINDS), 294–5, 301
nausea and vomiting, 160, 208, 230
necrosis, ischemic cell death, 7–9
neglect. *See* spatial neglect
neonates, CVT in, 233
nephrotoxicity, contrast agents, 45, 49
nervous tissue, energy metabolism, 12–14
neurobehavioral deficits, 236, 251–2
neuroborreliosis, 349–50
neurocysticercosis, 350
neurogenesis, ischemia-induced, 22
neurogenic regions, regeneration, 22
neurogenic swallowing disorder. *See* dysphagia
neurological complications, 311–12, 345
neuromuscular disorders, 149
neuronal activity, mapping, 70–1
neuronal plasticity, 74, 373
    functional imaging, 72–3
    post-ischemia, 7, 15
neurons, cell death, 7–9
neurontine, 334
neuroplasticity, 392
    induction and promotion, 373–6
    mechanisms, 371–3
    pharmacological interventions, 375–6
neuroprotection, 301
neuropsychological syndromes, 389–90
neurorehabilitation, 371, 392
    assessments, 378
    bladder dysfunction, 390–1
    brainstem syndromes, 390
    cognitive impairment, 389–90
    driving ability, 391
    dysphagia, 386–8
    goal-setting and assessments, 379–82
    medication, 377–8
    multidisciplinary team, 287, 371, 376–81
    neuroplasticity in, 371–6
    neuropsychological syndromes, 389–90
    physiotherapy concepts, 382
    physiotherapy techniques, 382–5
    post-stroke depression, 391
    post-stroke pain, 391
    sexual functioning, 391–2
    social problems, 392
    spasticity, 388–9
    speech disorders, 385–6
    therapy initiation and intensity, 378–9

neurosyphilis, 349–50
neurotransmitters, 12–13, 18–19
nimodipine, 213
NINDS (National Institute of Neurological Disorders and Stroke), 294–5
Nine Hole Peg Test (NHPT), 381
nitrendipine, 356–7
nitric oxide (NO) toxicity, 19
nocturnal paroxysmal hemoglobinuria, 275
non-bacterial thrombotic endocarditis (NBTE), 177, 345–7
non-cardiac-origin cerebral ischemia, 363–4
non-contrast CT (NCCT), 45–6
non-cruoric emboli, 276
non-invasive vascular ultrasound evaluation (NVUE), 92
non-valvular atrial fibrillation, 37–8
Nurses' Health Study
    diet, 124–5
    lifestyle, 119
    smoking, 122
nystagmus
    cerebellar artery lesions, 160–1
    posterior circulation infarcts, 159
    RVAO and stroke, 170–1
    Wallenberg syndrome, 160

OAC (oral anticoagulants). *See* anticoagulant therapy
obesity, 123, 132–3
obstructive sleep apnea (OSA), 132–3
OEF. *See* oxygen extraction fraction (OEF)
olfactory bulb, 22
omega 3 fatty acids, 125
onset to start of treatment times (OTT). *See* door-to-needle times
ophthalmic artery, 155
ophthalmic-distribution zoster infection, 179–80
ophthalmopathy, ischemic, 170
oral contraception (OC), 122, 277, 279
OSA (obstructive sleep apnea), 132–3
osmodiuretic drugs, 231
outcome prediction, motor deficits, 67
outcome probability scores, 65
outcomes. *See also* door-to-needle times
    international, 102–8
oxygen extraction fraction (OEF), imaging, 23–5
oxygen level measurement, in brain function, 71–2
oxygen, brain energy metabolism, 12–13

pain syndrome, thalamic, 164
pain, post-stroke, 391
palipsychism, 164
papillary fibroelastoma, 270
paradoxical embolism, 38, 147, 155
paradoxical steal effect, 11
paramedian arteries, 164
parasitic diseases
    similar to stroke, 351–2
    Taenia solium (tapeworm), 350
paroxysmal atrial fibrillation, 38, 131,
    140–2
passive smoking, 122
patent foramen ovale (PFO)
    cardioembolic stroke, 38
    closure, 363
    diagnosis, 146
    imaging, 269
    in young people, 269–70
    stroke risk, 147
    TCD in detection, 97
pathological conditions, stroke risk,
    127–34
pathological crying, 248–9, 390
patient criteria
    antithrombotic therapy, 93
    for thrombolysis, 57–8, 77
    multimodal imaging, 55–6
    revascularization trials, 54–6
    TCD monitoring of therapy, 93–8
    ultrasound screening, 92–3
PCAs. *See* posterior cerebral arteries
    (PCAs)
PCT. *See* perfusion computed
    tomography (PCT)
peak systolic velocities (PSV), 84–5, 98
penumbra, 12–14
    detection by PET, 23–4
    imaging, 14–16
    surrogate markers, 26–7
    volumetric studies, 25
Penumbra System, 315
Percutaneous Closure of Patent
    Foramen Ovale in Cryptogenic
    Embolism trial (PC-Trial), 363
percutaneous transluminal balloon
    angioplasty (PTA), 313
perfusion computed tomography (PCT)
    acute stroke, 45–8
    criteria for revascularization trials,
        54–5
    criteria for thrombolysis, 57
perfusion-weighted imaging (PWI),
    16, 49
    mismatch concept, 51–3
    penumbra and irreversible damage,
        26–7
pericytes, 11–12
peri-infarct spreading depression, 17–18

perimesencephalic SAH (PMSAH),
    214
perindopril, 356–7
peripartum cardiomyopathies, 270
peripheral nervous system, sprouting
    neurons, 373
personality changes, 250–1
PET. *See* positron emission
    tomography (PET)
PFO. *See* patent foramen ovale (PFO)
phenytoin, 230–1, 334
pH-weighted imaging (pHWI), 16
physical activity, effects, 109–10, 124
physical fitness training, 384–5
physiotherapy
    concepts, 382
    techniques, 382–5
PICA. *See* posterior inferior cerebellar
    artery (PICA)
PLAATO device, 142
plaques. *See also* atheromatous plaques
    Doppler ultrasonography, 83
    IMT measurement, 86
    sonographic detection, 83
Plasmodium falciparum, 352
Platelet Oriented Inhibition in New
    TIA (POINT) trial, 361
platelets, in thromboembolism, 2–3
pleasure, lack of, 250
pneumonia, post-stroke, 352–3, 387
polar (tuberothalamic) artery, 164
polycythemia vera, 172
pontine hemorrhages, 6, 189
pontine stroke syndromes, 161–3
positron emission tomography (PET),
    69–70, 72, 77
    MCA occlusion, 24
    motor and sensory deficits, 72–3
    neuronal activity mapping, 77
    penumbra detection, 16, 23–4
    plasticity mapping, 372–3
    regeneration from post-stroke
        aphasia, 386
    volumetric studies, 25
    with rTMS in aphasia, 75–7
postconditioning of ischemic injury,
    22
posterior cerebral arteries (PCAs), 155
    infarcts
        blind sight, 174–6
        in PSD prediction, 260
    occlusions, 89
    stroke syndromes, 163
posterior cerebral artery (PCA),
    proximal, 155
posterior choroidal artery (PChA),
    164–5
posterior circulation syndromes,
    158–60, 167, 170–2

posterior circulation, stenosis and
    occlusion, 89–90
posterior communicationg artery
    (PCoA), 155
posterior inferior cerebellar artery
    (PICA), 89, 160
posterior perireticular (PPr) area, 22
post-irradiation cervical
    arteriopathies, 272
postmenopausal hormone
    replacement therapy, 126–7,
    358
post-partum cerebral angiopathy, 274,
    296
post-stroke aphasia. *See* aphasia
post-stroke dementia (PSD).
        See dementia (post-stroke)
post-stroke fatigue. *See* fatigue (post-
    stroke)
post-traumatic stress disorder (PTSD),
    249
postural tone loss, 171
potassium, dietary, 125
preconditioning of ischemic
    injury, 22
pregnancy
    choriocarcinoma, 276
    CVT, 224, 232–3
    imaging in cerebral ischemia, 267
    post-stroke, 278–9
    stroke in, 266, 277
premonitory signs, of BA stroke, 161
prepontine SAH, 214
primary vasculitis, 274
PRoFESS trial, 357, 360
Prognosis on Admission of
        Aneurysmal Subarachnoid
        Haemorrhage (PAASH), 209
PROGRESS trial, 357
prosopagnosia, 244–5
prosthetic heart valves, 146
    anticoagulant management, 131
    IE risk, 343–5
    in cardioembolic stroke, 38
    post-surgery stroke, 146
    recurrence prevention, 361
protein synthesis, inhibition, 20
prothrombin complex concentrate
    (PCC), 201
proximal thrombectomy, 314–16
PSD (post-stroke dementia).
        See dementia (post-stroke)
pseudoaneurysm, 272
pseudo-occlusion, differentiation
    diagnosis, 311–12
PSV. *See* peak systolic velocities (PSV)
psychotic disorders, post-stroke,
    247–8
ptosis, 156

puerperium
    cardiomyopathies, 270
    cerebral angiopathy, 274, 296
    cesarean section, gas emboli, 276
    CVT, 224, 232–3
    eclampsia, 275
    emboli, 276
pure motor hemiparesis, 165, 173
pure sensory stroke, 165
pusher syndrome, 390
putaminal hemorrhages, 5, 189, 197
pyramidal tract, imaging, 66
pyrexia. See fever

QT prolongation, 144
quality of life (QoL) post-stroke,
    young people/children, 278

radiofrequency catheter ablation
    (RFA), 142–3
Raloxifene Use For the Heart (RUTH)
    trial, 126
ramipril, 356
Rankin Scale (modified), on ADLs,
    64–5, 297
reactive oxygen species (ROS), 19–20
reading impairment, 237–9
rebleeding prevention, 212
reboxetine, 375
recanalization, 322–3
    outcomes, 311, 327
recombinant factor VIIa (rFVIIa), 305
recombinant tissue plasminogen
    activator (rtPA), 96–7, 99,
    294–9
    contraindications, 298
    emergency treatment guidelines,
    286
    ESO treatment guidelines, 289, 291
    reperfusion trials, 56–7, 294–5
recovery assessments, imaging, 64–78
recurrent vascular events, young
    people/children, 278
red (hemorrhagic) infarctions, 4–5
regeneration, neurogenic regions, 22
regional cerebral blood flow (rCBF), in
    CVT, 223
rehabilitation, in stroke units, 290–1
RE-LY trial, 362
repetitive training, 384
repetitive transcranial magnetic
    stimulation (rTMS), 76, 374–9
    for neuroplasticity, 374–5
    for spatial neglect, 390
    in aphasia, 75–8, 386
research studies, animal models, 9–10
respiratory infections.
    See also pneumonia
    pre-stroke, 342

restrictive cardiomyopathy (rCMP), 148
retinal artery occlusion, 158
revascularization. See also
    thrombolysis
    key indicators for, 55–6
revascularization trials
    multimodal imaging, 56–7
    patient criteria, 54–8
Reveal XT, 141–2
RFA (radiofrequency catheter
    ablation), 142–3
rhythm disturbances, 140–4, 150
right hemisphere strokes
    agitation and delirium, 175–6
    aphasia, 75–7
    neglect, 239–40
right-to-left shunt, detection, 97
rivaroxaban, 132, 361–2
Rivermead Mobility Index (RMI), 380–1
robotics
    in gait training, 383
    upper limb rehabilitation, 383–4
ROCKET AF trial, 362
rotational vertebral occlusion
    (RVAO), 170–1
rTMS. See repetitive transcranial
    magnetic stimulation (rTMS)
rtPA. See recombinant tissue
    plasminogen activator (rtPA)
RVAO (rotational vertebral artery
    occlusion), 170–1

saccular aneurysms, 207
Safe Implementation of Thrombolysis
    in Strokes (SITS) data, 295
SAH. See subarachnoid hemorrhage
    (SAH)
SCA (superior cerebellar artery), 161
SCD. See sickle-cell disease (SCD)
secondary prevention, 356, 366–7
    Essen risk score, 360–1
    in PSD, 262
    risk factors treatment, 356–61
    strategies, 360
Secondary Prevention in Small
    Subcortical Strokes Trial
    (SPS3), 357, 360
secondary vasculitis, 273–4
seizures. See epileptic seizures
Seizures After Stroke Study (SASS), 333
selective estrogen receptor modulators
    (SERMs), 126–7
selective serotonin reuptake inhibitors
    (SSRIs), 247
sensorimotor stroke, 165
sensory deficits, 163–4, See also pure
    sensory stroke; sensorimotor
    stroke; visual disturbance
    imaging, 72–3

septic CVT, 223–5, 228
    therapy, 232
sexual functioning, 391–2
sickle-cell disease (SCD), 275
    blood hyperviscosity, 173
    TCD evaluation, 97
silent infarcts, 41, 259–60
SITS (Safe Implementation of
    Thrombolysis in Strokes) data,
    295
skin disorders
    secondary vasculitis, 273
    Sweet syndrome, 276
small-vessel disease (SVD), 3,
    See also lacunar stroke
    syndromes
    in CADASIL, 181
    in ICH, 192–3
    in young people, 271
    lacunar infarcts, 40–2
    later PSD risk, 259
smoking, 121–2
    ICH and, 192
    lifestyle risk factor, 109–10
    young people, 268
Sneddon syndrome, 274
social problems, 392
sodium, dietary intake, 125,
    See also Dietary Approaches to
    Stop Hypertension (DASH)
    trial
Solitaire FR Thrombectomy for Acute
    Revascularization (STAR trial),
    322
Solitaire FR, stent retriever, 318–19,
    321–2
somatosensory deficits, 77
SonoVue, contrast agent, 94–5
space perception disorders, 390
SPACE trial, 365
spasticity, 388–9, 392
spatial delirium, 248
spatial neglect, 239–40, 392
    cortical networks, 240
    rehabilitation, 389–90
    right hemisphere stroke, 239–40
speech disorders, 392, See also aphasia
    classification, 237
    focal paresis, 178
    frontal lobe lesions, 176–7
    rehabilitation, 385–6
speech disturbance, in mania, 250
speech fluency, 237
    in aphasia, 238
spot signs, 195–8
Staphylococcus aureus infection, 345
statin therapy, 129–30
    ICH and, 192
    secondary prevention, 357–8

steal phenomena
  anastomotic, 12
  paradoxical, 11
steal syndrome, subclavian stenosis, 172
stent recanalization, 316–17
stent retrievers, 320
  in recanalization, 317–22
Stenting versus Aggressive Medical
     Therapy for Intracranial
     Arterial Stenosis (SAMMPRIS)
     trial, 366
stenting, ICA stenosis, 364–5
stereotactic guidance with aspiration,
     199
stimulation. See brain stimulation;
     environmental stimulation
strength training, targeted, 385
stress. See post-traumatic stress
     disorder (PTSD)
stroke. See also acute strokes;
     hemorrhagic strokes; ischemic
     strokes
  defined, 102
Stroke Alarm protocol, hospital, 286
stroke classification, 9, 102
stroke hemodynamics, 10–12
Stroke Impact Scale (SIS), 381
stroke physiology, 27
stroke prediction, 112–14
stroke prevention. See also secondary
     prevention
  lifestyle factors, 133
Stroke Prevention by Aggressive
     Reduction in Cholesterol
     Levels (SPARCL), 358
Stroke Prevention in Reversible
     Ischemia Trial (SPIRIT), 364
stroke recovery. See neurorehabilitation
stroke recurrence. See secondary
     prevention
stroke research. See also individual
     trials by name
  animal models, 9–10
  clinical application, 23–7
stroke risk, 108–10, 114–16, 120
  after TIA, 110–12
  BP and, 128
  cigarette smoking, 121–2, 207
  diseases and pathological
     conditions, 133–4
  lifestyle patterns, 111, 113
stroke screening, prehospital, 286
stroke syndromes, 155, 166–7
  anterior circulation, 155–8
  classification, 162
  posterior circulation, 158–60
  uncommon, 169, 185–6
stroke treatment, prehospital, 285–6
stroke units, 285, 291–2

care infrastructure and quality,
     286–8
  clinical assessment, 288–9
  complications management, 291
  diagnostic procedures, 290
  facilities, 288–9
  intravenous thrombolysis in, 298–9
  monitoring and treatment
     guidelines, 290
  multidisciplinary team, 287, 371,
     376–81
  patient transport to, 285–6
  rehabilitation, 290–1
  secondary prevention, 290
  stroke management, 289–91
  structured neurorehabilitation,
     376–81
  treatment guidelines, 291
  treatment window, 286–8
structural imaging
  computed tomography (CT), 64–6
  magnetic resonance imaging (MRI),
     66–7
subarachnoid hemorrhage (SAH), 206
  aneurysmal, 208, 211
  clinical presentation, 207–8
  complications, 213–14
  diagnosis, 209–10
  epidemiology, 206
  grading scales/classification, 209
  memory defects, 241–2
  mortality rates, 206–7
  NCCT in identification, 45–6
  pathogenesis, 207
  prognosis, 206–7, 209
  risk factors, 206–7
  smoking and, 121–2
  treatment, 210–13
subclavian arteries, occlusions, 86
subclavian stenosis
  levels of evidence, 86–7
  steal syndrome, 172
subdural hematomas (SDHs),
     imaging, 54
subgranular zone (SGZ), neurogenic
     region, 22
subventricular zone (SVZ), neurogenic
     region, 22
suicidal thoughts, 250
superior cerebellar artery (SCA), 161
supratentorial lesions, 260
surgical interventions
  decompression in brain edema,
     303–4
  for ICH, 199, 305
  in IE, 347
Surgical Trial in IntraCerebral
     Hemorrhage (STICH), 199,
     305

susac/SICRET syndrome, 276
susceptibility-weighted imaging
     (SWI), 54
Sweet syndrome, 276
Sylvian artery. See middle cerebral
     artery (MCA)
synaptic plasticity, 373
syphilis
  and stroke, 349–50
  meningovascular, 180
systemic disorders
  secondary vasculitis in, 273–4
  stroke manifestations, 177–81
systemic lupus erythematosus, 179
systolic flow velocities, 84–5

T1/T2-weighted imaging, 49
tachycardia, 143–4
Taenia solium (tapeworm), 350
Takayasu disease, 273
Takotsubo cardiomyopathy (TTC),
     148–9
tamoxifen, 126–7
TCCD (transcranial color-coded
     duplex) sonography, 87–8, 90,
     98
TCD. See transcranial color Doppler
     (TCD) sonography
tDCS. See transcranial direct current
     stimulation (tDCS)
tea intake, 126
telmisartan, 356–7
temporal arteritis, 179
temporal herniation, 156
temporal lobe infarcts, 175
territorial infarcts, 3–4
thalamic aphasia, 158
thalamic bleeding, deep ICH, 188
thalamic dementia, 164
thalamic hand, 164
thalamic hematomas, 197
thalamic hemorrhages, 5, 189
thalamic infarcts, 175
thalamic nuclei, vascularization, 163
thalamic pain syndrome, 164
thalamic strokes, 241
thalamic-subthalamic artery, 180
thalamogeniculate arteries, 164
thalamus
  ischemia in, 163–5
  lesions in, 8–9
thiazide diuretics, 128
thrombectomy, 230, 314–16
thrombin inhibitors, 132
thromboangeiitis obliterans, 273
thromboembolism, 2–3
  avoidance, 305
thrombolic thrombocytopenic
     purpura, 275

thrombolysis, 294–9, 306,
    See also revascularization
  accelerated, 96–7
  BP and outcome, 327
  emergency treatment, 289–90
  in CVT, 230
  intra-arterial application, 312–13
  monitoring, 95–6
  patient criteria, 57–8
  treatment response, 48
Thrombolysis in Brain Ischemia
    (TIBI), 95–6
thrombophilias, 229–30, 275
  screening for, 227–8
thrombosis, infectious causes, 343–50
thrombus
  direct treatment, 312–13
  evaluation, 48–9
  MRI imaging, 226–7
  of the MCA, 10
thrombus disruption, 313–14
thrombus removal, mechanical, 313–22
TIAs. *See* transient ischemic attacks
    (TIAs)
tinnitus, 170–1
tissue acidosis, 11
TOAST classification, 33–4, 43, 155,
    162
top of the basilar artery, occlusion,
    173–4
torsades de pointes, 144
Toxoplasma gondii, differential
    diagnosis, 351–2
tracheostomy
  dysphagia management, 388
  evaluation by FEES, 388
transcallosal inhibition, 73
transcortical aphasia, 169, 176–7, 237
transcranial color Doppler (TCD)
    sonography, 98–9
  fast-track, 90
  in thrombolysis, 95–6, 298
  intracranial stenosis and occlusion,
    86–9
  MES detection, 90–4, 99, 103
  PFO detection, 269
  right-to-left shunt detection, 97
  rtPA and, 96–7
  SCD evaluation, 97
  vasomotor reactivity, 97
transcranial color-coded duplex (TCCD)
    sonography, 87–8, 90, 98
transcranial color-coded sonography
    (TCCS), accuracy, 87
transcranial direct current stimulation
    (tDCS), 374–9, 386
transcranial magnetic stimulation
    (TMS), 372–3
transcranial MCA occlusion
    (research), 9

transient ischemic attacks (TIAs)
  large artery embolism, 36
  limb-shaking TIA, 158, 170–1
  low CBF as cause, 169–72
  PCT data, 47
  posterior circulation, 158–9
  recurrence prevention, 358–63
  stroke risk score, 110–12
  transient hemiplegic, 173
transorbital MCA occlusion
    (research), 9
treadmill training, 382–3
Treatment of Hyperglycemia in
    Ischemic Stroke (THIS), 329
Trevo Pro retriever, 320–1
Trial of Org 10172 in Acute Stroke
    Treatment (TOAST), 33–4, 43,
    155, 162
triangle-shaped non-enhanced
    structure, 226
Trypanosoma cruzi infection, 348
TTC (Takotsubo cardiomyopathy),
    148–9
tuberculous meningitis, 180, 349
tuberothalamic artery, 164

ultrasound, 82–99
  fast-track, 90
  patient screening for therapy, 92–3
  prognostic value, 95–6, 99
  sensitivity, 82
  specificity, 82
ultrasound contrast agents (UCAs),
    94–5, 99
ultrasound thrombus disruption,
    313–14
unfractionated heparin (UFH), 228–9
uninhibited behavior, 242–3
  aggression, 247
  in mania, 250
unruptured intracranial aneurysm
    (UIA), 207–8
urinary tract infections (UTI), 342, 353

valproic acid, 230–1
valves. *See* heart valves
valvular heart disease, 145–6, 268
varicella zoster virus (VZV)
    vasculopathy, 179–80, 350
vascular dementia (VaD), 181, 255,
    260–1
vascular permeability, 5
vascular risk factors
  cognitive decline, 132–3
  for PSD, 258–9
vasculitis, 350–1
  primary, 274
  secondary, 273–4
vasculopathies, 177–80
vasogenic edema, 21

vasomotor reactivity, 97
vasopressors, 327
vasorelaxation, tissue acidosis, 11
vasospasm, 214
vegetable consumption, 124–5
ventricular aneurysms, embolic stroke,
    145
verbal comprehension, assessment, 237
vertebral arteries (VAs), 158
  dissection, 184
  Doppler analysis, 83
  occlusions, 86, 89, 170–2
  stroke syndromes, 160
  ultrasound screening, 92
vertebrobasilar insufficiency, 89
vertebrobasilar ischemia, drop attacks,
    171–2
vertebrobasilar stroke syndromes,
    158–60
vertigo, 160–1, 170–1
vicariation, in neuroplasticity, 372
videofluoroscopic swallowing study
    (VFSS)
  ultrasound screening, 387
vigilance reduction, 175
viral infections
  pre-stroke, 342
  vasculopathy, 179–80, 350–1
virtual reality (VR) devices, 384
visual agnosia, 243–6
visual disorientation, 169
visual disturbance. *See also* blind sight;
    blindness
  ischemic ophthalmopathy, 170
  posterior circulation infarcts, 159
visual field defects
  AChA infarcts, 158
  basilar artery occlusion, 173–4
  cerebral artery infarcts, 156, 163
  retinal artery occlusion, 158
  thalamic ischemia, 165
visual hallucinations, 248
visual stimuli, processing, 246
vitamin K antagonists
  long-term treatment, 229–30
  teratogenicity, 232
vitamin K antagonist-associated ICH
    (VKA-ICH), 200
vitamin supplements, 358
vomiting, 160
  AICA syndrome, 160–1
  ICH presentation, 197
  in SAH, 208
VZV (varicella zoster virus),
    vasculopathy, 179–80, 350

waist-to-hip ratio, 123
Wallenberg syndrome, 160
WARCEF trial, 362
warfarin

AF management, 131–2, 361–3
ASA compared, 366
hemorrhage risk assessment, 112
Warfarin Aspirin Recurrent Stroke
        Study (WARSS), 364
warning bleed, before SAH, 208
WASID-II study, 366
watershed infarcts (WS), 166
weakness, MCA infarcts, 157–8
Wernicke's aphasia, 157
white matter abnormalities.
        See also lobar (white matter)
        hemorrhages

in CADASIL, 181–2
   young person, 272
whole grain consumption, 125
word repetition, 237
World Health Organization (WHO)
   clinical signs of stroke, 102
   international mortality rates, 104
   MONICA study, 105–8
writing impairment, 237–9

young people
   cardioembolism in, 268–70
   diagnostic workup, 267–8

ischemic stroke, 266, 279–80
young people/children
   causes of stroke, 268–76
   epidemiology, 266
   history taking, 267
   mortality rates, 278
   outcome of strokes, 278–9
   risk factors for stroke, 269,
      277–8
   secondary prevention post-stroke,
      279

zinc toxicity, 19